PERIOPERATIVE MANAGEMENT

Michael J. Breslow, M.D.

Assistant Professor
Co-Director, Surgical Intensive Care Unit
Department of Anesthesiology and Critical Care Medicine
The Johns Hopkins Medical Institutions
Baltimore, Maryland

Clair F. Miller, M.D.

Assistant Professor
Department of Anesthesiology and Critical Care Medicine
The Johns Hopkins Medical Institutions
Baltimore, Maryland

Mark Rogers, M.D.

Chairman and Professor,
Department of Anesthesiology and Critical Care Medicine
The Johns Hopkins Medical Institutions
Baltimore, Maryland

with 142 illustrations

THE C. V. MOSBY COMPANY

St. Louis • Washington, D.C. • Toronto   1990

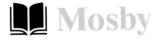 Mosby

Editor: George Stamathis
Developmental Editor: Elaine Steinborn
Project Manager: Suzanne Seeley
Production Editor: Jolynn Gower
Designer: Susan E. Lane

Printed in the United States of America

The C.V. Mosby Company
11830 Westline Industrial Drive, St. Louis, Missouri 63146

Library

Perioperative management / [edited by] Michael J. Breslow, Clair F.
    Miller, Mark C. Rogers.
        p.   cm.
    ISBN 0-8016-5049-6
    1. Therapeutics, Surgical.   I. Breslow, Michael J.   II. Miller,
    Clair F.   III. Rogers, Mark C.
        [DNLM: 1. Anesthesia.   2. Intraoperative Care—methods.
    3. Postoperative Care—methods.   4. Preoperative Care—methods.   WO
    178 P445]
    RD49.P46   1989
    617′.91—dc20
    DNLM/DLC
    for Library of Congress   89-13093
                                                                                                                      CIP

To
Seymour Breslow, Gerald Rosenberg,
and our families

Contributors

MARIA D. ALLO, M.D.
Chairperson
Department of Surgery
Santa Clara Valley Medical Center
San Jose, California

CHARLES BEATTIE, Ph.D., M.D.
Associate Professor
Director, Division of Critical Care Anesthesia
Department of Anesthesiology and Critical Care Medicine
The Johns Hopkins Medical Institutions
Baltimore, Maryland

THOMAS J. J. BLANCK, M.D.
Associate Professor
Department of Anesthesiology and Critical Care Medicine
The Johns Hopkins Medical Institutions
Baltimore, Maryland

SANDRALEE A. BLOSSER, M.D.
Fellow
Department of Anesthesiology and Critical Care Medicine
The Johns Hopkins Medical Institutions
Baltimore, Maryland

CECIL BOREL, M.D.
Assistant Professor
Co-Director, Neurosciences Critical Care Unit
Departments of Anesthesiology and Critical Care Medicine
and Neurology and Neurosurgery
The Johns Hopkins Medical Institutions
Baltimore, Maryland

DENNIS L. BOURKE, M.D.
Associate Professor
Director, Division of Regional Anesthesia
Department of Anesthesiology and Critical Care Medicine
The Johns Hopkins Medical Institutions
Baltimore, Maryland

BARRY BRASFIELD, M.D.
Assistant Professor
Department of Anesthesiology
Emory University
School of Medicine
Atlanta, Georgia

MICHAEL J. BRESLOW, M.D.
Assistant Professor
Co-Director, Surgical Intensive Care Unit
Department of Anesthesiology and Critical Care Medicine
The Johns Hopkins Medical Institutions
Baltimore, Maryland

STEPHEN A. DERRER, M.D.
Assistant Professor
Department of Anesthesiology and Critical Care Medicine
The Johns Hopkins Medical Institutions
Baltimore, Maryland

CLIFFORD S. DEUTSCHMAN, M.S., M.D.
Assistant Professor
Director, Anesthesia Trauma Services
Department of Anesthesiology and Critical Care Medicine
The Johns Hopkins Medical Institutions
Baltimore, Maryland

WILLIAM R. FURMAN, M.D.

Assistant Professor
Department of Anesthesiology and Critical Care Medicine
The Johns Hopkins Medical Institutions
Associate Director
Department of Anesthesiology
Francis Scott Key Medical Center
Baltimore, Maryland

LEE GOLDMAN, M.D., M.P.H.

Associate Professor
Vice-Chairman, Chief
Division of Clinical Epidemiology
Consolidated Department of Medicine
Brigham and Women's Hospital
Beth Israel Hospital
Harvard Medical School
Boston, Massachusetts

ANDREW P. HARRIS, M.D.

Assistant Professor
Chief, Obstetric Anesthesiology
Departments of Anesthesiology and Critical Care Medicine, and
    Gynecology/Obstetrics
The Johns Hopkins Medical Institutions
Baltimore, Maryland

LINDA S. HUMPHREY, M.D.

Assistant Professor
Department of Anesthesiology and Critical Care Medicine
Associate Chief
Division of Cardiac Anesthesia
The Johns Hopkins Medical Institutions
Baltimore, Maryland

MICHAEL HUMPHREY, M.D.

Instructor, Department of Anesthesiology
The Johns Hopkins Medical Institutions
Chief
Department of Anesthesiology
St. Agnes Hospital
Baltimore, Maryland

LUCILLE W. KING, M.D.

Clinical Instructor
Department of Medicine
The Johns Hopkins Medical Institutions
Chief, Endocrinology Division
Wyman Park Medical Associates
Baltimore, Maryland

THOMAS H. LEE, M.D.

Associate Professor of Medicine
Brigham and Women's Hospital
Boston, Massachusetts

MICHAEL LISH, M.D.

Assistant Professor
Department of Anesthesiology and Critical Care Medicine
The Johns Hopkins Medical Institutions
Baltimore, Maryland

TERI H. MANOLIO, M.D.

Medical Officer
Division of Epidemiology and Clinical Applications
National Institutes of Health
Bethesda, Maryland

JACKIE L. MARTIN, M.D.

Assistant Professor
Department of Anesthesiology and Critical Care Medicine
The Johns Hopkins Medical Institutions
Baltimore, Maryland

WILLIAM T. MERRITT, M.D.

Assistant Professor
Department of Anesthesiology and Critical Care Medicine
The Johns Hopkins Medical Institutions
Baltimore, Maryland

CLAIR F. MILLER, M.D.

Assistant Professor
Department of Anesthesiology and Critical Care Medicine
The Johns Hopkins Medical Institutions
Baltimore, Maryland

STEPHEN D. PARKER, M.D.

Assistant Professor
Department of Anesthesiology and Critical Care Medicine
The Johns Hopkins Medical Institutions
Baltimore, Maryland

PETER ROCK, M.D.

Assistant Professor
Department of Anesthesiology and Critical Care Medicine
The Johns Hopkins Medical Institutions
Baltimore, Maryland

BRIAN A. ROSENFELD, M.D.

Assistant Professor
Department of Anesthesiology and Critical Care Medicine
The Johns Hopkins Medical Institutions
Baltimore, Maryland

ALAN F. ROSS, M.D.

Associate Professor
Department of Anesthesiology
University of Iowa
Iowa City, Iowa

NEAL T. SAKIMA, M.D.

Senior Clinical Fellow
Department of Anesthesiology and Critical Care Medicine
The Johns Hopkins Medical Institutions
Baltimore, Maryland

CHARLES L. SCHLEIEN, M.D.

Assistant Professor
Departments of Anesthesiology and Critical Care Medicine
    and Pediatrics
Assistant Director
Pediatric Intensive Care Unit
The Johns Hopkins Medical Institutions
Baltimore, Maryland

MICHAEL J. SENDAK, M.D.

Assistant Professor
Department of Anesthesiology and Critical Care Medicine
The Johns Hopkins Medical Institutions
Chief
Department of Anesthesiology and Critical Care Medicine
The Homewood Hospital Center
Baltimore, Maryland

RICHARD M. SHAPIRO, M.D.

Assistant Professor
Department of Anesthesiology and Critical Care Medicine
The Johns Hopkins Medical Institutions
Staff Anesthesiologist
Director of Post-Anesthesia Care Unit
Homewood Hospital
Baltimore, Maryland

DOUGLAS S. SNYDER, M.D.

Assistant Professor
Department of Anesthesiology and Critical Care Medicine
The Johns Hopkins Medical Institutions
Baltimore, Maryland

DONALD R. TAYLOR, M.D.

Assistant
Department of Anesthesiology and Critical Care Medicine
The Johns Hopkins Medical Institutions
Baltimore, Maryland

PATRICIA A. TEWES, M.D., Ph.D.

Assistant Professor
Department of Anesthesiology and Critical Care Medicine
The Johns Hopkins Medical Institutions
Baltimore, Maryland

JOHN H. TINKER, M.D.

Professor and Head
Department of Anesthesia
The University of Iowa
Iowa City, Iowa

A. TERRY WALMAN, M.D.

Assistant Professor
Assistant Clinical Director
Department of Anesthesiology and Critical Care Medicine
The Johns Hopkins Medical Institutions
Baltimore, Maryland

Preface

This book is very much a personal statement. In it we address the various factors responsible for adverse outcomes in patients who present for surgery. The belief that clear-cut mistakes in either anesthetic or surgical technique are only rarely responsible for perioperative complications is central to this text. We believe that the end-organ effects of anesthetic drugs and the neurohumorally induced changes in physiologic function induced by surgical trauma interact with preexisting disease states to produce morbid events. While this statement seems simple, it runs counter to the standard manner of care for patients in the perioperative period. Historically, anesthesiologists have focused on adverse effects associated with the various anesthetic agents and techniques, surgeons have focused on complications as a function of specific surgical procedures, and internists have attempted to correlate various preexisting medical conditions with perioperative complications. These different perspectives in most institutions result in internists medically preparing patients for surgery and attesting to their readiness, anesthesiologists assuming responsibility for intraoperative care, and surgeons operating and delivering care postoperatively. We believe that this system is flawed; not only is care fragmented, but more importantly, it does not allow the multidisciplinary approach to patient care that is necessary for an optimal perioperative outcome. Rather, internists need to better understand the effects of anesthetics and surgery and follow patients beyond the double doors leading into the operating room. Anesthesiol-

ogists need to better appreciate how specific disease states alter responses to specific anesthetics, and how different management approaches affect the postoperative course. And surgeons must learn to appreciate differences in patient responses to surgical procedures as a result of specific preexisting medical conditions, and must increase their knowledge concerning the beneficial and adverse effects of different anesthetic practices.

This text presents a multidisciplinary approach to the care of the surgical patient. The first section consists of general concepts of preoperative, intraoperative, and postoperative care. The remainder of the book addresses specific medical problems, identifies ways in which they increase perioperative risk, and discusses how these factors necessitate alterations in standard anesthetic and surgical techniques. For each disease we have outlined what we believe to be the essential patient management issues, and have critically reviewed the relevant literature from the fields of medicine, anesthesia, and surgery. Where adequate studies are not available, this is clearly indicated. This is not a "how to" book. Rather we identify ways in which perioperative events interact with preexisting disease states. It is our conviction that only through this type of approach can we improve patient outcome.

Michael J. Breslow
Clair F. Miller
Mark C. Rogers

Contents

xiii

PART ONE

PREOPERATIVE EVALUATION

CHAPTER **1**

Preoperative Screening Tests

TERI A. MANOLIO

Preoperative screening tests are often ordered according to a standard checklist, with little consideration given to their indications or implications. While adequate preoperative evaluation is a necessary adjunct to a smooth perioperative course, adequacy is frequently confused with exhaustiveness. Traditional attitudes regarding preoperative tests are summarized in the 1976 edition of Collins' *Principles of Anesthesiology:*[7] "Certain laboratory procedures are necessary in the evaluation of any patient preoperatively. These procedures should be considered as screening tests and whenever a positive finding appears, it must be explored and further detailed examinations carried out." The reasons that such beliefs have been questioned, the rationale behind a more directed approach to preoperative testing, and the specifics of such an approach are the topics of this chapter.

REASONS TO LIMIT PREOPERATIVE TESTS
Accuracy of a Test and the Problem of False Positives

No diagnostic test is perfect, as everyone knows. The accuracy of a test can be defined as its ability to distinguish persons with a disease from persons without a disease. Various terms have been devised to characterize the accuracy of a test, such as its validity, reproducibility, precision, sensitivity, specificity, and predictive value. The latter three are most commonly used in the clinical setting and will be described here. Other sources offer a more detailed discussion of the clinical usefulness of a diagnostic test.[39]

The sensitivity of a test is the probability of a positive test result given that the patient has the disease being sought. It reflects the ability of the test

2

to detect the disease correctly. Specificity is the probability of a negative test result given that the patient does not have the target disease. It reflects the ability of the test to rule out the disease correctly. These terms are more easily understood in the context of a 2 × 2 table:

	Disease present	Disease absent	
Test positive	a	b	a + b
Test negative	c	d	c + d
	a + c	b + d	

Sensitivity is therefore equal to:

$$\frac{a \quad \text{(those with positive test results with disease)}}{a + c \text{ (all those with disease)}}$$

Specificity is equal to:

$$\frac{d \quad \text{(those with negative test results without disease)}}{b + d \text{ (all those without disease)}}$$

Cell c represents those persons who have the disease but whose test results were negative; they are referred to as "false negatives." The false negative rate of the test can be calculated as:

$$\frac{c \quad \text{(those with negative test results but with disease)}}{c + d \text{ (all those with negative test results)}}$$

Similarly, cell b represents those persons who do not have the disease but whose test results were positive; they are referred to as "false positives." The false positive rate of the test can be calculated as:

$$\frac{b \quad \text{(those with positive test results but without disease)}}{a + b \text{ (all those with positive test results)}}$$

Note that if the test were perfect, sensitivity and specificity would be 100% and there would be *no* false positives or false negatives. Cells b and c would both be empty.

Finally, the positive predictive value of a test is defined as the probability of having the disease given that the test is positive. It is equal to:

$$\frac{a \quad \text{(those with positive test results with disease)}}{a + b \text{ (all those with positive test results)}}$$

Similarly, the negative predictive value is the probability of being free of the disease given that the test is negative, or:

$$\frac{d \quad \text{(those with negative test results without disease)}}{c + d \text{ (all those with negative test results)}}$$

In clinical medicine, we most commonly use tests for their predictive value; that is, we obtain a test to rule in disease (relying on its positive predictive value) or rule out disease (relying on its negative predictive value). Although predictive value obviously varies with the accuracy of a test (as reflected by its sensitivity and specificity), what is not so obvious is that predictive value *also varies with disease prevalence*. Any test that has less than 100% sensitivity and specificity (almost all do) will lose predictive value as disease prevalance drops. The mathematical formulation of this concept is known as Bayes' theorem, and the understanding of it is critical in using and interpreting diagnostic tests. For a more detailed discussion of Bayes' theorem, the reader is referred to Ingelfinger et al.[17]

To illustrate the concept of dependence of predictive value on disease prevalence, consider the following three situations:

1. *You have a test that is 90% sensitive and 90% specific for detecting a disease. You apply this test in 1000 members of population A, which has a 70% prevalence of the disease. The following 2 × 2 table will be generated:*

	Disease present	Disease absent	
Test positive	630	30	660
Test negative	70	270	340
	700	300	

Positive predictive value = 630/660 = 95.5%
Negative predictive value = 270/340 = 79.4%

2. *Next, you apply the same test to a population with a 20% prevalence of disease:*

	Disease present	Disease absent	
Test positive	180	80	260
Test negative	20	720	740
	200	800	

Positive predictive value = 180/260 = 68.2%
Negative predictive value = 720/740 = 97.3%

Note that your positive predictive value has dropped considerably, although the negative predictive value is increased. Also notice that the number of false positives has almost tripled (from 30 to 80).

3. *Finally, you apply the test in a population with a 2% prevalence of disease:*

	Disease present	Disease absent	
Test positive	18	98	116
Test negative	2	882	884
	20	980	

Positive predictive value = 18/116 = 15.5%
Negative predictive value = 882/884 = 99.8%

Note now that the number of false positives (98) outnumbers the true positives by more than 5 to 1, leaving a positive predictive value of only 16%. This means that only 16% of those with a positive test will actually have the disease! Negative predictive value in this instance is quite good, at 99.8%, but it is really already known (from the 2% prevalence) that 98 out of 100 persons will be disease free.

Understanding the relationship between disease prevalence and sensitivity/specificity/predictive value is crucial to the rational application of diagnostic tests. The indiscriminate use of diagnostic tests can produce far more false positives than it identifies true cases of disease, particularly when you are screening for disease that is not evident by clinical examination and thus has a low prevalence. Investigation of these false positives in the preoperative period leads to needless delay, increased costs of further testing, and, worst of all, completely unnecessary anxiety on the part of the patient.

Costs of Preoperative Testing

The effects of routine preoperative screening tests on medical care costs are difficult to estimate. In addition to the cost of performing the test, one must consider the cost of delayed surgery and prolonged hospitalization because of false positive results and the cost of further testing to establish or exclude a diagnosis. Obviously, delays and increased costs may also result from failure to order a test, perhaps leading to complications from an unidentified disease. However, evidence that routine screening tests in an asymptomatic population have a beneficial effect on patient outcome is hard to produce.[4,9,20]

Perhaps the best study of the effects of routine screening comes from a controlled trial of multiphasic screening in a British hospital.[10] In this study, patients were assigned either to have their test results routinely reported back to their attending physicians, or to have the results withheld and available only upon request. Patients in whom results were routinely reported had 32% more requests for repeat testing than did patients in whom results were only available by request. The routine reporting group also had 15% more follow-up tests not included in the screening battery, and 25% more consultations for a second clinical opinion. There was no difference between groups in length of hospital stay, and no obvious difference in patient outcome. Testing charges were 64% higher in the routine reporting group, and total hospital charges were approximately 5% higher.

Diagnostic Versus Screening Tests

All this is not to say that no preoperative tests should be performed, nor that there are not valid indications for some screening tests in almost all preoperative patients. To determine which tests are indicated, one must first discriminate between screening tests designed to detect occult or asymptomatic disease not suggested by the clinical presentation and diagnostic or confirmatory tests performed in patients with obvious signs and symptoms. The latter category, often referred to as "indicated" tests, includes those performed for the following reasons:

1. To evaluate a known condition to choose appropriate surgical therapy; for example, metastatic work-up before pulmonary resection for lung cancer
2. To evaluate a known condition to choose appropriate anesthetic therapy; for example, pulmonary function tests before deciding on type of anesthesia in patients with lung disease
3. To monitor the status of a known condition: for example, blood glucose in a diabetic or blood gases in a patient with lung disease
4. To confirm diagnosis suspected on clinical grounds; for example, chest x-ray and sputum in a patient with signs of pneumonia or urinalysis in a patient with symptoms of urinary tract infection

Screening tests, on the other hand, are tests performed without signs and symptoms to detect preclinical or asymptomatic disease. Such tests in nonsurgical patients would include periodic screening for occult blood in stools, glucose in urine, or elevated cholesterol in serum. In the preoperative period, such screening should be designed to detect occult disease that could have a direct bearing on operative risk and outcome. Robbins and Mushlin have described five criteria for useful preoperative screening tests[34]:

1. *The condition tested for must be asymptomatic and not obvious on routine history and physical examination.*

That the history and physical examination establish far more diagnoses than any laboratory test has been demonstrated repeatedly. Crombie[8] showed that 88% of diagnoses were made following a history and physical examination. Sandler showed that correct diagnoses would be made in 57% of medical outpatients following the history alone, in a further 17% following the examination, and in only another 5% following routine laboratory tests. The clinical examination performed best in patients with cardiovascular and neurologic disease and poorest in endocrine and digestive diseases.[41] Similar results were obtained by Hampton et al, who established diagnoses in 71 of 94 conditions on the basis of the clinical examination alone.[14] Therefore, the most important and useful screening test is the attentive clinical examination. Recall from the previous discussion of disease prevalence that screening tests are of necessity low in predictive value and high in false positives, because of the low prevalence of most diseases in their clinically silent forms.

2. *The condition must significantly affect the morbidity or mortality of surgery or must represent a significant risk to those associated with the patient's care.*

Conditions with a known or suspected detrimental effect on surgical outcome include anemia, ischemic heart disease, cardiac arrhythmias, chronic obstructive pulmonary disease, diabetes, chronic nephritis, urinary tract infection, clotting disorders, thrombocytopenia, nephrotic syndrome, and chronic interstitial lung disease. Conditions that put those caring for the patient at risk include tuberculosis, viral hepatitis, and HIV infections. The ethics of routine HIV testing in preoperative patients are complex and hotly debated; such a discussion is beyond the scope of this chapter. The reader is referred to Kunkel for an in-depth discussion.[22]

3. *Preoperative diagnosis must be more beneficial to management than a diagnosis established in the perioperative or postoperative period, even though detection might not necessarily affect the outcome of surgery.*

Such conditions might include glaucoma, gonorrhea, hepatitis, hypercholesterolemia, malignancy, and urinary tract infection (in procedures not involving insertion of a foreign body). Patients undergoing surgery for a specific condition whose health maintenance has been irregular or poor in the past do present the opportunity to perform some routine testing that they might otherwise go without. Whether the surgeon or other members of the perioperative team are obligated to perform such testing within the limitations of a surgical encounter is a difficult issue; one must balance the long-term interests of the patient with the short-term goals of treatment of the surgical illness. Few would argue with a urologist's obligation to test stool for occult blood after performing a prostate examination in preparation for prostatic surgery. Less clear is the responsibility, for example, to screen for cervical or colon cancer in patients without surgical illness in those organ systems. A prudent approach, dictated more by experience than by hard evidence, is to recommend to the patient that routine health maintenance be performed at regular intervals (using the guidelines of the Canadian Task Force on the Periodic Health Examination[43] or the American College of Physicians Medical Practice Committee[25] and to offer such testing as is within the abilities of the perioperative team to perform. As long as the attending surgeon makes it clear that further management of any abnormalities detected must be carried out by another health care provider (one recommended by the surgeon, if the patient so desires), reasonable care can be provided at this "therapeutic opportunity" without delay or unreasonable expense. It should be strictly borne in mind, however, that whenever such testing is performed it is the ordering physician's legal and ethical responsibility to obtain the test results, inform the patient, and provide adequate follow-up.

4. *Tests must be sufficiently specific and sensitive to allow detection of the condition.*

As discussed in the preceding section, the performance of a test must always be considered before ordering it. This is such an obvious criterion that it often goes unstated; therefore, it may also often be overlooked. While no test is perfect, many of the preoperative tests currently ordered are quite inefficient at detecting their target diseases, or are ordered for persons in whom their interpretation may be difficult. The routine electrocardiogram is a good example of a widely used screening test for coronary artery disease that has a poor sensitivity (27%) and low specificity (81%).[24] Its interpretation may be further complicated by the use of digitalis or the presence of conduction blocks or electrolyte imbalance. While this does not mean that an ECG should never be ordered to detect occult coronary disease, it does mean that use of the test must be tempered by an understanding of the patient groups in which it performs the best.

5. *Prevalance of the condition must be high enough that efficient detection of an asymptomatic patient with the condition is possible.*

Even a test with almost perfect sensitivity and specificity will be of little use if the disease sought is vanishingly rare. A good example of such a test is the partial thromboplastin time to detect an asymptomatic bleeding disorder. Such disorders (in their totally asymptomatic form) have a prevalence of about 1 per 100,000. The test is 99% sensitive and 72% specific at detecting them, but at $10 apiece, $1 million in tests must be performed to detect one case.[34] That $1 million might more reasonably be spent in other ways.

YIELD OF FREQUENTLY USED PREOPERATIVE TESTS

Recommendations for routine preoperative tests most commonly include an electrocardiogram, serum electrolytes, glucose and urea nitrogen, complete blood count with differential, and a urinalysis. Chest x-ray examinations, liver function tests, and clotting times are often added as well. Each of these tests will be dealt with in turn.

Electrocardiogram

One of the most routinely ordered and frequently abnormal preoperative tests is the resting electrocardiogram (ECG).[6] In a study of 1410 admission electrocardiograms performed on the Duke University medical service, only 360 (26%) were totally normal.[26] Many of the abnormalities found were nonspecific, however, and when study members reviewed hospital records and ECGs, only 52 patients (4%) were deemed to have useful information added by the admission ECG. Because this was a medical population, often admitted for cardiac-related complaints, the yield in preoperative patients might be expected to be even lower. Of the more than 800 patients in the Duke study who had no evidence of a cardiovascular abnormality, the ECG provided added information in only eight patients, or less than 1%. The only factors associated with an increased yield of the test were the patients being over 45 years

of age and presence of a clinically evident cardiac abnormality. Moorman et al concluded that ". . . the routine admission ECG infrequently added new information to the clinical evaluation, but was useful when it did." Its estimated cost-effectiveness, while believed to be low, was comparable to that of many other accepted medical practices.

Fewer studies have addressed the use of routine ECGs in surgical patients, but one study of 1068 patients found a 19% prevalence of abnormalities, 56% of which were nonspecific repolarization abnormalities or left anterior fascicular block, which have little effect on the outcome of surgery.[12] The incidence of abnormalities was observed to increase steadily with patient age. A later series of 198 patients undergoing major noncardiac surgery showed that an abnormal preoperative electrocardiogram was independently associated with increased risk of perioperative course complicated by death, myocardial infarction, or myocardial ischemia. Both ST-T abnormalities and intraventricular conduction delays showed trends toward higher prevalence in patients with a complicated course versus those with an uncomplicated course, although only a minority of patients developed a complication.[3]

An interesting approach to decreasing the use of preoperative ECGs was developed by Paterson et al in Glasgow.[28] A simple six-item questionnaire was administered to 267 patients undergoing elective surgery and receiving preoperative electrocardiograms (see box on p. 7). Ninety-six patients (36%) gave one or more positive responses to the questionnaire, and 29 of them had a major abnormality on ECG (defined as ST depression less than 1 mm or T inversion, conduction defects, prior infarct, significant arrhythmia, or left ventricular hypertrophy). Only 5 patients with completely negative questionnaires had major abnormalities, and all were over 50 years of age. The authors recommended limiting routine ECGs to those over 50, and to those under 50 with signs or symptoms of heart disease. They estimate that adoption of these guidelines would lead to a 30% reduction in routine ECGs. It should be noted, however, that assessment of the effects of these recommendations on patient outcome, and the ability to generalize these findings to other centers, are not available.

The usefulness of the ECG in establishing a "baseline" has also been questioned. A study of 236 emergency room patients complaining of chest pain con-

---

Questionnaire to detect risk factors for abnormal ECG

1. Have you had any chest pain?   yes/no
2. Have you experienced breathlessness on exertion?   yes/no
3. Have you experienced breathlessness lying flat?   yes/no
4. Has any form of heart disease ever been diagnosed?   yes/no
5. Have you had rheumatic fever?   yes/no
6. Have you ever been found to have a heart murmur?   yes/no

From Paterson KR et al: The preoperative electrocardiogram: an assessment, Scott Med J 28:116-118, 1983.

---

cluded that a prior ECG would only have affected treatment decisions in 4.7%, and that in no case would it have helped to avoid an inappropriate discharge.[36] In the preoperative setting, 812 patients were studied who had an ECG recorded at some time in the past (mean of 24 months) followed by a routine ECG preoperatively.[30] Although 165 tracings showed new abnormalities, none of them led to delay or cancellation of surgery.[29] The probability of a new abnormality was greater in patients 60 years of age or older, in patients whose prior ECG had been obtained more than 2 years before the preoperative ECG, and in patients whose prior ECG was abnormal. Rabkin and Horne concluded that a preoperative ECG following a prior ECG had little impact on decisions related to surgical case delay and cancellation.

A problem in assessing the impact of any test such as the ECG on perioperative decisions is the difficulty of documenting its exact contribution. Rarely does a single test "make or break" a decision to operate or a choice of anesthesia, but more often it is used as contributing evidence in supporting one line of thought over another. Whether such decisions would be made in the absence of the ECG is almost impossible to assess.

Chest Radiography

The data on chest x-rays evaluations are somewhat clearer. Hubbell and colleagues looked at the prevalence of abnormalities in chest x-ray evaluations of 294 medical inpatients in a VA hospital (a population with a high prevalence of smoking and chronic obstructive pulmonary disease) and found abnormalities in 36%.[16] Nearly half of these abnormalities resulted from chronic obstructive lung disease or cardiomegaly, however, and the vast majority (81%) were considered to be chronic and stable. The investigators felt that the chest x-ray evaluation might have altered treatment in 12 of the 294 patients for whom admission films were ordered; however, only one serious disease would have been missed without the films, and the outcome in that case would not have changed.

A similar study of 6063 admission chest x-ray evaluations in patients on all services at Barnes Hospital showed 1001 (16.5%) to have a "serious" abnormality, the majority of which again resulted from cardiomegaly (50%) or chronic obstructive lung disease (34%). The prevalence of abnormalities increased steadily with patient age, from 0% in the newborn to 19 age-group to 43% in those over 70. The screening chest films were believed to add new diagnostic information in only 4% of patients, but the impact of this information on outcome could not be assessed.[40]

The use of screening chest x-ray evaluations in 10,619 patients undergoing nonacute, noncardiopulmonary surgery was studied in eight British hospitals by the Royal College of Radiologists.[35] The researchers concluded that the routine films ". . . did not seem to influence the decision to operate or the choice of anaesthetic; nor was there any evidence that preoperative chest radiography, at the levels of utilisation observed in this study, would be of much value as a baseline against which subsequent radiographs in patients with postoperative pulmonary complications could be judged."

A study of 1000 preoperative chest x-ray films in another British hospital showed only one significant new finding in 437 patients under the age of 30.[23] Of the 563 patients over age 30, 64 (11%) were felt to have significant findings. However, 44 of these findings were cardiac enlargement or emphysema. No data are given on the chronicity or stability of these findings (though the author states that most were not known beforehand) and there is no assessment of the effect of chest radiography on outcome. The conclusion of the author, that chest x-ray evaluations are essential in preoperative patients over the age of 30, does not seem to be supported by the data presented.[23]

A similar study of 667 preoperative chest films in Wales identified 126 significant abnormalities; 54% were because of cardiomegaly and 19% resulted from chronic respiratory disease. Of interest, 38% of these patients had had a chest x-ray examination within the preceding year, and the maximum recommended marrow radiation dose had been exceeded in 12.5%.[32] Thus not only is the yield of preoperative chest radiography low, but it may be exposing patients to potentially harmful effects of radiation.

In an attempt to limit the use of preoperative chest x-ray films, a hospital screened 872 patients admitted for surgery for the presence of clinically identifiable risk factors for abnormal chest x-ray films (see the box at right). Of the 368 patients without any risk factors, only one had an abnormal finding. This finding did not affect his surgical course and was not followed up. One hundred-fourteen serious abnormalities were identified in the 504 patients considered to be at risk, but the nature of the abnormalities and their effects on surgical course are not reported. The authors concluded that the chest x-ray film should not be used as a routine preoperative examination, but ". . . should be used as an adjunct to careful clinical evaluation of the patient in whom some reasonable expectation exists that the procedure will provide or confirm additional useful information."[37] Such advice is applicable to every laboratory test discussed here.

Complete Blood Counts and Hemostasis Tests

The major reasons for obtaining routine preoperative CBCs are to detect anemia, thrombocytopenia, and leukocytosis. Detection and quantitation of anemia have received the most attention in the preoperative patient, probably because mild degrees of anemia are common and relatively asymptomatic, and because severe anemia in the perioperative period can be life threatening. The minimum acceptable hemoglobin level in the preoperative patient, traditionally set at 9 to 10 g/dl,[21] is the subject of much discussion but little research. Hemoglobin is only one of several contributing factors determin-

---

> **Risk factors for abnormal chest roentgenogram**
>
> **Medical history**
> Cancer at any site
> Valvular heart disease
> Stroke
> Myocardial infarction
> Angina
> Asthma
> Tuberculosis
> Chronic obstructive pulmonary disease
> Cigarette smoking
> Occupational exposure (asbestos, fume, ores)
>
> **Review of systems**
> General: fever, chills, sweats, weight loss
> Paroxysmal nocturnal dyspnea
> Orthopnea
> Class 3 or 4 dyspnea
> Angina
>
> **Physical findings**
> Vital signs: fever, tachycardia, hypertension, tachypnea
> Chest: abnormal breath sounds, abnormal adventitial sounds, dullness
> Heart: severe murmurs, S3, or displaced PMI
> Abdomen: tenderness, organomegaly, or ascites
>
> From Rucker L, Frye EB, and Staten MA: Usefulness of screening chest roentgenogram in preoperative patients, JAMA 250:3209-3211, 1983.

---

ing oxygen supply to the tissues, the other major ones being cardiac output and determinants of the hemoglobin-oxygen dissociation curve. Level of hemoglobin, since it is the easiest to quantify, usually receives the most emphasis, but the other two factors are probably more important in determining the consequences and manifestations of anemia. Low hemoglobin levels that develop over a prolonged period are usually quite well tolerated, but compensatory mechanisms may not be able to accommodate further blood loss, especially that which develops acutely.

For these reasons, detection of modest degrees of anemia (< 9 to 10 g/dl) is important in patients undergoing procedures in which major blood loss is anticipated. Other factors that would necessitate detection of modest anemia include advanced age, reduced exercise tolerance, existing or previous myocardial or cerebral ischemia, and reduced arterial oxygen tension.[44] There is no evidence that detection and correction of milder degrees of anemia (< 11 to 12 g/dl) has any effect on surgical outcome. Furthermore, there is no evidence that early detection of mild or even modest anemia affects morbidity or mortality in asymptomatic members of the general population.[42]

The prevalence of clinically silent abnormalities of the CBC other than mild anemia is quite low. Asymptomatic thrombocytopenia is estimated to occur in 5 per 100,000 surgical patients,[34] making it extremely costly to detect. In addition, there is no evidence that detection and correction of asymptomatic thrombocytopenia affects surgical outcome. Asymptomatic leukocytosis or leukopenia are also uncommon and of unknown import in the perioperative period. Abnormalities of the differential white cell count, although common, are nonspecific and have little effect on surgical outcome.[33]

Abnormalities of the prothrombin and partial thromboplastin times are also rare in asymptomatic surgical patients. No abnormalities of these tests were detected in 201 patients undergoing preoperative screening, 77% of whom were felt not to have indications for such testing.[18] No evidence is available that detection of asymptomatic abnormalities in PT/PTT affect surgical outcome, and these tests are not recommended for routine screening.[11,18,34] Abnormal bleeding times are also rare in asymptomatic patients, and their effect on surgical outcome is unclear.[1] Abnormalities of PT/PTT, whole blood clot lysis and bleeding times, and fibrinogen level and platelet counts in 92 patients undergoing cardiac surgery were not associated with excess blood component transfusion.[31] Therefore, the performance of any of these tests in the preoperative period is difficult to justify.

Serum Chemistries

Abnormalities in six-factor automated analysis (electrolytes, BUN, creatinine) were detected in 41 of 514 preoperative patients, 176 of whom were felt not to have indications for the test.[18] Only one abnormality, a creatinine level of 1.8, was detected in the "unindicated" group. Effects of electrolyte abnormalities on surgical outcome were not detailed in this study. Blood glucose abnormalities were de-

tected in 5.4% of these patients, and again the impact of detection of these abnormalities is unclear. The remarkably low yield of significant abnormalities in this and other screening blood tests in preoperative patients is demonstrated in Figure 1-1.[18]

Extensive biochemical profiles (such as those including liver function tests, uric acid, and cholesterol) have a high prevalence of abnormalities in the asymptomatic patient.[27] Of 31,439 different measurements performed in 2071 patients, 10% were abnormal, but more than 40% of asymptomatic patients had at least one unexpected abnormal result.[45] This is really not surprising when one considers the way in which abnormal ranges are defined, and then applies the laws of probability. Abnormal ranges for most biochemical profiles are defined as those values falling more than two standard deviations beyond the mean in an ostensibly normal population. Because the interval defined by the mean ± 2 standard deviations contains 95% of a normal distribution, 5% of normal people will have values in the "abnormal" range for any one test. If multiple tests are performed, the probability that two unrelated tests will be normal is the product of the probability of each being normal, or $0.95 \times 0.95 = 0.90$. If 12 tests are performed, the probability that all will be normal is equal to 0.95^{12}, or only 54%. Thus 46% of ostensibly normal persons will have at least one test that lies outside the normal range on multiple screening. Further investigations of these abnormalities often fail to demonstrate any explanations for them, and many resolve on repeat testing[2] (the phenomenon of regression to the mean).[38] This led one author to conclude that ". . . in many cases the abnormal result persists and is evidently simply an idiosyncrasy of the individual concerned."[45] For these reasons, routine biochemical profiling is not recommended in preoperative patients. One should remember, however, that hypokalemia is not uncommon in patients on diuretic therapy, and hypokalemia may exacerbate ventricular arrhythmias in perioperative patients who become hypoxic or acidotic. Therefore, it is reasonable to obtain "screening" potassium levels in patients on diuretic therapy.

Urinalysis

Abnormalities of routine urinalysis are quite frequent and almost double in prevalence when the test is clinically indicated.[19] Of 1607 admission urinalyses performed at the Brooke Army Medical Center,

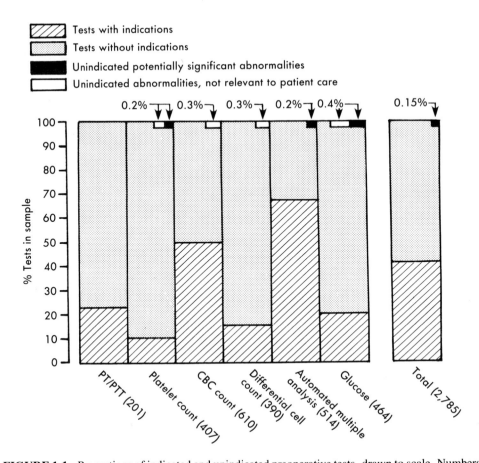

FIGURE 1-1. Proportions of indicated and unindicated preoperative tests, drawn to scale. Numbers in parentheses represent sample sizes used. *PT/PTT* indicates prothrombin time/partial thromboplastin time; *CBC*, complete blood cell. *Automated multiple analysis* is six factor.

From Kaplan et al: Preoperative laboratory screening, JAMA 253:3578, 1985.

861 were considered to be clinically indicated, of which 341 (40%) were abnormal. Eighteen percent of the unindicated urinalyses were abnormal. Of interest, two thirds of abnormalities in routine urinalysis were ignored by the treating physician, and only 1.3% had any potential impact on therapy. These findings are similar to those of Heimann et al, in which more than half of the urinalysis abnormalities in 400 medical patients were overlooked.[15] Few such studies have been performed in surgical patients, although one study on 3375 preoperative oral and maxillofacial surgery patients showed a prevalence of 2.7%.[13] The effect of detection of these abnormalities on patient outcome is not reported.

MEDICAL-LEGAL ISSUES

A frequent concern in attempting to limit preoperative testing involves the legal implications. The perception is that certain tests are obligatory because it would be negligent to allow patients to come through the hospital without screening for a variety of asymptomatic problems. This was dealt with somewhat in the discussion of preoperative diagnosis of unrelated, asymptomatic disease. It is difficult to find evidence of legal liability for failure to order a *routine*, otherwise unindicated preoperative test, although one would obviously be culpable for failure to order a test indicated by clinical examination. A far greater source of liability lies in abnormalities of routine screening that are detected and recorded by the appropriate laboratory, yet are not noted or followed up by the attending physician. Thus the medical-legal implications are much more serious when one is ordering a test and failing to follow up than in not ordering a *routine* test at all.

Which preoperative tests are indicated? Robbins recommends checking the hematocrit levels in patients who are otherwise healthy.[34] Considering the lack of evidence that detection of modest anemia affects perioperative outcome, this may be hard to justify in patients with no signs or symptoms. However, a finger-stick hematocrit is certainly an economical test, with almost 100% sensitivity and specificity, and it is an easy one to do.

Robbins also recommends routine urinalysis, primarily for detection of asymptomatic bacteriuria. This would be most important in the elderly (who have a high prevalence of this condition) and in patients scheduled to receive valve replacements, vascular grafts, or other foreign bodies or to undergo urinary tract instrumentation. Microscopic examination of the urine is accurate and inexpensive, and graft infection or sepsis are devastating complications of surgery that may be prevented by identification and treatment of urinary tract infection.

Considering the relatively poor sensitivity and specificity of the routine ECG for coronary artery disease, and the lack of obvious benefit from the baseline ECG, this test is difficult to justify in the asymptomatic preoperative patient. However, since cardiac complications are a major source of operative mortality and the interpreted preoperative ECG is such a traditional part of the preoperative examination, elimination of this routine test may be extremely difficult. If one feels compelled to order ECGs for patients at risk for coronary disease (and this is the only asymptomatic group in which one should consider performing them), the nonspecific nature of many ECG abnormalities must be kept in mind.

Few other tests can be justified in the asymptomatic preoperative patient. The only one to consider using on a routine basis would be pregnancy screening in women of child-bearing age, because exposure to anesthetic agents in the first trimester may have teratogenic effects. A beta-human chorionic gonadotropin assay is a reasonable part of the preoperative evaluation of a woman of child-bearing age undergoing elective surgery.

In summary, one must ask oneself several questions about any test ordered in the perioperative period.

1. *Is the test needed to confirm a suspicion formed on the basis of clinical findings?*

The best preoperative screening test is the clinical examination, and if a test is indicated from the history and physical findings, it is not a screening test but a confirmatory test.

2. *Is the abnormality occult but likely to carry a serious morbidity if undetected?*

In this category might fall screening for bacteriuria, or for hypokalemia in patients on diuretic therapy.

3. *Does a patient have a higher-than-average likelihood of having an abnormality?*

Since most asymptomatic abnormalities are rare, one should attempt to limit screening, if it must be performed, to patients at high risk for having an abnormality.

4. *Will a positive or negative result alter the management in any way?*

If one is not going to act on the results of the test, there is absolutely no reason to administer the test in the first place.

REFERENCES

1. Barber A et al: The bleeding time as a preoperative screening test, Am J Med 78:761–764, 1985.
2. Bradwell AR, Carmalt MHB, and Whitehead TP: Explaining the unexpected abnormal results of biochemical profile investigations, Lancet 2:1071–1074, 1974.
3. Carliner NH et al: The preoperative electrocardiogram as an indicator of risk in major noncardiac surgery, Can J Cardiol 2:134–137, 1986.
4. Catchlove BR et al: Routine investigations in elective surgical patients, Med J Aust 2:107–110, 1979.
5. Clarke JR and Eisenberg JM: A theoretical assessment of the value of the PTT as a preoperative screening test in adults, Med Decis Making 1:40–43, 1981.
6. Collen MF et al: Dollar cost per positive test for automated multiphasic screening, N Engl J Med 283:459–463, 1970.
7. Collins VJ: Principles of anesthesiology, Philadelphia, 1976, Lea & Febiger.
8. Crombie DL: Diagnostic process, J Coll Gen Practit 6:579, 1963.
9. Delahunt B and Turnbull PRG: How cost effective are routine preoperative investigations? NZ Med J 92:431–432, 1980.

10. Durbridge TC et al: Evaluation of benefits of screening tests done immediately on admission to hospital, Clin Chem 22:968–971, 1976.

11. Eisenberg JM, Clarke JR and Sussman SA: Prothrombin and partial thromboplastin times as preoperative screening tests, Arch Surg 117:48–51, 1982.

12. Ferrer MI: The value of obligatory preoperative electrocardiograms, J Am Med Wom Assoc 33:459–469, 1978.

13. Gold B and Wolfersberger WH: Findings from routine urinalysis and hematocrit on ambulatory oral and maxillofacial surgery patients, J Oral Surg 30:677–678, 1980.

14. Hampton JR et al: Relative contributions of history-taking, physical examination, and laboratory investigation to diagnosis and management of medical outpatients, Br Med J 2:486–489, 1975.

15. Heimann GA, Frohlich J, and Bernstein M: Physician's response to abnormal results of routine urinalysis, Can Med Assoc J 115:1094–1095, 1976.

16. Hubbell FA et al: The impact of routine admission chest x-ray films on patient care, N Engl J Med 312:209–213, 1985.

17. Ingelfinger JA et al: Biostatistics in Clinical Medicine, ed 2, New York, 1987, Macmillan Publishing Co, Inc.

18. Kaplan EB et al: The usefulness of preoperative laboratory screening, JAMA 253(24):3576–3581, 1985.

19. Kroenke K et al: The admission urinalysis: impact on patient care, J Gen Intern Med 1:238–242, 1986.

20. Korvin CC, Pearce RH, and Stanley J: Admissions screening: clinical benefits, Ann Intern Med 83:197–203, 1975.

21. Kowalyshyn TJ, Prager D, and Young J: A review of the present status of preoperative hemoglobin requirements, Anesth Analg 51:75–79, 1972.

22. Kunkel SE and Warner MA: Human T-cell lymphotrophic virus type III (HTLV-III) infection: how it can affect you, your patients, and your anesthesia practice, Anesthesiology 66:195–207, 1987.

23. Loder RE: Routine preoperative chest radiography, Anesthesiology 33:972–974, 1978.

24. Margolis JR, Kannel WB, and Feinleib M: Clinical features of unrecognized myocardial infarction—silent and symptomatic, eighteen year follow up, Framingham study, Am J Cardiol 32:1–7, 1973.

25. Medical Practice Committee, American College of Physicians: Periodic health examination: a guide for designing individualized preventive health care in the asymptomatic patient, Ann Intern Med 95:729–732, 1981.

26. Moorman JR et al: The yield of the routine admission electrocardiogram, Ann Intern Med 103:590–595, 1985.

27. Newman HF: Chemical screening in ambulatory adults, NY State J Med 14:2172–2175, 1978.

28. Paterson KR et al: The preoperative electrocardiogram: an assessment, Scott Med J 28:116–118, 1983.

29. Rabkin SW and Horne JM: Preoperative electrocardiography: effect of new abnormalities on clinical decisions, Can Med Assoc J 128:146–147, 1983.

30. Rabkin SW and Horne JM: Preoperative electrocardiography: its cost-effectiveness in detecting abnormalities when a previous tracing exists, Can Med Assoc J 121:301–306, 1979.

31. Ramsey G, Arvan DA, and Stewart S: Do preoperative laboratory tests predict blood transfusion needs in cardiac operations? J Thorac Cardiovasc Surg 85:564–569, 1983.

32. Rees AM et al: Routine preoperative chest radiography in non-cardiopulmonary surgery, Br Med J 1:1333–1335, 1976.

33. Rich EC, Crowson TW, and Connelly DP: Effectiveness of differential leukocyte count in case finding in the ambulatory care setting, JAMA 249:633–636, 1983.

34. Robbins JA and Mushlin AI: Preoperative evaluation of the healthy patient. From Symposium on Medical Evaluation of the Preoperative Patient, Med Clin North Am 63 (6):1145–1156, 1979.

35. Royal College of Radiologists: Preoperative chest radiology, Lancet 2:83–85, 1979.

36. Rubenstein LZ and Greenfield S: The baseline ECG in the evaluation of acute cardiac complaints, JAMA 244:2536–2539, 1980.

37. Rucker L, Frye EB, and Staten MA: Usefulness of screening chest roentgenograms in preoperative patients, JAMA 250:3209–3211, 1983.

38. Sackett DL: The usefulness of laboratory tests in health-screening programs, Clin Chem 19(4):366–372, 1973.

39. Sackett DL, Haynes RB, and Tugwell P: Clinical epidemiology: a basic science for clinical medicine, Boston, 1985, Little, Brown & Co, Inc.

40. Sagel SS et al: Efficacy of routine screening and lateral chest radiographs in a hospital-based population, N Engl J Med 291:1001–1004, 1974.

41. Sandler G: The importance of the history in the medical clinic and the cost of unnecessary tests, Am Heart J 100:928–931, 1980.

42. Shapiro MF and Greenfield S: The complete blood count and leukocyte differential count, Ann Intern Med 106:65–74, 1987.

43. Spitzer WO, chairman: Report of the Task Force on the Periodic Health Examination, Can Med Assoc J 121:1193–1254, 1979.

44. Watson-Williams EJ: Hematologic and hemostatic considerations before surgery. From Symposium on Medical Evaluation of the Preoperative Patient, Med Clin North Am 63(6):1165–1189, 1979.

45. Whitehead TP: Biochemical profiles for hospital patients, Lancet 2:1439–1443, 1974.

CHAPTER 2

Risk of Anesthesia

ALAN F. ROSS
JOHN H. TINKER

Difficulties in characterizing anesthetic risk
Errors in management versus toxicity of agents
Preoperative risk assessment
Trends in anesthesia risk
New horizons for risk studies
Summary

Anesthesia has been a major advance in medicine; it has enabled the physician to contest disease in its deepest hiding places within the body. Yet this advance has had a cost. The anesthetic that could overcome the body's most tenacious defenses could also be harmful. Are the drugs themselves dangerous, or is it the technique of administration? Are some patients at greater risk than others? A discussion of the risk of anesthesia must address the great potency of these agents, the patients who receive them, and the responsibility of the men and women who are charged with their control.

The definition of anesthetic risk is important for several reasons. First, patients need to understand the risks involved to make informed decisions. Patients need to be aware that all activities contain elements of risk and that anesthesia may involve risks that are separate from and in addition to their surgery. A thoughtful discussion will help the patient to make an informed decision and is thus likely to

relieve rather than increase any anxiety the patient may feel.

A second reason for determining the anesthetic risk is to allocate the appropriate resources for patient care. The patient who has suffered a recent myocardial infarction and who is admitted to the hospital for emergency repair of an abdominal aortic aneurysm will require specialized personnel and monitors in the operating room and the intensive care unit. When a patient is identified as high risk, such resources can be more focused. Medical care facilities that do not have such resources can assess their ability to care for such high-risk patients.

The third reason for assessing anesthetic risk is to identify ways to reduce the risk. Ideally, epidemiologic methods can identify factors that have a causal relationship to an adverse outcome. Therapy directed at the risk factor should improve the results. For example, the Goldman Cardiac Risk Index[8] (1976) lists nine factors that increase the risk of perioperative cardiac events. One of these factors is symptomatic aortic stenosis. The mechanism by which aortic stenosis contributed to the cardiac event was not immediately apparent, but it is now known that the hypertrophied ventricle can suffer ischemia even with normal coronary arteries.[21] This knowledge has suggested therapy to reduce the impact of this risk factor, namely, maintenance of coronary perfusion pressure,[15] control of heart rate, and correction of anemia.

This chapter examines some of the problems involved in characterizing anesthetic risk. Although it is helpful to know how many persons may die from anesthesia, it is much more important to try to determine *why* they died. Analysis of anesthetic risk is a tool used to make anesthesia safer.

DIFFICULTIES IN CHARACTERIZING ANESTHETIC RISK

A major problem in characterizing the risk of anesthesia is the difficulty of distinguishing it from surgical risk and the risk resulting from the patient's disease. Epidemiologic studies constantly face this type of problem. Cuyler Hammond, the pioneer in studies of cigarette smoking, had this to say regarding his work[12]:

I have said that there is abundant evidence of an association between death rates and antecedent amount of cigarette smoking. Perhaps I should have pointed out that this is probably true only under certain conditions . . . such as exist in human populations where death from infections and parasitic diseases is uncommon and where violence and accidents account for a relatively small proportion of all deaths.

Can anesthetic risk be studied in a population where the risk of death from surgery or patient disease is minimal? Perhaps healthy patients undergoing minor surgery would be such a group. Yet the healthy patient may tolerate a stress from anesthesia that an ill patient or a patient undergoing major surgery could not. Thus a healthy study population may lead to an underestimation of the risk of anesthesia. We are faced with the reality that illness and surgical trespass are characteristic of the population that receives anesthesia.

To separate mortality caused by anesthesia from mortality caused by surgery or patient disease, Edwards et al[6] (1956) analyzed 1000 reports of death associated with anesthesia that were voluntarily and anonymously submitted to the Council of the Association of Anaesthetists over a period of 5½ years ending in 1955. The cases were classified into eight categories based on the estimated cause of death (see the box below).

The Council determined that anesthesia contributed to the death (categories I, II and III) in 598 (59%) of the cases. Detailed descriptions of the circumstances of the 598 cases provided important information to anesthesia practitioners. However, the classification scheme itself was this paper's important contribution. Its attempt to distinguish the causes of death *not* resulting from anesthesia was a major step toward defining risk of anesthesia.

The difficulty of separating the risk of anesthesia from that of surgery is illustrated by the report of Lunn et al[20] in 1983. These authors evaluated 197 reports of death occurring within 6 days of anesthesia that were voluntarily and anonymously submitted from five regions in the United Kingdom. A questionnaire was sent to both the anesthetist and the

---

Deaths associated with anaesthesia

I.   Where it was reasonably certain that death was caused by the anaesthetic agent or technique of administration, or in other ways coming entirely within the anaesthetist's province.

II.   Similar cases, but in which there was some element of doubt as to whether the agent or technique was entirely responsible for the fatal result.

III.   Cases in which the patient's death was caused by both the surgical and anaesthetic techniques.

IV.   Deaths entirely referable to surgical technique, e.g. uncontrolled hemorrhage.

V.   Inevitable deaths, e.g. cases of severe general peritonitis in which the anaesthetic and surgical techniques were apparently satisfactory.

VI.   Fortuitous deaths, e.g. due to pulmonary embolism.

VII.   Cases that could not be assessed despite considerable data.

VIII.   Cases on which an opinion could not be formed on account of inadequacy of data.

From Edwards et al: Deaths associated with anaesthesia: a report on 1000 cases, Anaesthesia 11:194, 1956.

surgeon in each case. Both were asked to decide whether the contribution of anesthesia to the patient's death was none, some, or total. These responses and the cases were then reviewed by two independent assessors who made the final determination as to the contribution of anesthesia to the death. Not surprisingly, the surgeon's and the anesthetist's opinions frequently did not agree. A comparison of the opinions of the anesthetist and the surgeon in 32 cases, which were ultimately determined by the assessors to be totally the result of anesthesia, is given in Table 2-1.

Overall, the assessor agreed with the anesthetist alone 33% of the time, with the surgeon alone 29% of the time, with both 18.4% of the time, and with neither 19% of the time. This study emphasizes the need for several independent opinions to determine the significance of anesthesia to a patient's death.

ERRORS IN MANAGEMENT VERSUS TOXICITY OF AGENTS

Many medical discoveries have begun from the study of mortality in patients. Yet in the early years of anesthesia, anesthetic drugs were assumed to be safe. In 1948, a leader in anesthesia, Sir Robert MacIntosh, wrote[22]:

As I hold that there should be no deaths due to anaesthetics, I am very uneasy as to how far we are justified in testing new drugs when the correct administration of those already available to us will give excellent operating conditions to the surgeon at negligible risk to the patient.

This statement reminds us of the proposal by the Director of the U.S. Patent Office, circa 1890, to close down the office on the grounds that everything worthwhile had already been invented. However, in the early post–World War II period, improper administration of anesthesia was a major problem. Sir Robert MacIntosh wrote[22]:

My opinion that anaesthetic deaths are preventable . . . was confirmed during the war when I travelled around visiting RAF hospitals . . . I found that what might be described as stock accidents were happening all over.

Thus in those early days of anesthesia the emphasis on anesthetic risk was directed toward correcting errors in management rather than toward toxicity of the agents themselves or better standards of monitoring.

In a classic paper in 1979, Keats[17] found that many studies of anesthetic mortality exhibited the same bias expressed by MacIntosh in 1948, namely that anesthetic agents were inherently safe when administered properly and thus deaths resulting from anesthesia were the result of errors or mismanagement. Anesthesia study commissions were confining their efforts to a search for errors in management. Keats pointed out that adverse reactions to any drug must be expected on pharmacodynamic principles. Anesthetic drugs may have adverse responses even when correctly selected and administered. More importantly, Keats warned that such an emphasis on errors may prevent the recognition of toxicity of the agent. For example, the symptoms of cyanosis and hypercarbia during anesthesia may be attributed to an error in airway management. Yet these symptoms could also have been caused by an anesthetic toxicity, namely malignant hyperpyrexia. Similarly, the search for error would not have revealed the mechanisms of succinylcholine-induced hyperkalemia, genetic differences in plasma cholinesterase, or halothane hepatitis. Dr. Keats challenged the assumption that anesthetic death always resulted from error. Patient variability, adverse reactions, and toxicity of anesthetic agents must be considered to establish a cause and effect relationship for anesthetic risk. Recent evidence has confirmed Dr. Keats's proposals.

The study of errors can produce useful information. Cooper et al[4] asked anesthesiologists, residents, and nurse anesthetists to report on past and present incidents that involved a preventable human error or equipment failure. A critical incident was defined as "a human error that could have led (if not discovered

TABLE 2-1. Thirty-two cases of mortality determined by independent assessors to be entirely caused by anaesthesia

Contribution of anaesthesia to patient death	Anaesthetist opinion	Surgeon opinion
No contribution	5 cases	9 cases
Some contribution	21 cases	13 cases
Total contribution	5 cases	8 cases
(Blank)	1 case	2 cases
TOTAL	32 cases	32 cases

From Lunn et al: Anaesthesia related surgical mortality, Anaesthesia 38:1090, 1983.

TABLE 2-2.   Common critical incidents

Incident	Number of incidents
Breathing circuit disconnection	57
Syringe swap	50
Gas flow control technical error	41
Loss of gas supply	32
Intravenous line disconnection	24

From Cooper et al: An analysis of major errors and equipment failures in anesthesia management, Anesthesiology 60:34, 1984.

TABLE 2-3.   Common factors associated with critical incidents

Factor	Number of incidents
Failure to check	223
First experience with situation	208
Inadequate total experience	201
Inattention or carelessness	166
Haste encouraged by situation	131

From Cooper et al: An analysis of major errors and equipment failures in anesthesia management, Anesthesiology 60:34, 1984.

TABLE 2-4.   ASA physical status

Category	Description
I	Healthy patient
II	Mild systemic disease; no functional limitation
III	Severe systemic disease; definite functional limitation
IV	Severe systemic disease that is a constant threat to life
V	Moribund patient unlikely to survive 24 hours with or without operation

or corrected in time) or did lead to an undesirable outcome, ranging from increased length of hospital stay to death." A total of 1089 critical incidents were examined. The most common critical incidents are listed in Table 2-2, and the most common factors associated with critical incidents are listed in Table 2-3.

No correlation was found between frequently occurring errors and negative outcomes (longer hospital stay, cancelled procedure, cardiac arrest, or death). For example, the fifth most frequent critical incident, intravenous line disconnection, was not associated with any substantial negative outcome. However the twenty-third and twenty-fourth most frequent events, vaporizer drug overdose and intravenous drug overdose, were responsible for two and four substantial negative outcomes, respectively. The authors were unable to determine why some errors were promptly detected, whereas others led to adverse outcomes. Even so, this study was helpful in alerting anesthesiologists to common problems and strategies for prevention.

PREOPERATIVE RISK ASSESSMENT

One method of preoperative risk assessment addresses the overall condition of the patient. Since the ill patient has less physiologic reserve than the healthy patient, it is logical that such a patient would be less able to tolerate the stress of anesthesia and surgery. Thus the ASA physical status (Table 2-4) should predict perioperative mortality. Class III and IV patients would be expected to have greater mortality than class I and II patients. However, in the 1970 review by Goldstein and Keats[9] of deaths attributable to anesthesia, a total of 41% of deaths studied occurred in ASA class I or II patients. Their conclusion was that the ASA physical status was not

a sensitive predictor of anesthetic mortality. Vacanti et al[30] in 1970 collected 68,388 cases from 11 U.S. naval hospitals and reported that ASA physical status was somewhat predictive, at least of overall outcome.

Several explanations are possible. Extensive operations are not usually planned for the extremely ill patient. Instead, limited procedures are weighed against the patient's condition. These procedures may in fact prolong life (for example, drainage of septic abscess). Anesthetic drugs may be chosen that preserve the body's stress response. Sophisticated monitoring, more experienced physicians and postoperative recovery in the intensive care unit may also contribute to better than expected survival in class III and IV patients.

A different strategy for assessing preoperative risk is to examine one factor in detail. The best illustration is the risk of perioperative myocardial infarction. In 1977 Goldman[8] identified nine risk factors in 1001 patients that appeared predictive of postoperative cardiac events (see the box on p. 17). This study has been used to preoperatively evaluate a

TABLE 2-5. Incidence of perioperative myocardial infarction and stroke in patients undergoing coronary artery bypass surgery

	1971-1973	1974-1976	1977-1979	1980-1982	1983-1984
Perioperative infarction	4.5%	4.0%	1.9%	1.1%	0.8%
Stroke	1.8%	1.4%	1.8%	1.7%	1.3%

From Cleveland Clinic Foundation: Morbidity associated with myocardial revascularization. In Brest, A (editor): Cardiovascular clinics, Philadelphia, 1987, F A Davis Co.

Goldman preoperative cardiac risk factors

1. S$_3$ gallop or jugular venous distention
2. MI in preceding 6 months
3. Rhythm other than sinus
4. Premature ventricular contractions > 5/minute
5. Intraabdominal, intrathoracic, aortic surgery
6. Age greater than 70 years
7. Significant valvular aortic stenosis
8. Emergency operations
9. Poor general medical condition

Reprinted with permission from Goldman et al: Multifactorial index of cardiac risk in noncardiac surgical procedures, N Engl J Med 297:845, 1977.

---

patient's risk for surgery. However, Waters et al[31] prospectively tested the Goldman risk index and found it no more predictive than the subjective ASA physical status rating. Jeffrey et al[16] used the Goldman risk factors to predict perioperative cardiac events in patients undergoing abdominal aortic aneurysm repair. Their report found the Goldman index to markedly underestimate postoperative cardiac events in this high-risk patient group.

In 1978, Steen et al[29] further defined the relationship between prior myocardial infarction and perioperative reinfarction. In a large retrospective study, they showed that:

1. Patients with prior MI have overall reinfarction risk of about 6%.
2. Patients with a relatively recent (3 to 6 months) MI have approximately 15% reinfarction risk.
3. Patients with a recent MI (within 3 months) have an approximate risk of 30% reinfarction within 7 days of anesthesia and surgery.

However, myocardial infarction may occur without symptoms, making accurate timing of the event impossible. Furthermore, dangerously extensive coronary disease can exist without myocardial infarction. In 1985 Boucher et al[1] demonstrated that an objective (and noninvasive) indicator, the thallium dipyridamole scan, could accurately identify which patients were at increased risk for perioperative myocardial infarction.

TRENDS IN ANESTHESIA RISK

Risks may be expected to change as experience and techniques improve. Advances in surgical method, cardioplegia, monitoring, and cardiac anesthesia may have reduced the incidence of perioperative myocardial infarction associated with coronary artery bypass surgery. This trend is evident from the morbidity data from the Cleveland Clinic (Table 2-5). In contrast, there has been little apparent change in the incidence of cerebral injury. Either this risk has approached an "irreducible minimum" or, more likely, it needs more attention.

There is evidence that more attention directed at the high-risk patient will reduce the risk. In 1983, Rao et al[25] reported reduced risk of postoperative infarction in patients managed by invasive cardiovascular monitoring and inotrope/vasodilator pharmacology. They retrospectively examined 364 prior MI patients who underwent anesthesia and surgery from 1973 to 1977. They then examined 733 prior MI patients who underwent surgery from 1977 to 1982 with the benefit of invasive monitoring and vasoactive drugs. Patients in the 1977 to 1982 group had a considerably lower incidence of perioperative myocardial infarction than in all previous retrospective studies (Table 2-6).

Rao et al[25] attributed the lower reinfarction rates to the use of invasive hemodynamic monitoring, beta blockers, vasodilators, and postoperative intensive care unit management. However, these results have not been repeated elsewhere even though considerable time has elapsed. Anecdotal evidence suggests that such low risk is not the rule in the United States today.

TABLE 2-6.   Reduced reinfarction rates

Preoperative risk	1973-1976 Reinfarction rates (%)	1977-1982 Reinfarction rates (%)
MI 3-6 months before surgery	36	5.8
MI less than 3 months before surgery	26	2.3

From Rao et al: Reinfarction following anesthesia in patients with myocardial infarction, Anesthesiology 59:499, 1983.

TABLE 2-7.   Cases of anesthetic mortality

	1960-1969	1970-1980	1983-1985
Number of cases evaluated	961	1149	406
Number of cases in which anesthesia played a part in causing death	335	239	50
Percentages of cases evaluated	35%	21%	12.2%

From Holland: Anaesthetic mortality in New South Wales, Br J Anaesthesia 59:834-841, 1987.

There is evidence, however, that the risk from undergoing anesthesia has decreased in recent years. The most recent information is that reported by Holland[13] from New South Wales, Australia. Since 1960, a committee has investigated deaths occurring in relation to anesthesia. The percentage of deaths related to anesthesia in this series (Table 2-7) has declined from 35% (1960 to 1969) to 12.2% (1983 to 1985). By relating number of anesthesia deaths in a given year to the estimated number of anesthetics administered, an indication of anesthetic risk can be calculated (Table 2-8). The number of anesthetics administered increased, but the incidence of deaths related to anesthesia decreased. Holland concludes that it was at least five times safer to undergo anesthesia in 1987 than in 1960 in New South Wales.

The reasons for the apparent improvement are not certain. Are anesthetic drugs safer? Health care stan-

TABLE 2-8.   Estimated risk of death due to anesthesia

Year	Number of deaths	Estimated anesthetics	Deaths per number of anesthetics
1960	55	300,000	1 per 5500
1970	39	400,000	1 per 10,250
1984	24	550,000	1 per 26,000

From Holland: Anaesthetic mortality in New South Wales, Br J Anaesthesia 59:834-841, 1987.

TABLE 2-9.   Cases of anaesthetic mortality according to patient preoperative condition

Preoperative condition	1960-1969	1970-1980	1983-1985
Good	65(19.4%)	42(17.6%)	9(18%)
Fair	80(23.8%)	72(30.1%)	14(28%)
Poor	155(46.3%)	80(33.4%)	20(40%)
Desperate	35(10.4%)	45(18.8%)	7(14%)
TOTAL	335	239	50

From Holland: Anaesthetic mortality in New South Wales, Br J Anaesthesia 59:834-841, 1987.

dards may have been raised in response to anesthesia mortality studies and recommendations from commissions. Holland[13] discusses several changes that have occurred in New South Wales. Particularly there has been a trend toward administration of anesthetic by physicians specially trained in this field instead of nonspecialists. This led to a marked decrease in the number of deaths in low-risk patients from the 1960 to 1969 period to the 1983 to 1985 period.

Similarly, the nonanesthesia medical officer had been associated with anesthetic mortality in low-risk patients in the early years of 1960 to 1969. This led to a phasing out of the medical officer as a member of the anesthetic work force. An improvement was also noted in anesthesia trainee (registrar) performance. Despite a sixfold increase in the number of anesthesia trainees, their contribution to anesthetic mortality has not increased. Holland speculates this may be in part a result of better supervision.

The data from New South Wales, however, still leave questions to be resolved. When patients were classified according to preoperative condition (good,

TABLE 2-10. Common errors in anesthetic management

	Ranking in order of frequency in 1960-1969	Later ranking of same errors	
		1970-1980	1980-1983
Overdose	1st	7th	4th
Wrong choice	2nd	3rd	2nd
Inadequate preparation	3rd	1st	1st
Inadequate crisis management	4th	2nd	3rd

From Holland: Anaesthetic mortality in New South Wales, Br J Anesthesia, 59:834-841, 1987.

fair, poor, or desperate), it was clear that the absolute number of deaths had decreased but the percentage in each category had not. That is, 19.4% of the total deaths for 1960 to 1969 occurred in low-risk patients and 18% of the total deaths in 1983 to 1985 (Table 2-9). Questions also remain regarding the factors that contribute to adverse outcomes. Holland[13] notes that anesthetic overdose was the most common error in the 1960 to 1969 period (Table 2-10). While it has dropped to the fourth most common error in 1980 to 1983, preoperative management errors have increased in relative frequency. Furthermore, the top four error categories of 1960 to 1969 remain in the top four slots for 1983 to 1985 (although their order has changed). The persistence of mortality in low-risk patients and the persistent frequency of certain types of errors suggest areas for more attention.

NEW HORIZONS FOR RISK STUDIES

A major goal of anesthetic risk studies is to identify factors that can be treated to reduce risk. Some studies have concentrated on equipment malfunction and errors in management. By increasing our awareness of these dangers, such studies should help reduce anesthetic risk. However, as Keats[17] warned, studies concentrating on errors in judgment or administration may overlook risks resulting from the toxicity of the agent itself. Recently Caplan et al[2] have studied cases of cardiac arrest under spinal anesthesia from the ASA Closed Claims Study.[2] Their findings indicate that the margin of safety in the tolerance of spinal anesthesia may be considerably less than previously thought. Their findings substantiate Keats's view that careful review of the case circumstances can be more fruitful than a simple assignment to a category of mortality resulting from anesthesia.

During a review of 900 cases of major anesthetic mishaps from insurance company closed claims, Caplan et al[2] noted 14 cases of cardiac arrest under spinal anesthesia in healthy patients (ASA I or II). Despite prompt cardiovascular resuscitation, only four patients regained consciousness (three of these with neurologic deficits). This is in contrast to "out of hospital" cardiopulmonary resuscitation, which has been reported to result in 41% of patients recovering without neurologic deficit. Careful analysis of the cases revealed two patterns. The first pattern was the use of intraoperative sedation to produce a sleeplike state (seven cases). In six of these seven cases, cyanosis was one of the first clues of arrest. The authors postulated that unappreciated respiratory insufficiency may have been present. Perhaps a vasodilating effect from hypercarbia and hypoxia occurred and was additive to the sympathetic blockade from the spinal anesthetic. The combination of these factors may have led to hypotension and cardiac arrest.

The second pattern noted by the authors was an inadequate appreciation of the influence of spinal anesthesia on the mechanism of cardiopulmonary resuscitation. The authors postulated that the spinal sympathetic block may have shifted blood flow to peripheral tissues rather than the brain during CPR. Epinephrine was not administered until an average of 8 minutes of asystole had elapsed in these cases.

The authors of this study offered recommendations to reduce the risk of spinal anesthesia. When sedatives are used, pulse oximetry should be employed. Epinephrine should be considered early in the treatment of bradycardia, especially if atropine and ephedrine are ineffective. Upon recognition of cardiac arrest, a resuscitation dose of epinephrine should be given immediately.

In an editorial accompanying the Caplan study, Dr. Keats added to the authors explanation of risk of spinal anesthesia. He pointed out that knowledge of the respiratory effects of drugs has been obtained from healthy volunteer subjects. Perhaps the behavior of these agents is influenced by the state of spinal anesthesia. Keats also speculated on the delay in the use of vasopressor agents. This may be a product of modern teaching about the inverse relationship between cardiac output and systemic resistance and a belief that high systemic resistance must be avoided.

SUMMARY

In this review of anesthetic risk two somewhat diverse views have been presented. One view of anesthetic risk involves collection of mortality statistics with committee-type decisions as to anesthetic versus surgical risk. This method analyzes the events for errors in preparation, management of anesthesia, or equipment malfunction. The utility of such studies is to increase anesthesiologists' awareness of the problems and hopefully prevent their occurrence. The other perhaps more positive view of risk is that when searches for causation are exhaustive, sometimes new knowledge emerges. Perhaps we have been too self-flagellant in our incessant stridency about vigilance. By concentrating on errors as the cause of anesthetic risk, perhaps we have overlooked some physiologic answers to explain why the patients died.

Consider the Caplan[2] study of cardiac arrest under spinal anesthesia. Since the patients were healthy and the surgery minor, these cases probably would have been classified in the Edwards[6] classes I or II (death related to anesthesia). Since the death was placed in one of the anesthesia categories, a committee of experts would have been required to determine which error of management had been present. Of the 12 errors used in Holland's[13] reports, "inadequate intraoperative resuscitation," "inadequate crisis management," or "inadequate monitoring" categories would probably have accounted for these cases of cardiac arrest under spinal anesthesia. Thus the classification of the death would have ended the search for the cause. Caplan et al have demonstrated the search for cause must go further to truly determine the nature of anesthetic risk.

It may be that some of our most strongly held beliefs about anesthetic risk need to be reexamined. Consider the studies of perioperative myocardial in-farction. Despite apparent advances in hemodynamic monitoring, control of blood pressure, heart rate, and even myocardial ischemia itself, there still is a distressingly high and consistent number of perioperative myocardial infarctions. Could it be that we are missing something here also? While Slogoff and Keats[28] were able to relate intraoperative ischemic episodes to postoperative myocardial ischemic infarctions, only 7% of the ischemic patients had actual infarctions. Perhaps control of blood pressure and heart rate are not the root cause of infarction. Consider the recent success in treating acute myocardial infarction with streptokinase[32] and tissue plasminogen activator,[10] and the recent report of decreased myocardial infarction in patients who take aspirin.[24] Each of these major advancements involve the coagulation system. Could it be that anesthesia or surgery in some way in some patients alters the coagulation system and initiates the infarct? Perhaps the anesthetic enhances thrombosis. There is some evidence for this idea. General anesthesia and trauma does influence the activity of the coagulation system and the fibrinolytic system.[14,23] Levels of plasminogen and antithrombin III fall after general anesthesia and surgery.[27] A reevaluation of anesthesia and perioperative myocardial infarction may reveal a new mechanism for understanding anesthetic risk.

Most importantly, we must keep open minds and learn whatever we can from each new study. Some anesthetic deaths are certainly caused by errors in equipment use, drug use, preparation, and/or judgment. We must be aware of the occurrences, marshal our defenses against them, and help others avoid repeating the same mistakes. We must also be scientists and constantly research our ideas and beliefs. We hope these paths will lead to the continued reduction of anesthetic risk.

REFERENCES

1. Boucher CA et al: Determination of cardiac risk by dipyridamole-thallium imaging before peripheral vascular surgery, N Engl J Med 312:389-394, 1985.
2. Caplan RA et al: Unexpected cardiac arrest during spinal anesthesia: a closed claims analysis of predisposing factors, Anesthesiology 68:5-11, 1988.
3. Cleveland Clinic Foundation: Morbidity associated with myocardial revascularization. In Brest A (editor): Cardiovascular clinics, Philadelphia, 1987, FA Davis Co.
4. Cooper JB et al: An analysis of major errors and equipment failures in anesthesia management: con-

siderations for prevention and detection, Anesthesiology 60:34, 1984.

5. Dripps et al: Preanesthetic consultation and choice of anesthesia. In Introduction to anesthesia, ed 6, Philadelphia, 1982, WB Saunders Co.

6. Edwards G et al: Deaths associated with anaesthesia: report on 1000 cases, Anaesthesia 11:194, 1956.

7. Egbert LD et al: The value of the preoperative visit by an anesthetist, JAMA 185:553-555, 1963.

8. Goldman L et al: Multifactorial index of cardiac risk in noncardiac surgical procedures, N Engl J Med 297:845-850 1977.

9. Goldstein A et al: The risk of anesthesia, Anesthesiology 33:130, 1970.

10. Guerci A et al: A randomized trial of intravenous tissue plasminogen activator for acute myocardial infarction with subsequent randomization to elective coronary angioplasty, N Engl J Med 317:1613, 1987.

11. Hammond EC: The relationship between human smoking habits and death rates: a follow-up study of 187,766 men, JAMA 155:1316-1328, 1954.

12. Hammond EC: Remarks on smoking: evidence and ethics, CA 38(1):59-60, 1988.

13. Holland R: Anaesthetic mortality in New South Wales, Br J Anaesth 59:834-841, 1987.

14. Homann B et al: Effect of anaesthesia on blood coagulation factor XIII, Anaesthesist 33:145, 1984.

15. Jackson JM: Valvular heart disease. In Thomas, S (editor): Manual of cardiac anesthesia, New York, 1984, Churchill Livingstone.

16. Jeffrey CC et al: A prospective evaluation of cardiac risk, Anesthesiology 58:462, 1983.

17. Keats AS: What do we know about anesthetic mortality, Anesthesiology 50:387, 1979.

18. Keats AS: Anesthesia mortality—a new mechanism, Anesthesiology 68:2-4, 1988.

19. Longstreth WT et al: Prediction of awakening after out-of-hospital cardiac arrest, N Engl J Med 308:1378-1383, 1980.

20. Lunn JN et al: Anaesthesia related surgical mortality, Anaesthesia 38:1090, 1983.

21. Marcus M et al: A mechanism for angina pectoris in patients with aortic stenosis and normal coronary arteries, N Engl J Med 307:1363, 1982.

22. Macintosh RR: Deaths under anaesthetics, Br J Anaesth 21:107, 1948.

23. Modig J et al: Role of extradural and of general anesthesia in fibrinolysis and coagulation after total hip replacement, Br J Anaesth 55:625, 1983.

24. Relman AS: Aspirin for the primary prevention of myocardial infarction, N Engl J Med 318:245-246, 1988.

25. Rao TL et al: Reinfarction following anesthesia in patients with myocardial infarction, Anesthesiology 59:499, 1983.

26. Ruth HS: Anesthesia study commissions, JAMA 127:514, 1945.

27. Seyfer A et al: Coagulation changes in elective surgery and trauma, Ann Surg 193:210, 1980.

28. Slogoff S et al: Does perioperative myocardial ischemia lead to postoperative myocardial infarction? Anesthesiology 62:107-114, 1985.

29. Steen PA et al: Myocardial reinfarction after anesthesia in surgery, JAMA 239:2566, 1978.

30. Vacanti CJ et al: A statistical analysis of the relationship of physical status to postoperative mortality in 68,388 cases, Anesth Analg 49:564, 1970.

31. Waters J et al: Evaluation of cardiac risk in noncardiac surgical patients, Anesthesiology 55:A343, 1981.

32. White HD et al: Effect of intravenous streptokinase on left ventricular function and early survival after acute myocardial infarction, N Engl J Med 317:850, 1987.

CHAPTER 3

Cardiac Risk Assessment for Individual Patients

THOMAS H. LEE
LEE GOLDMAN

Clinical risk factors
  Ischemic heart disease
  Congestive heart failure
  Valvular heart disease
  Arrhythmias and conduction disturbances
  Type of surgery
  Noncardiac clinical variables

Specialized tests
Multifactorial risk assessment
Future directions

In the mid-1970s, when the first multifactorial index of cardiac risk in noncardiac surgery was being developed,[31] the risk of a myocardial infarction or cardiac death associated with general anesthesia and surgery was estimated to be about 0.2%.[53,66] In the years since, surgical procedures have become more ambitious. Furthermore, the aging of the population has led to a rise in the prevalence of chronic diseases such as angina, diabetes, and hypertension so that the condition of the surgical patient is often more complex. These changes have increased interest in perioperative risk assessment and evaluations made by anesthesiologic and medical consultants have become more important. For example, in one recent series of preoperative medical consultations, 47% of the patients had two or more chronic illnesses.[9]

Despite these trends toward higher risk in both procedures and patients, the rate of cardiac complications with surgery appears to have declined.[5,56,73]

For example, among 30,000 cases of major elective or emergent noncardiac operations at the Cleveland Clinic, 1980 through 1984, perioperative myocardial infarctions were identified in only 28 (0.1%) of the patients, and only 12 patients (0.04%) had cardiac deaths.[5] These circumstantial data suggest that cardiac risk in noncardiac surgery may have declined by as much as 50% in the last decade.

Several factors, including recent advances in surgical[4] and anesthetic[46a] techniques, may have contributed to this apparent improvement. In addition, anesthesiologists, surgeons, and medical consultants have been refining their ability to stratify cases according to risk since the publication of the American Society of Anesthesiologists' classification system[16,49] in the early 1960s. Settings in which the risks of surgery outweigh those associated with alternative treatments can now be more readily recognized, and management strategies that reduce surgical risk for individual patients can be planned.

However, the assessment of cardiac risk in surgical patients is clearly a field in the early stages of its development, and important clinical issues have not been explored. The optimal preoperative role of traditional diagnostic techniques such as the exercise tolerance test has not yet been defined, even as newer techniques, such as dipyridamole-thallium imaging,[6] become more available. Therefore, this chapter will first review the known clinical predictors of cardiac risk in noncardiac surgery and the available data on the diagnostic performance and incremental impact of specialized tests. It will then describe current approaches to multifactorial risk assessment and conclude with a summary of major problems that should be addressed by future clinical investigation.

CLINICAL RISK FACTORS
Ischemic Heart Disease

Recent myocardial infarction. While early studies of perioperative risk correctly identified ischemic heart disease as a major predictor of complications,[2,3,62,66,70] subsequent investigations have demonstrated that recent myocardial infarction is by far the most important single risk factor.* Analysis of pooled data from the 1960s and 1970s[31,64,66] shows that recurrent myocardial infarction or cardiac death occurred in about 30% of patients who underwent noncardiac surgery within 3 months after an acute myocardial infarction and about 15% of patients who underwent surgery 3 to 6 months after infarction.[28] After 6 months, the risk of recurrent infarction or death fell to and remained constant at about 5%. Patients who have had non-Q-wave myocardial infarction seem to have the same risk as those who have had Q-wave infarctions.[31,32]

More recent data suggest that the risk of surgery in patients who have had recent acute myocardial infarctions may have decreased since these studies were performed.[56,73] Wells and Kaplan[73] reported no infarctions in 48 patients who had surgical procedures within 3 months of an infarction, and in a series of patients who underwent perioperative invasive hemodynamic monitoring, Rao et al[56] found a reinfarction rate of 6% in patients who had surgery within 3 months of infarction and 2% in those who had surgery 3 to 6 months after infarction.

If, as we suspect, these data reflect true improve-

*References 2, 22, 31, 32, 64, 66, 70.

ments, the gains may be the result of a combination of improved surgical and anesthesia techniques, wider use of hemodynamic monitoring, and improved prognostic stratification of patients within the subpopulation with recent myocardial infarction. It seems reasonable to assume that the same factors that have proved useful in estimating overall prognosis for patients after acute myocardial infarction— for example, left ventricular function and the presence or absence of inducible ischemia[13]—are also the chief determinants of surgical risk for these patients.[72]

These data have led to recommendations[72] that purely elective surgery be delayed until 6 months after an acute myocardial infarction. When major emergency surgery is necessary, patients who have had more recent infarctions usually should undergo hemodynamic monitoring with a pulmonary artery catheter and arterial line, and fluctuations in left heart filling pressures or blood pressure should be treated promptly. When surgery is semielective, but prolonged delay may be deleterious, as in a patient with a potentially resectable malignancy, surgery can be considered 4 to 6 weeks after infarction if the patient is judged to be at low risk on the basis of his or her clinical course or performance on an exercise tolerance test. Higher-risk patients should be considered for coronary angiography and revascularization with either bypass graft surgery or percutaneous coronary angioplasty before their noncardiac operations.

Stable angina. Several investigators have found that patients with stable angina are not at substantially increased risk of cardiac complications with noncardiac surgery,[10,31,64] and therefore, neither aggressive evaluation of the extent of coronary artery disease, including angiography, nor bypass surgery has been recommended as routine in this setting. Nonrandomized data from the Coronary Artery Surgery Study (CASS) registry[20] indicate that patients with stable angina (for example, patients with New York Heart Association class I or II anginal symptoms) have lower mortality with noncardiac surgery if coronary artery bypass graft surgery has been performed (0.9% versus 2.4%). However, the operative mortality for bypass graft surgery in this population averaged 1.4%; thus the combination of cardiac and noncardiac surgery led to a total mortality rate of 2.3%, which was similar to the perioperative mortality associated with noncardiac surgery alone.

Consequently, instead of aggressive diagnostic workups, the perioperative evaluation of the patient with stable angina should emphasize the assessment of whether the patient's ischemic symptoms are truly stable. Physicians should not rely on the self-reported frequency of angina alone, because patients may voluntarily reduce their activity levels to avoid symptoms.[33] The exercise tolerance of the patient should be evaluated as well as possible from the patient's description of his or her daily activities. Classification systems such as the criteria of the Canadian Cardiovascular Society[7] or the Specific Activity Scale[33,34] may enhance the accuracy and reproducibility of these assessments. Patients who are class I or II by these scales generally tolerate most procedures well. In such cases, management should include the maintenance of an effective antianginal regimen during and after surgery, with substitution of topical and intravenous preparations of antianginal drugs for oral formulations.

Unstable angina. In contrast to stable angina, unstable angina probably represents an important risk factor for cardiac complications. Data directly addressing this issue are scanty, but unstable angina has been shown to indicate a poor prognosis for patients undergoing coronary artery bypass graft surgery,[48] and it is reasonable to expect that its impact on mortality associated with noncardiac surgery would be similar. Therefore, if possible, noncardiac surgery should be postponed in patients with new onset or worsening angina until their ischemia has been stabilized. If they are indicated, coronary angiography and revascularization procedures should precede the noncardiac operation.

If the noncardiac surgery cannot be delayed, the patient with unstable angina should undergo the procedure with full hemodynamic monitoring. In selected circumstances, consideration should be given to intraaortic balloon counterpulsation.[21]

For patients who require vascular operations such as carotid endarterectomy in the presence of coronary artery disease, an alternative strategy has been the simultaneous performance of the noncardiac operation and coronary artery bypass graft surgery.[12,18,59] Reported operative mortality with this combined approach has ranged from 5% to 10%, reflecting the high prevalence of severe coronary artery disease in such patients.[59] We recommend a combined procedure only when there is severe bilateral or currently symptomatic carotid disease associated with unstable angina, left main coronary disease, or severely symptomatic three-vessel disease.

Patients with prior coronary artery bypass graft surgery. Data from CASS and other investigators[20,47] demonstrate that patients who have undergone bypass graft surgery, and who are now asymptomatic or minimally symptomatic, tolerate noncardiac surgery well. In the CASS registry, perioperative mortality was 0.9% in patients who had had bypass surgery,[20] and no perioperative infarctions were found among 99 patients undergoing noncardiac surgery after bypass surgery in the series of Mahar et al.[47] As noted above, however, these data simply reflect the excellent prognosis of patients who have had bypass surgery, and do not provide support for performing bypass surgery routinely before noncardiac surgery in stable patients.

Patients with no history of ischemic heart disease. The risk of perioperative infarction or cardiac death in patients without previous evidence of ischemic heart disease is extremely low, and previous investigators have not been able to demonstrate an increase in this risk in the presence of coronary risk factors (that is, diabetes, smoking, hypertension, or hyperlipidemia) alone.[31] Therefore, when evaluating the patient who does not have a prior history of angina or infarction, the assessment should focus on trying to elicit any symptoms of previously undiagnosed ischemia.

This assessment should be especially thorough if the patient is undergoing surgery for peripheral vascular disease, since such patients have a 1% to 2% risk of perioperative cardiac death.[17,44,50] This higher risk reflects the greater prevalence of coronary disease in this population. For example, in a series of 68 patients with abdominal aortic aneurysms who underwent preoperative coronary angiography, only one (1%) had normal coronary arteries, while 32 (47%) had extensive coronary disease.[36] High rates of coronary disease have also been documented in patients with other types of peripheral vascular disease.[69]

Congestive Heart Failure

Despite the large volume shifts associated with surgery, patients with no prior history of congestive heart failure are at low risk for the development of postoperative pulmonary edema or new congestive heart failure (Table 3-1). Among 1001 patients who

TABLE 3-1. Correlation between preoperative clinical findings and postoperative heart failure

Preoperative findings	Number (Total = 1001)	Postoperative complications	
		Percent with pulmonary edema	Percent with new or worsened heart failure with or without pulmonary edema
No prior history of heart failure	853	2%	4%
History of heart failure but not evident on preoperative evaluation	87	6%	16%
Left-sided heart failure on preoperative examination or chest x-ray evaluation	66	16%*	26%*
Jugular venous distention	23	30%*	35%*
S₃ gallop	17	35%*	47%*
History of pulmonary edema	22	23%*	32%*
Preoperative New York Heart Association functional class for congestive heart failure			
I	935	3%	5%
II	15	7%	7%
III	34	6%	18%
IV	17	25%	31%

Adapted with permission from Goldman L, Caldera DL, Southwick FS, et al: Cardiac risk factors and complications in non-cardiac surgery, Medicine 57:357-370, 1978.
*$P < 0.01$ when comparing patients with finding to patients without it.

underwent surgery at Massachusetts General Hospital in the mid-1970s, new onset of congestive heart failure after surgery was rare except in patients over 60 years of age, patients with baseline electrocardiographic abnormalities, and patients undergoing major abdominal or thoracic operations.[32]

In this series, the risk of postoperative heart failure was greater if the patient had a history of heart failure, even in the absence of current volume overload, and was greater still if heart failure was evident during the preoperative evaluation. The rate of development of new or worsened heart failure or pulmonary edema was only 3% in patients with a normal functional status (that is, with a New York Heart Association class of I) but rose to 31% in patients with symptoms of congestive heart failure at rest (see Table 3-1).

Because the risk of postoperative heart failure is lower when congestive heart failure is controlled at the time of the preoperative evaluation, it is reasonable to assume that treatment of volume overload before surgery will help reduce the risk of subsequent worsening of heart failure. However, aggressive diuresis may be hazardous, because both spinal and general anesthesia induce peripheral vasodilation, which can lead to hypotension if the patient is volume depleted. Therefore, we recommend that preoperative diuresis should be vigorous enough to improve congestive heart failure without causing postural signs or symptoms.

Management of patients who are at high risk for postoperative pulmonary edema may be improved by perioperative hemodynamic monitoring with a pulmonary artery catheter,[40] usually continuing for about 24 to 48 hours after surgery. For patients with severe heart failure and low blood pressures, intra-arterial blood pressure monitoring may also help guide treatment.

Valvular Heart Disease

The most important valvular disease to detect before surgery is severe *aortic stenosis*, which is associated with a 13% risk of perioperative mortality[32] and is increasing in prevalence as the population ages. The narrowing of the aortic valve restricts the ability of the cardiac output to rise in response to vasodilation or volume loss, thus placing the patient at high risk for shock with surgery. In addition, the left ventricular hypertrophy that is induced by high wall stresses within this chamber leads to a decrease in ventricular compliance and impaired diastolic filling.[52] Consequently, these patients may tolerate hypovolemia, tachycardia, or the development of new atrial fibrillation[65] poorly.

When hemodynamically important aortic stenosis is suspected on the basis of clinical findings,[37] an echocardiogram, preferably supplemented with Doppler flow imaging, should be obtained before surgery. These tests are highly sensitive for aortic stenosis, and few patients without severe stenosis require cardiac catheterization to exclude the diagnosis. Doppler evidence of a gradient ≥ 50 mm Hg suggests that critical aortic stenosis may be present.

Clinical trials of optimal management strategies for noncardiac surgery in patients with aortic stenosis have not been performed, but most experts recommend performing an aortic valve replacement before the noncardiac surgery if the patient has any symptoms (angina, congestive heart failure, or syncope) resulting from the aortic stenosis.[28,57] If, on careful questioning, a patient with noninvasive evidence of aortic stenosis does not appear to have any of these symptoms despite a reasonable activity level, the patient may undergo most operations without a valve replacement; invasive hemodynamic monitoring should be initiated before surgery and continue for 24 to 48 hours postoperatively.[28] Occasionally a patient may have evidence of severe aortic stenosis but be asymptomatic, because noncardiac conditions greatly limit activity. If the cardiac stress of the planned general surgical procedure clearly exceeds the stress of the activities that the patient can perform, aortic valvuloplasty or valve replacement may be indicated even with no cardiac symptoms.

In patients with chronic *aortic regurgitation* and *mitral regurgitation,* the left ventricle is subjected to high volume loads that can lead to impairment of contractility. These patients are not as sensitive to subtle shifts in hemodynamic status as are patients with critical aortic stenosis, and, if they are not in congestive heart failure on their preoperative evaluation, they may be managed during the perioperative period without invasive hemodynamic monitoring. However, because left ventricular dysfunc-

tion may be present even if clinical evidence of congestive heart failure is absent, their volume status should be followed carefully.

In *mitral stenosis,* tachycardia associated with the stresses of surgery can lead to a precipitous fall in cardiac output and the development of pulmonary edema caused by a decrease in emptying time for the left atrium. Furthermore, fluid shifts that might be well tolerated by a patient without mitral stenosis may lead to major changes in cardiac output. High filling pressures are required to force blood across the stenotic valve, so blood loss or venodilation may decrease left ventricular filling and compromise output. However, vigorous volume replacement can lead to pulmonary edema. Therefore, patients with moderate or severe mitral stenosis may benefit from invasive hemodynamic monitoring if significant fluid shifts are expected with surgery. Supraventricular tachycardia should be treated with intravenous verapamil, digoxin, or a beta-adrenergic antagonist.

Patients with *hypertrophic obstructive cardiomyopathy* (HOCM) are also susceptible to pulmonary edema. The cause of elevated pulmonary venous pressures in this syndrome is left ventricular stiffness that leads to impaired diastolic filling and, in some patients, a subvalvular outflow gradient.[59] Drugs that increase myocardial contractility, such as beta-adrenergic agonists, should be avoided, whereas beta-adrenergic antagonists and calcium channel blocking agents may be useful in optimizing hemodynamics.[46] Because adequate left ventricular filling pressures are critical for maintenance of cardiac output, volume depletion, drug-induced venodilation, and new atrial fibrillation are hazardous for these patients. In this setting, spinal anesthesia must be used only with extreme caution,[67] and, if major fluid shifts are expected, a pulmonary artery catheter should be considered. Hypotension occurring during or after surgery should be promptly treated with volume expansion.

Patients with *prosthetic valves* are at risk of bacterial endocarditis and thromboembolic complications during the perioperative period. The rationale and recommendations for prophylaxis against endocarditis are discussed elsewhere in this book. Patients who take chronic anticoagulant therapy because of a nonbioprosthetic valve may have thromboembolic complications when anticoagulation is discontinued around the time of surgery, particularly when the older caged-disk prostheses have been used for mitral valve replacement.[39] These data are consistent with other studies showing that for patients with mechanical prosthetic valves the risk of thromboembolic complications is generally higher if the valves are in the mitral position than if they are in the aortic position.[35]

A reasonable strategy that balances the risk of thromboembolism against the risk of perioperative bleeding[39,72] is to discontinue oral anticoagulants 2 to 3 days before surgery in patients with prosthetic valves in the aortic position. Surgery can then proceed when the prothrombin time has fallen within 1 to 2 seconds of the control value. Once hemostasis is achieved postoperatively, usually at 12 to 24 hours, intravenous heparin is initiated and continued until anticoagulation with oral sodium warfarin (Coumadin) therapy is achieved. For patients with mechanical prostheses in the mitral position, we recommend a similar approach except that intravenous heparin should be initiated preoperatively as soon as sodium warfarin is discontinued and continued until about 6 hours before surgery. This approach, which reflects the higher embolic risk in such patients, necessitates admission about 2 days before surgery.

Arrhythmias and Conduction Disturbances

With either general or regional anesthesia, arrhythmias and conduction abnormalities occur commonly during the perioperative period, regardless of whether or not patients have underlying heart disease.[43,71] For example, in the course of monitoring 5013 patients during surgery, Vanik and Davis[72] found a 16% incidence of arrhythmias among patients with no known heart disease. Clinically significant arrhythmias were less frequent, occurring in only about 0.7% of patients with no history of cardiac disease. In the higher risk population of patients with a prior history of heart disease with or without arrhythmias, 174 (32%) of 551 patients had perioperative arrhythmias, including 14 (3%) who had clinically significant arrhythmias.

The high incidence of minor arrhythmias reflects the alterations in autonomic tone, metabolic disturbances, and pharmacologic interventions that accompany surgery, and even clinically significant perioperative arrhythmias do not necessarily have long-term prognostic importance for the patient. For example, in our experience, only 35 (4%) of 916 patients over 40 years of age developed new postoperative *supraventricular tachyarrhythmias*.[27] No

deaths were related to supraventricular tachycardias, and all treated patients had restoration of sinus rhythm. Only two (6%) required electrical cardioversion, and 14 (40%) converted back to sinus rhythm without specific cardiac therapy.

Risk factors for the development of supraventricular tachycardia that were identified in this study included people greater than 70 years of age, presence of preoperative rales, and intraabdominal, intrathoracic, or major vascular surgery.[27] Surprisingly, histories of cardiac or pulmonary disease or the presence of preoperative atrial premature contractions were not major independent correlates of the occurrence of supraventricular arrhythmias. However, the majority of patients with supraventricular arrhythmias had coexisting medical problems, including major infections, anemia, and metabolic derangements. In these 35 patients, the death rate was nearly 50%, but all deaths were because of the underlying medical problems, thus prompting recommendations to search for noncardiac disease in patients who develop supraventricular arrhythmias.

Patients with five or more *ventricular premature contractions* (VPCs) per minute at any time are at increased risk for perioperative cardiac complications.[31] However, the clinical importance of VPCs (and of supraventricular arrhythmias) appears to be as a marker for underlying myocardial dysfunction; in general, in patients without evidence of structural heart disease, the presence of complex VPCs is not associated with increased cardiac mortality or morbidity.[42] We believe that the significance of VPCs in otherwise healthy patients who are undergoing surgery is similarly limited.

The patient with ventricular arrhythmias *and* myocardial dysfunction is at higher risk for perioperative congestive heart failure and cardiac death, but this risk is mainly a reflection of the myocardial dysfunction. Prophylactic antiarrhythmic therapy will not correct the underlying dysfunction. Accordingly, we feel that such therapy should be reserved for patients with serious arrhythmias, such as those with histories of hemodynamically significant ventricular arrhythmias or sudden death.[72] The management of hemodynamically significant or high grade ventricular arrhythmias that develop perioperatively is described elsewhere in this book.

Similarly, we believe that prophylactic placement of a temporary pacemaker is rarely indicated for *conduction abnormalities* such as preoperative sinus bradycardia or chronic bifascicular heart block (that is, left bundle-branch block or complete right bundle-branch block with anterior or posterior fascicular block). Analysis of pooled data shows that only one of 339 patients with chronic bifascicular block developed perioperative complete heart block,[72] and, in this single case, the complete heart block developed during intubation and was transient.

When autonomic instability associated with intubation and surgery leads to second or third degree heart block or hemodynamically significant sinus bradycardia, intravenous atropine usually restores normal conduction and heart rate. Therefore, we feel that the morbidity and expense of temporary pacemaker placement are not warranted unless the patient has indications for a permanent pacemaker and it has not yet been placed (see the box at right).[23] If the planned surgery is elective, a permanent pacemaker can be placed beforehand. If the procedure is emergent or is likely to induce a transient bacteremia, a temporary pacemaker may be inserted preoperatively, and a permanent pacemaker can be placed subsequently.

An exception to this policy may be made for patients with preoperative left bundle-branch block who undergo perioperative placement of a pulmonary artery catheter. This procedure is associated with the development of a new right bundle-branch block in about 5% of the cases.[63] While a new right bundle-branch block may be well tolerated by most patients, in the presence of a left bundle-branch block, it may lead to development of complete heart block.[1,68] Therefore, a method for ventricular pacing should be available before right-sided heart catheterization in patients with a left bundle-branch block.

For *patients with permanent pacemakers,* a potentially fatal intraoperative problem is inhibition of demand pacemakers by electrocautery.[45] If electrocautery is used in patients with pacemakers, duration and frequency should be limited to 1 second bursts 10 seconds apart, the ground plate should be placed as far from the pacemaker pulse generator as possible, and cautery near the pacemaker should be minimized.[61] During periods of electrocautery, electrical activity may render the electrocardiogram useless as a monitor of heart rate; an alternative, such as direct palpation of the patient's pulse, should be planned. Placing a magnet over many pacemakers switches them into a mode in which the heart is paced

---

Indications for permanent pacemaker implantation

1. Complete heart block (permanent or intermittent) associated with:
   a. Symptomatic bradycardia
   b. Congestive heart failure
   c. Arrhythmia requiring drugs that will suppress escape rhythm
   d. Documented asystole ≥ 3 sec or escape rate < 40 bpm
2. Second degree atrioventricular block with symptomatic bradycardia
3. Bifascicular block with intermittent complete heart block with symptomatic bradycardia
4. Symptomatic bifascicular block with intermittent type II second degree atrioventricular block
5. Sinus node dysfunction with documented symptomatic bradycardia
6. Persistent, advanced, second degree atrioventricular block or complete heart block following acute myocardial infarction

Modified from Frye R et al: Guidelines for permanent pacemaker implantation, Circulation 70:331A-339A, 1984.

---

at a fixed rate (usually 72 beats per minute [bpm]) regardless of other electrical activity that is perceived by the pacemaker. Because pacemaker programming varies markedly, it is important that the pacemaker type and model number, its response to electrical interference, and the reprogramming methods be determined before surgery.[60]

Type of Surgery

All types of cardiac complications are more common after major intraabdominal, intrathoracic, or aortic operations—a reflection of the major volume shifts that are common in such procedures (Table 3-2).[31,32] Some data suggest[38] that, after adjusting for other clinical variables, the cardiac risk for patients undergoing abdominal aortic surgery may be about 40% greater than would be predicted by a multivariate risk index.[31] Similarly, emergency operations are associated with cardiac complication rates that are as much as four times higher than those found with elective procedures.[31,32,72]

TABLE 3-2. Major complications in patients over 40 years of age undergoing different types of operations

Complication	Intrathoracic, intraperitoneal, or aortic procedures (n = 437)	Other major noncardiac procedures (n = 564)
New perioperative supraventricular tachycardia	28 (6%)	13 (2%)
Pulmonary edema	23 (5%)	2 (0.4%)
Myocardial infarction	11 (2.5%)	7 (1%)
Death from cardiac causes	11 (2.5%)	8 (1%)

From Goldman L: Cardiac risks and complications of noncardiac surgery, Ann Intern Med 98:504-513, 1983.

Noncardiac Clinical Variables

While elderly patients have higher prevalences of cardiac disease and other conditions that may increase their surgical risk, multivariate analysis suggests that patients greater than 70 years of age have a higher risk of major cardiac complications even after adjusting for other clinical factors.[31] Various investigators have reported perioperative mortality rates of 5% to 6%[26,32] in geriatric populations, and Gerson et al found that risk was especially high in patients who were unable to perform low grade exercise (that is, pedal a bicycle in a supine position and raise heart rate to ≥ 100 bpm).[26] Thresholds for hemodynamic monitoring and other precautionary measures should be lower in this population.

Surgical risk is also elevated in patients with *poor general medical condition*,[31] a clinical finding that is more easily recognized than defined. In the original derivation of the multivariate risk index,[31] the following criteria were used:

1. Electrolyte abnormalities (potassium < 3.0 meq/L or HCO₃ < 20 meq/L)
2. Renal insufficiency (blood urea nitrogen > 50 mg/dl or creatinine > 3.0 mg/dl)
3. Abnormal blood gases (PO_2 < 60 mm Hg or PCO_2 > 50 mm Hg)
4. Abnormal liver status (elevated serum aspartate transaminase or signs at physical examination of chronic liver disease)
5. Any condition that has caused the patient to be chronically bedridden

Perioperative cardiac death occurred in 13 (4%) of 362 patients who met one or more of these criteria, prompting recommendations that elective procedures be delayed until these conditions are corrected, if possible.[72]

Obesity is also considered a potentially important risk factor in noncardiac surgery, but most postoperative deaths in such patients are caused by infection, compromised respiratory status, and pulmonary emboli.[51] However, massive obesity imposes hemodynamic stresses upon the heart that may lead to biventricular hypertrophy and myocardial dysfunction. Thus, evidence for congestive heart failure should be sought in such patients during the preoperative evaluation.

Hypertension does not appear to be a major independent risk factor for cardiac complications in noncardiac surgery.[31] Postponing elective surgery to achieve better control of hypertension has not been shown to reduce risk for patients with stable high blood pressure and diastolic pressures ≤ 110 mm Hg.[30] Conversely, for patients under treatment for hypertension, continuing medications up to and including the morning of surgery is safe and recommended.*

SPECIALIZED TESTS

Because patients with evidence of ischemia during *exercise tolerance tests* are at increased risk to develop cardiac complications with noncardiac surgery, several authors have recommended routine use of exercise testing to be followed by angiography and consideration of bypass graft surgery if the test is markedly positive.[11,24,25] However, it is unclear whether the exercise test adds information that is not

*References 19, 41, 54, 55, 72.

available through the routine clinical evaluation. Carliner et al studied 200 patients older than 40 years of age who underwent elective major noncardiac surgery with general anesthesia and found that the preoperative electrocardiogram was the most important independent clinical predictor of surgical risk.[8] After consideration of information from the electrocardiogram, exercise test data did not appear to improve risk stratification in this study. However, only 3% of the patients in this study had cardiac events, and, as noted by the authors, the unexpectedly low outcome rate limited their statistical power for detecting any incremental predictive value of the exercise test.

While future studies in larger series of patients may help define a role for the exercise test in risk stratification of surgical candidates, these tests are expensive and may be difficult to arrange on short notice before surgery. We currently feel that risk usually can be adequately assessed on the basis of the clinical evaluation. Exercise testing is generally most helpful in patients in whom the history is felt to be an unreliable index of functional status.[27] Patients with stable angina (New York Heart Association classes I and II) usually do well if angina is their only risk factor, and patients with severe symptoms of ischemic heart disease (New York Heart Association class III or IV) are generally candidates for catheterization and consideration of revascularization (angioplasty or coronary artery bypass graft surgery). In such cases, if noncardiac surgery is elective, it should be delayed until the cardiac evaluation is complete.

The low complication rate of the patients who underwent exercise testing in the series described by Carliner et al may reflect the good overall prognosis of patients who are capable of taking this test. As Gerson et al have reported, inability to exercise is an important predictor of poor outcomes,[26] and several investigators have recently been evaluating tests that may assist prognostic stratification within the high-risk population of patients for whom traditional exercise tolerance testing is unsuitable.

One new technology that has drawn considerable interest is *dipyridamole-thallium imaging*.[6,17,44] Dipyridamole induces vasodilation of portions of the coronary artery bed that are not affected by atherosclerosis, leading to a relative increase in flow in normal arteries in comparison with vessels with stenoses. Injected thallium reflects this distribution of

blood flow and shows areas of hypoperfusion in regions supplied by diseased coronary arteries. Subsequent reperfusion of these regions suggests that the local myocardium is viable but in jeopardy, while persistent defects are interpreted as indications of old infarctions. Thus, this test is analagous to a thallium stress test except that the stress is pharmacologic, not exertional.

Boucher et al performed dipyridamole-thallium imaging on 54 stable patients with suspected coronary artery disease who were scheduled to undergo surgery for peripheral vascular disease[6] and found that no cardiac events occurred among 32 patients whose scans were normal or showed only persistent defects. Among the 22 patients whose scans suggested myocardium in jeopardy, six patients underwent coronary angiography, which showed multivessel coronary artery disease in all six cases. The other 16 patients who had abnormal scans did not have angiography and underwent surgery; eight had cardiac events. Similar findings in subsequent studies suggest that this test has considerable promise for enhancing risk assessment in patients who are at high risk of complications on the basis of clinical data, but are unable to undergo exercise testing.[17,44]

In this setting, an alternative test that is more widely available is the resting *radionuclide angiogram*. Pasternak et al found no perioperative myocardial infarctions among 50 patients who underwent lower extremity revascularization procedures and who had preoperative ejection fractions greater than 55%.[50] In contrast, the rate of perioperative infarction was 19% among patients with ejection fractions 36% to 55% and 75% among those with ejection fractions 26% to 35%. Thus, low ejection fractions at rest appear to identify high risk patients, but it is unclear whether this test adds information beyond that available through a clinical assessment of congestive heart failure status.

MULTIFACTORIAL RISK ASSESSMENT

The first multifactorial index of cardiac risk in noncardiac surgery was published in 1977.[31] This index was based upon multivariate analysis of preoperative clinical data from 1001 consecutive patients 40 years of age or more who underwent noncardiac surgery at Massachusetts General Hospital in 1975 to 1976. In this population, the overall mortality was 5.9% and the cardiac mortality was 1.9%.

The nine clinical factors in the index were found

TABLE 3-3. Multifactorial index of cardiac risk in noncardiac surgery

Parameter	Points
HISTORY	
Myocardial infarction within six months	10
Age over 70 years	5
PHYSICAL EXAMINATION	
S_3 or jugular venous distention	11
Important aortic stenosis	3
ELECTROCARDIOGRAM	
Rhythm other than sinus or sinus plus APBs on last preoperative electrocardiogram	7
More than five premature ventricular beats/min at any time preoperatively	7
OTHER	
Poor general medical status*	3
Intraperitoneal, intrathoracic, or aortic surgery	3
Emergency operation	4
TOTAL	53

Reprinted with permission from Goldman L, Caldera DL, Nussbaum SR, et al: Multifactorial index of cardiac risk in noncardiac surgical procedures, N Engl J Med 297:845-850, 1977.

Abbreviation: APB = atrial premature beat.

*Electrolyte abnormalities (potassium < 3.0 meq/L or HCO_3 < 20 meq/L); renal insufficiency (blood urea nitrogen > 50 mg/dL or creatinine > 3.0 mg/dL); abnormal blood gases (PO_2 < 60 mm Hg or PCO_2 > 50 mm Hg); abnormal liver status (elevated serum aspartate transaminase or signs on physical examination of chronic liver disease); or any condition that has caused the patient to be chronically bedridden.

to have independent predictive value for risk of cardiac complications, and were weighted with "risk points" to allow a preoperative estimate of patient risk of perioperative cardiac mortality and morbidity (Table 3-3). Of some interest are factors that were *not* found to be independent risk predictors, such as hypertension, diabetes, stable angina, smoking, peripheral vascular disorders, and hypercholesterolemia. Common factors that are not included (for example, hypertension) presumably have little if any impact on risk after consideration of the variables that are included in the model. Less common factors (for example, unstable angina) may have occurred in too few patients to emerge in the analysis as important predictors; a larger study might have detected their true role.

The index is usually used by assigning patients to one of four classes according to level of risk (Table 3-4). For example, a 75-year-old patient (5 points) who had had a myocardial infarction within the previous 6 months (10 points), had evidence of congestive heart failure on examination including an S_3 gallop and jugular venous distention (11 points), was in atrial fibrillation (7 points), and required an emergency (4 points) cholecystectomy (3 points) would have a total score of 40 points, which would place him in class IV, the highest risk group.

If that operation could be deferred through medical treatment of the cholecystitis until more than 6 months had passed, the congestive heart failure had been well controlled, and sinus rhythm had been restored, the patient would then have only 8 points, which would place him in class II. The patient's risk would still be elevated, but would be much less than it had been.

Since this index was derived, it has been prospectively evaluated at other institutions in varying patient populations and has been shown to separate patients into risk groups reliably (see Table 3-4). Zeldin[74] performed preoperative classifications of 1140 consecutive patients whom he personally followed at several hospitals in Toronto; he noted complication rates very similar to those of the original series of Goldman et al, especially for patients in classes I through III. In the highest risk group, class IV, Zeldin found a complication rate of only 30%, compared with 78% in the original study. This difference may reflect improved management and greater selectivity of patients in this group.

Detsky et al have evaluated the index in a higher risk population of patients who were referred for preoperative medical consultation.[15] The overall risk of complications in their series of 268 patients was 10% (see Table 3-4), but even within this highly-selected patient subgroup, the index separated patients well according to risk. Similar findings have been reported by Jeffrey et al from a series of patients undergoing surgery for abdominal aortic aneurysms.[38]

The experience with the index in these higher risk populations demonstrates the importance of considering the patient's "prior probability" of complications when applying a prediction rule.[14] In the series of patients who were referred for medical consultations, the overall risk of cardiac complications was higher, partly because of factors that are not mea-

TABLE 3-4. Major complication rates in studies that have analyzed the multifactorial risk index

Class	Definition (points)	Goldman[31] unselected noncardiac surgery patients >40 years old		Zeldin[74] unselected noncardiac surgery patients >40 years old		Detsky[14] referrals for preoperative medical consultation		Jeffrey[38] abdominal aortic aneurysm surgery	
I	0-5	5/537	(1%)	4/590	(1%)	8/134	(6%)	4/56	(7%)
II	6-12	21/316	(7%)	13/453	(3%)	6/85	(7%)	4/35	(11%)
III	13-25	18/130	(14%)	11/74	(15%)	9/45	(20%)	3/8	(38%)
IV	≥26	14/18	(78%)	7/23	(30%)	4/4	(100%)	0	
All patients:		58/1001	(6%)	35/1140	(3%)	27/268	(10%)	11/99	(11%)

Adapted from Goldman L: Multifactorial index of cardiac risk in noncardiac surgery: ten-year status report, J Cardiothorac Anesth 1:237-244, 1987.

TABLE 3-5. Use of the multifactorial cardiac risk index in patient subgroups with different baseline risks of cardiac complications

Patient type	Approximate baseline risk for major cardiac complications	Adjusted cardiac complication risk using multifactorial index			
		I	II	III	IV
Minor surgery	1%	0.3%	1%	3%	19%
Unselected consecutive patients over age 40 years who have major noncardiac surgery	4%	1.2%	4%	12%	48%
Patients undergoing abdominal aortic aneurysm surgery or who are over 40 years of age and have high risk characteristics that generally generate medical consultations before major noncardiac surgery	10%	3%	10%	30%	75%

Adapted from Goldman L: Multifactorial index of cardiac risk in noncardiac surgery: ten-year status report, J Cardiothorac Anesth 1:237-244, 1987.

sured by the index. Therefore, while the index is successful in stratifying patients into risk groups, the complication rate within each group would be expected to be higher when the groups are part of a patient population with an overall higher risk.

One way to use the index is to separate the patients into three general groups with different baseline risks of perioperative cardiac complications (Table 3-5).[29] Then, patients can be assigned to a risk class on the basis of the index, and their approximate risk, as predicted by a Bayesian analysis, can be calculated.

Another refinement is a modification of the original index by Detsky et al[14] that uses slightly different point scores and includes factors to account for prior history of class III or class IV angina, remote myo-cardial infarction, and prior pulmonary edema. Prospective evaluations of this modified index have not yet been performed at other institutions.

FUTURE DIRECTIONS

The original multifactorial risk index is now more than a decade old. Although the stratification scheme itself still appears to be valid, advances in anesthesia have probably reduced the risk of cardiac complications in noncardiac surgery for any individual patient. Moreover, several new technologies, such as Doppler flow imaging, dipyridamole-thallium imaging, percutaneous coronary angioplasty, and external transthoracic pacemakers, and several older ones that have become more accessible or safer, such as exercise testing, coronary angiography, and echocardiography, may improve our ability to assess the surgical patient.

The major task at hand for clinical investigators is to determine what impact these technologies may have in the routine assessment of surgical patients. Of particular importance is identifying which patients may benefit from preoperative exercise testing, dipyridamole-thallium scanning, invasive monitoring, and prophylactic coronary artery revascularization procedures. Because these technologies are most likely to be beneficial to a small subpopulation of high risk patients, studies of these issues will require large numbers of patients. In the meantime, the multifactorial index remains a valuable means for assessing risk in general surgical patients.

REFERENCES

1. Abernathy WS: Complete heart block caused by the Swan-Ganz catheter, Chest 65:349, 1974.
2. Arkins R, Smessaert AA, and Hicks RG: Mortality and morbidity in surgical patients with coronary artery disease, JAMA 190:485-488, 1964.
3. Baker HW, Grismer JT, and Wise RA: Risk of surgery in patients with myocardial infarction, Arch Surg 70:739-747, 1955.
4. Baue AE: Surgery, JAMA 258:2289-2291, 1987.
5. Becker RC and Underwood DA: Myocardial infarction in patients undergoing noncardiac surgery, Cleve Clin J Med 54:25-28, 1987.
6. Boucher CA et al: Determination of cardiac risk by dipyridamole-thallium imaging before peripheral vascular surgery, N Engl J Med 312:389-394, 1985.
7. Campeau L: Grading of angina pectoris (letter), Circulation 54:522-523, 1972.
8. Carliner NH et al: Routine preoperative exercise testing in patients undergoing major noncardiac surgery, Am J Cardiol 56:51-58, 1985.
9. Charlson ME, Cohen RP, and Sears CL: General medicine consultation. Lessons from a clinical service, Am J Med 75:121-128, 1983.
10. Cooperman M et al: Cardiovascular risk factors in patients with peripheral vascular disease, Surgery 84:505-509, 1978.
11. Cutler BS: Assessment of operative risk with electrocardiographic exercise testing in patients with peripheral vascular disease, Am J Surg 137:484-489, 1978.
12. DeBakey ME and Lawrie GM: Combined coronary artery and peripheral vascular disease: recognition and treatment, J Vasc Surg 1:605-607, 1984.
13. DeBusk RF et al: Identification and treatment of low-risk patients after acute myocardial infarction and coronary artery bypass graft surgery, N Engl J Med 314:161-166, 1986.
14. Detsky AS et al: Cardiac assessment for patients undergoing noncardiac surgery: a multifactorial clinical risk index, Arch Intern Med 146:2131-2134, 1986.
15. Detsky AS et al: Predicting cardiac complications in patients undergoing non-cardiac surgery, J Gen Intern Med 1:211-219, 1986.
16. Dripps RD, Lamont A, and Eckenhoff JE: The role of anesthesia in surgical mortality, JAMA 178:261-266, 1961.
17. Eagle KA et al: Dipyridamole-thallium scanning in patients undergoing vascular surgery: optimizing preoperative evaluation of cardiac risk, JAMA 257:2185-2189, 1987.
18. Emery RW et al: Coexistent carotid and coronary artery disease: surgical management, Arch Surg 118:1035-1038, 1983.
19. Foex P and Prys-Roberts C: Anaesthesia and the hypertensive patient, Br J Anaesth 46:575-588, 1974.
20. Foster E et al: Risk of noncardiac operation in patients with defined coronary disease: the Coronary Artery Surgery Study (CASS) registry experience, Ann Thorac Surg 41:42-50, 1986.
21. Foster ED et al: Mechanical circulatory assistance with intra-aortic balloon counterpulsation for major abdominal surgery, Ann Surg 183:73-76, 1976.
22. Fraser JG, Ramachandran PR, and Davis HS: Anesthesia and recent myocardial infarction, JAMA 199:318-320, 1967.
23. Frye R et al: Guidelines for permanent pacemaker implantation, Circulation 70:331A-339A, 1984.
24. Fudge TL et al: Improved operative risk after myocardial revascularization, South Med J 74:799-801, 1981.
25. Gage AA et al: Assessment of cardiac risk in surgical patients, Arch Surg 112:1488-1492, 1977.
26. Gerson MC et al: Cardiac prognosis in noncardiac geriatric surgery, Ann Intern Med 103:832-837, 1985.
27. Goldman L: Supraventricular tachyarrhythmias in hospitalized adults after surgery: clinical correlates in patients over 40 years of age after major noncardiac surgery, Chest 73:450-454, 1978.
28. Goldman L: Cardiac risks and complications of noncardiac surgery, Ann Intern Med 98:504-513, 1983.
29. Goldman L: Multifactorial index of cardiac risk in noncardiac surgery: Ten-year status report, J Cardiothorac Anesth 1:237-244, 1987.
30. Goldman L and Caldera DL: Risks of general anesthesia and elective operation in the hypertensive patient, Anesthesiology 50:285-292, 1979.
31. Goldman L, Caldera DL, Nussbaum SR, et al: Multifactorial index of cardiac risk in noncardiac surgical procedures, N Engl J Med 297:845-850, 1977.
32. Goldman L, Caldera DL, Southwick FS, et al: Cardiac risk factors and complications in non-cardiac surgery, Medicine 57:357-370, 1978.

33. Goldman L, Cook EF, Mitchell N, Flatley M, Sherman H, and Cohn PF: Pitfalls in the serial assessment of cardiac functional status, J Chron Dis 35:763-771, 1982.

34. Goldman L, Hashimoto B, Cook EF, and Loscalzo A: Comparative reproducibilities and validities of systems for the assessment of cardiovascular functional class: advantages of a new specific activity scale, Circulation 64:1227-1234, 1981.

35. Hammermeister KE et al: Comparison of outcome after valve replacement with a bioprosthesis versus a mechanical prosthesis: initial 5 year results of a randomized trial, J Am Coll Cardiol 10:719-732, 1987.

36. Hertzer NR et al: Routine coronary angiography prior to elective aortic reconstruction, Arch Surg 114:1336-1344, 1979.

37. Hoagland PM et al: Value of noninvasive testing in adults with suspected aortic stenosis, Am J Med 80:1041-1050, 1986.

38. Jeffrey CC et al: A prospective evaluation of cardiac risk index, Anesthesiology 58:462-464, 1983.

39. Katholi RE, Nolan SP, and McGuire LB: Living with prosthetic heart valves: subsequent noncardiac operations and the risk of thromboembolism or hemorrhage, Am Heart J 92:162-167, 1976.

40. Katz JD et al: Pulmonary artery flow guided catheters in the perioperative period, JAMA 237:2832-2834, 1977.

41. Katz RL, Weintraub HD, and Papper EM: Anesthesia, surgery and rauwolfia, Anesthesiology 25:142-147, 1964.

42. Kennedy HL et al: Long term follow up of asymptomatic healthy subjects with frequent and complex ventricular ectopy, N Engl J Med 312:193-197, 1985.

43. Kuner J et al: Cardiac arrhythmias during anesthesia, Dis Chest 52:580-587, 1967.

44. Leppo J et al: Noninvasive evaluation of cardiac risk before elective vascular surgery, J Am Coll Cardiol 9:269-276, 1987.

45. Lerner SM: Suppression of a demand pacemaker by transurethral electrocautery, Anesth Analg 52:703-708, 1973.

46. Lorell BH et al: Improved diastolic function and systolic performance in hypertrophic cardiomyopathy after nifedipine, N Engl J Med 303:801-803, 1980.

46a. McKechnie, FB: Anesthesiology, JAMA 258:2272-2273, 1987.

47. Mahar LJ et al: Perioperative myocardial infarction in patients with coronary artey disease with and without aorta-coronary artery bypass grafts, J Thorac Cardiovasc Surg 76:533-537, 1978.

48. National Cooperative Study Group: Unstable angina pectoris: national cooperative study group to compare surgical and medical therapy. II. In hospital experience and initial follow-up results in patients with one, two and three vessel disease, Am J Cardiol 42:839-848, 1978.

49. New classification of physical status, Anesthesiology 24:111, 1963.

50. Pasternak PF et al: The value of the radionuclide angiogram in the prediction of perioperative myocardial infarction in patients undergoing lower extremity revascularization procedures, Circulation 72(suppl II): 13-17, 1985.

51. Pasulka PS et al: The risks of surgery in obese patients, Ann Intern Med 104:540-546, 1986.

52. Peterson K et al: Diastolic left ventricular pressure-volume and stress-strain relations in patients with valvular aortic stenosis and left ventricular hypertrophy, Circulation 58:77-89, 1978.

53. Plumlee JE and Boettner RB: Myocardial infarction during and following anesthesia and operation, South Med J 65:886-889, 1972.

54. Prys-Roberts C et al: Studies of anaesthesia in relation to hypertension. IV. The effects of artificial ventilation on the circulation and pulmonary gas exchanges, Br J Anaesth 44:335-339, 1972.

55. Prys-Roberts C, Meloche R, and Foex P: Studies of anesthesia in relation to hypertension. I. Cardiovascular responses of treated and untreated patients, Br J Anaesth 43:122-137, 1971.

56. Rao TLK, Jacobs KH, and El-Etra AA: Reinfarction following anesthesia in patients with myocardial infarction, Anesthesiology 59:499-505, 1983.

57. Rose SD: Cardiac risk factors in patients undergoing non-cardiac surgery. In Bolt RJ, editor: Medical evaluation of the surgical patient, Mount Kisco, NY, 1987, Futura Publishing Co, Inc.

58. Sanderson JE et al: Left ventricular filling in hypertrophic cardiomyopathy: an angiographic study, Br Heart J 39:661-670, 1977.

59. Schwartz RL et al: Simultaneous myocardial revascularization and carotid endarterectomy, Circulation 66(suppl I): 97-101, 1982.

60. Shapiro W et al: Intraoperative pacemaker complications, Anesthesiology 63:319-322, 1985.

61. Simon A: Perioperative management of the pacemaker patient, Anesthesiology 46:127-131, 1977.

62. Skinner JF and Pearce ML: Surgical risk in the cardiac patient, J Chronic Dis 190:485-488, 1964.

63. Sprung CL et al: Advanced ventricular arrhythmias during bedside pulmonary artery catheterization, Am J Med 72:203-208, 1982.

64. Steen PA, Tinker JH, and Tarhan S: Myocardial reinfarction after anesthesia and surgery, JAMA 239:2566-2570, 1978.

65. Stott DK et al: The role of left atrial transport in aortic and mitral stenosis, Circulation 41:1031-1041, 1970.

66. Tarhan S et al: Myocardial infarction after general anesthesia, JAMA 220:1451-1454, 1972.

67. Thompson RC, Liberthson RR, and Lowenstein E: Perioperative anesthetic risk of noncardiac surgery in hypertrophic obstructive cardiomyopathy, JAMA 254:2419-2421, 1985.
68. Thomson IR et al: Right bundle branch block and complete heart block caused by the Swan-Ganz catheter, Anesthesiology 51:359-362, 1979.
69. Tomatis LA, Fierens EE, and Verbrugge GP: Evaluation of surgical risk in peripheral vascular disease by coronary arteriography, Surgery 71:429-435, 1972.
70. Topkins MJ and Artusio JF: Myocardial infarction and surgery: a five year study, Anesth Analg 43:716-720, 1964.
71. Vanik PE and Davis HS: Cardiac arrhythmias during halothane anesthesia, Anesth Analg 47:299-307, 1968.
72. Weitz HH and Goldman L: Noncardiac surgery in the patient with heart disease, Med Clin North Am 71:413-432, 1987.
73. Wells PH and Kaplan JA: Optimal management of patients with ischemic heart disease for noncardiac surgery by complementary anesthesiologist and cardiologist interaction, Am Heart J 102:1029-1037, 1981.
74. Zeldin RA: Assessing cardiac risk in patients who undergo noncardiac surgical procedures, Can J Surg 27:402-404, 1984.

CHAPTER 4

Chronic Medications:
Implications in the Perioperative Period

STEPHEN D. PARKER

The components of modern anesthetic practice
Medications for cardiovascular disease
    Antihypertensive medications
    Beta-blockers
    Calcium channel blockers
    Digoxin

Psychotropic agents
Miscellaneous medications
Summary

The population of the United States is growing older.[57] It is estimated that 13% of the population will be greater than 65 years of age by the year 2000 and 20% by the year 2025. From data included in the 1980 census, it is estimated that 43% of Americans will reach 80 years of age and live for an average of 8 more years.[37] The prevalence of chronic diseases is high in this segment of the population, and a significant number of these patients will be taking chronic medications when they are admitted to the hospital for anesthesia and surgery. Symptomatic cardiovascular disease, for example is present in roughy 40% of the population greater than 80 years of age.[37a] Since the rate of surgical procedures also increases with age,[1] increasing numbers of surgical patients with complex and severe underlying multisystem disease require the expert management of anesthesiologists and other consultants throughout the perioperative period. This chapter discusses the implications for anesthetic and perioperative care of several classes of commonly used chronic medications.

Recent information from the U.S. Food and Drug Administration[58] finds that cardiovascular drugs were the most frequently prescribed drugs in 1986, with antibiotics and psychotherapeutic drugs being the second and third most frequently prescribed, respectively. In the elderly population (older than 65), cardiovascular agents, diuretics, antiinfectives, and analgesics were the most frequently prescribed medications, together accounting for over 50% of prescriptions in this age-group. Since antibiotics are not usually long-term medications, they will not be considered further in this chapter. The medications selected for discussion here have provoked controversy in the literature or in my practice. Further discussion of drug interactions with respect to anesthesiology can be found in reference textbooks.[34,52]

It is important for nonanesthesiologists to have a feel for the components of modern anesthesiology, so that they will not regard the intraoperative period as a "black box" from which the patient emerges, but rather as an integral part of the preoperative, intraoperative, and postoperative continuum of care that our patients require.

THE COMPONENTS OF MODERN ANESTHETIC PRACTICE

Anesthetic objectives may vary somewhat, depending on the type of case and the type of anesthesia used (regional versus general), but generally include the maintenance of physiologic stability, analgesia, a "quiet" surgical field, and amnesia and/or unconsciousness. Although these objectives can at times be accomplished through the use of a single anesthetic agent, more often the use of a single agent to produce these diverse effects leads to undesirable side effects, particularly in older patients with chronic underlying medical conditions that reduce the margin of safety (therapeutic index) of any one anesthetic agent. For example, halothane is an excellent inhalation anesthetic agent but few anesthesiologists would consider using it as the sole agent in a patient with congestive heart failure because the required concentrations would produce negative inotropic effects undesirable in such a patient. The current practice in anesthesiology is to use specific agents to produce specific effects, thereby decreasing the total amount of any particular agent needed. Thus narcotics are used as analgesics, short-acting barbiturates (or other drugs) and potent inhalation agents are used to induce and maintain unconsciousness, respectively, and muscle relaxants are enlisted to produce muscle relaxation. The dosages of each of these drugs can be titrated to effect so that potential toxicity is minimized in patients with underlying medical disease.

This principle of specificity may also lead the anesthesiologist to choose a different set of drugs for the different perioperative periods: preoperative, induction, maintenance, and early postoperative. However, the advantages of using multiple drugs must be weighed against the potential for adverse interactions between these drugs and other chronic medications the patient may be taking. Some interactions may in fact be beneficial and are commonly used in the practice of anesthesiology. For example, there is the synergistic relation between nondepolarizing muscle relaxants and the potent inhalation anesthetic agents. Other interactions are, of course, potentially detrimental.

The remainder of this chapter will discuss some of the issues of interactions between chronic medications and anesthetic agents.

MEDICATIONS FOR CARDIOVASCULAR DISEASE

Cardiovascular diseases are the most common serious conditions affecting elderly Americans. Hypertension and ischemic heart disease are prevalent in this group of patients, and many of the medications used to treat one or both of these conditions are of concern in the perioperative period. The following discussion will review the use of antihypertensive medications, beta-blockers, calcium channel blockers, and digoxin.

Antihypertensive Medications

The availability of increasingly effective antihypertensive therapy over the past 3 decades is responsible for the improved prognosis of hypertensive patients today.[36] The preoperative assessment of patients with hypertension is directed toward determining the degree and severity of end-organ dysfunction, that is, the presence and significance of the renal, cerebrovascular, and cardiac sequelae of hypertension. However, the medications that the patient is taking can be equally important. Soon after effective and life-saving antihypertensive therapy became available in the 1950s, reports began to appear suggesting that such therapy was dangerous in patients undergoing anesthesia and surgery, causing hemodynamic lability in the perioperative period. It became standard practice to discontinue all antihypertensive medications 2 weeks preoperatively. Many years passed before controlled studies demonstrated that hypertensive patients who were treated throughout the perioperative period suffered no more hemodynamic instability than those in whom therapy was discontinued preoperatively.[24] In addition, Prys-Roberts et al[42] suggested that continuation of treatment for hypertension up to the day of surgery decreased perioperative morbidity. Later studies by Goldman and Caldera[18] did not confirm this observation, but both studies support the current recommendation to continue antihypertensives up to and including the morning of surgery. Most antihypertensive medications have effects that are potentially detrimental perioperatively. These interactions are reviewed below.

Reserpine blocks the uptake of catecholamines into storage vesicles and depletes norepinephrine stores, thereby making the patient less responsive to indirect-acting vasopressors. If vasopressors are required during the anesthetic course, direct-acting vasopressors, such as neosynephrine, should be used. However, reserpine-induced denervation hypersensitivity may increase the sensitivity to direct-acting agents, and careful titration of the drugs to desired endpoints is required. Reserpine also apparently decreases anesthetic requirements for inhalation agents in animals,[9] but the clinical relevance of this in humans is unclear. Guanethidine also depletes peripheral norepinephrine stores and has effects similar to those of reserpine, except that anesthetic requirements are not altered. Vasodilators such as hydralazine and minoxidil also reduce sensitivity to all classes of vasopressors. Converting enzyme inhibitors, such as captopril, may attenuate the expected hemodynamic response to acute volume depletion, but this potential effect does not seem to be a problem in practice.[31]

Diuretic agents, such as thiazides and furosemide, may produce hypovolemia and hypokalemia but recent evidence suggests that preoperative hypokalemia is not associated with increased perioperative morbidity.[21] These agents also prolong nondepolarizing neuromuscular blockade,[35] but this effect does not result in clinically important paralysis if muscle relaxants are carefully titrated to effect.

Clonidine is a centrally acting alpha-2 agonist that is associated in some patients with severe rebound hypertension when abruptly withdrawn because of marked increases in plasma catecholamine levels.[22] This drug should be continued preoperatively up to and including the day of surgery. Transdermal clonidine has recently become available and can be substituted for oral clonidine to ensure maintenance of therapeutic drug levels during the perioperative period. Transdermal preparations should be started 48 hours before surgery (time to steady state) and are of particular value in patients likely to have postoperative gastrointestinal absorptive defects. No intravenous form of the drug is currently available in the United States. Although the hypotensive effects of clonidine may be additive with those of other antihypertensive and anesthetic agents, it does not appear to predispose patients to any particular hemodynamic instability intraoperatively, provided anesthetic agents are titrated to desired effect.[17] There is evidence that suggests that preoperative clonidine may decrease intraoperative and postoperative hemodynamic lability in certain groups of high-risk patients through a reduction in sympathetic nervous system activity.[14,29]

To summarize, most of the potential interactions of commonly used antihypertensives with anesthetic agents and drugs typically used during anesthesia can be understood if the primary mechanisms of action are kept in mind. Available evidence suggests that it is prudent to continue antihypertensive therapy up to and including the day of surgery.

Beta-Blockers

The current perioperative use of beta-blockers represents a significant change in practice since their introduction in the early 1970s. Although beta-blockers were initially used to treat patients with angina, indications for their use have expanded to include hypertension, hyperthyroidism, migraine, glaucoma, arrhythmias, and myocardial infarction. Initially, it was widely feared that these drugs would potentiate hemodynamic instability intraoperatively by impairing the patient's ability to tolerate blood loss and by augmenting the myocardial depression caused by anesthetic agents.[60] Consequently, it became standard practice to discontinue beta-blockers 2 weeks before elective surgery and to avoid their use during and after surgery. However, abrupt discontinuation of beta-blocker therapy was soon discovered in nonsurgical settings to precipitate a withdrawal syndrome characterized by a hyperadrenergic state caused by an increase in the number and sensitivity of beta-receptors. Patients with ischemic heart disease or hypertension who were being treated with beta-blockers often developed myocardial infarction, unstable angina, ventricular tachycardia, or sudden death after abrupt withdrawal.[16,35,38] While abrupt withdrawal of beta-blockers in nonsurgical patients was discouraged, the proper management of surgical patients who were treated with beta-blockers awaited further study.

Numerous studies demonstrate that modern anesthetic agents do not potentiate beta-blockade[50] and intraoperative hemodynamics are quite stable in patients receiving beta-blockers.[25] One large prospective study demonstrated that aortocoronary bypass patients abruptly withdrawn from propranolol had a higher incidence of intraoperative arrhythmias and ischemia when compared to patients who received their regular dosage just before surgery.[51] In addition, hypotension and bradycardia occurred with equal frequency in both groups, suggesting that propranolol does not contribute to increased intraoperative hemodynamic instability as was previously feared. In the early 1970s Prys-Roberts and Foex suggested that the tachycardia, hypertension, and myocardial ischemic episodes occasionally associated with endotracheal intubation were greatly diminished in beta-blocked patients.[41] Slogoff and Keats have recently shown that preoperative beta-blockade markedly decreases the incidence of ischemic episodes caused by tachycardia in patients undergoing coronary artery bypass operations.[49] Since perioperative ischemic episodes appear to predict the occurrence of postoperative myocardial infarction,[48] it seems reasonable to assume that careful perioperative heart rate control can decrease the incidence of perioperative infarction. A study that was done recently also suggests that a single oral dose of a beta-blocker preoperatively may reduce the risk of perioperative ischemia in untreated hypertensive patients.[54]

A variety of beta-blockers are available for use in the United States, each with a different duration of action and beta-1 selectivity (Table 4-1). Patients taking atenolol, for example, may require only their usual dose on the morning of surgery to maintain an acceptable degree of beta-blockade, while patients taking propranolol may require intravenous supplementation during lengthy surgery. Mixed alpha-blockers and beta-blockers, such as labetolol, can be used both to maintain a degree of beta-blockade

and to control blood pressure on emergence from anesthesia in the early postoperative period.[28] With the advent of short acting beta-blockers, such as esmolol, it is now possible to acutely beta-block patients during especially stressful portions of a surgical procedure.[8,43] This can be done to blunt the reflex-mediated increase in sympathetic activity often seen during laryngoscopy and intubation, skin incision, sternotomy, and emergence. Esmolol is useful as a continuous intravenous infusion, allowing initiation or continuation of beta-blockade during the intraoperative and early postoperative periods.[19,44]

In patients with reactive airway disease selective beta-blockers may be tolerated better than nonselective beta-blockers, but cardioselectivity is dose-dependent and individual responses can be highly variable.[32] Intravenous beta-blockers should always be carefully titrated to the desired effect. It has been noted that patients maintained on topical beta-blockers for the treatment of glaucoma may be at some risk for the side effects of systemic beta-blockade, such as bradyarrythmias and heart block.[46]

Approaches to the perioperative use of beta-blockers have thus come full circle since the debut of these drugs almost 20 years ago. They are now regarded by most anesthesiologists as valuable adjuncts in the perioperative hemodynamic management of the complex patient, especially since the degree of beta-blockade can be instantaneously controlled with short-acting agents such as esmolol. Although current evidence is inferential, preoperative beta-blockade may be protective in patients at high risk for perioperative myocardial ischemia.[45,54]

Calcium Channel Blockers

The first calcium blocker was described in 1964,[15] but these drugs have been widely used clinically only

TABLE 4-1. **A comparison of some commonly used beta-blockers**

Drug	Beta-blockade potency ratio (propranolol = 1.0)	Relative beta-1 selectivity	Intrinsic sympathomimetic activity
Atenolol	1.0	+	0
Metoprolol	1.0	+	0
Nadolol	1.0	0	0
Pindolol	6.0	0	+
Propranolol	1.0	0	0
Timolol	6.0	0	0

TABLE 4-2. In vivo cardiovascular effects of calcium channel blockers

	Negative inotropy	Slowing of AV conduction	Systemic vasodilation
Nifedipine	0	0	+ + +
Diltiazem	+	+	+ +
Verapamil	+ +	+ + +	+ +

in the past 10 years. Calcium channel blockers were initially intended for treatment of ischemic heart disease but they are now used to treat an ever expanding variety of disorders such as arrhythmias (predominately supraventricular), hypertension, and congestive heart failure. Other potential uses include cerebrovascular disease, esophageal motility disorders, and reactive airway disease.[26] The physiologic and pharmacologic actions of these drugs have been recently reviewed.[39,61] Verapamil, diltiazem, and nifedipine all act to impair the passage of extracellular calcium into cells, but each drug has a variable effect in relaxing vascular smooth muscle, their dominant site of action. The three drugs variably dilate coronary and peripheral arterioles, decrease myocardial contractility, and slow atrioventricular (AV) conduction (Table 4-2). Nifedipine is the more potent vasodilator, while verapamil predominantly affects the AV conduction system. Optimal management during anesthesia and surgery of patients who require treatment with calcium channel blockers must account for potential adverse interactions between these and other commonly used perioperative drugs.

The potent inhalation anesthetic agents (halothane, enflurane, and isoflurane) are, to varying degrees, myocardial depressants. Although the mechanism of the negative inotropic effect that these agents produce is not completely understood, it may be mediated by altered intracellular calcium kinetics.[4] Interactions between inhalation anesthetic agents and calcium channel blockers have been evaluated in animal models receiving intravenous calcium channel blockers,[7] but clinical studies to assess these effects and to guide clinical management have been few. Shulte-Sasse et al examined the hemodynamic effects of intravenous verapamil administered during halothane anesthesia to patients who had received preoperative beta-blockers but in whom

preoperative left ventricular function was normal.[47] Halothane decreased cardiac index (23%), mean arterial pressure, and left ventricular contractility as measured by dP/dT. Intravenous verapamil infusion (0.15 mg/kg over 10 min) caused a further reduction in peak dP/dT and mean arterial pressure by 16% and 12%, respectively. Cardiac index was unchanged secondary to a fall in systemic vascular resistance. Patients tolerated these changes well, with no overt evidence of myocardial ischemia.

Concomitant use of calcium channel blockers and beta-blockers may augment the myocardial depressant and AV slowing effects of each of these classes of drugs. While their combined use is efficacious in the treatment of chronic stable angina,[55,62] the incidence of hemodynamic or electrophysiologic abnormalities with the combination of verapamil and beta-blockade is approximately 14% in a nonsurgical population.[27] The risk of an adverse interaction tends to increase in patients with poor left ventricular function or intrinsic conduction system disease.[61] A propranolol/nifedipine combination may entail the least risk in these patients, while a propranolol/diltiazem combination may produce fewer adverse effects in other patients.[23] Patients on combined calcium and beta antagonist therapy who require anesthesia may be at risk for intraoperative hemodynamic deterioration, since most inhalation anesthetics also slow AV conduction and depress myocardial contractility. Severe intraoperative and postoperative conduction disturbances have been reported in these patients, and some authors question whether continuation of all antianginal medications until the time of surgery is indicated.[49] In the absence of definitive data from large trials, it seems prudent to continue combined antianginal treatment until the time of surgery unless preoperative evaluation suggests signs of congestive heart failure or EKG evidence of conduction system delay. The anesthesiologist must be ready to intervene intraoperatively, either pharmacologically or with transvenous pacing, should this become necessary.

Animal studies suggest that both depolarizing and nondepolarizing motor blockade can be prolonged by calcium channel blockers.[11] This prolongation should not produce any clinical problems so long as the degree of neuromuscular blockade is monitored and the muscle relaxants are titrated to effect.

Digoxin

Many patients who require anesthesia and surgery are being treated with one or another digitalis preparation (digoxin is the most commonly used). While it is often difficult to determine the exact indication for long-term digoxin therapy, its use may be a clue to otherwise occult myocardial dysfunction or supraventricular rhythm disturbances. The digitalis glycosides have a very low therapeutic index, and it has been estimated that about 20% of patients who take these drugs will at some time exhibit some toxic reaction.[53] The fall in creatinine clearance that occurs with age makes the elderly particularly prone to develop toxicity. Common perioperative events may predispose to toxicity, primarily as a result of the hypokalemia or interactions with other medications. Hypokalemia is common in the perioperative period and may be exacerbated by hyperventilation, metabolic alkalosis, and increased catecholamine levels. Perioperative Holter monitoring has confirmed an increased incidence of ventricular ectopy in digitalized patients, but these arrythmias do not correlate with the serum potassium level.[21] Concomitant administration of other medications such as quinidine and calcium channel blockers, may predispose to digitalis toxicity. The mechanism by which serum digoxin levels are increased is unclear, but increases on the order of 40% to 77% may occur with concomitant administration of verapamil.[40] Serum digoxin levels and clinical signs of digoxin toxicity should be monitored closely when these drugs are used together. Finally, animal studies suggest that general anesthetics do not predispose to digitalis toxicity, but whether or not they are protective is controversial.[2]

Optimal perioperative management of the patient taking digoxin requires a careful preoperative search for the sometimes subtle signs of digitalis toxicity. The elderly and those with impaired renal function are at greatest risk. Serum digoxin levels may be helpful, but increased levels alone do not indicate toxicity. Patients taking digoxin for the control of atrial fibrillation, for example, may require high serum levels to achieve an appropriate ventricular response. If the drug is not being used for arrhythmia control, it is probably safe to omit it on the morning of surgery. Far better inotropic agents are available for use intraoperatively, should the need arise.

PSYCHOTROPIC AGENTS

Tricyclic antidepressants are used extensively for the treatment of severe depression and may also be used in the treatment of chronic pain and certain anxiety disorders. Amitriptyline and imipramine are the most commonly used agents, but other drugs in this class include amoxapine, maprotiline, trazodone, doxepin, nortriptyline, and desipramine. All of these drugs block the uptake of neurotransmitters presynaptically and increase central adrenergic tone.[1] Most of these drugs also produce moderate anticholinergic effects. A quinidine-like effect on cardiac conduction is produced by the tricyclic antidepressants (slowing of AV conduction), so that patients with preexisting delayed ventricular conduction should be observed closely when taking these drugs.[10] These properties pose several problems for perioperative management of patients who are treated with these drugs.

Chronically reduced noradrenergic catecholamine stores result in hypersensitivity to direct acting sympathomimetic agents, and the usual dosages of phenylephrine, norepinephrine, and epinephrine must be carefully titrated to avoid serious hypertensive responses.[5] Animal studies suggest that tricyclics interact with halothane and pancuronium to produce serious ventricular arrhythmias.[12] Presumably tricyclic pretreatment enhances the sympathomimetic effect of pancuronium on the myocardium, which is already sensitized by halothane to the arrhythmogenic effects of catecholamines. Central anticholinergic effects of tricyclics may be additive with the anticholinergic effects of other drugs used in the perioperative period, an effect which may produce delirium, particularly in the elderly. If anticholinergic agents are necessary, noncentrally acting agents such as glycopyrolate should probably be used. The effects of tricyclic antidepressants to slow AV conduction may augment similar effects on cardiac conduction of beta-blockers, calcium channel blockers, and inhalation anesthetic agents, but no such reports have appeared in the literature. Current information suggests that tricyclic antidepressants may be continued until the time of surgery, but clinicians should be aware of the potentially adverse interactions.

The monoamine oxidase (MAO) inhibitors such as phenelzine, pargyline, isocarboxazide, and tranylcypromine bind to intracellular MAO and increase intraneuronal levels of neurotransmitter amines. While the use of these drugs declined after the introduction of tricyclic antidepressants, it seems now to be increasing since these drugs may be efficacious in some patients unresponsive to the tricyclics. MAO inhibitors predispose the patient to exaggerated hypertensive responses to indirect-acting sympathomimetics such as ephedrine, which is commonly used intraoperatively. Meperidine may, through unknown mechanisms, interact with MAO inhibitors to produce agitation, hyperpyrexia, hypertension, rigidity, and convulsions; it is best avoided in the perioperative period. Conventional recommendations that MAO inhibitors be discontinued for 2 to 3 weeks before anesthesia and surgery have been challenged.[59] One case report describes two patients undergoing urgent cardiac procedures who were managed with high-dose fentanyl anesthesia without complications related to MAO inhibitor therapy.[33] Another more controlled study[13] examined a group of patients, treated with MAO inhibitors, who were undergoing electroconvulsive therapy (ECT). There were no differences in heart rate, blood pressure, or body temperature after ECT between this group and a similar group who were not taking MAO inhibitors preoperatively. Further uncontrolled observations of 14 patients on chronic MAO inhibitors who underwent a variety of surgical procedures under general anesthesia revealed no adverse reactions attributable to MAO-inhibitor therapy. None of the patients in these reports were given indirect-acting sympathomimetics or meperidine perioperatively, nor were patients who had recently started MAO-inhibitor therapy (within 1 month) evaluated. The authors concluded that discontinuation of long-term MAO-inhibitor therapy is unnecessary and suggested that postsynaptic adrenergic down-regulation may account for the apparent safety of these drugs. However, the management of perioperative MAO inhibitors remains controversial. If there are no major psychiatric risks in discontinuing therapy, it would make sense to do so 2 weeks before elective surgery. For patients in whom discontinuation of antidepressant therapy is ill advised, or for those requiring emergency surgery, the risk of adverse reactions is probably less than previously thought. The patient recently started on MAO inhibitors may be at an increased risk.

Lithium is often used chronically to treat patients with manic-depressive illness but has effects that may complicate the perioperative course. Mental confusion occasionally develops during lithium therapy, and this effect can complicate the differential diagnosis of postoperative delirium, especially in elderly patients and in those with extracellular volume contraction. Although case reports have appeared relating lithium to prolongation of neuromuscular blockade, this relation appears to be of little clinical significance.[30] Evidence linking lithium to disturbances in cardiac rhythm and function is controversial. T-wave changes may occur, but their clinical significance is uncertain. Chronic lithium use has been associated with cardiac conduction abnormalities, but Brady et al have stated that "the prevalence and clinical significance of these changes remains to be established."[6] Currently there is no reason to discontinue lithium therapy before elective surgery.

Antipsychotic drugs including phenothiazines, thioxanthenes, and butyrophenones are dopaminergic blockers, but also have varying antiadrenergic and anticholinergic effects. Accordingly they may enhance the sedation and hypotensive effects of anesthetic agents. Careful titration of anesthetic agents to desired effect should minimize these interactions. Dopaminergic blockade does not appear to cause clinically important complications and there is no compelling evidence to suggest that antipsychotic drugs should be discontinued preoperatively.

The various psychotropic agents discussed above have engendered much concern about possible adverse effects in the perioperative period. With the possible exception of MAO inhibitors, however, they may be continued up to and including the day of surgery.

MISCELLANEOUS MEDICATIONS

Chronic medications required to treat patients with pulmonary or neuromuscular disease are reviewed in other chapters. Chronic glucocorticoid therapy is useful for a variety of inflammatory disorders and for patients with severe asthma. Suppression of the hypothalamic-pituitary-adrenal (HPA) axis is a predictable effect following steroid therapy, and patients who have been on steroids for more than a few weeks are assumed to be suppressed.[3] HPA suppression may last up to 1 year after treatment is discontinued, so that supplementary steroids are required perioperatively during this period (see Chapter 21). HPA axis recovery occurs quickly (days) in patients given steroids for 1 week or less. Inhaled steroids are often used in asthmatics to decrease the side effects of chronic oral therapy. It has been determined that up to 1 mg of beclamethasone per day may be given before HPA suppression begins to occur.[56] If HPA status is uncertain and there is no time for diagnostic evaluation, a short course of steroids should be administered perioperatively; few side effects are likely.

SUMMARY

It is rarely necessary to interrupt a patient's medication regimen preoperatively, and most medications should be continued up to and including the morning of surgery. An accepted, although debatable, exception is monoamine oxidase inhibitors. It is also important to continue necessary medications in the postoperative period, substituting parenteral forms when it is impractical for the patient to resume oral intake in the early postoperative period. A parenterally available alternative drug may have to be used if the patient's usual medication is not available in parenteral form. Postoperative ileus may prevent adequate absorption of oral medications.

It is quite important for clinicians providing perioperative care to be aware of the pharmacology and potential interactions of chronic medications with the potent pharmacologic agents that are commonly used in anesthesiology. This importance increases as the population ages and new medications are introduced into clinical practice.

REFERENCES

1. Anderson BO: Long term prognosis in geriatric surgery: 2-17 year follow-up of 7922 patients, J Am Geriat Soc 20:255-258, 1972.
2. Atlee J, Pammendrup M, and Malkinson C: Halothane and hypocapnia: effects on electrically stimulated atrial arrhythmias in digitalized dogs, Anesth Analg 60:302-305, 1981.
3. Axelrod L: Side effects of glucocorticoid therapy. In. Schliemer RP et al (editors): Antiinflammatory steroids: basic and clinical aspects, New York, 1987, Academic Press.
4. Blanck TJ and Thompson M: Calcium transport by cardiac sarcoplasmic reticulum: modulation of halothane action by substrate concentration and pH, Anesth Analg 60:390-394, 1981.
5. Boakes AJ et al: Interactions between sympathomimetic amines and antidepressant agents in man, Br Med J 1:311-315, 1973.
6. Brady HD and Gargan JH: Lithium and the heart: unanswered questions, Chest 93:166-169, 1988.
7. Chelly JE et al: Cardiovascular effects of and interaction between calcium blocking drugs and anesthetics in chronically instrumented dogs. I. Verapamil and Halothane, Anesthesiology 64:560-567, 1986.
8. Covinsky J: Esmolol: a novel cardioselective, titratable, intravenous beta blocker with ultra-short half life, Drug Intell Clin Pharm 21:316-321, 1987.
9. Craig D and Bose, D: Drug interactions in anaesthesia: chronic antihypertensive therapy, Can Anaesth Soc J 31:580-588, 1986.
10. Drugs for psychiatric disorders, The Medical Letter 28(725):99-105, 1986.
11. Durant WN, Nguyes A, and Briscoe JR: Potentiation of neuromuscular blockade by verapamil, Anesthesiology 60:298-303, 1984.
12. Edwards RP et al: Cardiac responses to imipramine and pancuronium during anesthesia with halothane and enflurane, Anesthesiology 50:421-425, 1979.
13. El-Ganzouri AR et al: Monoamine oxidase inhibitors: should they be discontinued preoperatively? Anesth Analg 64:592-596, 1985.
14. Flacke J et al: Reduced narcotic requirement by clonidine with improved hemodynamic and adrenergic stability in patients undergoing coronary bypass surgery, Anesthesiology 67:11-19, 1987.
15. Fleckenstein A: Die Bedeutung der energiereichen Phosphosphate für Kontraktilität und Tonus des Myokards, Verh Deutsch Ges Inn Med 70:81-99, 1964.
16. Frishman W: Beta-adrenergic blocker withdrawal, Am J Cardiol 59:26F-32F, 1987.
17. Ghignone M, Calville O, and Quintin L: Anesthesia and hypertension: the effect of clonidine on perioperative hemodynamics and isoflurane requirements, Anesthesiology 67:3-10, 1987.
18. Goldman L and Caldera D: Risks of general anesthesia and elective operation in the hypertensive patient, Anesthesiology 50:285-292, 1979.
19. Gray RJ: Managing critically ill patients with esmolol, an ultra short-acting beta adrenergic blocker, Chest 93(2):398-403, 1988.
20. Hartwell BL and Mark JB: Combinations of beta-blockers and calcium channel blockers: a cause for malignant perioperative conduction disturbances? Anesth Analg 65:905-907, 1986.
21. Hirsch I et al: The overstated risk of preoperative hypokalemia, Anesth Analg 67:131-136, 1988.
22. Hobt A et al: Withdrawal syndromes and the cessation of antihypertensive therapy, Arch Intern Med 141:1125-1127, 1981.
23. Johnson DL et al: Clinical and hemodynamic evaluation of propranolol in combination with verapamil in exertional angina pectoris: a placebo controlled

double blind randomized crossover study, Am J Cardiol 55:680, 1985.

24. Katz RL, Weistraub HD, and Papper EM: Anesthesia, surgery, and rauwolfia, Anesthesiology 25:142-147, 1964.

25. Kopriva C, Brown A, and Pappas G: Hemodynamics during general anesthesia in patients receiving propranolol, Anesthesiology 48:28-33, 1978.

26. Larach D and Zelio R: Advances in calcium blocker therapy, Am J Surg 151:527-537, 1986.

27. Leon MB et al: Combination therapy with calcium channel blockers and beta-blockers for chronic stable angina pectoris, Am J Cardiol 55:69B-80B, 1985.

28. Leslie JB et al: Intravenous labetolol for treatment of postoperative hypertension, Anesthesiology 67 (3):413-416, 1987.

29. Longnecker D: Alpine anesthesia: can pretreatment with clonidine decrease the peaks and valleys? Anesthesiology 67:1-2, 1987.

30. Martin B and Kramer P: Clinical significance of the interaction between lithium and a neuromuscular blocker, Am J Psych 139:1326-1328, 1982.

31. Martin D and Kammerer W: The hypertensive surgical patient: controversies in management, Surg Clin North Am 63(5):1017-1033, 1983.

32. McDewitt D: Pharmacologic aspects of cardioselectivity in a beta-blocking drug, Am J Cardiol 59:10F-12F, 1987.

33. Michaels I et al: Anesthesia for cardiac surgery in patients receiving monoamine oxidase inhibitors, Anesth Analg 63:1041-1044, 1984.

34. Miller RD (editor): Anesthesia, ed 2, New York, 1986, Churchill Livingstone.

35. Miller R, Sobn Y, and Matteo R: Enhancement of tubocurarine neuromuscular blockade by diuretics in man, Anesthesiology 45:442-446, 1976.

36. Moses M: Historical perspective on the management of hypertension, Am J Med 80(5B):1-11, 1986.

37. National Center for Health Statistics: United States life tables: U.S. decennial life tables for 1979-1981, Vol 1, No 1, Washington, DC, 1988, Government Printing Office.

37a. National health interview survey 1983-1985, Hyattsville, Md, 1986, National Center for Health Statistics.

38. Nattel S, Rangro R, and VanLoon G: Mechanism of propranolol withdrawal phenomena, Circulation 59:1158-1164, 1979.

39. Opie LH: Calcium ions, drug action and the heart with special reference to calcium antagonist drugs, Pharm Ther 25:271-295, 1984.

40. Piepho R, Culbertson V, and Rhodes R: Drug interactions with the calcium entry blockers, Circ 75(Suppl IV):V181, 1987.

41. Prys-Roberts C and Foex P: Studies of anesthesia in relation to hypertension. V. Adrenergic beta receptor blockade, Br J Anaesth 45:671-681, 1973.

42. Prys-Roberts C, Melocke R, and Foex P: Studies of anesthesia in relation to hypertension 1. Cardiovascular responses of treated and untreated patients, Br J Anaesth 43:122-137, 1971.

43. Reves JG and Flegzane P: Perioperative use of esmolol, Am J Cardiol 56:57F-62F, 1985.

44. Reynolds RD and Gorczaski RJ: Pharmacology and pharmacokinetics of esmolol, Clin Pharmacol 26 (suppl A):A3-A14, 1986.

45. Roizen M: Should we all have a sympathectomy at birth? Or at least preoperatively? Anesthesiology 68:482-484, 1988.

46. Samuels ST and Maze M: Beta-receptor blockade following the use of eye drops, Anesthesiology 52:369-370, 1980.

47. Shulte-Sasse U et al: Combined effects of halothane anaesthesia and verapamil on systemic hemodynamics and left ventricular myocardial contractility in patients with ischemic heart disease, Anesth Analg 63:791-798, 1984.

48. Slogoff S and Keats A: Does perioperative ischemia lead to postoperative myocardial infarction? Anesthesiology 62:107-114, 1985.

49. Slogoff S and Keats A: Does chronic treatment with calcium entry blocking drugs reduce perioperative myocardial ischemia? Anesthesiology 68:676-680, 1988.

50. Slogoff S et al: Failure of general anesthesia to potentiate propranolol activity, Anesthesiology 47:504-508, 1977.

51. Slogoff S, Keats A, and Ott E: Preoperative propranolol therapy and aortocoronary bypass operation, JAMA 240:1487-1490, 1978.

52. Smith N and Corbascio A (editors): Drug Interactions in Anesthesia, Philadelphia, 1986, Lea & Febiger.

53. Smith TW and Haber E: Digitalis, (4 parts), N Engl J Med 285:1125, 1973.

54. Stone JG et al: Myocardial ischemia in untreated hypertensive patients: effect of a single small oral dose of a beta-adrenergic blocking agent, Anesthesiology 68:495-500, 1988.

55. Subramanin VB et al: Combined therapy with verapamil and propranolol and chronic stable angina, Am J Cardiol 49:125, 1982.

56. Togood JH and Moote DW: Steroid therapy and allergic reactions. In Kaplan AP (editor): Allergy, New York, 1985, Churchill Livingstone.

57. U.S. Department of American Bureau of the Census: Statistical abstract of the United States 1986, ed 106.

58. U.S. Food and Drug Administration, U.S. Department of Commerce: Drug utilization in the U.S.—1986, eighth annual review, 1987, National Technical Information Service.

59. Viegas OJ: Psychiatric illness. In Stoelting RK and Deerdorf SF (editors): Anesthesia and co-existing disease, New York, 1983, Churchill Livingstone.

60. Viljoen JF, Estefanous FG, and Kellner GA: Propranolol and cardiac surgery, J Thorac Cardiovasc Surg 64:826-830, 1972.

61. Winniford MD and Hollis LD: Calcium antagonists in patients with cardiovascular disease, current perspectives, Medicine (Baltimore) 64:61-73, 1985.

62. Winniford MD, Huxley RL, and Hillis DL: Randomized, double-blind comparison of propranolol alone and a propranolol-verapamil combination in patients with severe angina of effort, J Am Coll Cardiol 1:492-498, 1983.

CHAPTER 5

Role of the Consultant

THOMAS H. LEE
LEE GOLDMAN

Function
Availability
    Factors associated with the effectiveness of
       consultations
    Recommendations

Both internists and anesthesiologists are being called on more frequently to act as consultants for surgical patients. The need for such consultations has grown partly because the success of modern surgical techniques has encouraged surgeons to undertake ambitious procedures in an aging patient population with multiple medical problems such as diabetes, ischemic heart disease, and malignancies. Thus the cases on the operating room schedule are increasingly complex. In addition, the fields of surgery, anesthesiology, and medicine have become so sophisticated that the interfaces between are areas requiring special skills.

A growing literature reflects the evolution of a specific body of knowledge for internal medicine consultants,[8] and residency programs at many teaching hospitals have started general medical consultative services primarily for the care of surgical patients.[2,3,14,17] Similarly, anesthesiology training programs have emphasized the anesthesiologist's role in both preoperative evaluation and postoperative follow-up.

Preoperative consultation often emphasizes prognostic stratification for surgical candidates, as described in the other chapters of this volume. However, the essence of consulting is communication; no matter how sound the consultant's clinical judgment, it will contribute to care of the patient only if it is communicated effectively. Considerable data suggest that there is room for improvement in the art of consultation.* When we interviewed consultants and the physicians who requested consultations in 156 cases at a teaching hospital, we found that in 14% of the cases they completely disagreed on both the reason for the consultation and the principal clinical issue.[12] When communication between consultant and consultee is so tenuous, it is not surprising that reported rates of compliance with the recommendations of consultants are only 54% to 77%.[1,10,20] Compliance rates for recommendations from preoperative consultations have been found to be significantly lower than compliance rates associated with consultations in other settings.[10]

This chapter focuses not on the clinical assessment performed by consultants but on the context in which this assessment is performed. We describe the function of the consultant in the perioperative period and the basic requirements for following patients. Investigations into the determinants of the effectiveness of consultations are summarized, and we conclude with a list of recommendations that we have

*References 1, 10, 12, 16, 20.

previously described as the "Ten commandments for effective consultations."[7]

FUNCTION

While consultants are frequently asked to "clear" a patient for surgery, the guarantee of a good outcome that "clearance" implies is, of course, impossible to provide. All patients, no matter how stable, are at some risk when they undergo anesthesia and surgery. All consultations for surgical patients, even if the consultation request is simply for "clearance," must address the following issues:

1. Estimation of cardiac and noncardiac risk of surgery
2. Comparison of surgical risk to the risk of medical therapy
3. Identification of management strategies that minimize risks
4. Anticipation of complications that might occur during the perioperative period

The consulting roles of anesthesiologists and internists may be different in different institutions. Input from an internist is required when the patient has an unstable medical problem (for example, myocardial ischemia precipitated by an acute surgical condition), an uncertain medical status (a hip fracture caused by a new syncopal event), or multiple chronic diseases (diabetes or congestive heart failure). The internist can help not only in the preoperative assessment but also for the duration of the postoperative course. Familiarity with the past history and the baseline condition of the patient will greatly aid management. Anesthesiologists, however, are most competent to evaluate questions on intraoperative physiology, complications, and management.

Because many patients who are scheduled for surgery may never have been evaluated by an internist, the internal medicine evaluation must include a comprehensive gathering of primary data. The consultant should not rely on an old chart to exclude a history of symptoms of congestive heart failure or ischemic heart disease, or on the vital signs obtained by other health care personnel. The internal medicine consultant may be the first physician to check a patient's blood pressure in both arms, thus unmasking undetected hypertension, or the only clinician to check a patient's stools for the presence of blood before that patient undergoes heparinization in the course of cardiopulmonary bypass.

Whereas the medical or anesthesiologic consultant must approach the patient clinically as if the patient were his or her own, the patient's true primary physician is the surgeon who called the consultation, and the consultant must respect this relationship. Thus the consultant should be circumspect in interactions with the patient; both honesty and discretion are required. For example, a consultant might answer questions about a patient's diabetes mellitus, but should not engage the patient in lengthy discussions on whether the surgery is indicated or likely to succeed. Telling a patient that surgery should be canceled without first discussing this opinion with the surgeon would obviously be an extreme breech of etiquette.

The consultant has a responsibility to the patient, but this responsibility can almost always be fulfilled through the consultant's primary relationship with the surgeon. Competition for the respect and loyalty of the patient is inappropriate. In our experience, direct discussions with the surgeon or surgical housestaff can almost always resolve differences of opinion on management strategies.

In these interactions with surgical staff, the consultant has a teaching role, but this role must be exercised with tact and sensitivity to the surgeon's needs. Opinions should be expressed concisely and without condescension, and reprints of references should be shared selectively. Whereas a table listing a differential diagnosis is often helpful, long intellectual discussions in the medical record are unlikely to be read and may alienate the surgeon who called the consultation.

In addition to this role as a teacher, the consultant also has a role as a student, because consultations offer an unusual opportunity to learn about new approaches in other specialties. This form of continuing medical education enriches the clinician's skills in both internal medicine and consultative medicine.

AVAILABILITY

Consultants must be available to the patient and surgeon at several key points of the perioperative period. Because rising health care costs have created pressures for increased efficiency in the health care system, the first of these key points may occur before the hospitalization. Many surgeons now commonly refer patients who are scheduled for elective surgery to internists and anesthesiologists for outpatient visits a week or more beforehand.

These preadmission evaluations offer several important advantages over the more traditional in-hospital evaluation on the day before surgery. Hasty consultations are avoided and consultants have an opportunity to obtain baseline tests and, if necessary, pursue abnormal values or arrange further testing (for example, an exercise tolerance test) without disrupting the surgical schedule or prolonging the hospitalization. By seeing a patient twice before surgery (both before and after admission), the consultant becomes more familiar with the patient's baseline mental status and physical examination. This approach facilitates outpatient surgery and same-day surgical programs in which patients are admitted on the morning of their operation. Early scheduling depends on a good working relationship between individual consultants and surgeons, and in turn can strengthen that relationship.

Whether or not a preadmission evaluation is performed, the consultant should examine the patient in the hospital before surgery. Although surgeons have a responsibility to produce timely requests for evaluations (before or shortly after admission), occasionally a consultant must see the patient late in the evening on the day of admission or very early the next morning because the request for consultation has not been transmitted promptly. When such communication failures occur, the consultant should resist the temptation to punish the surgeon who has requested the consultation (and the patient) by delaying surgery. Instead, he or she should seek to develop a system for earlier consultations in the future. Because operating room time is one of the most expensive hospital resources, disruptions of the surgical schedule should be avoided in the interest of efficiency.

Another key point in the consultation process is in the recovery room, where the patient may be least stable as a result of arrhythmias, hemodynamic shifts, and clouded mental status. For example, postoperative hypertension usually occurs within 30 to 60 minutes after the end of anesthesia.[4] Particular attention should be paid to the patient's volume status and fluid orders to prevent hypotension or congestive heart failure. An early evaluation of a postoperative electrocardiogram may lead to detection of ischemia. A rule used by many experienced internal medicine consultants is "Never go home before the patient is out of the operating room."

Once the surgery and the immediate postoperative period have passed, the consultation does not end. Because intravenous fluids given perioperatively may be mobilized slowly, a second high-risk time for myocardial infarction, hypertension, and congestive heart failure occurs 24 to 48 hours after surgery.[5] Ischemic heart disease may also be exacerbated by increasing activity at this point in the hospitalization, making it prudent to evaluate a second electrocardiogram 3 to 5 days after surgery in high-risk patients. Patients with known ischemic heart disease should be followed daily for a minimum of 6 days if they remain hospitalized after surgery.

Thus perioperative consultation requires an intense evaluation and a commitment lasting at least several days. However, the internal medicine consultant's role is limited for the few hours that the patient is in the operating room, when the anesthesiologist's role is greatest. Although internists may be interested in the surgical techniques and type of anesthesia used, making unsolicited recommendations in these areas is usually inappropriate. Most internists are not sophisticated in their understanding of the events that occur in the operating room and may not understand how intraoperative physiologic changes may alter the usual therapeutic approach to common problems. The expertise of surgeons and anesthesiologists should not be underestimated, and trite suggestions such as "Avoid hypotension" are unlikely to be appreciated.

Factors Associated with the Effectiveness of Consultations

The art of consultation is basically effective communication.[11] As noted, we have found that disagreement between the consultant and the primary physician on the issues of a consultation occur in 14% of cases.[12] At another university hospital, no specific question was asked in 24% of preoperative diabetic consultations, and consultants ignored the stated question in another 12%.[19] When such breakdowns in communications occurred in our study, the primary physicians had significantly lower opinions of the impact of the consultation than the consultants.[12] Obviously, oral communication between the consultant and the primary physicians before the consultation is likely to prevent such misunderstandings; similarly, direct contact with the physicians who requested the consultation within 24 hours after

> **Factors associated with compliance with consultants' recommendations**
>
> Direct contact between consultant and physician ordering the consultation[16]
> Limited number of recommendations[16,20]
> Identification of high priority recommendations[20]
> Specification of drug dosage, route, and duration[9]
> Continued follow-up of patients[9,13,19]

the consult has been associated with high compliance rates (see box at right).[16]

Several investigators have identified other factors associated with effectiveness, which can be summarized as brevity, clarity, persistence, and specificity. For example, Sears and Charlson found that compliance decreases as the number of recommendations increases.[20] In their series of 202 general medicine consultations, compliance was highest when five or fewer recommendations were made, regardless of the severity of illness of the patient. Other data suggest that a long list of suggestions decreases the likelihood that any of them will be followed, including the crucial ones.[13]

The tendency to formulate long lists of recommendations reflects the value placed on completeness and compulsiveness in internal medicine training, and may also result from a need on the part of the consultant to justify his or her "expert" status. These forces can result in, for example, long lists of recommendations for mild anemia discovered on preoperative screening studies. In our series at Brigham and Women's Hospital, the total charges for the additional tests or procedures suggested by medical consulting services were approximately $300 (1981 dollars) per case, but the perceived value of the consultation, according to the requesting physician, was not correlated with the amount of recommended testing.[12]

One way to reduce the number of recommendations is to eliminate trivial suggestions or tests that are already planned. In the series of medical consultations performed for surgical colleagues reported by Ballard et al,[1] 122 (12%) of 1016 recommendations were judged to be "insulting" by the reviewer, a surgical chief resident. Many of these suggestions were considered "elementary and obvious,"

such as "Maintain hematocrit > 30." An additional 61 (6%) of the 1016 recommendations were judged to be nonessential.

Conversely, clear identification of important recommendations leads to a higher rate of compliance. Pupa et al found that labeling recommendations as "crucial" led to greater than 90% compliance even if they were contained in a long list of other suggestions.[16] Obviously, communication of the priority of recommendations is most effective when the consultant and surgeon talk with one another directly.

Another tactic is to give the recommendations serially over several days while continuing to follow the patient. Several investigators have shown that suggestions are more likely to be followed if consultants write periodic follow-up notes with recommendations.[9,13,19] Thus, Horwitz et al[9] found that when more than one follow-up note was left, the consultation had an effect on diagnosis in 92% of cases and an effect on management in 84% of cases. When one or no follow-up note was left, effects on diagnosis were detected in only 74% of cases (p <0.001), and effects on management were found in only 56% of cases (p <0.001).

Many problems can be evaluated more fully and appropriately during the follow-up period than before surgery. For example, postponing surgery to achieve better blood pressure control in patients with stable hypertension and diastolic blood pressures of 110 mm Hg or less does not reduce perioperative risk.[6,15] Thus a consultant might delay recommendations for an etiologic workup (for example, 24-hour collections for urinary catecholamines) or major changes in the therapeutic regimen until after surgery. Similarly, delaying recommendations for the evaluation of a problem such as newly discovered mild asymptomatic hypercalcemia may enhance the chances that the surgeons will note the recommendation for postoperative cardiac enzyme sampling.

A consultant's recommendations should also be as specific as possible so that a surgeon who may not be familiar with the latest antiarrhythmic agents or cephalosporins may copy the recommendations directly into the order book. Horwitz et al found that when recommendations for drug therapy included both the dose and duration 100% of the recommendations were followed, but compliance fell to 85% when only one was specified, and to 64% when neither was described explicitly (p <0.001).[9]

Recommendations

Because most physicians learn how to perform consultations through trial and error, there is considerable variability in consultative skills. As a result, some consultants are sought by surgical colleagues, whereas others have difficulty translating their expertise into effective consultations.[18] We have previously described some basic principles of effective consultation that have been derived from the investigations described above and from observing respected consultants in our own clinical experience, and we have presented them as "Ten commandments for effective consultations" (see box at right).[7]

1. *Determine the question.* Often the primary physician has not clearly communicated the question, whereas in other cases the consultant may overlook it. When the issue has not been clearly stated, direct contact can help avoid consultations that do not address the primary physician's needs.

2. *Establish urgency.* While consultation requests may be transmitted via mail or a call from a ward clerk, the consultant should determine whether a consultation is emergent, urgent, or elective, and respond promptly in critical situations.

3. *Look for yourself.* Historical and physical examination data should be gathered independently.

4. *Be as brief as appropriate.* A long discussion is unlikely to be read, and a long list of recommendations is unlikely to be followed.

5. *Be specific.* The surgeon should be able to copy recommendations directly into the order book if he or she agrees.

6. *Provide contingency plans.* Initial recommendations may prove irrelevant within a few hours. Thus, the consultant should try to anticipate potential problems and provide brief descriptions of management strategies that can be invoked should they arise.

7. *Honor thy turf.* (Or, thou shalt not covet thy neighbor's patient.) While the consultant may have more day-to-day contact with a surgical patient than the surgeon, the consultant plays a subsidiary role. The surgeon is the patient's physician, and the consultant is the surgeon's adviser.

8. *Teach . . . with tact.* Expertise and insight

Ten commandments for effective consultations

1. Determine the question
2. Establish urgency
3. Look for yourself
4. Be as brief as appropriate
5. Be specific
6. Provide contingency plans
7. Honor thy turf
8. Teach . . . with tact
9. Talk is cheap . . . and effective
10. Follow-up

From Goldman L, Lee T, and Rudd P: Ten commandments for effective consultations, Arch Intern Med 143:1753-1755, 1983.

---

should be shared without condescension.

9. *Talk is cheap . . . and effective.* There is no substitute for direct personal contact.

10. *Follow-up.* Because perioperative complications can occur several days after surgery, the consultant's role does not end when the operation is over. Furthermore, the postoperative period provides an opportunity to address other internal medicine issues that may arise.

REFERENCES

1. Ballard WP, Gold JP, and Charlson ME: Compliance with the recommendations of medical consultants, J Gen Intern Med 1:220-224, 1986.
2. Burke GR and Corman LC: The general medicine consult service in a university teaching hospital, Med Clin North Am 63:1353-1357, 1979.
3. Charlson ME, Cohen RP, and Sears CL: General medicine consultation. Lessons from a clinical service, Am J Med 75:121-128, 1983.
4. Gal TJ and Cooperman LH: Hypertension in the immediate postoperative period, Br J Anaesth 47:70-74, 1975.
5. Goldman L: Cardiac risks and complications of noncardiac surgery, Ann Intern Med 98:504-513, 1983.
6. Goldman L and Caldera DL: Risks of general anesthesia and elective operation in the hypertensive patient, Anesthesiology 50:285-292, 1979.
7. Goldman L, Lee T, and Rudd P: Ten commandments for effective consultations, Arch Intern Med 143:1753-1755, 1983.
8. Gross R and Kammerer W: Medical consultation on surgical services. An annotated bibliography, Ann Intern Med 95:523-529, 1981.

9. Horwitz RI, Henes CG, and Horwitz SM: Developing strategies for improving the diagnostic and management efficacy of medical consultations, J Chron Dis 36:213-218, 1983.

10. Klein LE et al: The preoperative consultation: response to internists' recommendations, Arch Intern Med 143:743-744, 1983.

11. Lee TH and Goldman L: Principles of effective communication in consultative medicine. In Bolt RJ (editor): Medical evaluation of the surgical patient, Mt. Kisco, New York, 1987, Futura Publishing Co, Inc.

12. Lee TH, Pappius EM, and Goldman L: Impact of inter-physician communication on the effectiveness of medical consultations, Am J Med 74:106-112, 1983.

13. MacKenzie TB et al: The effectiveness of cardiology consultations: concordance with diagnostic and drug recommendations, Chest 79:16-22, 1981.

14. Moore DA et al: Consultations in internal medicine: a training program resource, J Med Educ 52:323-327, 1977.

15. Prys-Roberts C: Hypertension and anesthesia—fifty years on (editorial), Anesthesiology 50:281-284, 1979.

16. Pupa LE et al: Factors affecting compliance for general medicine consultations to non-internists, Am J Med 81:508-514, 1986.

17. Robie PW: The service and educational contributions of a general medicine consultation service, J Gen Intern Med 1:225-227, 1986.

18. Rudd P: Contrasts in academic consultations, Ann Intern Med 94:537-538, 1981.

19. Rudd P, Siegler M, and Byyny RL: Preoperative diabetic consultation. A plea for improved training, J Med Educ 53:590-596, 1978.

20. Sears CL and Charlson ME: The effectiveness of a consultation: compliance with initial recommendations, Am J Med 74:870-876, 1983.

CHAPTER 6

Legal Considerations of Perioperative Care

A. TERRY WALMAN

This chapter discusses the medicolegal aspects of perioperative evaluation and management. Specific legal advice and pronouncements regarding the practice of medicine are avoided, but a general overview of legal principles that relate to medical practice are presented. All references to health care personnel are restricted to physicians for purposes of simplicity and convenience, but these are often applicable to other health care providers. The perioperative period is notable for the team concept involving medical practitioners from many different specialities and backgrounds. Most legal concepts apply similarly to the relationship between the patient and each of the various health care providers that are involved in this complex and highly organized interaction.

THE PHYSICIAN-PATIENT RELATIONSHIP

The physician-patient relationship is the cornerstone for understanding the rights and responsibilities at issue in any discussion of the legal aspects of medical practice.[1] The perioperative period is no exception. When a physician (or other health care provider) provides care to a patient, exercise of reasonable skill and diligence on behalf of the patient is expected.[2] In the eyes of the law, this is the provision of a service and the relationship is contractual. Each of the two contracting parties have duties and responsibilities to the other as a result.[3]

The Law of Contract

Contracts may be either expressed or implied in law, and they may be either in written or oral form. Implied oral contracts are generally just as valid and enforceable as expressed written agreements. The difference under law is that the existence of expressed written agreements is easier to prove.[4] Most often in medical practice and hospital care, the agreements between doctor and patient are neither written nor expressed. The interaction is typically oral in character and the patient may or may not articulate in detail the specific care desired. Arrival of a patient at a medical care facility usually implies that care is desired, and the expectation is that a physician will provide medical expertise for the patient. Thus, a contractual relationship may begin entirely by implied agreement without any words ever spoken— as with the arrival of an unconscious patient to the emergency department. Mere existence of a facility that accepts patients for emergency medical admission impliedly states to the public that appropriate medical care will be provided.[5] The act of a patient's arrival (by whatever means) implies a willingness to accept diagnostic intervention and appropriate medical treatment unless the patient states otherwise. The law presumes that any reasonable person would enter into such a contractual agreement for the purpose of protecting life and health.[6] Hence, the valid initiation of the physician-patient relationship.

Under law, contractual arrangements are voluntary and undertaken in mutual consent. Because it is voluntary, physicians are not forced to care for patients with whom they do not wish to become involved.[7] The purpose for recognizing contracts under law is to provide individual parties with a framework for conducting their private arrangements in advance, and for enforcement of the agreement upon which each party has come to rely.[8] The formal elements of a contract include an offer by one party to provide goods or services, and acceptance of the offer by the other party. Something of value must be exchanged from one to the other (valuable consideration).[9] In the case of medical services, the physician offers to provide (valuable) medical care services to the patient, and the patient agrees to cooperate with the physician and to pay for medical services. It does not matter whether the patient or the physician initiates the offer.[10]

Solicitation. It has long been considered improper for physicians to solicit patients, but solicitation is an ethical impropriety, not a legal one. Contractual arrangements are binding regardless of which party initiated the offer. However, an offer by one party must be accepted by the other to effect an agreement. Thereafter, it is the responsibility of each contracting party to fulfill the terms of the agreement.[11] If either party is dissatisfied, contract law allows that a lawsuit may be initiated by the aggrieved party to compensate for damages suffered as a result of unfulfilled obligations. The award to the aggrieved is limited to the reasonable expecta-

tions of the parties under the actual terms of the contract.[12] However, solicitation of patients may be used as evidence that certain expectations of the patient were not unreasonable.

Guarantee of outcome. Physicians should never promise a satisfactory result when caring for patients. Because of individual biological variations, such warranties cannot be assured. In the view of law, such promises may constitute breach of contract if the outcome is worse than predicted.[13] A famous case in American contract law, *Hawkins v McGee*, illustrates this point.[14] Dr. Hawkins, a surgeon, offered to operate on McGee's deformed hand and promised to make it "perfect." The patient was excited at the prospect of having a normal functioning hand and readily agreed to the procedure. Surgery was performed carefully according to standards of medical care for the time, but the result was not as successful as Dr. Hawkins and the patient had hoped. Both parties agreed that the hand was worse after the operation than before. McGee sought redress in a lawsuit against Dr. Hawkins for violation of their agreement. Although it was agreed that Dr. Hawkins had not committed malpractice, the patient noted that he had been solicited by Dr. Hawkins as a patient, and contended that it was Dr. Hawkins' promise to make the hand "perfect" that convinced him to undergo the operation. In ruling for patient McGee in this breach of contract dispute, the court found that Dr. Hawkins had guaranteed a perfect result. It decreed that the amount of money awarded for damages should reflect the extent of postoperative functional impairment compared to a normal hand, rather than comparing the postoperative deformity to that which was present when Dr. Hawkins undertook treatment. The court reasoned that McGee had contracted for a normal hand, not just good medical care. The rule that emerges from this case is clear: never promise more than can reasonably be delivered. There should be no expectation of a certain outcome of diagnosis or treatment in medical practice. To promise more than careful and skillful medical care is to open oneself to unnecessary and probably uninsurable liability.

Termination of the Physician-Patient Relationship

Contracting parties are normally considered as equals in their ability to deal with the other. However, the law recognizes that one participant may be more powerful or knowledgeable and the other party inherently more vulnerable and dependent.[15]

This is the case in the typical physician-patient relationship. The physician is presumed to be in a stronger position than the patient because of extensive training and medical knowledge; the patient is presumed to be weaker and more vulnerable because of illness and lack of medical knowledge. This inequality is most noticeable when dissolution of the physician-patient relationship is undertaken.[16]

Whereas either party may initiate the physician-patient relationship, only the patient may terminate the relationship at will—without notice and without incurring further responsibility.[17] The patient may simply decide to ignore further payments and/or appointments; however unpaid medical bills and broken appointments do not constitute notification that the patient wishes to terminate the doctor-patient relationship. As long as the patient reasonably expects the physician to provide medical services, the physician remains obligated to do so.[18] Of course, the physician's responsibility to provide care extends only to that area of medicine in which the physician claims to be proficient.[19] For example, if the physician is an internist, the patient may not reasonably expect surgical services or opinions. However, it is reasonable for the patient to expect referral to a qualified specialist. In other words, no matter how noncompliant a patient may be, the physician-patient relationship (contract) remains intact. By virtue of the patient's more vulnerable position relative to the professional, such behavior may be reasonable under law. The physician is expected to be available to the patient until such time as the physician-patient relationship is actually terminated.[20]

Written notification from a patient would terminate the relationship under any circumstances, but the physician is not at liberty to terminate the relationship unilaterally.[21] The needs of the patient take precedence over the doctor's need and desires. The relationship is properly terminated by the physician only if the patient no longer needs the kind of care the physician is able to provide, or if the withdrawing physician is replaced by an equally qualified physician. Withdrawal from care under any other circumstance constitutes abandonment.[22] If the physician wishes to terminate the relationship and avoid patient claims of wrongful abandonment, the patient must be given: (1) written notice, (2) adequate time to seek other medical care providers, and ideally (3) referral to another equally qualified practitioner of the same medical specialty.[23] Identification of another physician who is equally qualified and who agrees to take over the care of a properly notified patient fulfills all responsibilities of the withdrawing physician and protects against any claim of abandonment by the patient.[24]

CIVIL VERSUS CRIMINAL LAW

Legal guidelines for medical practice fall under the broad category of civil law. Civil law is often confused with criminal law, but important differences exist between the two. Civil law traditionally consists of the law of contract (discussed above), the law of property, and tort law (the law of negligence and product liability).

Under criminal law, the government acts on behalf of the citizenry (prosecutor) to bring actions against an individual defendant charged with violating a specific statute that defines the alleged crime and sets guidelines for penalties. The purposes of criminal law are: (1) to punish the wrongdoer for intentional or reckless behavior that society usually (through the legislature) finds unacceptable and (2) to deter criminal behavior by the defendant or other individuals in the future. The defendant, if convicted, is punished with monetary fines, loss of liberty (incarceration), or both. Monetary fines are received by the government. Traditionally the victim of criminal behavior has received no compensation.

Under civil law, the victim initiates a lawsuit as the plaintiff and states a claim for losses suffered because of an alleged wrongdoing (breach of contract, for example). The defendant in a civil action may be an individual, a group of individuals, a corporation, or a governmental body. The plaintiff seeks compensation for losses (damages or injury), rather than a determination that the defendant acted unlawfully and thus suffer some punishment at the hands of the state.

Monetary compensation under civil law is received by the plaintiff in an attempt to "make the victim whole again."[25] In a breach of contract decision for the plaintiff, the victim of the broken agreement is entitled to compensation equal to the benefit that the unbroken contract would have yielded. Punitive damages may be added to the plaintiff's award to punish the civil wrongdoer for intentional improper behavior. Most wrongdoing under civil law is accounted unintentional, whereas criminal behavior is usually intentional. Although deterrence is not a primary function of civil law, large damage awards often dramatically alter the behavior of others who are in a position similar to that of a losing defendant.

TORT LAW AND MEDICAL MALPRACTICE

Most lawsuits in the medical care setting are civil suits filed under tort law. Tort is French for "wrong"; in Latin it means "twisted." Tort law covers both unintentional wrongdoing (negligence and product liability) and some intentionally wrong behaviors that are also addressed under criminal law.[26]

Intentional Tort Wrongs

The perpetrator of an assault and battery could be prosecuted and convicted by the state under criminal statutes. In addition to pressing charges and cooperating with the public prosecutor in the criminal proceeding, the victim of the assault and battery could file a civil claim arising from the same incident against the same defendant for damages to be compensated under tort law. The likelihood of prevailing in the tort case would be greater than in the criminal case because of a lower standard of proof required in civil cases. Because civil law provides monetary compensation rather than loss of liberty (incarceration), proof of the defendant's liability requires only a "preponderance of the evidence" (greater than 51% likelihood that the claim is factually true).[27] Criminal law requires that the defendant be found guilty of the charges on the evidence "beyond a reasonable doubt."[28] Therefore, a defendant might escape conviction and punishment for assault in a criminal proceeding, but the same evidence may lead to the finding of civil liability in a tort action under civil law.

For intentional tort interference such as assault and battery, actual injury need not be shown for the plaintiff to win the lawsuit. It is only necessary to prove that the defendant intentionally acted in an unauthorized manner. Compensatory damages will be limited if harm is not proven, but commission of the act itself may lead to a judgment against the defendant, and in egregious cases punitive damages may be awarded. In this regard, intentional tort law is similar to criminal law. Although the standard of proof is easier to meet in the civil action, punishment for having committed the act is intended both to make a social policy statement against the behavior and to deter further similar behavior. Punitive dam-

ages however would be awarded to the victim of the civil (intentional) wrong rather than to the state.

Unintentional Tort Wrongs: Negligence

Most cases of medical malpractice are directed against unintentional, but careless, unreasonable behavior that directly and proximately results in harm to a victim. Punitive damages are not allowed under the legal theory of negligence even though injury is proven, because the purpose of monetary awards is to compensate the victim rather than to punish the negligent wrongdoer. Although announcement of awards for compensatory damages often influence future behavior, deterrence is not a specific purpose of damage awards for negligent behavior. Under unintentional tort law (negligence), the fact of negligent action is not enough to justify compensation for damages that may have occurred. Damages claimed by a plaintiff must be shown to actually have been caused by the negligent behavior. The plaintiff must not only prove that negligent medical care occurred, but must also prove that negligent medical behavior resulted in the injuries that are claimed.

The Four-Part Test for Negligence

Proof of negligence requires that each of the four separate components of the test for negligence be proven by a preponderance of the evidence. The four components of the test for negligence are (1) injury (2) caused by (3) breach of a (4) duty. If any one of these four parts is less than 51% likely to be true as determined by the judge or jury, the plaintiff cannot succeed in a negligence claim.[29]

Injury. There must be actual injury to the plaintiff and/or his family. It is compensation expressed in terms of a money award for damages suffered that is the object of every malpractice suit. Compensation may be expressed in terms of "special damages" to pay for money losses suffered as a result of injury—such as actual expenses incurred and lost income.[30] Additionally, nonmonetary losses incurred such as pain and suffering, mental anguish, scarring, and deformity may be sought under the designation of "general damages."[31] The loss or injury must be measurable by some criterion for conversion into a monetary award that the plaintiff seeks to be "made whole again." If the injuries claimed do not add up to be a significant award for damages that may be recovered, it is unlikely that a medical negligence lawsuit will be worth the significant investment in time and expenses to satisfy most plaintiff's attorneys threshold interest in pursuing the lawsuit.

Causation. Negligence cases require the plaintiff prove that the defendant's negligent conduct actually caused the plaintiff's injuries. Causation is a complex legal and philosophical concept. It is not enough that the tortious conduct preceded the victim's injury. The claimed unreasonable behavior on the part of the defendant must be shown to have directly and proximately resulted in the claimed injury to the plaintiff. Causation is often difficult to prove in a given medical malpractice case, and it will predictably be hotly contested when the other elements of the case are not in dispute: where injury is severe (such as when death occurs), and the breach of duty is not contested; or where no one responded to a patient's alarm to the nurses' station. Thus causation may be the only real issue in a negligence claim. For example, if autopsy reveals that the patient suffered a massive saddle embolus to the pulmonary outflow tract of the right ventricle, then the defendant in a negligence lawsuit would likely argue that despite the lack of medical intervention, there was no good medical therapy that any responding medical personnel could have employed. The absence of a response to the patient's alarm did not cause the patient to suffer a bad outcome, because even if a complete resuscitation had been undertaken, massive pulmonary embolism is almost uniformly fatal. Under these circumstances, the patient's poor outcome could not be said to be a direct and proximate result of the failure of medical expertise to respond at the patient's bedside.

Breach of duty. In the medical care setting, duty is not usually hard to prove. If a physician-patient relationship exists, responsibility for the doctor to provide medical expertise in a manner similar to any ordinary prudent physician under the same or similar circumstances is expected.[32] This concept is in keeping with the "reasonable man" standard that applies to negligence cases in general. The standard for expected behavior in any situation is defined as conduct that any "reasonably prudent" individual might pursue in the same or similar situation. Formulation of hypothetical scenarios assists in determining which of various possible responses to an analogous situation of fact are reasonable. For ordinary behavior that can easily be understood by the lay public, a jury determines reasonableness from the facts presented by drawing on their own individual life experiences.[33]

In the medical care setting, however, a judge or jury is not likely to understand the complex medical and scientific factors that are involved in physician behavior during delivery of medical care. Therefore, the law provides for experts to educate the factfinder in the relevant issues that may be involved. These experts actually become witnesses and present evidence for consideration by the factfinder.[34] One might contend that the best way for the factfinder to become educated in medical cases would be to find a neutral expert to advise them in the matters at issue. However, the adversarial nature of American law does not require the court to seek outside neutral advice on their own. The conduct and outcome of a lawsuit is entirely dependent on hearing both the claims made by the plaintiff in the pleadings and the response formulated by the defense. Each side in the controversy is expected to find its own experts who will testify on its behalf, and the experts are likely to disagree with the testimony of the other. It is the job of the jury to hear both sides and determine which version of facts to believe.

Expert witnesses are different from the usual "fact witnesses" in a legal proceeding. Testimony of fact witnesses is limited to events that were actually seen, heard, or otherwise perceived through the senses to be true. Expressions of opinion as to what might have happened or what would have been proper behavior are not permitted.[35] Expert witnesses, in contrast, may testify to facts in the medical record even though they were neither present at the time nor participated in the patient's care. Expert witnesses may express opinions about particular fact situations.[36]

In allowing experts to give opinions, courts are asking for assistance in understanding complicated issues of medical care. In fact, courts request opinions from expert medical witnesses to educate the court regarding: (1) the prevailing standards of care applicable to the specific medical specialty in question (duty), (2) whether or not there was breach of duty, and (3) whether or not negligent behavior actually caused the injuries claimed. Opinions of expert witnesses are also occasionally sought to determine whether or not an injury actually exists. When injuries are readily apparent even to lay persons, expert opinion is often needed to evaluate the extent and limitation of the injury. Nonmedical statisticians and actuaries may be called upon for expert opinions regarding the amount of monetary compensation required to restore the quality of life that existed before the negligent activity (make the plaintiff whole again). Both plaintiff and defendant attempt to persuade the factfinder that its own expert witness is more credible than the other. Inability to enlist expert testimony could result in failure of the case because of lack of merit if the opposing side has uncontested expert testimony in its behalf. Thus opinions by witnesses are powerful instruments in law. For this reason, ordinary fact witnesses are prohibited from rendering opinions.[37]

Failure to provide care that meets minimum professional standards is the legal definition of the term negligence.[38] Failure to give an appropriate level of care occurs frequently in complicated activity such as the practice of medicine. Negligence is committed by good physicians who are practicing high quality medical care, and everyone who practices medicine (or any other profession) is negligent at one time or another. Fortunately, most acts of negligence do not cause harm, because they are either insignificant or are discovered before injury occurs.

The law of negligence reflects this reality. For legal liability to result from negligence, it must be shown that the injury was directly and proximately caused by negligent acts. Thus, the preponderance of evidence must indicate that injury was caused by breach of physician duty to establish legal responsibility and liability for negligent behavior.[39]

SPECIAL PERIOPERATIVE PROBLEMS
Emergency Versus Elective Care

Many perioperative problems require urgent management. Appropriate perioperative evaluation and management for elective repair of an aneurysm of the abominal aorta may not be appropriate for emergency repair of a leaking abdominal aortic aneurysm. Management of elective versus emergency cases would be appropriately different in the hands of the same internist, anesthesiologist, or surgeon. Therefore, legal review of medical care properly begins with questions such as "What was the patient's condition? What was the diagnosis? Was the medical setting an emergent one?" Many legal considerations are resolved with the answers to these questions. The professional standards of care (what a reasonably prudent qualified physician would do in the same or similar circumstances) regarding the amount of information that should be gathered to confirm a diagnosis, the quality of disclosure of information to the patient, and even the technical aspects of a surgical procedure may be less stringent in an emergency than in an elective situation.

Consent to Treatment

A major requirement of the physician-patient relationship is that physicians respect the right of each patient to safeguard the integrity of his or her own body. Self-determination is a basic societal concept that has been recognized in American law for many years. In 1891, the United States Supreme Court commented[40]:

No right is held more sacred or is more carefully guarded by the common law than the right of every individual to the possession and control of his own person, free from all restraints of interference by others, unless by clear and unquestionable authority of law.

In the absence of an emergency, consent of a patient is required to undertake any diagnostic or therapeutic endeavor. The legal foundation for this requirement derives from the law of battery. While court decisions as early as 1905 assert this theory,[41] the most eloquent statement of the principle was expressed by Justice Benjamin Cardozo in what has since become a maxim[42]:

Every human being of adult years and sound mind has the right to determine what shall be done with his own body; and a surgeon who performs an operation without his patient's consent commits an assault for which he is liable in damages . . .

As originally applied in the 1914 decision of Schoendorff *v* New York Hospital, patient consent required agreement between the physician and patient regarding the proposed treatment plan. A Mrs. Schoendorff had consented to an examination under anesthesia, but specifically withheld consent to an invasive surgical operation. When she awoke, she discovered that a tumor had been excised from her abdomen, (and she suffered additional injury to an unrelated part of her body). A patient's refusal of therapy is grounds for an intentional tort action if such therapy is given despite the patient's objections. Unauthorized nonemergency care (even when it benefits the patient) may be grounds for intentional tort liability under the claim of battery. If a patient has not specifically consented to a surgical procedure on a particular body part, proceeding with surgery may be judged to constitute an intentional unauthorized contact.[43] However, an individual who consents to bodily contact by another cannot later claim battery. Valid consent of the person touched is a complete defense against a claim of battery [44] even though the touching may have caused harm.

Even when consent is obtained, a negligence action can be claimed based on "negligent nondisclosure." The claim of negligent nondisclosure asserts that insufficient information was provided by the physician to properly inform the patient about the risks of and alternatives to a medical treatment that would otherwise have been refused.[45] The patient contends that the physician's duty to inform about the treatment was unfulfilled. Rather than claiming that the care itself was negligent, the patient contends that given better quality information, he would likely have refused to consent. As with any negligence claim, the plaintiff must prove actual injuries as a direct result of the medical intervention. However, under a negligent nondisclosure theory, the injuries need only be expected complications that the patient could have avoided with enough knowledge to have refused the procedure.

The amount of information required for a patient to make a fully informed choice may be viewed from either the perspective of the physician or of the patient.

Most jurisdictions require the plaintiff to establish by expert testimony that the prevailing professional practice standard for information disclosure was not met.[46] Other states have adopted a "reasonable patient" standard. This standard states that the information disclosed must be of a nature and quantity that would allow the ordinary "reasonable patient" to make an intelligent and informed decision. Thus, although expert medical witnesses are necessary to provide information regarding risks, outcome, complications, and alternative treatments, the amount and kind of information necessary to meet the "reasonable patient" standard is determined by a judge or lay jury, rather than by expert testimony. One frequently cited case declares that even serious complications that occur with only a 1% incidence must be disclosed for patient consideration for the consent to be truly informed.[47]

A few states have even gone beyond the patient-based disclosure standard and require the judge or jury to determine what information the individual patient-plaintiff in the medical malpractice case should have been told to make a properly informed decision. This subjective disclosure standard is extremely difficult for physicians to meet. Clearly, the intent of subjective patient disclosure standards is to put the plaintiff-patient in a more equal position with the medical specialist who is perceived as being too powerful and controlling. Fortunately, it has been embraced in only a few jurisdictions.

Consent for ordinary versus extraordinary medical care. The informed consent doctrine applies equally to non-invasive (conservative) and invasive medical care, and all patients must consent to any treatment.[48] Consent may be oral, written, expressed, or implied. For routine noninvasive care, the law assumes that the patient would discontinue medical care if the risks, benefits, and alternatives were not understood. Consent in these circumstances is oral and often implied. It is assumed that the physician informs and educates the patient through normal communication, explanation, and answering of questions. The ideal physician-patient relationship discloses important information routinely as part of everyday care. In contrast, invasive or extraordinary care requires expressed and documented consent.[49] Unfortunately, the process of obtaining written informed consent is often viewed as a procedural ritual than a conscientious effort to educate the patient to the risks and benefits of the medical intervention. Care must be taken to provide appropriate information.

Surgical consent forms versus a note in the chart. Written consent for medical treatment can be documented in a special consent form or in a specific note in the medical record. Both methods are meaningful and legally acceptable if they are undertaken with sincerity. Most hospitals use a standard preprinted form, but the information on many of these forms is overly broad and not specific to the individual patient. Most forms have a significant amount of fine print, and the print size becomes smaller as the form becomes more detailed. The patient's signature on a consent form indicates that the information has been read, and that the risks and alternatives of the procedure have been explained to the patient's satisfaction.

A written note in the medical record is another method to document informed consent. The physician first speaks with the patient about the proposed procedure, risks, and alternatives. After a detailed explanation that is satisfactory to the patient, the physician writes a note in the medical record to document that such a discussion took place. The physician may then ask the patient to countersign the note to verify that consent was given, that it was informative, and that the patient took part in the decision. Although this procedure is time consuming, it overcomes the broad inclusive nature of standardized forms, eliminates the fine print, and provides evidence that informed consent appropriate to the individual patient was obtained.

Consent for procedures that are not surgical. The law does not require written consent for many invasive procedures such as central venous and arterial cannulations, and the decision whether or not to obtain specific consent depends on the desires of the individual physician or requirements of the hospital. However, any therapy or procedure that is outside the ordinary realm of medical care because of invasiveness, the need for patient cooperation, or significant risk of complication should be thoroughly explained to the patient. Experimental therapies and research protocols should be similarly explained. Documentation in the patient's chart that consent was obtained after satisfactory explanation of the risk, benefits, and alternatives is advised.

Withdrawal of consent by the patient. The presence of a written express consent is not irretrievably binding, and a change of decision must be respected by the medical staff. Withdrawal of consent, whether oral, written, expressed, or implied, invalidates the previous decision by the patient. The patient's autonomy to give consent in the first place is retained when that decision is altered; signing a piece of paper does not revoke the ability to exercise free choice.

Consent obtained after premedication. Obtaining consent for elective surgical procedures after the patient has been treated with sedative, hypnotic, or tranquilizing premedicants is incompatible with free choice and autonomy. The purpose of such drugs is to sedate the patient and to relieve anxiety; it is well known that these drugs interfere with cognitive processes. Proceeding with elective surgical procedures under such "tainted" consent cannot be justified if delay of operation until mental status returns to normal will not interfere with the patient's underlying condition. For the same reason, postponement of elective surgery is also indicated if consent is withdrawn by the patient regardless of whether or not premedication was given.

Consent for emergency treatment. As a general rule, the law finds implied consent in situations of emergency where the patient is unable to express themselves and there is no one who is authorized to

speak on the patient's behalf.[50] Conditions that require immediate medical treatment for the protection of the life or health have been held to justify the implication of consent because it is generally assumed that a competent, reasonable adult under similar circumstances would consent to the necessary treatment (if it were at all possible) to maintain life and health.[51]

The general rule of implied consent for emergency treatment applies to the treatment of minors as well as adults.[52] The same principle applies when the minor's parents or legal guardian is unavailable to consent when emergency treatment is necessary to prevent serious harm to life or health—for example, a reasonably prudent parent or guardian would consent under similar circumstances, therefore consent is implied. Documentation of attempts to contact the minor patient's parents/guardian is always advised.

Incompetent patients and consent. Adults are presumed to be competent to consent to proposed medical treatment unless they are shown to be otherwise. An adult patient who is incapacitated by mental or physical illness such that they are unable to understand the nature and consequences of proposed medical treatment is unable to give a valid informed consent. In such instances, consent must be obtained from someone who is authorized to speak on the patient's behalf.[53] If a court has determined that a patient is incompetent to give consent for medical treatment, then it likely will have appointed a guardian or conservator to act on the patient's behalf. However, many times the physician will determine that the patient lacks capacity to understand and consider medical treatment choices. In these circumstances, it is acceptable to solicit consent from the patient's next of kin unless the patient or relative cannot agree with the physician or with each other. In the absence of an emergency, disagreements over consent for nonessential medical care should be adjudicated by a court.

Patients with do not resuscitate orders. Patients with do not resuscitate (DNR) orders are almost always terminally ill. A decision not to resuscitate a dying patient who has suffered a cardiopulmonary arrest is viewed more favorably than a decision to withhold or withdraw other forms of medical care. Open discussion of this issue has lead many hospitals to develop formal policies to govern DNR orders. These policies address issues of patient competency and suggest methods for applying the principle of substituted judgement that are consistent with ethical principles of autonomy and beneficence.[54] Criteria to guide DNR decisions in individual patients and procedural frameworks to effect these decisions are also provided in most formal DNR policies.

Unfortunately, much confusion is still generated by DNR orders. Surveys at both primary and referral hospitals indicate that DNR orders are interpreted variably and with uncertainty,[55] especially in situations where physicians are cross-covering for one another while the physician responsible for writing the DNR order is not available.[56]

For the majority of DNR patients, operative care is not warranted. Emergency procedures of almost any kind are not considered because of DNR status. Occasionally, elective surgical procedures are warranted for palliative care to improve efficiency of nursing care or to relieve pain. Perioperative care of these patients is often controversial.

Iatrogenic complications of palliative care such as cardiac or pulmonary complications from anesthesia or surgery are not the natural consequences of underlying disease, and practitioners must define the level of support that is appropriate for perioperative care of DNR patients. Preoperative discussion with the patient or surrogate is necessary to establish limitations of therapy for the perioperative period. A patient's desire not to be resuscitated in order not to prolong the dying process does not translate into a wish to receive no therapy for an easily reversible iatrogenic process that is associated with a palliative intervention.[57]

Jehovah's Witnesses and other religious limitations. Just as it has been clearly established at common law that every adult patient of sound mind has the right of self-determination in medical matters, it is a constitutionally guaranteed right that "Congress shall make no law respecting an establishment of religion, or prohibiting the free exercise thereof . . . "[58] This means that all adult citizens are free to practice their own religious beliefs so long as they do not infringe on the rights of others, and that neither laws nor persons are entitled to force religious beliefs on unwilling participants. Therefore, religious beliefs of patients that impose limitations of medical care are to be respected by physicians in the same manner as patient decisions to withhold consent for medical intervention on nonreligious grounds. Whether or not the physician may

agree with a religiously motivated withholding of consent for certain kinds of medical treatment, it is clear that patients such as Jehovah's Witness believers or Christian Scientists have the legal right to refuse overall treatment, or any part of medical treatment that they choose.

There is quite a lot of case law on the issue of blood transfusion refusal by Jehovah's Witness patients. Even when administration of blood would be lifesaving, the competent adult patient's decision to forego transfusion on religious principle is accepted as long as preservation of the individual patient's life is the only issue. Courts have usually recognized individual autonomy as superior to all other interests. However, where innocent third parties may be adversely affected—such as minor children at home who are dependent on the patient for support, courts have intervened to force blood transfusions for the parent on the theory that the state has an interest in protecting the dependent children from abandonment.[59]

Where the patient is a minor, intervention by judicial action is assured. The juvenile courts will not allow a parent to refuse consent for necessary treatment of a minor child: "Parents may be free to become martyrs themselves, but it does not follow they are free in identical circumstances to make martyrs of their children."[60] Therefore, when the patient is a minor child and the parents refuse to consent to blood transfusion that is deemed necessary for survival of the child, the hospital legal department should be notified to seek court intervention. If the circumstances are emergent and the child's immediate health/life are threatened, the physician may administer blood to the child over the parent's objection. It is highly unlikely that court approval will be denied in the setting of a true emergency.

If the patient is an adult and presents as a life-threatening emergency whose status as a Jehovah's Witness practitioner is not evident to the treating physician—that is, the patient is incapable of refusing blood transfusion by reason of his medical condition—then the principle of implied consent for emergency treatment, in general, applies. Lacking the patient's informed refusal of blood products, the physician may proceed to treat the patient as an emergency victim who could otherwise be assumed to desire life-saving therapy. However, if the patient is known to the physician or hospital to be a practicing Jehovah's Witness who refuses blood product therapy, then even life-threatening illness in need of emergency treatment cannot be assumed to override the patient's refusal.

CONSULTATION AND REFERRAL

While a patient is under the care of a physician, the need occasionally arises to involve other practitioners in evaluation and treatment of a medical condition. The terms consultation and referral are often used interchangeably by both physicians and lay people to express two different concepts in shared patient care. Consultation is distinguished from referral by identification of the individual responsible for continued care of the patient.[61]

Consultation is a request for both opinion regarding patient status, and recommendation for approaches to therapy. The opinion and recommendation of the consulting specialist may be used or rejected by the physician who requested consultation. Patient care remains the sole responsibility of the primary physician.[62] In contrast, referral implies that one practitioner requests that another take over management of a particular aspect of a patient's care. After acceptance of referral, both physicians may be accountable for the care of the patient.

The concept of shared responsibility is important in the perioperative setting. When more than one physician provides care to a patient, each has a duty to exercise reasonable skill and diligence on the patient's behalf. If negligent activity of two or more doctors results in a single, inseparable result, all physicians that are involved may be liable to the injured patient for damages. In law this concept is known as joint and several liability. The successful plaintiff can collect part of a judgement from each, or the entire sum may be collected from any one physician who has the assets (or insurance) to pay. It is the responsibility of the codefendant doctors who are jointly and severally liable to work out final accounting as to what proportion of proven damages each is responsible for. While shared responsibility for patient care is complicated by the legal doctrine of joint and several liability, appropriate referral of patients should not be avoided. Failure of a physician to refer a patient to a specialist implies expertise in all areas of medical care.[63]

SUMMARY

Some of the important legal principles involved in the practice of medicine in general and the peri-operative period in particular have been presented. Most of these principles address the unique respect for individual autonomy and self-determination that characterize English common law and American democractic institutions. The physician-patient relationship is a reflection of these deep-seated values and the cornerstone for understanding physician responsibilities and patient expectations. Generally, in American Law, the professional participant in this relationship is held to be in a stronger position by virtue of extensive training and knowledge than the inherently vulnerable and dependent patient who seeks to benefit from the physician's skill and expertise. This inequality is addressed in law and is expressed as increased requirement for professional behavior in areas such as informed consent, standards of care, and termination of the physician-patient relationship. A more thorough understanding of these fundamental concepts should help physicians to be less fearful of the liability that arises from modern medical practice, and the perioperative period in particular.

REFERENCES

1. *Kennedy v. Parrot*, 243 N.C. 355, 90 S.E. 2d 754 (1956).
2. *Price v. Neyland*, 320 F2d 674 (D.C. Cir. 1963).
3. 1.7 ALR 4th, 132.
4. Farnsworth EA, Contracts— § 6.12, Boston, 1982, Little, Brown and Co.
5. *Wilmington General Hospital v Manlove*, 54 Del. 15, 1974 A.2d 135 (1961).
6. 61 Am. Jur. 2D Physicians and Surgeons S 159 (1972).
7. *Childs v. Weis*, 440 S.W. 2d 104 (Tex. 1969).
8. *Osborne v. Frazor*, 425 S.W. 2d 768 (Tenn. 1968).
9. *Farnsworth, supra* §§ 2.3 and 3.3.
10. *Hoover v. Williams*, 203 A.2d 861 (1964).
11. *Hankerson v. Thomas*, 148 A2d 583 (D.C. 1959).
12. *Farnsworth, supra* § 12.8.
13. *Guilmet v. Campbell*, 188 N.W. 2d 601 (1971).
14. *Hawkins v. McGee*, cite
15. *Farnsworth, supra* § 4.20.
16. 99-ALR 3d 303.
17. Annas GJ, *The Rights of Hospital Patients*, New York, 1975, Avon Books.
18. *Rule v. Cheeseman*, 317 p.2d 472 (Kan. 1957).
19. *Brandl v. Grubin*, 329 A2d 82 (1972).
20. Annas GJ, *Id*.
21. Annas GJ, *Id*.
22. *Stohlman v. Dans*, 220 N.W. 247 (Neb. 1928).
23. Annas GJ, *Your Money or Your Life: "Dumping"*

Uninsured Patients from Hospital Emergency Wards,
76 AM. J. PUB. HEALTH 74, 1986.

24. *Sibert v. Boger,* 260 S.W. 2d 569 (Mo. 1953).

25. Prosser and Keeton, The Law of Torts, 5th Ed., Chapter 1 § 1, 1984, St. Paul, Minn, West Publishing Co.

26. Prosser and Keeton, *Id.* Chapter 1, § 2.

27. Cleary EW, *McCormick on Evidence,* 3rd Ed., Chapter 36, § 339, St. Paul, Minn, 1984, West Publishing Co.

28. *Id.* at 341.

29. *Prosser and Keeton, supra* at Chapter 5, § 30.

30. *Myers v. Stephens,* 43 Cal. Rptr. 420.

31. *Twin Coach Co. v. Chance Vought Aircraft,* Inc, 163 A2d 278 (1961).

32. *Price v. Neyland,* 320 F2d 674 (D.C. Cir. 1963).

33. *McCormick on Evidence, Supra* at Chapter 36, § 339.

34. Federal Rules of Evidence for United States Court and Magistrates Article VII, Rule 702 (1987).

35. *Id.,* Rule 701.

36. *Id.,* Rules 702, 703, 704, 705.

37. *Id.,* Rule 701.

38. *Prosser and Keeton, supra* at Chapter 5, § 30.

39. *Id.*

40. *Union Pacific Railroad Co v. Botsford,* 141 U.S. 250 (1891).

41. *Pratt v. Davis,* 118 Ill App 161 (1905), aff'd 224 Ill. 300 (1906).

42. *Schoendorff v. Society of New York Hospital,* 211 N.Y. 125 (1914).

43. *Mohr v. Williams,* 95 Minn 261 (1905).

44. *Prosser and Keeton, supra* at Chapter 4, § 18.

45. *Salgo v. Leland Stanford, Jr.,* University Board of Trustees 154 Cal App 2d 560 (1957).

46. *Aiken v. Clarey,* 396 S.W. 2d 668 (Mo. 1965).

47. *Canterbury v. Spence,* 464 F. 2d 772 (D.C. Cir. 1972).

48. *Nathanson v. Kline,* 186 Kan. 393 (1960).

49. American Medical Association Medicolegal Forms (1976).

50. *Dunham v. Wright,* 423 F 2d 940 (1970).

51. *Pratt v. Davis,* 224 Ill. 300 (1906).

52. *Sullivan v. Montgomery,* 17 N.E. 2d 446 (1935).

53. *Lester v. Aetna Casualty and Surety Co,* 240, F 2d. 676(1957).

54. President's Commission for the Study of Ethical Problems in Medicine and Biomedical and Behavioral Research: Appendix I: Orders Against Resuscitation: Selected Policy Statements in Deciding to Forego Life-Sustaining Treatment. Government Printing Office, 1983, pp 493–545.

55. Levy M.R., Lambe M>E>, Shear CL, *Do-Not-Resuscitate orders in a county hospital,* 140 WEST J. MED. 111 (1984).

56. Evans AL and Brody BA *The Do-Not-Resuscitate Order in Teaching Hospitals,* 253 JAMA 2236, (April, 1985).

57. Bedel SE and Delbanco TL, *Choices about cardiopulmonary resuscitation in the hospital: When do physicians talk with patients?* 310 NEW ENGL. J. MED. 1089 (1984).

58. U. S. Constitution, 1st Amendment (1791).

59. Application of the President and Directors of Georgetown College, Inc., 331 F 2d 1000 (1964).

60. *Prince v Commonwealth of Massachusetts,* 321 U.S. 158 (1944).

61. Higdon JH, *Medical/Legal Status of Consultants* J. LEGAL MED. 35 (1976).

62. Holder A: *Duty to Consult* 225 JAMA 125 (1974).

63. *Id.*

PART TWO

MANAGEMENT OF PATIENTS DURING SURGERY

CHAPTER 7

Monitoring Modalities

WILLIAM T. MERRITT

The production of unconsciousness in itself, has, and always will have, an element of danger to it.

SO GOLDMAN, 1901.[29]

Risks associated with anesthetic practice have been acknowledged since the introduction of anesthetic agents in the 1840s.[12] Recognizing this, a number of studies have attempted to identify and quantify these risks, but the lack of uniformity of design and definition makes it difficult to recommend definitive strategies to improve the safety of anesthetic delivery.* Somewhat surprisingly, objective physiologic monitoring to detect deviations from baseline function and presumably improve patient safety perioperatively has only recently been incorporated into routine use. Although some anesthesiologists began to measure and record pulse and blood pressure during surgical procedures at the turn of the century, in most hospitals intraoperative monitoring for the first

*References 5, 19, 31, 36, 53.

100 years of anesthesia involved little more than assessing the depth of anesthesia by observing patterns of respiration, muscle tone, pupillary changes, movement, and skin color. Physiologic variables could not be manipulated because they were not measured. These limitations contributed to relatively unsafe practice when judged by today's standards. It is not surprising that a British judge could state in 1953: "It is a fact that to anaesthetise a human being, to deprive him of consciousness outright, is to take a considerable step along the road to killing him."[34]

Risk prevention in anesthetic practice has focused upon the detection and elimination of preventable untoward events. There is however, no universally accepted definition of "preventable mishap." Moreover, there is considerable controversy over the modalities of physiologic monitoring that are appropriate for intraoperative use. A discussion of monitoring at the International Symposium on Preventable Anesthetic Morbidity and Mortality in 1984 was summarized[37]:

The workshop on monitoring during anesthesia generated heated discussions, and in no other area were the differences between national practice patterns more in evidence. Clearly, the availability of a plethora of monitoring devices and the malpractice climate in the United States have created pressures for their use. Anesthesiologists in the United States have yielded to these pressures. An attempt to list monitors in terms of their importance to optimal anesthesia care elicited little agreement, primarily because their contribution to care never has been measured. The need for such study was apparent, since any contribution must be weighed against potential downside risks of decreased vigilance, equipment failure, and erroneous information. A clearly expressed concern, and here was ready consensus, was the legal implications of establishing a standard of minimal acceptable monitoring during anesthesia, particularly in the absence of supporting data.

In spite of those difficulties, the Department of Anesthesiology at Harvard published its own monitoring standards in 1986,[22] and similar minimal standards were adopted by the American Society of Anesthesiologists (ASA) shortly thereafter[21] (see box below).

The primary emphases of these standards for basic monitoring are to ensure that (1) qualified personnel be physically present throughout all anesthetic care and (2) oxygenation, ventilation, circulation, and temperature be continually (repeated regularly and frequently) or continuously (without interruption) evaluated. The guidelines do not mention specific assessments of renal function, cardiovascular pump function, oxygen utilization, neuromuscular blockade, CNS function, anesthetic gas concentration, or appropriate laboratory support, despite their intuitively apparent usefulness.

This chapter covers the minimal standards adopted by the ASA, additional options beyond minimal monitoring, and newer monitoring modalities for specific purposes. All the monitoring modalities to be discussed are either already commonly used outside the operating room or they can be readily adapted for use during anesthesia.

PERIOPERATIVE MONITORING

Surgical procedures involving anesthesia are almost as varied as the patients on whom they are performed, and choices for intraoperative monitoring are varied accordingly. Table 7-1 presents an overview of common intraoperative clinical events with a list of potentially useful monitoring modalities that may be employed in addition to the basic recommended standards.

Intravascular Pressures

Intravascular pressures are measured routinely during anesthetic practice. Arterial pressure is mea-

---

American Society of Anesthesiologists
Standards for basic intra-operative monitoring

These standards apply to all anesthesia care although, in emergency circumstances, appropriate life support measures take precedence. These standards may be exceeded at any time based on the judgement of the responsible anesthesiologist. They are intended to encourage high quality patient care, but observing them cannot guarantee any specific patient outcome. They are subject to revision from time to time, as warranted by the evolution of technology and practice. This set of standards addresses only the issue of basic intra-operative monitoring, which is one component of anesthesia care. In certain rare or unusual circumstances, (1) some of these methods of monitoring may be clinically impractical, and (2) appropriate use of the described monitoring methods may fail to detect untoward clinical developments. Brief interruptions of continual† monitoring may be unavoidable. *Under extenuating circumstances, the responsible anesthesiologist may waive the requirements marked with an asterisk (*): it is recommended that when this is done, it should be so stated (including the reasons) in a note in the patient's medical record.* These standards are not intended for application to the care of the obstetrical patient in labor or in the conduct of pain management.

†Note the "continual" is defined as "repeated regularly and frequently in steady succession" whereas "continuous" means "prolonged without any interruption at any time."

Continued on next page.

Standard I

Qualified anesthesia personnel shall be present in the room throughout the conduct of all general anesthetics, regional anesthetics and monitored anesthesia care.

OBJECTIVE Because of the rapid changes in patient status during anesthesia, qualified anesthesia personnel shall be continuously present to monitor the patient and provide anesthesia care. In the event there is a direct known hazard, e.g., radiation, to the anesthesia personnel which might require intermittent remote observation of the patient, some provision for monitoring the patient must be made. In the event that an emergency requires the temporary absence of the person primarily responsible for the anesthetic, the best judgement of the anesthesiologist will be exercised in comparing the emergency with the anesthetized patient's condition and in the selection of the person left responsible for the anesthetic during the temporary absence.

Standard II

During all anesthetics, the patient's oxygenation, ventilation, circulation and temperature shall be continually evaluated.

Oxygenation

OBJECTIVE To ensure adequate oxygen concentration in the inspired gas and the blood during all anesthetics.

METHODS 1. Inspired gas: During every administration of general anesthesia using an anesthesia machine, the concentration of oxygen in the patient breathing system shall be measured by an oxygen analyzer with a low oxygen concentration limit alarm in use.*

2. Blood oxygenation: During all anesthetics, adequate illumination and exposure of the patient is necessary to assess color. While this and other qualitative clinical signs may be adequate, there are quantitative methods, such as pulse oximetry, which are encouraged.

Ventilation

OBJECTIVE To ensure adequate ventilation of the patient during all anesthetics.

METHODS 1. Every patient receiving general anesthesia shall have the adequacy of ventilation continually evaluated. While qualitative clinical signs such as chest excursion, observation of the reservoir breathing bag and auscultation of breath sounds may be adequate, quantitative monitoring of the CO_2 content and/or volume of expired gas is encouraged.

2. When an endotracheal tube is inserted, its correct positioning in the trachea must be verified. Clinical assessment is essential and end-tidal CO_2 analysis, in use from the time of endotracheal tube placement, is encouraged.

3. When ventilation is controlled by a mechanical ventilator, there shall be in continuous use a device that is capable of detecting disconnection of components of the breathing system. The device must give an audible signal when its alarm threshold is exceeded.

4. During regional anesthesia and monitored anesthesia care, the adequacy of ventilation shall be evaluated, at least, by continual observation of qualitative clinical signs.

Circulation

OBJECTIVE To ensure the adequacy of the patient's circulatory function during all anesthetics.

METHODS 1. Every patient receiving anesthesia shall have the electrocardiogram continuously displayed from the beginning of anesthesia until preparing to leave the anesthetizing location.*

2. Every patient receiving anesthesia shall have arterial blood pressure and heart rate determined and evaluated at least every five minutes.*

3. Every patient receiving general anesthesia shall have, in addition to the above, circulatory function continually evaluated by at least one of the following; palpation of a pulse, auscultation of heart sounds, monitoring of a tracing of intra-arterial pressure, ultrasound peripheral pulse monitoring, or pulse plethysmography or oximetry.

Body temperature

OBJECTIVE To aid in the maintenance of appropriate body temperature during all anesthestics.

METHODS There shall be readily available a means to continuously measure the patient's temperature. When changes in body temperature are intended, anticipated or suspected, the temperature shall be measured.

Approved by House of Delegates on October 21, 1986
From Anesthesia Patient Safety Foundation Newsletter 2:1-3, 1987, with permission.

TABLE 7-1. Generalized monitoring considerations, in addition to basic standards, for various anesthetic and surgical procedures

Procedures	Potential clinical events	Monitoring considerations *(other than basic standards)* R-recommended; U-potentially useful
Any MAC	Over sedation, toxic effects of local injections, inadequate local anesthesia or sedation, hypertension, arrhythmia	None
Any RA	Inadequate anesthesia, excessive spread of anesthesia, systemic CV or respiratory toxicity, oversedation	U-automated BP, MLECG
Any GA	Overdose of inhalational agent, inadequate ventilation or improper intubation	U-agent specific end expiratory concentration of inhaled agents, MLECG
Intrathoracic	Vascular and cardiac manipulation or compromise; hemorrhage; oxygenation/ventilation diff; pneumothorax; arrhythmias	R-IA-BP, MLECG U-CVP vs PA cath vs Doppler CO
Cardiac	As above, unstable patient, anticoagulation, use of cardiopulmonary (CP) bypass	R-IA-BP, MLECG, CO assessment, ability to externally pace U-CVP
Major arterial vascular	Rapid changes in BP, systemic vascular resistance (SVR), CV stress with cross clamp, effects of distal ischemia, reperfusion effects, anticoagulation, hemorrhage, CV and pulmonary compromise	R-IA-BP, MLECG, CO assessment U-MVO$_2$
Major venous vascular	Loss of preload with clamp, major nonpulsatile hemorrhage, reperfusion effects	R-IA-BP, MLECG, CVP vs CO measurement U-MVO$_2$
Cerebrovascular	Baroreceptor responses to art clamp, arrhythmias, cerebral ischemia, +/− postsurgical deficit, CV instability	R-IA-BP, CVP vs CO assessment U-EEG vs EP
Intracranial	Inaccessability of head during surgery, rapid changes in BP, arrhythmias, air emboli, changes in intracranial compliance, hemorrhage; controlled hypotension may be necessary	R-IA-BP zeroed to head, if seated; CVP vs CO measurement, Doppler air detector U-ICP monitoring, end-tidal N$_2$ assessment
Major abdominal	Large losses of fluid secondary to evaporation and 3rd' space, +/− requirement for postoperative ventilation	R-Depends on patients CV/PULM status U-automated BP, CVP

MAC, monitored anesthesia care (local anesthetic with sedation); RA, regional anesthesia; GA, general anesthesia; BP, blood pressure; CO, cardiac output; CV, cardiovascular; CVP, central venous pressure; IA-BP, intraarterial blood pressure; ICP, intracranial pressure; MLECG, multilead electrocardiogram; MVO$_2$, mixed venous O$_2$ saturation; EP, evoked potential monitoring; PULM, pulmonary.

sured by both noninvasive and invasive means, whereas central venous pressure measurements are only practical via invasive methodology. The anesthesiologist has a variety of devices and methods to choose from (see box on p. 68). The invasive ones can be adapted to a particular vascular bed to assist surgical decision-making; for example, measure-ment of pre-porto-systemic and post-porto-systemic shunt venous pressures.

Arterial blood pressure

Noninvasive. Indirect methods of arterial pressure measurement include sphygmomanometry (Riva Rocce/Korotkoff), oscillotonometry, Doppler ultrasound, and plethysmography. Some instruments

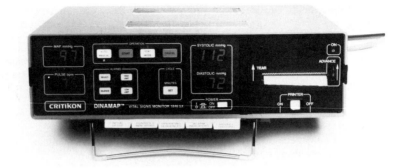

FIGURE 7-1. Noninvasive automatic blood pressure monitoring using oscillometric technology. Artifact rejection is relaxed in the "STAT mode" to allow for accelerated determinations.

Courtesy of Dinamap/Critikon, Tampa, Fla.

Intravascular pressure measurement

Arterial pressure measurement

Noninvasive/indirect
  Sphygmomanometry (manual, automated)
    Riva Rocce/Korotkoff auscultation
    Oscillotonometry
    Doppler ultrasound
  Plethysmography
    Penaz
Invasive/direct
  Intraarterial catheter, transducer system

Venous pressure measurement

Invasive/direct
  Central venous pressure measurement
  Pulmonary artery pressure measurement

---

combine several of these principles with electronic and computerized algorithms for automated pressure determinations. Sphygmomanometry (manual and auscultated) is the standard for noninvasive monitoring of systolic and diastolic pressures, but other methods are faster, more automated, or are capable of determining mean arterial blood pressure, and thus may be preferable in certain settings (Figure 7-1). Unfortunately, all noninvasive methods lose accuracy during periods of hemodynamic instability. Several devices for automated blood pressure rec-

ording have a STAT mode that permits rapid measurements during abrupt changes in blood pressure. Artifact rejection, however, may not be optimal in this mode. For example, during normal cuff deflation, internal algorithms search for two or more consecutive pressures of similar value before continuing to lower pressure. If similar pressures are not found, the search for a blood pressure is either terminated or the device defaults to a lower cuff pressure after a preset amount of time with loss of accuracy. Other units start in an auscultatory mode to detect systolic and diastolic measurements in a normal range, but switch to oscillotonometric means for periods of hypotension. One model looks for low-frequency components of the Korotkoff sounds that presumably allow more accurate measurements during periods of decreased blood pressure. Unfortunately, none of the currently available automated devices offer a quick way to switch to a "manual"/auscultatory mode to verify the electronic readings.

A relatively new method of noninvasive blood pressure measurement is based on photoelectric measurement of pressure and volume in the finger. As described by Penaz (Figure 7-2), a small pneumatic finger cuff is inflated to a pressure equal the arterial transmural pressure. An infrared transmission plethysmograph signal on one side of the finger and a photoelectric detector on the opposite side track the relative arterial volume instantaneously. Computerized algorithms allow the small cuff to maintain

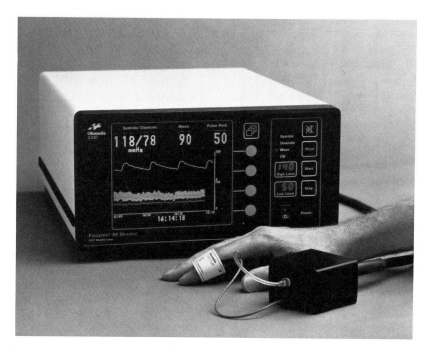

FIGURE 7-2. Continuous real time noninvasive blood pressure monitoring using the Penaz technique.

Courtesy of OHMEDA/FINAPRES, Madison, Wis.

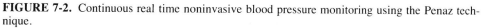

Indications for direct blood pressure measurement

Potential for instantaneous or rapid changes in blood pressure as a result of the nature of underlying heart disease and/or the intended surgical procedure

Need to frequently assess arterial blood gases intraoperatively or postoperatively

Underlying patient condition—hypotension; modest to severe hypertension; CV or CNS ischemia

---

transmural pressure at zero so that cuff pressure then equals arterial blood pressure. The plethysmogram produced by these measurements is then displayed on a monitor screen closely resembles an arterial waveform. Initial evaluations of this method have shown that it tends to underestimate systolic, diastolic, and mean arterial pressures in comparison with other methods. Cuffs come in several widths

and the ratio of cuff width to finger circumference must be adjusted for each patient. Proper alignment with the arteries is important and the thumb may be the preferred digit. Low peripheral temperature, hypovolemia, emaciation, low cardiac output, proximal arterial constriction, and the use of vasoconstrictors may make the readings unreliable. However, if the limitations can be overcome, this form of monitoring could become of major intraoperative value.[9]

Invasive. Direct invasive blood pressure monitoring is necessary when either the general health of the patient or anticipated perioperative problems dictate the need for continuous accurate blood pressure data (see box above, left). Most arterial lines are placed in the nondominant radial or ulnar artery. If the patient is to be in the lateral position, the dependent arm is often used to avoid artifactual changes in arterial waveform. Assessment of palmar arch flow is probably not necessary before placement.[59] If blood pressure in one arm is higher, that arm should be used. Other insertion sites include the dorsalis pedis, axillary, and femoral arteries, but the arterial line should not be placed distal to intended arterial clamping or ligation. Placement near the aortic arch increases the risk of air emboli during flushing maneuvers, especially with axillary lines or arterial lines in infants.

Because of the potential for line-site infection and bacteremia with arterial lines inserted by surgical cutdown, percutaneous insertion is preferred.[2] Techniques of insertion vary greatly. I favor a wide-area skin prep with tincture of iodine or clorhexidene. Insertion at a narrow angle to the skin increases the likelihood of establishing access with a "single hole" or "first-pass" technique. "Through and through" techniques allow blood extravasation from the deeper arterial hole and increase the potential for hematoma formation, nerve compression, and loss of vessel patency after the line is removed.[4,30,40] The risks of short-term arterial cannulation must be considered when arterial monitoring is undertaken.[59]

The accuracy of direct blood pressure measurements depends on the transformation of pressure energy in the arterial catheter into an electronic signal, which is then processed and displayed.* There were no mandated standards for physiological pressure transducers until 1986 when the American National Standard for Blood Pressure Transducers was developed by the Association for the Advancement of Medical Instrumentation.[1] Transducers should be linear over a pressure range of -30 to $+300$ mm Hg, accurate within 2% or 1 mm Hg, and exhibit hysteresis (lag in the direction of previous reading) less than 2% or 1 mm Hg. The device should tolerate normal wear and tear, withstand defibrillator discharge, and not pose a current-leak hazard to the patient.[48] Disposable transducers are available that meet all recommended standards and yield accurate and reproducible results.[20]

Because electronic signal processing, amplification, and display is different for each manufacturer, understanding the calibration and display procedures for the unit in use is essential. Many processing and display units provide internal electronic signal calibration functions. Nevertheless, in our program calibration to a mercury manometer is considered mandatory before each patient use.

---

*References 11, 26, 27, 49, 56.

> **Indications for CVP measurement**
>
> Dynamic assessment of volume status
> Central drug administration
> Air embolism aspiration
> Pacer insertion
> PA catheter flotation
> Poor venous access
> Hyperalimentation

Central venous pressure. Indications for establishing central venous access are varied (see box above). Central venous pressure (CVP) is most often used to assess intravascular volume status and the adequacy of right ventricular filling. However, changes in venous capacitance may alter the measured CVP. While these changes probably reflect parallel changes in ventricular filling, they may not indicate the absolute magnitude to which intravascular volume has been altered. As with all intravas-in ventricular pressure-volume relationships make precise assessment of ventricular volume impossible. Furthermore, in settings of increased intrapleural pressure (for example, during positive pressure ventilation), the extent to which these pressures are transmitted to the heart is variable and depends on the compliance characteristics of the lung. Accordingly, responses to fluid challenge may be required to assess ventricular filling status. Finally, in patients with right ventricular dysfunction or increased pulmonary artery pressure (as may occur in COPD), right ventricular pressure measurements may not reflect left ventricular filling. In spite of these drawbacks, most clinicians rely on changes in central venous pressure to make preliminary assumptions about vascular volume and ventricular function in normal patients.[6,61] When serious questions arise, other estimations of ventricular filling are in order.

Pulmonary artery and occlusion pressures. Perioperative measurements of pulmonary artery and pulmonary artery occlusion pressures are used to assess right ventricular afterload and ventricular preload, respectively. The limitations of CVP measurements discussed above also apply to measurements obtained from pulmonary artery catheters. In addition, accurate assessment of left ventricular preload requires correct placement of the PA catheter in zone 3 lung regions. Absence of both pulmonary venous obstruction and mitral valve disease in a setting of constant left ventricular compliance are also required for accurate measurements.[51] Information obtained from the PA catheter combined with measurements of cardiac output can be used to derive indices of pulmonary and systemic vascular resistance. A modified thermodilution catheter to evaluate ejection fraction is being developed and may prove to be practical for perioperative use.

Cardiac Monitoring

Electrocardiography. Anesthesiologists have recognized the importance of intraoperative ECGs for many years, and the ASA has stated that "every patient receiving anesthesia shall have the electrocardiogram continuously displayed from the beginning of anesthesia until preparing to leave the anesthetizing location."[21] In addition to rhythm disturbances, the ECG can be useful for detection of electrolyte abnormalities and myocardial ischemia. The ECG should have five leads and a monitor that allows selection of either standard (I, II, III), augmented (aVR, aVL, aVF), or precordial leads. Occasionally the site of surgery will require alteration in lead placement, or an unusual patient position may alter the electrical axis of the heart. The ECG should be recorded before and just after these alterations to establish a new baseline for detecting subsequent waveform changes. Either Lead V5 (anterior) or lead II (inferior) is commonly monitored routinely, but both leads should be observed simultaneously in patients with heart disease to maximally increase the ability to detect ischemia by ECG. Other leads may occasionally offer better information and esophageal leads may be useful in diagnosing supraventricular arrythmias.

ST-segment changes may not be the first sign of myocardial ischemia. Regional wall motion abnormalities,[60] altered ventricular compliance and lactate production often occur before ECG changes, but these changes require special monitors to detect. Nevertheless, approximately 90% of intraoperative myocardial ischemia is detected by lead V5 alone, and the availability of other leads improves on this. Since perioperative ischemia is common in patients with coronary artery disease and asymptomatic ischemia is often recognized in patients with and without known heart disease, ECG is an inexpensive and

---

Indications for intraoperative assessment of cardiac output
Recommended
Severe underlying cardiac disease (e.g.: unstable angina; EF < 30%; significant valvular disease; CHF; cardiomyopathy, pericardial disease, recent myocardial infarction)
Cardiac or major vascular surgery
Severe pulmonary hypertension
Liver transplantation
Potentially useful
Symptomatic heart disease (e.g.: angina)
Surgical procedures with major fluid shifts (e.g.: Whipple)
Sepsis hemodynamics
Surgical procedures requiring deliberate hypotension

---

diagnostically useful tool for ischemia detection in all patients undergoing anesthesia and surgery.

Computer-assisted ST-segment trending devices are available that may improve the sensitivity for perioperative ischemia detection. However, despite electronic filters to reduce the amplitude of interfering electronic frequencies, phase shifts can distort the recorded signal, artifactually depress the ST-segment, and provide falsely positive evidence for ischemia.

Ventricular function

Cardiac output. Cardiac outputs (CO) are obtained to assess the effects of anesthetic agents or surgical manipulation on the heart, and to monitor the status of underlying cardiovascular disease (see box above). Several methods for perioperative CO determinations are available that are based on either the Fick principal, Doppler methods, echocardiography, or combinations of these.

The original direct Fick method involved inhaled physiological gases (O_2 and CO_2) as indicators, but measurements were unreliable in the presence of volatile anesthetic agents. Injectable indicators such as dye and thermal dilution techniques are more adaptable to anesthetized patients. Dye dilution requires a central venous line for indocyanine green injections and a peripheral arterial line for sampling through a densitometer (peak absorption at wavelength 805 nm). The thermodilution method requires a PA catheter with built-in thermistor to sense

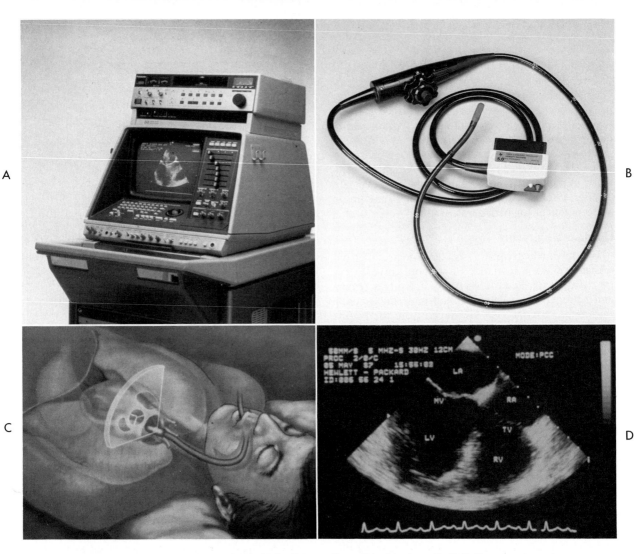

FIGURE 7-3. A, Hewlett-Packard (H-P) Echocardiographic Monitor. **B,** H-P Transesophageal Echocardiographic Transmitting and Receiving "Scope." **C,** Artists' depiction of "scope" in position with fan-shaped signal pattern. **D,** Actual ECHO with scope positioned to show all four chambers.

Courtesy Hewlett-Packard, Waltham, Mass.

changes between injectate and blood temperature. Iced injection may be more reproducible, and the test injection should be made rapidly (<4 sec) while the thermal output curve is observed. Both random and end-expiratory indicator injections have been recommended. Measurement errors may occur during periods of rapid infusion of room-temperature crystalloid solutions.[64] Dye dilution techniques may be more reproducible in this situation since blood temperature is not a measured variable. Slowing of the heart rate may occur during cold injection,[33,46] but the hemodynamic effects of these changes have not been evaluated. Catheter-associated thrombus around the distal thermistor may also decrease CO measurements.[7]

Echocardiography. Noninvasive evaluation of perioperative cardiac performance and ischemia detection by echocardiography (ECHO) is becoming more widespread. ECHO has recently become available in a practical transesophageal form (Figure

7-3). **M**-mode ECHO is limited to one dimension and may miss abnormal ventricular wall motion. In contrast, two dimensional echocardiography (2d-ECHO) measures both systolic and diastolic cardiac dimensions from which estimates of cardiac output, ventricular volume, ejection fraction, and pulmonary artery occlusion pressure can be made. ECHO readily demonstrates dose-dependent cardiovascular depression caused by halogenated anesthetic agents and the positive and negative inotropic effects of administered drugs. The ability to detect regional wall motion abnormalities makes 2d-ECHO a more sensitive indicator of myocardial ischemia than the ECG or changes in pulmonary artery occlusion pressure and cardiac output.[52,60] For a thorough discussion of ischemia detection in the perioperative time see Chapter 17. ECHO is also useful in the detection of intracardiac shunts, venous air embolism, and the adequacy of intracardiac air removal following cardiopulmonary bypass.

Doppler ultrasound. Doppler ultrasound is also used to assess ventricular function by measuring the change in frequency between emitted and reflected signals from moving red blood cells. Doppler CO measurements correlate highly with those obtained by thermodilution.[25,57] Doppler probes are available for external and transesophageal use (Figure 7-4). For uncertain reasons, accuracy of Doppler CO measurements after cardiopulmonary bypass is greatly decreased when thermodilution is used as a reference. Recently, both Doppler and 2d-ECHO transducers have been incorporated into the same esophageal probe. High-amplitude waves, reflected from the cardiac structures and detected by 2d-ECHO, yield a cardiac image. Lower-amplitude waves, reflected from the erythrocytes and detected by doppler shifts, give blood velocity (see Figure 7-3). This blood flow can be "color mapped" to allow determination of the direction, magnitude, velocity, and turbulence of blood flow.[18] Transesophageal ECHO with or without Doppler may be useful in the perioperative management of patients with valvular lesions, cardiomyopathies, ischemic heart disease, pericardial tamponade, and congenital heart disease.

RESPIRATORY MONITORING
Oxygenation

Adequate oxygenation is essential during all anesthetics; hypoxia accounts for the majority of deaths associated with anesthesia. Cyanosis is an unreliable

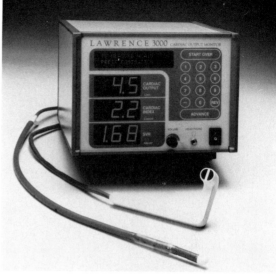

FIGURE 7-4. Noninvasive cardiac output monitor. The angular probe is used to determine a reference ascending aortic blood velocity externally from the suprasternal notch by Doppler ultrasonographic shift. The esophageal (internal) probe similarly determines descending aortic blood velocity continually. With ascending and descending aortic cross sectional areas known or estimated, stroke volume and cardiac output can be estimated.

Courtesy of Lawrence Medical Systems, Inc, Camarillo, Calif.

marker for arterial hypoxemia,[14,15,62] and a number of monitoring devices are currently used to assess the adequacy of oxygenation throughout the perioperative time. All anesthesia machines in current use are required to have in-line inspired O_2 concentration analyzers (polarographic electrode) with audible alarms to alert the anesthesiologist to hypoxic gas delivery (Figure 7-5). Newer anesthesia machines have flow-driven and pressure-driven proportioning valves that either prevent the delivery of a hypoxic (<21% FiO_2) mixture or sound an alarm if one is generated. Since tissue hypoxia can occur despite an adequate FiO_2, attention has been recently directed toward monitoring the adequacy of tissue oxygenation using transcutaneous oxygen saturation, transcutaneous oxygen tension, mixed venous oximetry or intraarterial blood gas measurements.

Pulse oximetry. Continuous pulse oximetry measures the oxygen saturation of hemoglobin. It re-

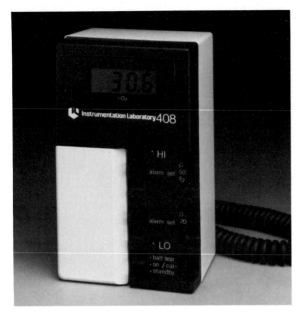

FIGURE 7-5. Oxygen analyzer for monitoring inspired oxygen concentrations using a polarographic electrode.

Courtesy of Instrumentation Laboratory, Inc, Lexington, Mass.

quires no site preparation, and there is no risk of cutaneous burns (Figure 7-6). Results accurately reflect direct measurements of arterial blood oxygen saturation. The usefulness of pulse oximetry may be limited by motion artifact, conditions with no pulse (cardiac arrest, nonpulsatile cardiopulmonary bypass, and placement below an inflated blood pressure cuff), low hemoglobin values, intravenous dyes, fiberoptic and infrared light sources, electrocautery, and in settings where venous flow has a pulsatile quality, as with tricuspid regurgitation.[45] Although wide swings in PaO_2 can occur within the 100% hemoglobin saturation range, pulse oximetry has proven to be the best oxygenation monitor to date. At greater than 70% saturation pulse oximetry is accurate to within 2% of in vitro methods, and is only slightly less accurate at lower saturations. Methemoglobin and carboxyhemoglobin are ignored by the oximeter. High concentrations of either will lead to overestimation of the O_2 saturation.[3a,30a] Pulse oximetry has led to cost savings by decreasing the need for measurement of arterial blood gases. Studies are

also beginning to show improved recognition of hypoxemic and near-hypoxemic events in the perioperative time.[13,15,39,42] Errors, however, are present in most monitors during profound hypoxia. Fortunately, they tend to underestimate the actual saturation value.[54a]

Transcutaneous oxygen tension. Transcutaneous oxygen tension ($PtcO_2$) techniques also assess blood oxygenation continuously and noninvasively. However, $PtcO_2$ sensors must heat the skin to arterialize local flow, which occasionally results in skin burns. A warm-up time of 5 to 10 minutes is required before reliable results are available. Whereas $PtcO_2$ measurements are highly correlated with direct measurements of arterial oxygen tension, the ongoing quality control is highly dependent on the skill and experience of the operator, and the device requires frequent intermittent calibration.[39,45]

Mixed venous oxygen saturation. Invasive monitoring of mixed venous O_2 saturation (SvO_2) combined with blood gas monitoring and cardiac output measurement permits calculation of oxygen delivery, peripheral oxygen extraction, and total body oxygen consumption (Figure 7-7). Normal SvO_2 is approximately 60% to 75%. Higher values may be a result of high FiO_2, left to right shunt, increased CO, sepsis, decreased temperature, cellular enzymatic poisoning, and arterialized samples from a wedged catheter. Lower values can be caused by cardiac failure, increased O_2 consumption, and lactic acidosis.

Continuous arterial blood gases. Continuous in vivo measurement of blood gases is under active investigation.[55a,60a] By use of fluorescent fiberoptic sensors that employ several fluorescent dyes covalently bonded with cellulose gels, the photoluminescent properties of the dyes can be used to measure PO_2, PCO_2, and pH individually. Three sensors and a thermocouple are bonded into a 0.024 inch diameter fiber designed to fit inside a 20-gauge arterial catheter used for blood pressure monitoring. It appears that problems with thrombogenicity have been resolved. Accuracy is good, but the use of these devices for PaO_2 measurements requires further refinement.[55a] To be truly useful in the OR and ICU, these devices should not be affected by anesthetic agents, should not decrease the life of the arterial line, and should remain accurate for the life of the arterial line.[3,28] Miniaturized Clark (polarographic) electrodes for continuous intraarterial measurements

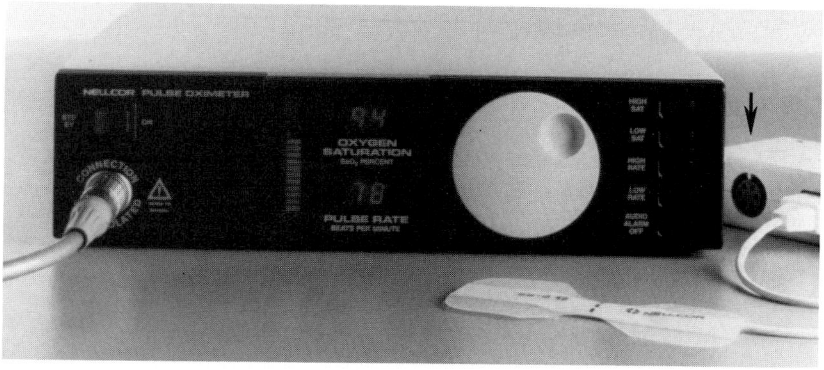

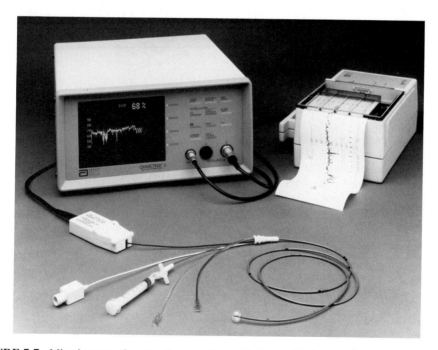

FIGURE 7-6. Pulse oximetry. The finger probe combines the principles of photoelectric plethysmography and oximetry. The ratio of absorbance of oxygenated to reduced hemoglobin at two monochromatic wavelengths (660 and 940 nm) allows calculation of the percent saturation of hemoglobin. This model, (*arrow* points to ECG input jack), in addition, tracks the electrocardiogram, permitting somewhat improved detection of arterial pulsation.

Courtesy of Nellcor, Hayward, Calif.

FIGURE 7-7. Mixed venous O_2 saturation monitor, with thermodilution cardiac output capability.

Courtesy of Abbott Critical Care/Oximetrix, Mountain View, Calif.

of PO_2 are also under development, but these devices are not yet available.[10]

Ventilation

The adequacy of ventilation must be continually evaluated for all patients in the perioperative time. Continuous auscultation of breath sounds and visual assessment of chest wall movement is mandatory in the anesthetized patient. In addition, the measurement of the end-tidal concentration of carbon dioxide is recommended for a breath-by-breath assurance of adequate ventilatory support, intraoperatively as well as postoperatively.

Infrared sensitive filters and photocells can be used to detect CO_2 in expired gas (Figures 7-8 and 7-9). Since expired gas includes gas from anatomic dead space and the alveoli, end-tidal CO_2 ($PETCO_2$) is diluted by gas from poorly ventilated lung areas. In normal awake persons, this arterial-to-end-tidal CO_2 difference is small, but because of increased ventilation-to-perfusion mismatching during anesthesia, the difference may increase to approximately 5 mm Hg. Patients with intrinsic lung disease may experience greater widening. Interindividual variability in arterial-to-end-tidal CO_2 differences and variations in the same patient during a single operation may limit the usefulness of continuous end-tidal CO_2 monitoring.[50] However, $PETCO_2$ gives first-breath and sustained confirmation of proper endotracheal tube placement, and this alone could justify its usefulness and cost. It also gives added protection against partial or complete airway disconnection ($PETCO_2$) and can detect air or particulate pulmonary emboli (Figure 7-10). $PETCO_2$ measurements may become a standard for noninvasive assessment of ventilatory effort during CPR.[24] Additionally, observation of an electronically displayed waveform adds information on parameters such as spontaneous breathing efforts by the patient.

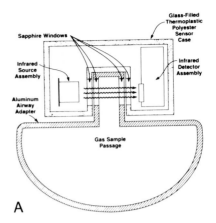

A

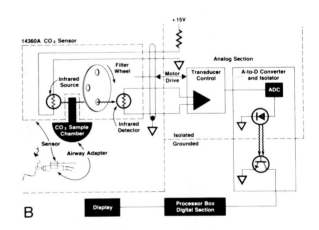

B

FIGURE 7-8. Infrared CO_2 detection system using a breathe-through sample chamber. **A,** Cross section schematic of breathe-through sample chamber and clip-on sensor. **B,** Simplified diagram of internal electronics.

Courtesy of Hewlett Packard, Waltham, Mass, with permission.

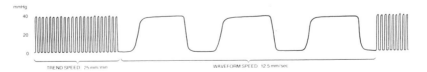

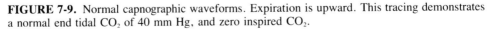

FIGURE 7-9. Normal capnographic waveforms. Expiration is upward. This tracing demonstrates a normal end tidal CO_2 of 40 mm Hg, and zero inspired CO_2.

Courtesy of Hewlett-Packard, Waltham, Mass.

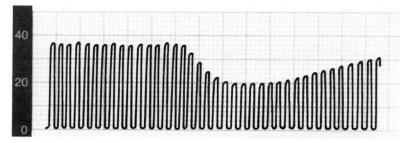
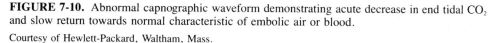

FIGURE 7-10. Abnormal capnographic waveform demonstrating acute decrease in end tidal CO_2 and slow return towards normal characteristic of embolic air or blood.

Courtesy of Hewlett-Packard, Waltham, Mass.

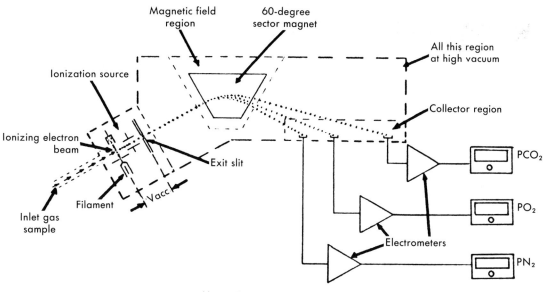

Magnetic mass spectrometer

FIGURE 7-11. Mass spectroscopy. A small gas sample is passed through an ionizing electron beam, focused into an ion beam, and then directed through a magnetic field. This field deflects components of the beam proportional to their charge-to-mass ratio, allowing for component-specific detection.

Courtesy of PPG/SARA Medical Systems, St Louis, Mo.

End-tidal samples of respiratory gases including nitrogen, oxygen, and carbon dioxide can be analyzed at the bedside by mass spectroscopy (Figures 7-11 and 7-12) or Raman spectroscopy (Figure 7-13). While these modalities are highly accurate and provide valuable on-line information, widespread use has been hampered by added costs for purchase and upkeep. However, pulse oximetry and end-tidal CO_2 monitoring are widely used, and the accuracy of these modalities can be validated intermittently with direct measurements of oxygen and CO_2 in arterial blood.

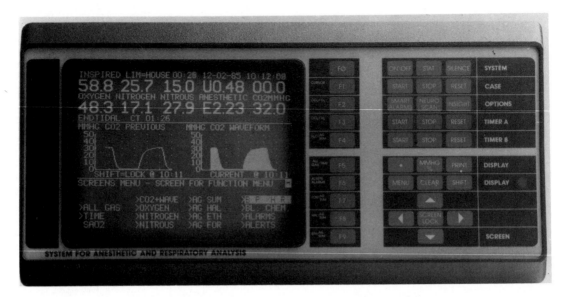

FIGURE 7-12. Typical monitor display for mass spectrometer. Capnographic waveform as well as O_2, N_2, N_2O, and halogenated agent are displayed.

Courtesy of PPG Biomedical Systems, Lenexa, Kan.

Central Nervous System

Patients with cerebrovascular, intracranial, or spinal cord disease may benefit from monitoring of central nervous system parameters in the perioperative time. This section briefly reviews indices of CNS function that can be clinically assessed, including cerebral blood flow and metabolism, electrical activity, and intracranial pressure measurements. Unfortunately, these measurements are difficult to obtain and interpret, indications for their use are not well defined, and controlled studies to document improved outcome with their use are infrequently reported.

Cerebral blood flow and metabolism. Cerebral blood flow (CBF) in the normal awake human adult remains constant at 50 to 60 ml/100 g/min over a wide range of arterial blood pressures. A critical threshold for ischemia as determined by EEG dysfunction appears to exist at CBF values of 15 ml/100 g/min, and irreversible neuronal cell death occurs at flow less than 10 to 15 ml/100 g/min. Monitors to directly detect either globally reduced CBF during hypotension or cardiopulmonary bypass, or regional reductions during interruption of carotid or vertebral artery flow require complicated computer-assisted indicator washout or dilution techniques that are available only on a research basis. The adequacy of collateral flow during carotid occlusion has been historically assessed indirectly by either ipsilateral ocular plethysmography or measurement of ipsilateral intraarterial pressure distal to the surgical clamp (stump pressure). However, neither of these techniques correlate well with simultaneous electrical recordings of CNS activity and have largely been abandoned.

Measurements of jugular venous oxygen tension and other enzymatic indicators of ischemia have been investigated during known ischemic insults. However, intracranial mixing of venous blood may lead to inaccurracies in these determinations. Positron emission tomography provides reliable data regarding relationships between CBF and metabolism, but this method is experimental, cumbersome, and too expensive for routine perioperative use. At this time there is no consensus regarding standards to detect intraoperative CNS ischemia.

Cerebral electrical activity. Continuous perioperative recordings of the electroencephalogram (EEG) or evoked potentials (EP) may be the most reliable means available to detect either ischemic

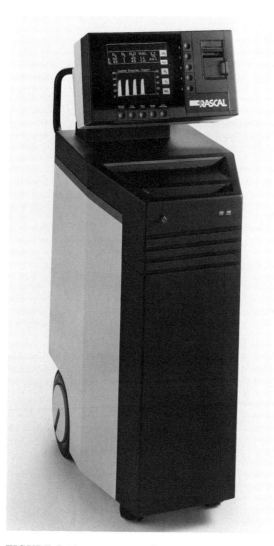

FIGURE 7-13. The Raman spectroscopy gas analyzer (Rascal) can detect O_2, CO_2, N_2, ethrane, halothane, isoflurane, H_2O, and argon. The argon laser beam photons are "scattered" by these respiratory gasses. Each gas produces a specific frequency shift in photon energy, measured by a complex photon multiplier and counting system.

Courtesy of Albion Instruments, Salt Lake City, Utah.

insults or dangerous surgical manipulations such as traction of the brainstem during posterior fossa craniotomy.

EEG. Changes in EEG activity have been correlated with blood flow changes, and EEG may thus be a reliable indicator of ischemia. New computer-processed EEG techniques are portable and use fewer electrodes than standard EEG. However, loss of sensitivity with these modalities may make them less reliable than unprocessed EEG signals for ischemia detection.[38] The EEG may not be an adequate indicator of new ischemic changes in patients with major preoperative changes in EEG resulting from previous cerebral infarction. Additionally, EEG requires extensive user training and experience for accurate and reproducible recordings and interpretation.

Evoked potentials. EP monitoring is used primarily to evaluate functional integrity during procedures in which injury to sensory pathways may occur. Loss of function may result from surgical manipulation, awkward positioning, or progression of underlying disease. EP monitoring should be established before induction of anesthesia and maintained throughout the surgical procedure. Somatosensory evoked potential (SEP) recording monitors the dorsal column of the spinal cord and cortical and subcortical areas of the brain. Direct insult to the dorsal (sensory) column will usually indicate the potential for anterior (motor) column injury during spinal cord surgery. If a question arises, intraoperative awakening may be necessary to evaluate motor function. In addition, since the anterior and posterior circulation of the spinal cord are not totally isolated, SEP's are useful monitors of neural function during surgery on the descending aorta as well.[35] Brainstem auditory EP monitoring is useful for monitoring eighth nerve and brainstem function during posterior fossa procedures. Cortical EP monitoring can be used to identify changes affecting the cerebral cortex and sensorimotor area whether caused by surgical retraction or interruption of blood flow. It is important to remember that electrical monitoring may be affected by both intravenous and inhaled anesthetic agents as well as temperature changes, which may obscure (false negative) or mimic (false positive) true physically induced changes in neuronal function.

Intracranial pressure. In patients with known or suspected intracranial hypertension, it may be useful to measure intracranial pressure (ICP) since it is a major determinant of downstream pressure controlling cerebral blood flow. Intraventricular catheter and subarachnoid bolts can be used to directly measure cerebrospinal fluid pressure. Only the intraventricular catheter, however, offers a practical method for intermittent withdrawal of cerebrospinal fluid (CSF) to acutely decrease ICP, if necessary. Infectious complications are common and often severe, especially for intraventricular catheters. Dural or brain tissue may contact the proximal end of the subarachnoid devices, resulting in artifactually low measurements. External tubing should be free of bubbles and leaks. Automatic flushing systems should not be used since marked increases in intracranial volume and ICP may inadvertently occur. Extradural monitors, which do not penetrate the dural membrane, are also used to estimate ICP. These devices are difficult to calibrate and do not allow aspiration of CSF. They do have a lower incidence of infection.

Use and interpretation of ICP monitors requires experience and training. Nonuniformity of pressure transmission in the supratentorial space and pressure gradients between the two hemispheres can be large. ICP should be monitored on the side of the lesion. The transducer should be positioned and zeroed at the level of the external ear canal. This is nearly the same as the level of the right atrium in the supine position, but much higher when the head is elevated. To accurately determine cerebral perfusion pressure when the head is elevated, the arterial line should also be zeroed to the level of the head.

Venous Air Embolism

Venous air embolism may occur during any procedure in which the site of surgery is higher than the right atrium. The negative pressure gradient created can entrain air through open intravascular venous channels. The incidence of venous air embolism in seated surgical patients is estimated to be 10% to 60%.[43,44] Monitoring for and detection of venous air embolism allows early intervention to prevent further emboli and to treat any changes already created. The precordial Doppler is the most sensitive monitor to detect intravascular air before significant physiologic changes occur. A pulmonary artery catheter will detect increased pulmonary artery pressure, and end-tidal gas monitoring will detect decreased expired CO_2 tensions (see Figure 7-10) or increased expired nitrogen concentration if air emboli are sufficiently large to obstruct a major portion of the pulmonary arterial tree. By the time CVP is elevated and cardiac output decreased, hypotension, ECG abnormalities, acidosis, and physiologic collapse are imminent. It is only during this late stage that the classic "mill wheel" murmur is heard by precordial or esophageal stethoscope.[55] Detection of air emboli should prompt closure of open veins or flooding of the surgical field with saline to prevent further occurrence. Air can sometimes be aspirated through a multiple-orifice right atrial line. About one fifth to one third of adult patients have a probe-patent foramen ovale, and are at risk of paradoxical arterial air embolism if right atrial pressure exceeds left atrial pressure (approximately 50% of seated patients develop RA pressure > LA pressure intraoperatively).[47] Transesophageal ECHO is a sensitive monitor for detection of both arterial and venous air emboli.[16] The only known treatment for symptomatic arterial air emboli is hyperbaric oxygen.

Miscellaneous Monitors

Temperature. Monitoring of body temperature is a recommended standard of the ASA, and temperature is routinely monitored throughout the perioperative time.[21] An increase in body temperature intraoperatively may signal the presence of malignant hyperthermia, which is a lethal metabolic derangement triggered by anesthetic agents in approximately 1 of 12,000 children and 1 of 40,000 adults. More common is hypothermia resulting from anesthetic-induced alterations in thermoregulatory mechanisms,[32] exposure of serosal surfaces to cool ambient temperature, and infusion of room-temperature intravenous solutions. Raising the temperature of the operating suite, warming administered fluids, use of heating lamps, warming blankets, and plastic or metallic coverings may preserve body temperature. Temperature is commonly monitored in the rectum, esophagus, mouth, nose, or axilla. In addition, core body temperature may be more accurately assessed by measurement of tympanic membrane or blood temperature. Skin temperature can be monitored for short procedures by liquid crystal thermometry, but cutaneous thermometry correlates poorly with core temperature as either an absolute value or as a trend indicator.[63]

Renal function. Intraoperative assessment of renal function is largely restricted to measurement of urine output as an index of renal perfusion and intravascular volume status. Reversible depression of renal function intraoperatively may result from direct effects of anesthetic agents on renal blood flow and tubular function, but indirect effects of circulatory and sympathetic nervous system changes also contribute. These changes may persist into the postoperative time. In addition, hemorrhage, positive pressure ventilation, and surgical stress result in increased antidiuretic hormone secretion. These changes reversibly decrease urine output intraoperatively regardless of intravascular volume or renal perfusion status. Nevertheless, severe or prolonged reduction in urine output may indicate the presence of significant renal injury.[41]

Neuromuscular blockade. The neuromuscular blockade can be monitored safely by observation of clinical response alone, but nerve stimulation and recording devices are often employed. Depolarizing and nondepolarizing muscle relaxants elicit distinctly different patterns of muscle contraction to either single twitch or sustained supramaximal tetanic electrical stimulation. If neuromuscular reversal cannot be demonstrated either clinically or electrically, the patient should remain intubated and artificially ventilated until complete reversal is demonstrated.

Anesthetic depth. In addition to monitoring of cardiovascular, respiratory, and pupillary changes, objective assessment of the depth of anesthesia is occasionally desirable. Continuous EEG is cumbersome and not widely used. Recently, changes in lower esophageal contractility during anesthesia have been proposed as an objective index of anesthetic depth (Figure 7-14). The smooth muscle of the lower esophagus is not paralyzed by muscle relaxants and is able to contract in response to external stimuli. Esophageal contractility may also be useful in assessing the presence or absence of brain death in other settings.[23,58] However, motor activity of the esophagus is controlled primarily by brain stem nuclei via vagal pathways. A better understanding of the effects of disease states and pharmacologic agents on these pathways and on the muscle cells themselves is necessary before this technique gains wide clinical acceptance.

THE COST OF MONITORING PATIENTS

It is estimated that more than 2000 healthy (ASA classification I-II) Americans die annually during anesthesia (approximately 0.01% of surgical cases). According to some estimates, more than half of these

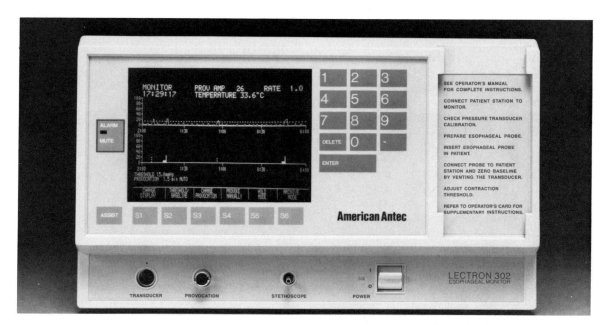

FIGURE 7-14. Lower esophageal contractility (LEC) monitor. A double-balloon esophageal probe (not shown) allows assessment of both provoked and spontaneous LEC as a measure of anesthetic depth.

Courtesy of American Antec, Valencia, Calif.

deaths could have been prevented. As mentioned above, however, there is no general agreement on the definition of "preventable" death, so estimates for preventable deaths range from 10% to 90%.[17] High-risk patients, in whom major systemic illnesses contribute to the undesirable effects of anesthesia, are estimated to have five times this number of deaths. Many more patients, presumably, experience a degree of morbidity associated with anesthesia and/or surgery, and certainly much of this morbidity is preventable as well. But prevented by what means and at what cost?

One of the most often quoted principles regarding prevention of untoward medical events comes *not* from a major medical center or a respected medical consultant, but rather from the legal profession. This rule of Judge Learned Hand states: "Negligence occurs whenever it would cost less to prevent a mishap than to pay for the damages predicted to result from it. More explicitly, the cost of preventing a mishap must be less than the probability that it will occur multiplied by the loss suffered when it does occur."[54] Or, because it is not possible to prevent all untoward outcomes, "negligent behavior is the failure to invest resources up to a level that equals the anticipated saving in damages."[54]

Recently, others have addressed the financial aspects of monitor acquisition and maintenance in terms of savings in hospital malpractice premiums. From a number of assumptions based on nationwide practice, it has been estimated that an investment of as much as $116,000 in monitors for *each* operating room would be fully compensated for by a 50% reduction in anesthetic malpractice losses.[8,65] This sort of reasoning should go a long way toward enlightening hospital administrators and improving budgetary support for anesthesia departments. Recent reviews also discuss the pros and cons of various equipment acquisition strategies aimed at achieving the broadest possible safety net.[8,65]

SUMMARY

Many physiologic variables can be measured perioperatively. While it seems, intuitively, that the safety and outcome of surgical patients should be improved by increased monitoring, this hypothesis has not been rigorously examined. Indeed, there is controversy within the leadership of the ASA about what physiologic parameters should be routinely measured during administration of anesthesia. Sophisticated electronic monitors cannot substitute for bedside observation by physicians and nurses. A patient who "looks bad" will require evaluation even when an electronic monitor has failed to sound an alarm. Many costly devices require considerable time to set up and calibrate. Data from them can be difficult to interpret. "Monitoring the monitor" may distract from monitoring the patient. Nevertheless, selection of monitoring modalities according to specific patient needs can yield goal-directed information that should decrease perioperative risk and improve outcome.

REFERENCES

1. American National Standard for Blood Pressure Transducers, General, ANSI/AAMI BP 22:1-22, 1986.
2. Band JD and Maki DG: Infections caused by arterial catheters used for hemodynamic monitoring, Am J Med 67:735, 1979.
3. Barker SJ et al: Continuous fiberoptic arterial oxygen tension measurements in dogs, J Clin Monitor 3:48-52, 1987.
3a. Barker SJ et al: The effects of carbon monoxide inhalation on noninvasive oxygen mointoring, Anesth Analg 65:512, 1986.
4. Bedford RF: Invasive blood pressure monitoring. In Monitoring in anesthesia and critical care medicine, New York, 1985, Churchill Livingstone.
5. Beecher HK and Todd DP: A study of the deaths associated with anesthesia and surgery: based on a study of 599,548 anesthesias in ten institutions 1948-1952, inclusive, Ann Surg 140:2-34, 1954.
6. Benumof JL: Monitoring: anesthesia for thoracic surgery, Philadelphia, 1987, WB Saunders Co.
7. Bjoraker DG and Ketcham TR: Catheter thrombus artifactually decreases thermodilution cardiac output measurements, Anesth Analg 62:1031-1034, 1983.
8. Block FE: A proposed standard for monitoring equipment: what equipment should be included, J Clin Monitor 4:1-4, 1988.
9. Boehmer RD: Continuous, real time, non-invasive monitor of blood pressure: Penaz methodology applied to the finger, J Clin Monitor 3:282-287, 1987.
10. Bratanow N et al: Continuous polarographic monitoring of intra-arterial oxygen in the perioperative period, Crit Care Med 10:859-860, 1985.
11. Bruner J et al: Comparison of direct and indirect methods of measuring arterial blood pressure, Med Instrum 15:11-21, 1981.
12. Clark AJ: Aspects of the history of anaesthetics, Brit Med J 2:1029-1034, 1938.
13. Cohen DE, Donnes JJ, and Raphaely RC: What difference does pulse oximetry make? Anesthesiology 68:181-183, 1988.

14. Comroe JH and Botelho J: The unreliability of cyanosis in the recognition of arterial hypoxemia, Am J Med Sci 214:1-6, 1947.

15. Coté CJ et al: A single-blind study of pulse oximetry in children, Anesthesiology 68:184-188, 1988.

16. Cucchiara RF et al: Detection of air embolism in upright neurosurgical patients by 2-D transesophageal echocardiography, Anesthesiology 59:A388, 1983.

17. Deaths during general anesthesia: technology related, due to human error, or unavoidable? Tech for Anesthesia (ECRI), 5:1-11, 1985.

18. deBruijn NP, Clements FM, and Kisslo JA: Intraoperative transesophageal color flow mapping. Initial experience, Anesth Analg 66:386-390, 1987.

19. Dinnick OP: Deaths associated with anaesthesia. Observations on 600 cases. Anaesthesia 19:536-556, 1964.

20. Disposable Pressure Transducers. Health Devices (ECRI) 17:75-94, 1988.

21. Eichhorn JH: ASA adopts basic monitoring standards. Anesthesia Patient Safety Foundation Newsletter, Park Ridge, Ill, 1987, Anesthesia Patient Safety Foundation.

22. Eichhorn JH et al: Standards for patient monitoring during anesthesia at Harvard Medical School, JAMA 256:1017-1020, 1986.

23. Evans JM, Davies WL, and Wise CC: Lower oesophageal contractility: a new monitor of anaethesia, Lancet ii:1151-1154, 1984.

24. Falk JL, Rackow EC, and Weil MH: End-tidal carbon dioxide concentration during cardiopulmonary resuscitation, N Engl J Med 318:607-611, 1988.

25. Freund PR and Padavich CA: A comparison of cardiac output techniques: transesophageal doppler vs thermodilution cardiac output during general anesthesia in man, Anesthesiology 63:A191, 1985.

26. Fung YC: Blood flow in arteries. In Fung YC: Biodynamics, New York, 1984, Springer-Verlag.

27. Gardner RM: Direct blood pressure measurement— dynamic response requirements, Anesthesiology 54: 227-236, 1981.

28. Gehrich JL: Optical fluorescense and its application to an intravascular blood gas monitoring system, IEEE Transactions on Biomedical Engineering BME 33:117-132, 1986.

29. Goldman SO: Anesthetization as a specialty: its present and future, Am Med 2:101-104, 1901.

30. Gravenstein JS and Paulus DA: Arterial pressure. In Clinical monitoring practice, ed 2, New York, 1987, JP Lippincott Co.

30a. Gravenstein JS and Paulus DA: Monitoring ventilation and gases. In Clinical monitoring practice, ed 2, New York, 1987, JP Lippincott Co.

31. Hamilton WK: Unexpected deaths during anesthesia: wherein lies the cause? Anesthesiology 50:381-383, 1979.

32. Hammel HT: Anesthetics and body temperature regulation, Anesthesiology 68:833-835, 1988.

33. Harris AP et al: The slowing of sinus rhythm during thermodilution cardiac output determinations and the effect of altering injectate temperature, Anesthesiology 63:540-541, 1985.

34. Hawkins WG: Medicolegal hazards of anesthesia, JAMA 163:746-748, 1957.

35. Kaplan BJ et al: Somatosensory evoked potential monitoring of spinal cord ischemia during aortic operations, Neurosurgery 19:82-90, 1986.

36. Keats AS: What do we know about anesthetic mortality? Anesthesiology 50:387-392, 1979.

37. Keats AS and Siker ES: Report on the International Symposium on Preventable Anesthetic Morbidity and Mortality. Boston, Massachusetts, October 8-10, 1984, Anesthesiology 63:349-50, 1985.

38. Levy WJ: Processed EEG: a machine and a number are not enough, J Cardiothoracic Anesthesia 2:121-122, 1988.

39. MacKenzie N: Comparison of a pulse oximeter with an ear oximeter and an in-vitro oximeter, J Clin Monitor 1:156-160, 1985.

40. Marshall G, Edelstein G, and Hirshman CA: Median nerve compression following radial arterial puncture, Anesth Analg 59:953-954, 1980.

41. Mazzei RI: Renal physiology and the effects of anesthesia. In Miller RD: Anesthesia, ed 2, New York, 1986, Churchill Livingstone.

42. Mendelson Y et al: Simultaneous comparison of three non-invasive oximeters in healthy volunteers, Med Instrum 21:183-188, 1987.

43. Michenfelder JD, Miller RH, and Gronert GA: Evaluation of an ultrasonic device (Doppler) for the diagnosis of venous air embolism, Anesthesiology 36:164-167, 1972.

44. Miller RA: Neurosurgical anesthesia in the sitting position, Anaesthesia 44:493, 1980.

45. New W: Pulse oximetry, J Clin Monitor 1:126-129, 1985.

46. Nishikawa T and Dohi S: Slowing of heart rate during cardiac output measurement by thermodilution, Anesthesiology 57:538, 1982.

47. Perkins-Pearson NAK, Marshall WK, and Bedford RF: Atrial pressures in the seated position: implication for paradoxical air embolism, Anesthesiology 57:493-497, 1982.

48. Physiological pressure transducers, Health Devices (ECRI), 8:199-217, 1979.

49. Prys-Roberts C: Invasive monitoring of the circulation. In Saidman LJ and Smith NT: Monitoring in Anesthesia, ed 2, Boston, 1984, Butterworth Publishers.

50. Raemer DP et al: Variation in PCO_2 between arterial blood and peak expired gas during anesthesia, Anesth Analg 62:1065-1069, 1983.

51. Raper R and Sibbald WJ: Misled by the wedge? The Swan-Ganz catheter and left ventricular preload, Chest 89:427-434, 1986.

52. Roizen MF et al: Monitoring with two-dimensional transesophageal echocardiography: patients undergoing supraceliac aortic occlusion, J Vasc Surg 1:300-305, 1984.

53. Ruth HS, Haugen FP, and Grove DD: Anesthesia study commission. Findings of eleven years' activity, JAMA 135:881-884, 1947.

54. Schwartz WB and Komesar NK: Doctors, damages, and deterence. An economic view of medical malpractice, N Engl J Med 298:1282-1289, 1978.

54a. Severinghaus JW, Naifeh KH, and Koh SO: Errors in 14 pulse oximeters during profound hypoxemia, J Clin Monit 5:72-81, 1989.

55. Shaprio HM: Monitoring in neurological anesthesia. In Saidman LJ and Smith NT: Monitoring in Anesthesia, ed 2, Boston, 1984, Butterworth Publishers.

55a. Shapiro BA et al: Preliminary evaluation of an intraarterial blood gas system in dogs and humans, Crit Care Med 17:455-460, 1989.

56. Shinozaki T, Deane RS, and Mazuzan JE: The dynamic responses of liquid-filled catheter systems for direct measurements of blood pressure, Anesthesiology 52:498-504, 1980.

57. Shuster AH and Nanda NC: Doppler echocardiographic measurement of cardiac output. Comparison with a non-golden standard, Am J Cardiol 53:257-259, 1984.

58. Sinclair ME and Suter PM: Lower oesophageal contractility as an indicator of brain death in paralyzed and mechanically ventilated patients with head injury, Br Med J 935-936, 1987.

59. Slogoff S, Keats AS, and Arlund C: On the safety of radial artery cannulation, Anesthesiology 59:42-47, 1983.

60. Smith JS et al: Intraoperative detection of myocardial ischemia in high-risk patients: electrocardiography versus two-dimensional transesophageal echocardiography, Circulation 72:1015-1021, 1985.

60a. Tremper KK and Barker SJ: The optode: next generation in blood gas measurement, Crit Care Med.

61. Teplick RS: Measuring central venous pressures: a surprisingly complex problem, Anesthesiology 67:289-291, 1987.

62. Tyler IL et al: Continuous monitoring of arterial oxygen saturation with pulse oximetry during transfer to the recovery room, Anesth Analg 64:1108-1112, 1985.

63. Vaughan MS, Cork RC, and Vaughan RW: Inaccuracy of liquid crystal thermometry to identify core temperature trends in postoperative adults, Anesth Analg 61:284, 1982.

64. Wetzel RC and Latson TW: Major errors in thermodilution cardiac output measurement during rapid volume infusion, Anesthesiology 62:684-687, 1985.

65. Whitcher C et al: Anesthetic mishaps and the cost of monitoring: a proposed standard for monitoring equipment, J Clin Monitor 4:5-15, 1988.

CHAPTER **8**

Pharmacology of Anesthetic Agents and Muscle Relaxants

STEPHEN A. DERRER

Induction agents
Inhalation agents
Opioid analgesics
Muscle relaxants
Conclusions

Appropriate anesthetic care cannot be provided without a detailed understanding of the pharmacology of anesthetic agents and muscle relaxants. In addition, this knowledge is necessary to appreciate the rationale behind current anesthesia practice. Here I will endeavor to describe the pharmacology of agents relatively specific to the practice of anesthesiology, and to demonstrate how this knowledge is incorporated into the synthesis of an anesthetic plan. The drugs discussed here are the intravenous induction agents, the inhalational anesthetic agents, narcotics, and muscle relaxants.

INDUCTION AGENTS

Although general anesthesia can be induced with an inhalation agent or any of the narcotics, induction is usually accomplished with a rapid and short acting intravenous agent. A number of agents, with considerable biochemical and pharmacologic heterogeneity, are useful almost exclusively in this role. The most popular induction agents are the ultrashort acting barbiturates.

Thiopental

Thiopental (Figure 8-1) is easily the standard of comparison for induction agents. It is an ultrashort acting thiobarbiturate that is highly lipid soluble. The usual induction dose of 3 to 5 mg/kg results in unconsciousness within seconds when given intravenously, and a peak effect is reached by 1 to 2 minutes. Aqueous solutions of thiopental sodium, although quite alkaline, are not irritating upon intravenous injection, and most patients find induction not at all unpleasant. This rapid, smooth production of the anesthetic state is quite desirable clinically; the interval between loss of consciousness and anesthetic depth adequate for airway or other manipulation is best shortened for reasons of patient safety.

After a typical induction dose of thiopental, consciousness usually returns in 5 to 10 minutes. The

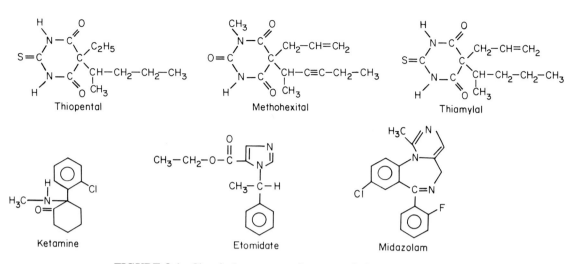

FIGURE 8-1. Chemical structures of nonnarcotic intravenous agents.

TABLE 8-1. Pharmacokinetic parameters of intravenous agents*

| | Distribution | | Elimination | |
	T½ π	T½ α	T½ β	References
Thiopental	2.5-8.5	38-62	306-719	20,36,49,73
Methohexital	5.6	58.3	234	49
Ketamine	11-17	150-186	150-186	24,113
Etomidate	28-32	230-270	230-270	3,108
Midazolam	7.2	78-150	78-150	17,41

*All times are in minutes.

effect of the drug after a single bolus is lost at that time because of rapid redistribution (T ½ π, see Table 8-1). Metabolism and final elimination are considerably slower (T ½ α 5 to 10 hours)[20,36,49,73] and duration of action becomes longer with multiple boluses or continuous infusion.

Usual induction doses of thiopental, although producing sleep, do not completely blunt hemodynamic and airway reflexes to pain or laryngeal manipulation. Accordingly, immediate addition of other analgesic, anesthetic, or relaxant agents is usually necessary. Higher doses of thiopental, 20 to 30 mg/kg, can produce an isoelectric EEG[106]; such conditions are certainly unnecessary for anesthetic induction.

Induction of anesthesia with thiopental is generally accompanied by mild cardiovascular depression with falls in blood pressure and cardiac contractility in the absence of stimulation. This depression can be exaggerated in the elderly, debilitated, or hypovolemic individual, and in such cases dose reduction (0.5 to 1.5 mg/kg) or use of an alternative agent may be desirable. Induction with thiopental is also associated with modest respiratory depression and the inability to maintain a patent airway, so ventilatory and airway support are often indicated.

A number of other ultrashort acting barbiturates are useful as induction agents. Thiamylal, an isomer of thiopental, is practically indistinguishable clinically. Methohexital is approximately twice as potent as thiopental and, because of a shorter elimination half life (T ½ β of 1.5 to 4 hours),[49] may be shorter acting in some settings, particularly when multiple doses are given. Methohexital has the annoying tendency to produce hiccoughing during induction.

All the barbiturates are specifically contraindicated in certain porphyrias, most notably the acute intermittent variety.[79] The action of the barbiturates on hepatic enzyme activity may precipitate life-threatening acute episodes in affected individuals.

Ketamine

Ketamine (see Figure 8-1) is a fascinating agent, its effect on the CNS being quite unlike that of the narcotics, barbiturates, or inhalation agents. Although ketamine anesthesia produces amnesia, analgesia, and immobility, it is also accompanied by nystagmus, nonpurposeful myotonic movements, swallowing, and occasional vocalization. The anesthetic state produced is called "dissociative anesthesia" because there is the appearance of considerable CNS activity despite adequate anesthesia. This is supported by measurement of increased cerebral blood flow and cerebral oxygen consumption ($CMRO_2$).[102] After recovery patients may have recall of vivid dreams or hallucinations occurring during the drug-induced state.

After a 1 to 2 mg/kg intravenous induction dose of ketamine, unconsciousness occurs in 1 to 2 minutes and returns in 10 to 15 minutes, although complete recovery often takes longer (0.5 to 1.5 hours). Clinical recovery depends upon redistribution (see Table 8-1); metabolism and elimination require more time (T ½ β 2 to 3 hours).[24,113] Larger doses (5 to 10 mg/kg) are suitable for induction when given intramuscularly.

Induction doses of ketamine produce minimal respiratory depression, and airway reflexes are less blunted than with any other agent. Airway patency is typically well maintained spontaneously, but this cannot be relied upon, and loss of patency or aspiration may occur in the improperly managed airway.

Probably the single most important quality of ketamine induction is the absence of apparent cardiovascular depression. Although ketamine has direct cardiac depressant effects,[107] these are generally obscured by direct and indirect sympathomimetic stimulation, so blood pressure and cardiac output usually increase or are unaffected. This property is most useful in the patient who is in shock or hypovolemic with shock potential. Ketamine may also be a useful induction agent in individuals with congenital heart lesions in whom vasodilation and hypotension upon induction can augment a right to left shunt and precipitate profound hypoxia.[78] Ketamine promotes bronchodilation both by direct effects and by increasing sympathetic activity.[63] Ketamine is thus useful in some asthmatic individuals as an induction agent.

Several circumstances may contraindicate the use of ketamine. Because of its effect on cerebral blood flow and metabolism, it is contraindicated in patients with intracranial masses or intracranial hypertension. The sympathomimetic effects of ketamine may be harmful to patients with coronary artery disease or cerebrovascular disease.

Ketamine is a unique agent with a limited but useful role in current practice routines. The greatest hindrance to more widespread use of the drug is that it occasionally produces unpleasant psychological side effects.

Etomidate

Etomidate is a rapidly acting intravenous anesthetic chemically unrelated to any other (see Figure 8-1). In onset and duration of action of a typical induction dose (0.3 mg/kg), it is comparable to thiopental. The elimination half-life is considerably shorter (1.2 to 4 hr)[3,108] because of ester hydrolysis (see Table 8-1).

The effects of etomidate on cerebral function, metabolism, blood flow, and EEG are similar to those of thiopental.[37,52,89] Etomidate may have somewhat less effect upon respiratory drive than a comparable dose of thiopental; the difference, however, is not of sufficient magnitude to be clinically important.

The principal advantage of etomidate over thiopental is its lack of cardiovascular effect at usual doses. Etomidate has been recommended by some for induction of individuals with cardiac disease. Because of its poor aqueous solubility, etomidate is marketed in an ethanol-propylene glycol-water solvent. Pain is common when the drug is given, and thrombophlebitis may occur from the irritation. Another annoying characteristic of etomidate is the production of myotonic movements, which are at times strong enough to interfere with airway management. Nausea and vomiting also seem to be more common after etomidate than after thiopental.[48]

Prolonged use of etomidate has been shown to produce adrenal suppression.[109] This is unlikely to be a problem when the drug is simply used for induction of anesthesia. Because of etomidate's drawbacks (for example, pain on injection and myotonus) and only subtle advantages (that is, lack of cardiovascular depression), etomidate is not as useful as thiopental as a routine induction agent. Although, like ketamine, it is a useful agent in a limited role.

Midazolam

Midazolam (see Figure 8-1) is a water-soluble benzodiazepine. Although the drug is frequently used as a perioperative sedative, its development as an agent for induction of anesthesia has been hindered because of its slower onset and longer duration of action than thiopental, etomidate, or ketamine. Sedative doses (0.02 to 0.07 mg/kg) provide more impressive amnesia than thiopental at a comparable dose, and although larger doses (0.1 to 0.25 mg/kg) will produce unconsciousness in an unstimulated patient, analgesia and muscle relaxation are lacking. At doses greater than 0.1 mg/kg, sedation is sufficiently long lived so that postoperative recovery is often delayed. Thus midazolam is rarely used for induction, despite producing less cardiovascular depression than thiopental.

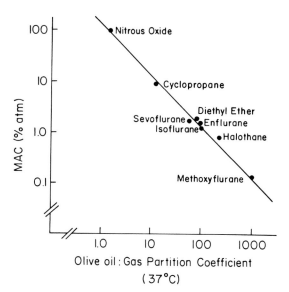

FIGURE 8-2. Relationship between anesthetic potency and lipid solubility.

Cook TL et al: Anesthesiology 43:70-77, 1975; Cromwell TH et al: Anesthesiology 35:365-373, 1971; Larson CP, Jr: Br J Anaesth 36:140-149, 1964; Hornbein TF et al: Anesth Analg 61:553-556, 1982; Katoh T and Ikeda K: Anesthesiology 66:301-303, 1987; and Koblin DD et al: Anesthesiology 54:314-317, 1981.

Other Agents Used for Induction

Many other drugs have been used for induction of anesthesia, including benzodiazepines (diazepam, lorazepam), barbiturates (secobarbital), steroids (alphadolone, alphaxalone), and other miscellaneous intravenous agents (propanidid, diisopropylphenol). Specific indications for any of these agents are uncommon.

INHALATION AGENTS

The inhalation agents produce all the obvious clinical effects usually associated with the definition of general anesthesia. These effects include unconsciousness, immobility, insensitivity to pain, abolition of reflexes, reversibility of the drug-induced state, and inability to recall events occurring during the drug-induced state.

A useful measure of clinical potency of an inhalation agent is the minimum alveolar concentration (MAC). This is the MAC of an agent observed to be associated with immobility in 50% of subjects in response to a noxious stimulus (that is, tail clamp in animal models, abdominal incision in humans). Thus MAC is essentially an ED_{50}, convenient for its relative ease of measurement and reproducibility. MAC is ordinarily expressed as percent concentration at one atmosphere pressure. It is common to express varying concentrations of anesthetic agents as multiples of MAC for purposes of comparison; for example, 0.5 MAC, 1.3 MAC, and 2.0 MAC. The relationship between MAC and oil/gas partition coefficient is featured in Figure 8-2.

Gas Uptake, Distribution, and Elimination

An important characteristic of any inhalation agent is the rate at which it appears at the site of action, and its subsequent rate of elimination. The ability to deliver an agent promptly to the brain facilitates onset of action with minimal excitation and allows titrability of the anesthetic effect. Rapid elimination of an agent minimizes risks inherent in drug-induced depression during the postanesthetic period.

For a volatile anesthetic to have its effect, it must pass from the breathing circuit to the lungs, from the lungs to the blood, and finally from the blood to the brain. The rate and direction of movement of anesthetic agents is dictated by the partial pressure gradients between these various compartments. Each step can be considered separately. First eventual attainment of an effective partial pressure of the agent will be accelerated if higher inspired concentrations are used. (The partial pressure of the anesthetic agent in the inspired mixture is equal to the inspired concentration, which is expressed as percent, and is multiplied times ambient pressure. It is approximately one atmosphere or 760 mm Hg.) Next, minute ventilation will determine the rate of rise in alveolar concentration. The uptake of agent from the lung and eventual equilibration of alveolar and blood concentrations are dependent upon the solubility of the agent in blood. If an anesthetic is relatively insoluble in blood, less of it dissolved in blood will be needed to reflect its partial pressure; blood will become saturated to the alveolar concentration relatively quickly. For a more soluble agent, more of the drug must be taken up until blood partial pressure reflects alveolar partial pressure. More time is required to take up a greater amount of the anesthetic. We can now describe the blood/gas partition coefficient:

Blood/gas partition coefficient

$$= \frac{\text{concentration (wt/vol) in blood}}{\text{concentration (wt/vol) in gas phase}}$$

Blood/gas partition coefficients for clinically important agents are listed in Table 8-2.

It must be clear that low blood/gas partition coefficient indicates low blood solubility, rapid uptake from the lungs, rapid distribution to the brain, and shorter time to anesthetic effect. Tissue/blood partition coefficients have also been described for various tissues, including brain, as a measure of uptake from blood and eventual equilibration. Basically, this ratio is closer to unity, exhibits less interagent variation than blood/gas partition coefficient, and correlates poorly with any clinical parameter.

The inhalation agents are taken up by all tissues at rates and total quantities dependent upon tissue blood flow and lipid content. Lean tissue with high blood flow (for example, the brain) will equilibrate with blood (and lung) more quickly than fatty tissue with low blood flow (for example, adipose tissue). High lipid content in a tissue would correspond to high anesthetic solubility in that tissue, and consequently more anesthetic must be taken up before equilibrium with blood is achieved.

While all the inhalation agents are metabolized to some extent, and very small amounts are lost through the skin and urine, the predominant mode for their elimination is via the respiratory tract. The sequence for elimination is the reverse of that described in anesthetic uptake, but the principles are the same. When inspired anesthetic concentration is reduced, the partial pressure gradients then favor elimination of the agent from alveoli, blood, and then tissue, including brain, as before. Those factors favoring rapid uptake and distribution also enhance elimination and excretion. Blood solubility is even more of a factor in elimination of an agent than in its initial uptake. The uptake of an agent can be enhanced by increasing the inspired concentration, even to inspired levels that would be lethal if equilibration were to occur. The potential to do this may be particularly useful in dealing with a very soluble agent because adequate blood concentrations would otherwise be slowly achieved. However, when recovery from anesthesia is desired, inspired anesthetic concentration cannot be reduced below zero, and the pressure gradient that can be achieved is limited. The limiting step becomes the movement of drug from blood to the lungs for elimination from lean, vascular tissues, such as the brain.

Nitrous Oxide

Of the agents notable in the early history of anesthesia development, only nitrous oxide (N_2O) has survived. Its success has been based on its nonflammability and its relative lack of systemic tox-

TABLE 8-2. Physical and clinical properties of inhaled anesthetic agents

	MAC (% atm)	Blood/gas partition coefficient	Vapor pressure (mm Hg; 20° C)	Oil/gas partition coefficient	References
Nitrous oxide	104	0.47	38,516	1.4	30,32,47
Halothane	0.74	2.3	243.3	224	32,81,88
Enflurane	1.68	1.9	175	96.5	30,56,81
Isoflurane	1.15	1.41	238	98	27,30,81

icity. At ambient temperature and pressure, it is a gas; its boiling point at 1 atmosphere pressure is $-88.5°$ C. Its critical temperature (that is, the temperature above which the substance is a gas despite any degree of compression) is $36.5°$ C. At room temperature, it is stored as a liquid in steel cylinders at a pressure of approximately 760 lb/in^2 (equal to 51 atmospheres or 40,000 mm Hg, the vapor pressure of nitrous oxide at room temperature). The gas is odorless, colorless, and nonirritating upon inhalation.

Several properties of nitrous oxide make it unique among currently used inhalation agents. First, as mentioned, it is a gas at room temperature; the other drugs in this class are volatile liquids. Also, it is an inorganic substance; the other agents are halogenated organic compounds. It is the least potent of the agents useful in clinical practice. The MAC of nitrous oxide is generally quoted as 105%, which represents an alveolar partial presence of approximately 805 mm Hg and is clearly not obtainable at ambient pressure. It is this low potency that most hindered the role of nitrous oxide in the early development of anesthesia. Finally, nitrous oxide is the least soluble of the inhalation agents (blood/gas partition coefficient 0.47); it is this property that has carved out a lively role for nitrous oxide in modern anesthesiology practice. The limited solubility of nitrous oxide results in a rapid increase in blood partial pressure and rapid delivery to tissues. Conversely, nitrous oxide is rapidly eliminated from the brain when its administration is discontinued.

The low solubility of nitrous oxide and its low potency make apparent several clinically important properties of inhaled agents, properties that become particularly significant in a consideration of nitrous oxide anesthesia. These include the concentration effect, the second gas effect, diffusion hypoxia, and the effect of an inhaled agent upon a closed gas space in the body.

Increasing the inspired concentration of an inhalation agent will accelerate the development of equilibrium with blood and tissues; this is the concentration effect. Consider that for nitrous oxide several liters can be taken up from the lung during the first few minutes of anesthetic administration in an adult. The uptake of this volume from the alveoli will bring more of the gas mixture into the lungs, further increasing the amount of nitrous oxide presented to the blood. Clearly, raising the inspired concentration

of the agent will enhance its initial blood uptake (increased Δ P) and increase the volume entrained into the lungs; thus the concentration effect.

Similar to the concentration effect is the second gas effect. To visualize this, presume two inhaled agents of different blood solubility administered together. Again, nitrous oxide is ideally considered here because its blood/gas partition coefficient is markedly different from other currently available agents, and nitrous oxide, because of its low potency, is frequently used in combination with another agent. The rapid initial uptake into blood of large volumes of the "first gas" (here nitrous oxide) will also augment the delivery of the second gas to the lungs, contributing thereby to accelerated uptake, distribution, and effect of the second gas.

Diffusion hypoxia is a phenomenon representing the undoing of the second gas and concentration effects. When administration of nitrous oxide is discontinued, the agent diffuses from the blood into the lungs, again moving in the direction of the concentration gradient. The appearance of nitrous oxide in the lungs will dilute the oxygen content there. A patient exposed to room air who has taken up nitrous oxide during the course of an anesthetic could conveivably become hypoxic by this dilution. While understanding diffusion hypoxia contributes to an appreciation of gas uptake and elimination, it is essentially relegated to hypothetical interest because most patients receive supplemental oxygen after the discontinuation of nitrous oxide (or any other inhalation anesthetic) to avoid hypoxia.

While the rapid movement of nitrous oxide from lungs to tissues and back is a major factor in the popularity of nitrous oxide, it also leads to some of the contraindications to nitrous oxide. This arises in the circumstance of a patient with trapped gas spaces in the body. For example, a patient having a pneumothorax may suffer considerably when breathing a mixture containing nitrous oxide. During initial uptake, the nitrous oxide is distributed rapidly and will quickly begin to enter the trapped air pocket, movement being directed by the large concentration gradient between the blood and the trapped air. Nitrous oxide is able to enter the trapped space far faster than nitrogen in the trapped space can diffuse into blood and out of the space; consequently the trapped space enlarges, or alternatively the pressure in the space increases. This phenomenon may occur with air trapped in the cranium, intestine, or even the inflated cuff of an endotracheal tube. This latter phenomenon can lead to increased pressure on the tracheal mucosa or cuff rupture.[94]

When used in general anesthesia, nitrous oxide is usually employed at 40% to 80% inspired concentrations, although lower concentrations may be useful as an analgesic in a conscious individual. In clinically useful concentrations in fit individuals the circulatory effects of nitrous oxide are minimal. The intrinsic cardiac and circulatory depressant effects are balanced by increased sympathetic outflow, suggesting central nervous system excitement; cerebral blood flow and intracranial pressure are minimally affected.[85,86]

Because of its low potency, nitrous oxide is practically never used alone in fit individuals to produce general anesthesia. Nitrous oxide will potentiate the cardiac and circulatory depressant effects of other inhalation agents. The presence of other central nervous system depressants will also unmask the intrinsic negative inotropic properties of nitrous oxide by suppressing central sympathetic outflow.[33] Similarly, the circulatory depressant effects of nitrous oxide may not be tolerated in the hemodynamically unstable patient.*

Despite the concern that the use of nitrous oxide limits the achievable inspired oxygen concentration, it is probably the most commonly used agent in current practice.

Halothane

Halothane is 2-bromo-2-chlor-1,1,1-trifluoroethane (see Figure 8-1). It is the oldest of the halogenated agents still in use. It was introduced in 1956 and widely accepted immediately because of its nonflammability. It is a volatile liquid at ambient temperature and pressure. Halothane is unstable when exposed to light and is marketed in amber bottles. Thymol 0.01% is added to the commercial product for stability and accumulates over time in vaporizers necessitating periodic flushing of vaporizers used for halothane. It is both the most potent (MAC 0.74%) and most soluble (blood/gas partition coefficient 2.3) of agents currently in use (see Table 8-2).

Despite producing a modest decrease in cerebral metabolism as measured by cerebral oxygen con-

sumption ($CMRO_2$), halothane is a potent cerebral vasodilator and increases cerebral blood flow under clinical circumstances.[105] It must therefore be used cautiously when increased intracranial pressure and decreased intracranial compliance are concerns.

Halothane has appreciable negative inotropic properties, generally increasing end-diastolic volume and pressure and decreasing stroke volume, cardiac output, dP/dt, and blood pressure.[93] It has minimal effect on peripheral vascular resistance. Halothane clearly must be used with caution in patients with diminished cardiac reserve.

Halothane is a hydrocarbon derivative. Patients anesthetized with halothane are more susceptible to ventricular arrhythmias than patients receiving other agents.[57] Arrhythmogenicity is markedly enhanced by increased endogenous or exogenous catecholamines; modest hypercarbia frequently contributes to the occurrence of halothane-induced arrhythmias. Ectopy can be seen commonly in individuals with healthy myocardium, and even bigeminy and ventricular tachycardia may be tolerated well in this setting. These arrhythmias are typically self-limiting, are rapidly responsive to antiarrhythmics, or may disappear with hyperventilation, although even in fit individuals disasters can occur.

Halothane is a potent bronchodilator, and has been used therapeutically in refractory asthma.[38] It is the least irritating to the airways of the potent inhalation agents (potent in this context meaning more potent than nitrous oxide), particularly in unanesthetized or lightly anesthetized subjects. Inspired concentration can usually be rapidly increased during induction of anesthesia without provoking coughing and choking. This quality is perhaps halothane's greatest feature in current anesthetic practice.

As with other available inhalation agents, halothane depresses ventilation, mainly via its general depressant effects on brainstem centers. As described elsewhere, there are some important differences in the central respiratory depression between the inhalation agents and the narcotics (see Figure 8-5).

Halothane is mainly eliminated unchanged via exhalation, although it is biotransformed to a considerably greater extent than enflurane or isoflurane. The toxicologic implications of this are discussed elsewhere.[4]

Although the use of halothane has been diminishing as newer agents and techniques have appeared,

---

*References 5, 43, 90, 91, 98.

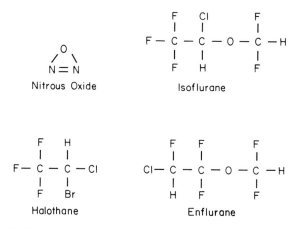

FIGURE 8-3. Chemical structures of inhalational anesthetic agents.

it is certainly an acceptable agent in most circumstances and some of its properties (for example, little systemic vasodilation, absence of airway irritation) suggest that it will remain a useful agent.

Enflurane

Enflurane (see Figure 8-3) is a substituted methyl ethyl ether (2 choloro-1,1,2 trifluoroethyl difluoromethyl ether). It is a volatile liquid, more stable than halothane and requiring no preservative. It is less potent than halothane (MAC 1.68%) and less soluble (blood/gas partition coefficient 1.91). While enflurane's lower solubility facilitates more rapid uptake, distribution, and elimination relative to halothane, enflurane vapor is more irritating to the airways than halothane. Initial uptake by an awake individual is thus limited somewhat by the advisability of slowly increasing the inspired enflurane concentration over several minutes to prevent coughing or laryngospasm. This obstacle can be circumvented by using other drugs (for example, an intravenous induction agent) to diminish responsiveness. After induction, enflurane is a potent bronchodilator comparable to halothane.[45] The central depression of ventilatory centers by enflurane exceeds that by halothane.[21,75]

Enflurane is apparently unique among inhalation agents in its ability to produce an EEG pattern resembling seizure activity, which may be accompanied by muscle twitching in some instances. This phenomenon is usually seen with high inspired enflurane concentrations and, like epileptic seizures, is more apparent during hyperventilatiion.[23,34] Despite the observation that this phenomenon is apparently no more likely in seizure-prone patients, and its significance is unknown, it is common practice to avoid enflurane in individuals with seizure disorders.

In the absence of seizures, enflurane depresses cerebral metabolism more than halothane and causes less cerebral vasodilation than halothane.[67,115] Cerebral blood flow is thus increased less with enflurane than halothane, although caution is again required if there is intracranial pathology.

Unlike halothane, enflurane produces considerable peripheral vasodilation.[21] Thus cardiac output may be better preserved than with halothane under some circumstances, although myocardial contractility is depressed as much or more by enflurane.[18,21] Enflurane does not sensitize the myocardium to catecholamines and therefore, lacks the substantial arrhythmogenic potential of halothane.

Isoflurane

Isoflurane is 1-chloro-2,2,2, trifluoroethyl difluoromethyl ether (see Figure 8-3), an isomer of enflurane. Like enflurane, it is chemically stable and nonflammable. The MAC of isoflurane is 1.15. The blood/gas partition coefficient is 1.4; it is the least soluble of the potent agents available (see Table 8-2).

Uptake, distribution, and elimination are enhanced by the low solubility of isoflurane as compared to halothane or enflurane. Like enflurane and unlike halothane, there can be considerable airway irritation in the lightly anesthetized individual. Isoflurane is also a potent bronchodilator,[46] and can be used therapeutically in refractory asthmatics without the degree of arrhythmia potential associated with the halothane-sensitized myocardium when other bronchodilators (for example, beta-adrenergic agonists) are simultaneously used. The central ventilatory depressant effect of isoflurane is similar to that of halothane.[1]

Isoflurane is the most profound depressant of cerebral metabolism of the inhalation agents. An isoelectric EEG can be achieved by concentrations tolerated in hemodynamically fit patients, accompanied by decreased cerebral oxygen consumption ($CMRO_2$).[55] Isoflurane produces less cerebral vasodilation than halothane or enflurane,[31,77,100,105] thus cerebral blood flow is increased only minimally in the normal patient. Again, in individuals with increased intracranial pressure or decreased intracranial compliance, care must be taken when isoflurane is administered.

Isoflurane is the most potent systemic vasodilator of the inhalation anesthetics. It is the least myocardial depressant of the potent agents; the decrease in cardiac output and dP/dt and the increase in filling pressure and end-diastolic left ventricular volume are significantly less pronounced with isoflurane.* There is frequently a modest increase in heart rate, although myocardial oxygen consumption generally falls.[82]

Isoflurane produces more coronary artery dilatation than halothane or enflurane.[82] The significance of this effect is a subject of controversy; that is, is there significant shunting of blood away from potentially ischemic myocardium in the patient with coronary artery disease (coronary steal)?[22,82,103] While this is debated, isoflurane seems to have a wider margin of cardiovascular safety than halothane or enflurane.

Isoflurane is biotransformed to a lesser extent than either halothane or enflurane.[44] While it has achieved fairly widespread use since its introduction in 1981, the cost of the agent has prevented the displacement of the older agents in many clinical circumstances.

Choice of Agent

For clinical purposes, the selection of an inhalation mixture (agent or agents plus oxygen) can be viewed in two stages: (1) to use or not use nitrous oxide, and in what concentration? and (2) which of the potent agents to use, and in what concentration?

Some practitioners avoid the first question by never using nitrous oxide. This practice is usually based on the satisfaction of giving very high inspired oxygen concentration undiluted by an impotent agent. A more common practice is to use nitrous oxide routinely at inspired concentrations up to about 70%, adjusted as tolerated by the patients' oxygenation, except when specific contraindications exist (for example, pneumothorax, poor pulmonary function requiring high FiO_2, or an uncertain airway with risk for fluctuating oxygenation). This approach permits the use of enough nitrous oxide in most anesthetics to benefit from the unique properties of this agent, specifically rapid induction and emergence,

and decreases the requirement for other longer lasting depressants.

Although there is considerable work done exploring and debating the differences among halothane, enflurane, and isoflurane, they are far more alike than they are different, and in most clinical situations, when administered with sufficient knowledge and skill, are practically interchangeable. There are of course some real differences in the circulatory, cerebral, and metabolic impact of these agents, but these can usually be compensated for by skillful administration. Selection of a specific agent in a particular circumstance is often based as much on familiarity as on the pharmacologic differences.

OPIOID ANALGESICS

An understanding of the pharmacologic basis of current anesthesiology practice without consideration of the narcotics is practically inconceivable. Although used for thousands of years, the role of these drugs intraoperatively has evolved tremendously in just a few decades. Not only have the opioids found a place in modern practice, but in some respects practices and techniques have arisen around the unique properties of these drugs.

The major clinical effects of the opioid analgesics (synonymous to narcotics) are mediated by their action on specific receptors. These opioid receptors are present in many different tissues, but are most concentrated and have been most intensively studied in the central nervous system (CNS), specifically in certain gray matter structures.[35,59] Numerous endogenous polypeptide agonists for these sites have been identified, termed endorphins, enkephalins, and dynorphins.[26,39,51] The physiologic role of these endogenous agonists and their receptors remains uncertain, although many of these endogenous substances exert effects similar to the narcotics.[40]

Various types and subtypes of the opioid receptor have tentatively been identified.[53] The drugs that will be considered here in detail, those with the most important roles in anesthesiology, are all apparently pure agonists at a specific receptor type,[53] judging by the similarities of their actions. The clinical differences among these drugs exist in their potency, pharmacokinetics, and side effects.

Morphine

Despite the development and popularization of synthetic narcotic agonists for anesthesiology, mor-

---

*References 29, 82, 89, 97, 101, 104.

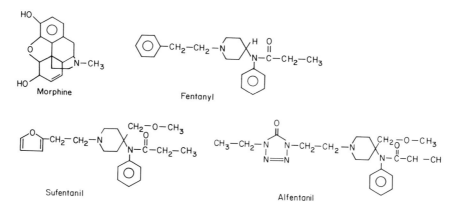

FIGURE 8-4. Chemical structures of narcotic agents used in anesthesia.

TABLE 8-3. **Pharmacokinetic parameters of intravenous narcotics**

	T½ α (min)	T½ β (min)	References
Morphine	9.0-19.8	177	28,76,96
Fentanyl	13.4	219	12
Sufentanil	13.7	164	13,64
Alfentanil	11.6	94	14

phine (Figure 8-4) remains a popular agent and the standard of comparison for other narcotics used in anesthesiology.

Intraoperatively, morphine is most commonly used to supplement the anesthesia provided by an inhalation agent (Table 8-3). In this context an initial dose of 0.1 to 0.25 mg/kg may be used. Supplemental boluses, or continuous infusion, of 0.05 to 0.1 mg/kg/hr may be desirable. Morphine in these doses facilitates the use of lower concentrations of inhalation anesthetics, hopefully providing less cardiovascular depression, more rapid emergence, postoperative analgesia, and adequate anesthesia. This desirable set of conditions can be frequently achieved, sometimes using nitrous oxide as the sole inhalation agent.

Morphine in much higher doses (1 to 4 mg/kg) has been used alone as an anesthetic when it is desirable to avoid all cardiac depressants, most frequently during procedures requiring cardiopulmonary bypass. Such high-dose narcotic anesthesia provides unconsciousness and obtundation of most reflexes. Immobility is usually achieved by addition of appropriate muscle relaxants. Amnesia is not as-

sured with this technique, and most practitioners will include an additional amnestic supplement, such as scopolamine or benzodiazepine.[10,62,95]

Morphine, like the other opioid agonists, produces dose-dependent respiratory depression of a type different from that of the inhalation anesthesics. This difference is apparent from inspection of the CO_2 response curves (Figure 8-5). While narcotics shift the dose response curve, inhalation agents additionally blunt the slope of the curve.

A major clinical difference between morphine and other agents in this class is the degree of histamine released by the drug. The increased circulating histamine levels produced by morphine, in turn, cause increased cardiac index, decreased vascular resistance, and decreased arterial pressure.[74] There is considerable individual variation in the amount of histamine released and in the secondary hemodynamic response. The magnitude of the response is influenced by the rate of morphine administration, and is often most dramatic with initial doses. Hence, when large doses of morphine are used, induction is usually prolonged by the desirability of slow initial dosing of the drug. Although true allergy to mor-

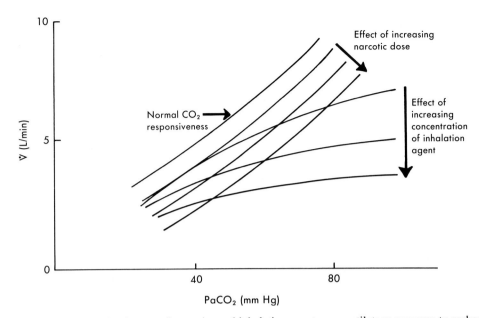

FIGURE 8-5. Relative impact of narcotics and inhalation agents on ventilatory response to carbon dioxide.

phine is quite uncommon, the drug should not be used thoughtlessly in asthmatics or in individuals who have demonstrated past sensitivity to narcotic-induced histamine release.[84,111]

Morphine is far less lipid soluble than other narcotics used in anesthesia. This characteristic slows drug entry into the brain across the blood-brain barrier, and likely slows egress from the central nervous system also. At comparable doses, morphine thus has a slower onset and longer duration than fentanyl or its relatives.

Small amounts appear in the urine and feces unchanged.[116] Morphine is extensively metabolized by the liver to the glucuronide, which is excreted by the kidney.[19,114,116]

Fentanyl

Fentanyl is a synthetic opioid agonist approximately 50 times as potent as morphine. Doses of 1 to 2 mcg/kg may be used to supplement the inhalation agents for surgical anesthesia. Six to ten mcg/kg may be used to supplement agents used for induction of anesthesia and apparently helps to blunt the hemodynamic responses to induction and endotracheal intubation. Much higher doses of fentanyl

have been used as a sole anesthetic. Thirty mcg/kg typically produces unconsciousness. Anesthesia for cardiac surgery can be achieved by 75 to 150 mcg/kg. Higher doses, up to 250 mcg/kg, have been said to blunt neuroendocrine stress responses to surgery, but are rarely used clinically.[117]

When high-dose narcotic anesthesia is desired to avoid cardiac depression, fentanyl is generally preferred to morphine because of its lack of histamine release and associated secondary effects, such as hypotension or vasodilatation. High doses of fentanyl can be administered faster than high doses of morphine, and induction is thus facilitated.

Fentanyl is far more lipid soluble than morphine. This accelerates fentanyl entry into the brain, further enhancing rapid onset of the narcotic effect. Similarly, fentanyl can leave the brain more quickly when blood levels are falling and fentanyl has a shorter duration of action than a roughly comparable dose of morphine, despite similar distribution and elimination kinetics for the two drugs (see Table 8-3).

The duration of the effect of a single dose of fentanyl is quite dependent upon the dose. The analgesic effect of a 1 to 2 mcg/kg bolus may last 1 to 1.5 hours, while 100 mcg/kg may cause analgesic and respiratory depressant effects significant for 12 hours or more. This is because the action of a smaller dose usually ends with redistribution. As compartment saturation occurs with larger doses, the duration becomes dependent upon the slower elimination time. This difference is significant for all the narcotics, but is most pertinent to the consideration of fentanyl because of the wide range of dosages used.

Fentanyl elimination is dependent primarily upon hepatic metabolism. Fentanyl apparently has no active metabolites.[50]

Sufentanil

Sufentanil is a synthetic opioid structurally related to fentanyl. It is approximately 10 times as potent as fentanyl. Sufentanil is the most lipid soluble of the narcotics used routinely in anesthesiology and thus has a very rapid onset. Although time required for sufentanil redistribution (T ½ β) is similar to that for fentanyl, the elimination half-life (T ½ β) is shorter for sufentanil (see Table 8-3). Therefore, while the duration of action of sufentanil in small doses is comparable to that of fentanyl, large doses of sufentanil (as used in unsupplemented narcotic anesthesia) have a shorter duration of action than fentanyl. Sufentanil has minimal effect on the cardiovascular system and, unlike morphine, does not increase circulating histamine levels.

Alfentanil

Like sufentanil, alfentanil is a synthetic opioid structurally related to fentanyl. It is approximately one fourth as potent as fentanyl, and similarly has very little potential for histamine release and secondary cardiovascular change. Both the T ½ α redistribution half-life and the T ½ β elimination half-life are significantly shorter for alfentanil (see Table 8-3) and alfentanil has a much shorter duration of its narcotic effect at both low and high dosages. Although experience with this newly released drug is limited, it would appear to be most useful when used as a continuous infusion.

Other Narcotics

Other opioid agonists and agents with mixed agonist-antagonist actions have been used successfully as supplemental agents in clinical anesthesia; among these are the agonists, (meperidine, alphaprodine, and hydromorphone), and the agonist-antagonists (butorphanol, pentazocine, and nalbuphine).

The agonists differ from morphine, fentanyl, sufentanil, and alfentanil in terms of potency, duration, and cardiovascular side effects, but none offer any particular advantages that cannot be realized with the more popular narcotics used in anesthesia.

The mixed agonist-antagonist agents differ from the others in that high doses produce a diminishing analgesic return, compared to pure agonists. On the other hand, the same ceiling phenomenon is seen in their respiratory depression; the mixed agonist-antagonist agents are not capable of producing the profound respiratory depression seen with high doses, or overdosage, of the pure opioid agonists. Thus they are less versatile than the agonists. Although, when they are administered by experienced individuals, the agonist-antagonist agents may be satisfactory supplements to the inhalation agents.

Role of Narcotics in General Anesthesia

With their effects mediated by specific receptors at multiple levels in the nervous system, the narcotics are clearly different clinically from the inhalation agents, which produce generalized depression. The different actions of the two classes of drugs tend to complement each other so most general anesthetics currently administered employ both classes of agents. The choice of which narcotic and what dose is based upon the type and duration of procedure, coexisting medical problems, anticipation of postoperative pain, the desirability of postoperative mechanical ventilation, and other factors, as well as the familiarity and experience of the anesthesiologist with a particular drug in a particular circumstance. Again, in skilled hands, there is rarely a simple right or wrong choice of agent.

The role of narcotic anesthesia without inhalation agent supplementation is currently limited largely to cardiac surgery, major trauma, and other procedures in hemodynamically unstable patients. Whether this technique will become more popular as shorter acting narcotics agents, such as alfentanil, become more widely available is uncertain.

MUSCLE RELAXANTS

Since their importation from the Amazon rain forests, the muscle relaxants have had a wonderful influence on the safety and conduct of general anesthesia. Introduced into clinical practice in the 1940s, this class of intravenous agents has had perhaps the greatest influence in the development of modern practice.

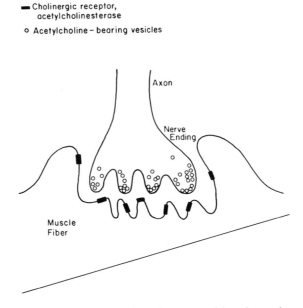

FIGURE 8-6. Schematic representation of myoneural junction and synaptic cleft.

Neuromuscular Physiology

An appreciation of normal neuromuscular transmission contributes to an understanding of the pharmacologic issues associated with the clinical use of muscle relaxants. The term "muscle relaxants" is used here to mean those drugs which cause skeletal muscle relaxation by their effects at the neuromuscular junction.

The neuromuscular junction consists of the unmyelinated terminal portion of a motor nerve, a 20 to 30 nM gap (synaptic cleft), and the motor endplate, the highly folded receptor portion of the muscle fiber. The presynaptic nerve terminal contains vesicles bearing the neurotransmitter acetylcholine, which is released upon depolarization of the distal nerve membrane. Across the synaptic cleft are appropriate receptors, nicotinic cholinergic receptors somewhat different from both the nicotinic receptors of autonomic ganglia and the muscarinic receptors of the autonomic nervous system. Coupling of released acetylcholine to the receptor initiates depolarization of the muscle membrane, and leads to muscle contraction. In the synaptic cleft, the enzyme acetylcholinesterase hydrolyzes the transmitter to acetic acid and choline. The state of the postsynaptic membrane is thus determined by the balance between acetylcholine release and breakdown, in a system with a considerable role for ionic and nonionic modulators and second messengers (Figure 8-6).

The primary mechanism of action of most of the skeletal muscle relaxants used in current practice is blockade of the cholinergic receptors on the postsynaptic membrane. This blockade is reversible and competitive, the degree of blockade (and subsequent muscle relaxation) is thus dependent upon the concentration of relaxant and the concentration of acetylcholine. Only succinylcholine works via a different mechanism.

Succinylcholine

Simply, succinylcholine looks like acetylcholine and acts like acetylcholine but is not metabolized like acetylcholine (Figure 8-7). Succinylcholine is the only clinically important member of a class of drugs termed depolarizing neuromuscular blocking agents.

After reaching the synaptic cleft, succinylcholine is able to occupy cholinergic receptors and, like acetylcholine, produces local depolarization of the muscle membrane, which can be propagated along the muscle fiber. Unlike acetylcholine, succinylcholine is not hydrolyzed by acetylcholinesterase; the drug

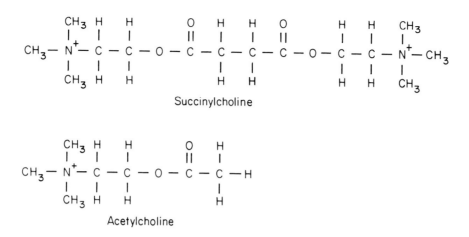

FIGURE 8-7. Chemical structures of acetylcholine and succinylcholine.

lingers near and at the cholinergic receptor, and the membrane cannot repolarize because of continuous receptor stimulation. The muscle fiber itself exhibits a brief period of activity, clinically evident as fasciculation, followed by flaccidity. If the exposure of the end-plate to succinylcholine is brief, the drug will soon diffuse out of the synaptic cleft, and the postsynaptic membrane will repolarize to its usual responsive, resting state. If the succinylcholine is allowed to persist at the membrane, because of either continued administration or altered drug clearance, the postsynaptic membrane will gradually repolarize, but remains blocked. This latter state is referred to as a "phase II block," "dual block," or "desensitized block"—the former circumstance (that is, the initial reaction to succinylcholine) being termed a "depolarized" or "phase I" block. Phase II block is of clinical significance because, although it is similar to a nondepolarized or competitive block in some respects, its response to reversal attempts and its temporal resolution may be unpredictable.[60,61]

Despite some significant drawbacks, succinylcholine has achieved popularity primarily because of its unique biotransformation. The drug is rapidly hydrolyzed by the plasma enzyme pseudocholinesterase to choline and succinic acid. This enzyme is so fast and efficient that only a fraction (5% to 10%) of an administered bolus of succinylcholine is ordinarily available at the site of action, and the duration of the blockade is quite brief, typically about 5 minutes. Because of the need to give a large initial dose to deliver an effective dose to the site of action,

the onset is also very rapid, with complete paralysis achievable in less than 60 seconds. This combination of rapid onset and brief duration was made succinylcholine the agent of choice in some settings in which intubation must be accomplished rapidly. Many practitioners also consider succinylcholine the agent of routine use for most intraoperative intubations.

Succinylcholine is associated with certain clinical hazards unique to this muscle relaxant. Some individuals have a genetically determined inability to metabolize succinylcholine as a result of an atypical pseudocholinesterase. On this basis approximately 1 in 3200 patients will develop paralysis that may last several hours from a usual intubating dose. Proper therapy for this condition, when encountered, is supportive; that is, ventilatory support, reassurance, and perhaps sedation, because conscious paralysis from any of these drugs can be a decidedly unpleasant experience. Approximately 1 in 480 individuals is heterozygous for the gene expressing atypical pseudocholinesterase, and may exhibit paralysis for up to 20 minutes after a usual intubating dose. This is rarely a significant clinical concern.[112]

Several varieties of atypical pseudocholinesterase have been identified. The most common of these is termed the dibucaine-resistant variant. In a standardized assay, normal pseudocholinesterase is markedly inhibited (by approximately 80%) by a given concentration of dibucaine. The dibucaine-resistant variant is inhibited by only about 20% in the same setting. The "dibucaine number" is thus the percent inhibition in the test setting by dibucaine, and is a common determination if there has been an exaggerated response to succinylcholine. Besides the dibucaine-resistant variant, other varieties of atypical pseudocholinesterase have been identified (for example, the fluoride-resistant and silent variants) that may lead to substantially prolonged effects.[112]

It has also been observed that certain drugs, liver disease, cancer, and pregnancy can reduce the level or activity of normal pseudocholinesterase, although in these situations the effect of succinylcholine is rarely prolonged beyond 10 to 20 minutes. This is rarely of clinical concern.[112]

Succinylcholine causes the release of potassium from muscle cells. Serum potassium levels routinely increase transiently by 0.5 to 1.0 meq/L. While this increase is ordinarily well tolerated, the presence of hyperkalemia, or the possible presence of hyperkalemia as in renal failure, must be weighed in the decision to use succinylcholine. There are several pathologic states in which the increase in serum potassium is markedly exaggerated, and cardiac arrest may occur. These include neurologic injury, particularly spinal cord trauma, major trauma, and burns. In these circumstances the muscles seem to be more sensitive to the effects of succinylcholine either because of increased cell membrane sensitivity or because of proliferation of the cholinergic receptors, as in denervated muscle.[42]

Another problem with succinylcholine is the production of diffuse postoperative myalgia.[15] This is most commonly a complaint in patients who have undergone procedures such as bronchoscopy or cystoscopy who are not subject to incisional pain. It is uncertain whether the myalgia is a consequence of the fasciculation produced by succinylcholine or the result of the same subtle injury that causes release of potassium from muscle fibers.

Significant cardiovascular effects of succinylcholine are uncommon. Sinus bradycardia, occasionally profound, may occur with repeated boluses over a short time.[99] This is predominantly a muscarinic effect and may be prevented by prior administration of an anticholinergic.[87]

Increase in intragastric[71] and intraocular[80] pressure may occur with succinylcholine. The advisability of either using or avoiding succinylcholine is quite controversial in patients with eye injury or risk of gastric aspiration (for example, hiatal hernia, pregnancy, or full stomach). When the use of succinylcholine is

elected under such circumstances, precautions are advised.

Some of the hazards of succinylcholine administration may be reduced in intensity by prior intravenous use of a small dose of a nondepolarizing agent such as pancuronium. Unfortunately this practice is most effective in prevention of nuisance effects (for example, fasciculation, postoperative myalgia) but totally unreliable for serious complications such as hyperkalemia and cardiac arrest in the paraplegic patient.*

Despite many undesirable features, succinylcholine is a valuable agent in anesthesiology practice, owing to its unique metabolism and consequent rapid onset and short duration. The usual intubating dose providing complete motor paralysis is typically 0.5 to 1.0 mg/kg, increased to 1.5 to 2.0 mg/kg if a nondepolarizing agent is first given to modify side effects. Smaller doses of succinylcholine (0.1 to 0.25 mg/kg) may be used when a lesser degree of relaxation is adequate, as in the treatment of laryngospasm.

It is hoped and anticipated that there will eventually be developed a nondepolarizing muscle relaxant with sufficiently rapid onset time and duration short enough to replace succinylcholine.

Nondepolarizing Muscle Relaxants

As discussed earlier, these drugs work by occupation of cholinergic receptors on the motor endplate, and preventing occupation of the receptor by acetylcholine. Binding is reversible and competitive and does not result in membrane depolarization, hence the designation competitive or nondepolarizing agents. Several drugs of this class have been developed and incorporated into clinical use. They differ in potency, duration, side effects, and mode of elimination, and are discussed here separately.

d-Tubocurarine

d-Tubocurarine (dTC, Figure 8-8) was introduced into clinical practice in the 1940s, the first muscle relaxant used as a supplement to anesthesia. Despite concerns then as now that the use of this drug, or any other muscle relaxant, interferes with the assessment of anesthetic depth, so that a patient may be awake and paralyzed, the ability to produce immobility in the unconscious individual by means

*References 11, 58, 66, 68, 110.

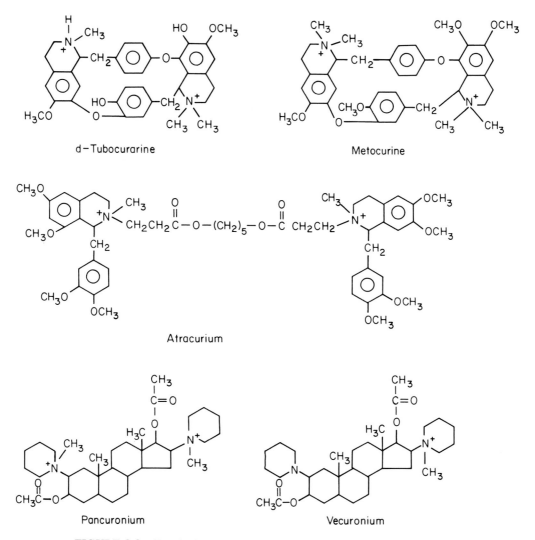

FIGURE 8-8. Chemical structures of the nondepolarizing muscle relaxants.

other than very deep anesthesia is frequently invaluable.

Administration of dTC produces a dose-dependent fall in blood pressure, caused primarily by histamine release, but there is a contribution by blockade of autonomic ganglia.[65] Because of this hypotensive effect, dTC is rarely used in doses large enough to provide relaxation for endotracheal intubation. dTC may be particularly useful however in hypertensive patients during other phases of an operative procedure.

An administered dose of dTC will typically begin to wear off in approximately 20 minutes, although there remains considerable residual effect after 2 to 4 hours. The drug is primarily excreted unchanged in the urine. Variable amounts of the drug are metabolized or excreted in bile. Biliary excretion is enhanced in renal failure and dTC is a reasonable agent in that setting, although its duration of action will be somewhat prolonged. Redistribution is slow, contributing only modestly to the waning of the agent's effect.

TABLE 8-4. Dosage schedules for nondepolarizing muscle relaxants*

	Relative potency[a]	Precurarization dose (mg/kg)	Intubation dose (mg/kg)	Maintenance dose (mg/kg/hr)
Pancuronium	1	0.01-0.02	0.08-0.15	0.01-0.02
Vecuronium	0.9	0.01-0.02	0.07-0.15	0.02-0.04
d-tubocurarine	7	0.04-0.1	b	0.08-0.15
Metocurine	3	0.03-0.06	0.025-0.5	0.03-0.08
Atracurium	20	0.15-0.25	0.5-0.6	0.15-0.3

*These doses represent approximations only. Actual dose requirements should be ascertained on clinical grounds.
[a] Dose equipotent to 1 mg pancuronium.
[b] Rarely used for this indication because of side effects.

Typical dosing for dTC is described in Table 8-4.

Pancuronium

Pancuronium is a steroid derivative (see Figure 8-8). Its duration of action is similar to that of dTC; among nondepolarizing agents it is considered a long acting agent. It does not exhibit histamine release or ganglionic blockade, and lacks the hypotensive tendencies of dTC. Pancuronium does have modest vagolytic properties and can produce an increase in heart rate. The degree of tachycardia produced is infrequently a problem, even in the dosage range required to achieve adequate conditions for intubation. In patients for whom increased heart rate may be hazardous, pancuronium may not be the best available agent when muscle relaxation is required.

Pancuronium is more dependent upon renal excretion than dTC. It is metabolized to a greater extent than dTC, but its metabolites possess significant neuromuscular blocking effect.[69] Pancuronium is probably best avoided in patients with renal insufficiency unless postoperative mechanical ventilation is planned.

Metocurine

Metocurine (see Figure 8-8) is a methylated derivative of dTC. Its potency is intermediate between those of pancuronium and dTC (see Table 8-4). Its duration of action is similar to that of dTC.

Metocurine is devoid of vagolytic tendencies. It does produce some release of histamine from tissues, but to a lesser extent than dTC. At doses used clinically, it lacks the ganglionic blocking effect of dTC.

Administration of metocurine can lower arterial pressure, although even doses sufficient for intubation are usually adequately tolerated. The absence of the tachycardia that can be produced by pancuronium may be quite desirable under some circumstances (for example, patients with coronary artery disease).

Metocurine is dependent upon renal function for excretion[16] and, like pancuronium, its use in patients with renal failure should not be undertaken lightly.

Atracurium

Atracurium (see Figure 8-8) is a nondepolarizing agent with a duration of action considerably shorter than that of pancuronium; it is considered to be of "intermediate" duration because it lasts longer than succinylcholine. A dose sufficient for intubation is largely worn off in 35 to 45 minutes. The drug is thus valuable for shorter surgical procedures. Atracurium owes its abbreviated effect to plasma hydrolysis. At least two different routes are involved, hydrolysis by plasma esterase and nonenzymatic breakdown.[70] Consequently, atracurium is useful in patients with renal insufficiency.

Atracurium does cause some release of histamine.[8] The hypotensive effect of an intubating dose is comparable to that seen with metocurine and is infrequently problematic. Atracurium produces no vagal or ganglionic blockade.

The onset of action of atracurium is a bit slower than that of the other nondepolarizing agents[83] even when larger doses are used, necessitating patience on the part of the practitioner when the drug is used to facilitate intubation. Despite this drawback, the unique metabolism of atracurium and its consequent abbreviated duration of action make it a useful agent in some settings.

Vecuronium

Vecuronium is a relaxant of intermediate duration of action, structurally quite similar to pancuronium (see Figure 8-8). Its potency is nearly identical to that of pancuronium also. The considerably shorter duration of action of vecuronium is mainly attributed to more rapid redistribution.[70,92] Vecuronium is extensively metabolized to less active metabolites than those of pancuronium. Vecuronium is less dependent upon renal excretion than pancuronium, a considerable portion ordinarily being eliminated in bile.

Vecuronium is devoid of cardiovascular side effects.[7] This feature contributes to its desirability in a variety of clinical circumstances.

Other Nondepolarizing Agents

Gallamine, alcuronium, and fazadinium are three other long acting nondepolarizing agents. Gallamine and fazadinium both produce substantially more tachycardia than pancuronium and are devoid of redeeming features. Alcuronium produces a degree of tachycardia similar to that of pancuronium, and is a mild ganglionic blocker as well. Of these agents, only gallamine has ever been commercially available in the United States and it is rarely used today.

Dosage and Monitoring

Although typical dosage requirements for clinical use of the muscle relaxants is indicated in Table 8-4, accurate titration is desirable to prevent excessive dosing and possible prolonged effect, or underdosing and patient movement intraoperatively. For this reason, monitoring the degree of neuromuscular blockade is recommended. This is readily accomplished with any of a number of marketed electrical nerve-stimulating devices. The techniques involved are described elsewhere.[2]

Reversal of Neuromuscular Blockade

The ability to reverse residual effects of muscle relaxants at the end of a surgical procedure contributes to the safety and convenience of these drugs. Because the nondepolarizing agents work by competitively blocking the cholinergic receptor, neuromuscular transmission can be enhanced by increasing the availability of acetylcholine in the synaptic cleft. This is ordinarily accomplished by administering an agent that inhibits acetylcholinesterase. Several such agents are available.

The most popular of the cholinesterase inhibitors is neostigmine. At a dosage of 0.03 to 0.08 mg/kg, the onset of its effect is usually seen in 3 to 5 minutes, with peak reversal apparent at 8 to 10 minutes. At the dosage used for reversal of blockade, the muscarinic stimulation produced is impressive and may be devastating (for example, profound heart block, asystole); oral secretions are greatly increased. Therefore, neostigmine, when used for reversal, should always be accompanied by an anticholinergic agent. Atropine 0.010 to 0.018 mg/kg is adequate. Glycopyrrolate 0.005 to 0.010 mg/kg is also good and is associated with less initial tachycardia than atropine.[6,72]

Edrophonium and pyridostigmine are other cholinesterase inhibitors useful in the reversal of neuromuscular blockade. Edrophonium has the advantage of very rapid onset, often apparent in 90 seconds. It is one tenth to one twentieth as potent as neostigmine. Edrophonium has the potential disadvantage of a duration of action that may be exceeded by that of the relaxants themselves, although reappearance of neuromuscular blockade after adequate reversal with any of the cholinesterase inhibitors is decidedly uncommon. Pyridostigmine has a slower onset and longer duration of action than neostigmine, and is approximately one fourth as potent. It reportedly produces fewer muscarinic side efects than neostigmine, but caution nevertheless dictates that it should not be given without a muscarinic inhibitor (for example, atropine).

CONCLUSIONS

Besides the agents discussed here, a complete text of pharmacological principles in anesthesiology would need to include discussions of drugs from many other classes, including major and minor tranquilizers, local anesthetics, antiarrhythmics, sympathomimetics, alpha-adrenergic and beta-adrenergic blockers, vasodilators, anticholinergics, and others. Agent selection is only part of an anesthetic plan and is rarely a critical part of anesthetic management. Success of an anesthetic plan and ease of immediate postoperative management, however, are greatly facilitated by a thorough understanding of the pharmacology of the agents involved.

REFERENCES

1. Alageson K et al: Comparison of the respiratory depressant effects of halothane and isoflurane in routine surgery, Br J Anaesth 59:1070-1079, 1987.
2. Ali HH and Miller RD: Monitoring of neuromuscular function. In Miller RD (editor): Anesthesia, ed 2, New York, 1986, Churchill Livingstone.
3. Ambre JJ et al: Pharmacokinetics of etomidate, a new intravenous anesthetic, Fed Proc 36:997, 1977.
4. Baden JM and Rice SA: Metabolism and toxicity of inhaled anesthetics. In Miller RD (editor): Anesthesia, ed 2, New York, 1986, Churchill Livingstone.
5. Bahlman SH et al: The cardiovascular effects of nitrous oxide-halothane anesthesia in man, Anesthesiology 35:274-285, 1971.
6. Baraka A et al: Glycopyrrolate-neostigmine and atropine-neostigmine mixtures affect post-anesthetic arousal times differently, Anesth Analg 59:431-434, 1980.
7. Barnes PK et al: Comparison of the effects of ORG NC45 and pancuronium bromide on heart rate and arterial pressure in anesthetized man, Br J Anaesth 54:435-439, 1982.
8. Basta SJ et al: Histamine-releasing potencies of atracurium, dimethyl-tubocurarine, and tubocurarine, Br J Anaesth 55:105-106S, 1983.
9. Beaupre PN et al: Isoflurane, halothane, and enflurane depress myocardial contractility in patients undergoing surgery, Anesthesiology 59:A59, 1983.
10. Bennett GM, Loeser EA, and Stanley TH: Cardiovascular effects of scopolamine during morphine-oxygen and morphine-nitrous oxide-oxygen anesthesia in man, Anesthesiology 46:225-227, 1977.
11. Birch AA et al: Changes in serum potassium response to succinylcholine following trauma, JAMA 210:490-493, 1969.
12. Bovill JG et al: The pharmacokinetics of sufentanil in surgical patients, Anesthesiology 61:502-506, 1984.
13. Bovill JG et al: Kinetics of alfentanil and sufentanil: a comparison, Anesthesiology 55:A174, 1981.
14. Bovill JG et al: The pharmacokinetics of alfentanil (R39209): a new opioid analgesic, Anesthesiology 57:439-443, 1982.
15. Brodsky JB, Brock-Unte JG, and Samuels SI: Pancuronium pretreatment and post-succinylcholine myalgias, Anesthesiology 51:259-261, 1979.
16. Brotherton WP and Matteo RS: Pharmacokinetics and pharmacodynamics of metocurine in humans with and without renal failure, Anesthesiology 55:273-276, 1981.
17. Brown CR et al: Clinical, electroencephalographic, and pharmacokinetic studies of a water soluble benzodiazepine, midazolam maleate, Anesthesiology 50:467-470, 1979.
18. Brown BR and Crout JR: A comparative study of the effects of five general anesthetics on myocardial contractility. I. Isometric conditions, Anesthesiology 34:236-245, 1971.
19. Brunk SF and Della M: Morphine metabolism in man, Clin Pharmacol Ther 16:51-57, 1974.
20. Burch PG and Stanski DR: The role of metabolism and protein binding in thiopental anesthesia, Anesthesiology 58:145-152, 1983.
21. Calverley RK et al: Ventilatory and cardiovascular effects of enflurane during spontaneous ventilation in man, Anesth Analg 57:610-618, 1978.
22. Cason BA et al: Effects of isoflurane and halothane on coronary vascular resistance and collateral myocardial blood flow: their capacity to induce coronary steal, Anesthesiology 67:665-675, 1987.
23. Clark DL and Rosner BS: Neurophysiologic effects of general anesthetics. I. The electroencephalogram and sensory evoked responses in man, Anesthesiology 38:564-582, 1973.
24. Clements JA and Nimmo WS: Pharmacokinetics and analgesic effect of ketamine in man, Br J Anaesth 53:27-30, 1981.
25. Cook TL et al: Renal effects and metabolism of servoflurane in Fischer 344 rats: an in-vivo and in-vitro comparison with methoxyflurane, Anesthesiology 43:70-77, 1975.
26. Cox BM et al: A peptide-like substance from pituitary that acts like morphine. Purification and properties, Life Sci 16:1777-1782, 1975.
27. Cromwell TH et al: Forane uptake, excretion, and blood solubility in man, Anesthesiology 35:365-373, 1971.
28. Dahlström B et al: Morphine kinetics in children, Clin Pharmacol Ther 26:354-365, 1979.
29. Dolan WM et al: The cardiovascular and respiratory effects of isoflurane-nitrous oxide anesthesia, Can Anaesth Soc J 21:557-568, 1974.
30. Dorsch JA and Dorsch SE: Understanding anesthesia equipment: construction, care, and complications, ed 2, Baltimore, 1984, Williams & Wilkins.
31. Drummond JC et al: Brain surface protrusion during enflurane, halothane, and isoflurane anesthesia in cats, Anesthesiology 59:288-293, 1983.
32. Eger EI and Larson CP, Jr: Anesthetic solubility in blood and tissues: values and significance, Br J Anaesth 36:140-149, 1964.
33. Eisele JH et al: Myocardial performance and N_2O analgesia in coronary artery disease, Anesthesiology 44:16-20, 1976.
34. Fleming DC et al: Diagnostic activation of epileptogenic foci by enflurane, Anesthesiology 52:431-433, 1980.
35. Franz DM, Hare BD and McCloskey KL: Spinal sympathetic neurons: possible sites of opiate with-

drawal suppression by clonidine, Science 215:1643-1645, 1982.

36. Ghoneim MM and Van Hamme MJ: Pharmacokinetics of thiopentone: effects of enflurane and nitrous oxide anesthesia and surgery, Br J Anaesth 50:1237-1242, 1978.

37. Ghoneim MM and Yamada T: Etomidate: a clinical and electroencephalographic comparison with thiopental, Anesth Analg 56:479-485, 1977.

38. Gold MI and Helrich M: Pulmonary mechanics during general anesthesia. V. Status asthmaticus, Anesthesiology 32:422-428, 1970.

39. Goldstein A et al: Porcine pituitary dynorphin: complete amino acid sequence of the biologically active heptadecapeptide, Proc Natl Acad Sci USA 78:7219-7223, 1981.

40. Goldstein AL: Opioid peptides (endorphins) in pituitary and brain, Science 193:1081-1086, 1976.

41. Greenblatt DJ et al: Automated gas chromatography for studies of midazolam pharmacokinetics, Anesthesiology 55:176-179, 1981.

42. Gronert GA and Theye RA: Pathophysiology of hyperkalemia induced by succinylcholine, Anesthesiology 43:89-99, 1975.

43. Hill GE et al: Cardiovascular response to nitrous oxide during light, moderate and deep halothane anesthesia in man, Anesth Analg 57:84-94, 1978.

44. Holaday DA et al: Resistance of isoflurane to biotransformation in man, Anesthesiology 43:325-332, 1975.

45. Hirshman CA and Bergman NA: Halothane and enflurane protect against bronchospasm in an experimental asthma dog model, Anesth Analg 57:629-633, 1978.

46. Hirshman CA et al: Mechanism of action of inhalational anesthesia on airways, Anesthesiology 56:107-111, 1982.

47. Hornbein TF et al: The minimum alveolar concentration of nitrous oxide in man, Anesth Analg 61:553-556, 1982.

48. Horrigan RW et al: Etomidate vs. thiopental with and without fentanyl—a comparative study of awakening in man, Anesthesiology 52:362-364, 1980.

49. Hudson RJ, Stanski DR, and Burch PG: Pharmacokinetics of methohexital and thiopental in surgical patients, Anesthesiology 59:215-219, 1983.

50. Hug LL and Murphy MR: Tissue redistribution of fentanyl and termination of its effects in rats, Anesthesiology 55:369-375, 1981.

51. Hughes J et al: Identification of two related pentapeptides from the brain with opiate agonist activity, Nature 258:577-579, 1975.

52. Ingram GS, Payne JP and Perry IR: Electroencephalographic patterns during anesthetic induction with etomidate, Br J Clin Pharmacol 3:35-37S, 1976.

53. Iwamato ET and Martin WR: Multiple opioid receptors, Med Res Rev 1:411-440, 1981.

54. Katoh T and Ikeda K: The minimum alveolar concentration (MAC) of sevoflurane in man, Anesthesiology 66:301-303, 1987.

55. Kavan EM and Julien RM: Central nervous system effects of isoflurane (Forane), Can Anaesth Soc J 21:390-402, 1974.

56. Koblin DD et al: Minimum alveolar concentrations and oil/gas partition coefficients of four anesthetic isomers, Anesthesiology 54:314-317, 1981.

57. Koehntop DE, Liao JC, and Van Bergen FH: Effects of pharmacologic alterations of adrenergic mechanisms by cocaine, tropolone, aminophylline, and ketamine on epinephrine-induced arrhythmias during halothane-nitrous oxide anesthesia, Anesthesiology 46:83-93, 1977.

58. Konchigeri HN, Lee YE, and Venugopal K: Effect of pancuronium on intraocular pressure changes induced by succinylcholine, Can Anaesth Soc J 26:479-481, 1979.

59. Kuhar MJ, Pert CB, and Snyder SH: Regional distribution of opiate receptor binding in monkey and human brain, Nature 245:447-450, 1973.

60. Lee C: Dose relationships of phase II, tachyphylaxis and train-of-fade in suxemethonium-induced dual neuromuscular blockade in man, Br J Anaesth 47:841-845, 1975.

61. Lee C and Katz RL: Neuromuscular pharmacology. A clinical update and commentary, Br J Anaesth 52:173-188, 1980.

62. Lowenstein E: Morphine "anesthesia"—a perspective, Anesthesiology 35:563-565, 1971.

63. Lundy PM, Gowdy CW, and Calhoun FH: Tracheal smooth muscle relaxant effect of ketamine, Br J Anaesth 46:333-336, 1974.

64. McClain DA and Hug CC, Jr: Intravenous fentanyl kinetics, Clin Pharmacol Ther 28:106-114, 1980.

65. McCullough LS et al: The effects of d-tubocurarine on spontaneous post-ganglionic sympathetic activity and histamine release, Anesthesiology 33:328-334, 1970.

66. Meyers EF et al: Failure of nondepolarizing neuromuscular blockers to inhibit succinylcholine-induced increased intraocular pressure, a controlled study, Anesthesiology 48:149-151, 1978.

67. Michenfelder JD and Cucchiaria RF: Canine cerebral oxygen consumption during enflurane anesthesia and its modification during induced seizures, Anesthesiology 40:575-580, 1974.

68. Miller RD: The advantages of giving d-tubocurarine before succinylcholine, Anesthesiology 37:568-569, 1972.

69. Miller RD et al: The comparative potency and pharmacokinetics of pancuronium and its metabolites in

anesthetized man, J Pharmacol Exp Ther 207:539-543, 1978.

70. Miller RD et al: Clinical pharmacology of vecuronium and atracruium, Anesthesiology 61:444-453, 1984.

71. Miller RD and Way WL: Inhibition of succinylcholine-induced increased intragastric pressure by nondepolarizing muscle relaxants and lidocaine, Anesthesiology 34:185-188, 1971.

72. Mirakhur RK, Dundee JW, and Clarke RSJ: Glycopyrrolate-neostigmine mixture for antagonism of neuromuscular block: comparison with atropine-neostigmine mixture, Br J Anaesth 49:825-829, 1977.

73. Morgan DJ et al: Pharmacokinetics and plasma binding of thiopental. I. Studies in surgical patients, Anesthesiology 54:468-473, 1981.

74. Moss J and Rosow CE: Histamine release by narcotics and muscle relaxants in humans, Anesthesiology 59:330-339, 1983.

75. Munson ES et al: The effects of halothane, fluroxene, and cyclopropane and ventilation: a comparative study in man, Anesthesiology 27:716-728, 1966.

76. Murphy MR and Hug CC, Jr: Pharmacokinetics of morphine in patients anesthetized with enflurane-nitrous oxide, Anesthesiology 54:187-192, 1981.

77. Newberg LA, Milde JH, and Michenfelder JD: The cerebral metabolic effects of isoflurane at and above concentrations that suppress cerebral cortical activity, Anesthesiology 59:23-28, 1983.

78. Nudel DB, Berman MA, and Talner NS: Effects of acutely increasing systemic vascular resistance on oxygen tension in tetrology of Fallot, Pediatrics 58:248-251, 1976.

79. Parikh RK and Moore MR: Effect of certain anesthetic agents on the activity of rat hepatic delta-aminolaevulinate synthetase, Br J Anaesth 50:1099-1103, 1978.

80. Pandey K, Gadola RP, and Dumar S: Time course of intraocular hypertension produced by suxemethonium, Br J Anaesth 44:191-196, 1972.

81. Quasha AL, Eger EI II, and Tinker JH: Determination and applications of MAC, Anesthesiology 53:315-334, 1980.

82. Reiz S et al: Isoflurane—a powerful coronary vasodilator in patients with coronary artery disease, Anesthesiology 59:91-97, 1983.

83. Robertson EN et al: Clinical comparison of atracurium and vercuronium (ORG NC45), Br J Anaesth 55:125-129, 1983.

84. Rosow CE et al: Histamine release during morphine and fentanyl anesthesia, Anesthesiology 56:93-96, 1982.

85. Sakabe T, et al: Cerebral effects of nitrous oxide in the dog, Anesthesiology 48:195-200, 1978.

86. Sakabe T et al: Cerebral responses to the addition of nitrous oxide to halothane in man, Br J Anaesth 48:957-962, 1976.

87. Schoenstadt DA and Witcher CE: Observations on the mechanism of succinyldicholine-induced cardiac arrhythmias, Anesthesiology 24:358-362, 1963.

88. Secher O: Physical and chemical data on anesthetics, Acta Anaesthesiol Scand 42S:1-95, 1971.

89. Shulte AM et al: The influence of etomidate and thipentone on the intracranial pressure elevated by nitrous oxide, Anaesthetist 29:525-529, 1980.

90. Smith NT et al: Impact of nitrous oxide on the circulation during enflurane anesthesia in man, Anesthesiology 48:345-349, 1978.

91. Smith NT et al: The cardiovascular and sympathomimetic responses to the addition of nitrous oxide to halothane in man, Anesthesiology 32:410-421, 1970.

92. Sohn YJ et al: Pharmacokinetics of vecuronium in man, Anesthesiology 57:A256, 1982.

93. Sonntag H et al: Left ventricular function in conscious man and halothane anesthesia, Anesthesiology 48:320-324, 1978.

94. Stanley TH, Kawamura R, and Graves C: Effects of nitrous oxide on volume and pressure of endotracheal tube cuffs, Anesthesiology 41:256-262, 1974.

95. Stanley TH and Webster LR: Anesthetic requirements and cardiovascular effects of fentanyl-oxygen and fentanyl-diazepam-oxygen anesthesia in man, Anesth Analg 57:411-416, 1978.

96. Stanski D, Greenblatt DJ, and Lowesnstein E: Kinetics of intravenous and intramuscular morphine, Clin Pharmacol Ther 24:52-59, 1978.

97. Stevens WC et al: The cardiovascular effects of a new inhalation anesthetic, Forane, in human volunteers at constant arterial carbon dioxide tension, Anesthesiology 35:8-16, 1971.

98. Stoelting RK and Gibbs PS: Hemodynamic effects of morphine and morphine-nitrous oxide in valvular heart disease and coronary artery disease, Anesthesiology 38:45-52, 1973.

99. Stoelting RK and Peterson C: Heart-rate slowing and junctional rhythm following intravenous succinylcholine with and without intramuscular atropine preanesthetic medication, Anesth Analg 54:705-709, 1975.

100. Stulken EH et al: The non-linear response of cerebral metabolism to low concentrations of halothane, enflurane, isoflurane, and thiopental. Anesthesiology 46:28-34, 1977.

101. Sybert PE et al: Effects of volatile anesthetics on the regulation of coronary blood flow, 59:A24, 1983.

102. Takeshita H, Okuda Y, and Sari A: The effects of ketamine on cerebral circulation and metabolism in man, Anesthesiology 36:69-75, 1972.

103. Tarnow J, Markschies-Horning A, and Schulte-Sasse U: Isoflurane improves the tolerance to pacing-induced myocardial ischemia, Anesthesiology 64:147-156, 1986.

104. Theye RA and Michenfelder JD: Individual organ contributions to the decrease in whole body $\dot{V}O_2$ with isoflurane, Anesthesiology 42:35-40, 1975.

105. Todd MM and Drummond JC: A comparison of the cerebrovascular and metabolic effects of halothane and isoflurane in the cat, Anesthesiology 60:276-282, 1984.

106. Todd MM, Drummond JC, and U HS: The hemodynamic consequences of high-dose thiopental anesthesia, Anesth Analg 64:681-687, 1985.

107. Traber DL, Wilson RD, and Priano LL: Differentration of the cardiovascular effects of CI-581, Anesth Analg 47:769-778, 1968.

108. Van Hamme MJ, Ghoneim MM, and Ambre JJ: Pharmacokinetics of etomidate, a new intravenous anesthetic, Anesthesiology 49:274-277, 1978.

109. Wagner RL et al: Inhibition of adrenal steroidogenesis by the anesthetic etomidate, N Engl J Med 310:1415-1420, 1984.

110. Walts LF and Dillon JB: Clinical studies of the interaction between d-tubocurarine and succinylcholine, Anesthesiology 31:39-52, 1969.

111. Watkins J: Anaphylactoid reactions to IV substances, Br J Anaesth 51:51-60, 1979.

112. Whittaker M: Plasma cholinesterase variants and the anaesthetist, Anaesthesia 35:174-197, 1980.

113. Wieber J et al: Pharmacokinetics of ketamine in man, Anaesthetist 24:260-263, 1975.

114. Wolff WA, Riegel C, and Fry EG: The excretion of morphine by normal and tolerant dogs, J Pharmacol Exp Ther 47:391-410, 1933.

115. Wollmann H, Smith AL, and Hoffman JC: Cerebral blood flow and oxygen consumption in man during electroencephalographic seizure patterns induced with ethrane, Fed Proc 28:356, 1969.

116. Yeh SY: Urinary excretion of morphine and its metabolites in morphine dependent subjects, J Pharmacol Exp Ther 192:201-210, 1975.

117. Zurick AM et al: Comparison of hemodynamic and hormonal effects of large single-dose fentanyl anesthesia and halothane/nitrous oxide anesthesia for coronary artery surgery, Anesth Analg 61:521-526, 1982.

CHAPTER 9

Regional Versus General Anesthesia

CHARLES BEATTIE

While the discovery and development of anesthesia have been embraced enthusiastically by modern society, there continues to be concern about the risks of anesthetic procedures. Morbidity and mortality secondary to anesthesia are viewed more critically, perhaps, than incidents within other medical specialties because the practice of anesthesia is not usually considered to be therapeutic. Complications are perceived as especially tragic, and risk assessment and minimization are of paramount importance.

Efforts to reduce risk fall into two categories: (1) the development of equipment, agents, and techniques for routine use to lessen morbidity in otherwise healthy persons presenting for elective surgery and (2) the creation of specialized methodology to enable seriously ill persons, clearly at "high risk" for perioperative difficulties, to undergo necessary surgery safely. The first category includes introduction of improved anesthetic agents with high therapeutic indices, medications to reduce acidity and volume of stomach contents (aspiration prophy-

laxis), and development of pulse oximetry and end-tidal CO_2 monitoring to enable immediate assessment of oxygenation and ventilation. In the second category are advanced techniques of invasive and noninvasive monitoring (thermodilution pulmonary artery catheters, echocardiography) combined with hemodynamic manipulations by means of potent cardiovascular agents.

Many surgical procedures can be performed with some form of neural conduction blockade, commonly called "regional" anesthesia, as either an adjunct to general anesthesia or as the sole anesthetic technique. Often the regional block can be limited to the anatomic location of surgery and thus intuitively, it may seem less dangerous than general anesthesia, which resembles a globally toxic state.[47] It is possible, therefore, that regional anesthesia could contribute to both categories of risk minimization. The relative safety of regional versus general anesthesia has been vigorously debated within the specialty of anesthesia[30,88] and remains a matter of concern for internal medicine and cardiology consultants who are called on to render presurgical evaluations. The anesthesia literature is replete with investigations comparing specific end-points in groups undergoing the two types of anesthesia, but they have not led to a common understanding among practitioners. Interestingly, there is least agreement concerning "high-risk" patients who arouse the most concern.

A major cause for the failure to resolve this issue lies in the nature of anesthetic practice. In spite of great advances within the specialty of anesthesia and stringent controls on anesthesia education imposed by the American Board of Anesthesiology, the practice of anesthesia (as with most other areas of medicine) encompasses a wide range of procedural latitude. There is little agreement on management issues such as indications for invasive monitoring, use and manipulation of measured or derived hemodynamic parameters, appropriate limits for blood pressure and heart rate, the "style" of induction, maintenance and emergence, the need for intraoperative pulmonary toilet, methods of temperature control, maintenance of oxygenation and ventilation postoperatively, and methods of postoperative pain relief. With rare exceptions, clinical investigations in anesthesia either fail to mention or give only the most superficial details of anesthetic management. Since all of these aspects of clinical care vary greatly from practitioner to practitioner, it is difficult to determine whether outcome differences in studies comparing regional anesthesia with general anesthesia are universally applicable or only obtain in the investigators' institution.

In this chapter we outline the fundamental methodologic differences between and within the two classes of anesthetic techniques. We also review the literature and present studies that have compared regional and general anesthesia with respect to various end-points including morbidity and mortality. It will be seen that with very few and rather specialized exceptions, broad statements regarding the advisability of one type of anesthesia over another are unwarranted.

GENERAL ANESTHESIA
Principles

This section summarizes the major features of general anesthesia, including the pharmacologic agents employed in its routine delivery. Other medications used in special cases to manipulate physiologic mechanisms are also discussed. Techniques of modern anesthetic care, including invasive monitoring as well as the traditional anesthesia procedures such as endotracheal intubation and mechanical ventilatory support, are reviewed.

The physiologic state of general anesthesia may be defined as a reversible condition of unconscious unresponsiveness to noxious stimuli caused by pharmacologic agents acting throughout the nervous system. This definition implies specific and distinguishable goals: (1) unconsciousness—absence of purposeful movement associated with verbal or mild tactile stimulation (usually assumed to include amnesia) and (2) unresponsiveness—originally defined as lack of movement in response to a painful stimulus, but in modern anesthesia care it also includes blunting or elimination of cardiovascular and pulmonary responses. There are many ways of producing the several elements that, in aggregate, constitute the anesthetic state. Immobility, common to both end-points, is clearly important to enable surgery to proceed and is often adequately achieved by inhalational and intravenous medications that are not primarily paralytic.[75] More complete, controlled paralysis, produced by neuromuscular blockers, may be required. Competitive inhibitors of the motor endplate are useful adjuncts to central nervous system agents to ensure a completely quiescent surgical field. However, they have disadvantages including masking inadequate or "light" general anesthesia. Postoperative recall of surgical events has been reported.[100] Some muscle relaxants have direct cardiovascular effects (vagotonic, vagolytic, and vasodilatory), and long-acting agents often require reversal with competitive antagonists, which can produce disturbances of cardiac rhythm, conduction, and rate.

The cascade effect, wherein an intervention is associated with consequences that in turn necessitate subsequent therapies, is particularly dramatic in the practice of anesthesia. Accordingly, it is well to consider all conceivable options when tailoring a plan that will be appropriate for an individual patient.

Adequate ventilation and oxygenation are essential regardless of the anesthetic agents and techniques employed. The additional requirement of preventing pulmonary aspiration of stomach contents has made endotracheal intubation an inevitable accompaniment to general anesthesia in the minds of many.

Some investigators include intubation as part of the general anesthesia regimen without mention of alternative methods of airway management.[33,72] The benefits of intubation, however, must be viewed in light of its drawbacks and the real indications for the procedure kept in mind. Direct laryngoscopy with intubation is a stress probably equal to a major surgical incision.[37] It requires administration of potent sedatives or analgesics and, usually, a short-acting muscle relaxant. Intubation is also associated with complications such as oral and laryngeal trauma[87] and esophageal intubation. Since most patients presenting for elective surgery are presumed to have "empty" stomachs and are not otherwise at risk for aspiration, it is frequently feasible to administer general anesthesia while managing the airway with a mask and controlling or assisting ventilation. If the nature of the surgical procedure leaves this possibility open, then numerous drugs and stressors may be avoided.

The issues of muscle relaxation and intubation are germane to the goal of this chapter. An informed consultant and effective practitioner must have a sense of the options of anesthetic practice and not be forced into rigid assumptions that limit the ability to minimize risk on a case-by-case basis. Further, interpretation of clinical studies may only fairly and critically proceed when the implications of the methodology are understood.

Anesthetic agents are treated in Chapter 8, but important features are summarized here. Currently used potent volatile inhalational agents (halothane, enflurane, and isoflurane) are easy to deliver, render patients unconscious, are fairly rapidly eliminated, and are well tolerated by most patients. They blunt cardiovascular and pulmonary responses to noxious stimuli, but only at concentrations higher than those necessary to produce simple unconsciousness. Because volatile agents are all direct myocardial depressants, they are commonly portrayed as deleterious.[46] However, this functional depression is accompanied by decreased metabolic rate (oxygen consumption) of both the heart and the total body. Thus it has been proposed that inhalational anesthesia may be "protective" of the organism.[70,92] Inhalational agents can produce a degree of muscle relaxation, and they are often used as complete anesthetic agents. However, this practice is not always advisable, since the depth of anesthesia necessary to prevent response to a forthcoming noxious stimu-

lation may cause hypotension to unacceptable levels. This situation can be circumvented or treated with fluids, vasoconstrictors, or inotropes, illustrating a fundamental principle of general anesthesia: that cardiovascular stability in this state is always a dynamic balance between stimulation and depression. As stimulation varies with changes in surgical or other noxious activity, blood pressure and heart rate will increase or decrease, depending on the anesthetic level existing at that moment and on whether the stimulation is intensifying or abating. Thus anesthetic depth or infusions of direct-acting cardiovascular medications must be adjusted continuously. Since the effect of such adjustments is not instantaneous, hemodynamic fluctuations are inevitable. This phenomenon is less apparent in regional techniques, as described in following sections.

Nitrous oxide is frequently used as a supplement to both the volatile agents and the intravenous drugs discussed below. It contributes to both hypnosis (sleep) and analgesia and is particularly valuable for its rapidity of onset and elimination. Although inappropriate as the sole anesthetic, when used as an adjunct it reduces the amounts required of other agents while usually exerting minimal systemic effects.

The use of intravenous narcotic analgesics is becoming more widespread. The newer synthetic agents (fentanyl, sufentanil) are intensely analgesic and minimally perturb the cardiovascular system. When used in small doses, they are short-acting, easily titratable, and only mildly sedating. When used in very large doses they can cause unconsciousness, but amnesia is not reliably produced.[50] Because of the intense analgesia, most cardiovascular responses to noxious stimuli are abolished and "high-dose" narcotic techniques have become widespread in cardiac surgery. Negative effects of this technique include (1) occasional serious blood pressure or heart rate "breakthroughs,"[63] (2) patient recall,[63] and (3) prolonged emergence (6 to 24 hours) and time-to-extubation.

Between the extremes of pure inhalational agent or pure narcotic lies the balanced use of selections from both categories with or without nitrous oxide.[88] A stable intraoperative course, followed by a spontaneously breathing and comfortable postoperative patient, is most likely achieved by a combination of these agents,[41] in addition to clinical maneuvers to be discussed.

Sedative hypnotics, such as the short-acting barbiturates (Pentothal [thiopental sodium] and Brevital [methohexital sodium]) are commonly used for induction of anesthesia. Their properties include rapid obtundation of consciousness but analgesia is produced only in the sense that all cerebral functions are depressed. Brevity of action caused by rapid drug redistribution is a useful property. Although most patients tolerate nominal standard doses of the short-acting barbiturates, extreme lowering of blood pressure occurs occasionally. These drugs are direct myocardial depressants and decrease central sympathetic tone. In fact, virtually all currently used general anesthetic agents relax efferent autonomic tone[79] and thus render normal individuals *relatively* hypovolemic after induction. To combat hypotension it is common practice to infuse several hundred milliliters of fluid before and during induction of anesthesia. Whereas such fluid administration is generally well tolerated, patients with congestive heart failure or renal compromise may require other means of blood pressure support. We will reconsider the matter of fluid administration in the Regional Anesthesia section of this chapter.

Plainly, general anesthesia is not just one "thing"—not a solo instrument. It is a complex combination of devices, drugs, procedures, and judgments composed to fit the surgical procedure and patient condition. In the next section we discuss aspects of that composition. Although much of the material will apply to routine anesthetic care, we will be particularly concerned with the special needs of the severely ill.

Case Conduct

The conduct of general anesthesia may be functionally separated into the following periods: induction (transition from conscious to unconscious state), maintenance (intraoperative manipulations and adjustments) and emergence (end-of-case return to independent pulmonary and reflex function). The selection of agents, choice of monitoring, and style of anesthesia are all discretionary over an extraordinarily broad range of possibilities, and different clinicians will conduct the same case differently. Ideal clinical care achieves both an adequate anesthetic state and a stable physiologic condition. Just as the first can be accomplished with many different regimens, the second is also successfully achieved in diverse ways. This variability results from several

features of clinical care. First, legitimate treatment options exist for dealing with a given physiologic perturbation (for example, hypotension could be corrected by decreasing anesthetic depth, administering a vasopressor, or infusing fluid). Second, no real agreement exists concerning physiologic bounds, the transgression of which should require treatment. There has been no definition by well-performed studies of appropriate limits of blood pressure, heart rate, filling pressures, blood gases, or electrolytes (much less the more oblique parameters of cardiac index, stroke work index, and systemic vascular resistance). Thus clinicians have collected personal "rules-of-thumb" that govern their practice. Finally, most patients have sufficient physiologic reserve to survive both undertreatment and overtreatment without apparent consequence. These aspects of clinical care have contributed to the development of myriad acceptable management styles but have simultaneously confounded attempts to investigate the issue of relative risk in a methodical fashion.

We make no attempt to delineate specific management guidelines here. In general, however, in the delivery of general anesthesia to marginally stable individuals, anesthetic agents should be chosen carefully, administered slowly, and titrated to effect. When drugs are delivered in this manner it is usually possible to safely induce and smoothly maintain remarkably fragile patients. Moreover, judicious use of invasive hemodynamic monitoring has permitted still another dimension of anesthetic care. Strict hemodynamic control can be achieved when inotropes, vasodilators, vasoconstrictors and fluid therapy are used intelligently in response to information provided by monitors of anesthetic depth, multiple-lead ECG, heart rate, cardiac output, blood pressure, right atrial pressure, pulmonary artery pressure, and pulmonary capillary wedge pressure. Calculated parameters, including left ventricular stroke work index and systemic vascular resistance can provide additional useful information. Control of the cardiovascular system can alleviate myocardial ischemia, optimize organ perfusion, and treat pulmonary edema while both anesthesia and surgery are in progress.[69] This control is accomplished by adjusting the major determinants of myocardial oxygen supply and demand, which results in the simultaneous altering of contractility, heart rate, and loading conditions. The overall cardiovascular status of patients may improve dramatically in response to these acute manipulations. Such management allows successful completion of anesthesia and surgery and can be carried through into the postoperative period. Thus the range of physiologic control exercised by the modern anesthesiologist has extended the tolerable limits of patient infirmity within which anesthesia and surgery may be reasonably and safely performed.

Emergence from general anesthesia is a dynamic and complex stage seldom addressed in clinical investigations. As the level of anesthesia lightens, central nervous system depression dissipates, autonomic tone returns, and arterial and venous pressures and heart rate increase. Extubation must await reversal of muscle relaxants and adequate return of respiratory drive, muscular tone, and reflex responsiveness, but inappropriate delay causes stimulation that can result in hypertension, myocardial ischemia, and bronchospasm. These issues can extend to the recovery area if postoperative pain relief has not been included as a part of the anesthetic plan. Hypercarbia and hypoxia are not uncommon postoperatively and may contribute to arrhythmias, whereas hypothermia may lead to shivering and increased oxygen demands.

Emergence problems are challenging and require fast, appropriate action. There are no universally accepted management methods, and clinical studies *never* specify how emergence difficulties are to be handled. One approach is to give large doses of narcotics and muscle relaxants near the end of a procedure and return the patient to the recovery facility to receive mechanical ventilation over a prolonged postoperative period. This strategy simply transfers responsibility for anesthetic emergence to the recovery staff. While there are circumstances where this approach is specifically indicated and entirely correct, when it is employed without discretion the patient may be subjected to unnecessary risks. The presence of an endotracheal tube and the accompanying suctioning procedures constitute an ongoing source of stimulation and, perhaps, infection. Even in high-technology intensive care units, the level of sensitivity of medical personnel to the seriousness of this stress may not be sufficient to avoid morbidity. Other methods of emergence can usually achieve extubation, freedom from pain, and adequate ventilation even after major surgery on marginally stable patients. Fluid status, oxygen carrying capacity, and body temperature must be maintained, in-

traoperative pulmonary toilet should be performed, and provisions should be made for immediate postoperative pain relief. The latter can be accomplished by titrating intravenous narcotics to balance amelioration of pain with respiratory drive while alternate techniques include central neuraxis intrathecal or epidural narcotics. (See Chapter 13.)

The conduct of general anesthesia is seen to extend far beyond the controlled administration of "sleep" producing agents. In the next section we consider analogous aspects of regional anesthesia in preparation for an evaluation of comparative clinical studies.

REGIONAL ANESTHESIA
Principles

Regional anesthesia may be thought of as any method whereby neural impulses (specifically pain) from an operative site are prevented from reaching higher levels of the nervous system. It includes the use of local anesthetic agents for skin infiltration, specific peripheral nerve blocks, or major conduction blockade in the form of spinal (subarachnoid) or epidural drug administration. Acupuncture and transcutaneous electrical neural stimulation (TENS) might be classified as regional anesthesia. It is helpful to distinguish between those procedures that are likely to partially or completely block the thoracolumbar sympathetic outflow, causing hemodynamic changes, and those lesser techniques that do not.

When regional techniques are used that do not involve perturbations in the autonomic nervous system, morbidity is limited to (1) direct complications of the procedure, (2) toxicity of the agents, and (3) pain and anxiety during injection or surgery. Procedural complications occur with a predictable frequency, which is inversely proportional to the experience of the operator, and consist of nerve damage resulting from intraneural injection or to needle penetration of a vital body part such as lung or blood vessel.[12] The local anesthetic agents used to effect neural blockade are of two general classes based on their molecular form and degradative pathways: (1) amides, which include lidocaine and bupivacaine, and (2) esters such as cocaine, chloroprocaine, and procaine (Novocaine). These drugs actually have a low rate of common medical side effects such as true allergic reactions. Many patients who believe they have allergies have had symptoms caused by epinephrine, which is frequently added to prolong block duration. True allergies have, however, been reported.[35a] In some regional techniques the total amount of agent used is quite large. If a significant portion is inadvertently injected intravascularly, serious systemic effects may be observed, including grand mal seizure activity,[74] severe myocardial depression, and conduction defects.[36] Recent reports indicate that resuscitation may be impossible when overdose with bupivacaine (a popular local anesthetic agent) has occurred.[3,40]

Pain and anxiety during establishment of a regional block or later during surgery are annoying to the patient and can be dangerous. Sedation during performance of a block is desirable, since frequent needle passes may be necessary and impingement on bone can occur. Furthermore, the pain of local anesthetic injection can be intense. Individuals with coronary artery disease may experience myocardial ischemia at this time. Techniques that require blockade of several nerves can result in "patchy" or inadequate analgesia requiring augmentation with intravenous or inhalational agents or conversion to general anesthesia. A 10% to 17% incidence is given for this circumstance.[32,61]

While the above concerns are serious, they are manageable, and the nonsympathetic blocking techniques (from local skin infiltration to nerve blocks) have a respected place in the armamentarium of anesthesiologists, surgeons, and dentists.[35] Spinal and epidural anesthesia can be associated with similar problems as well as some that are more physiologically complex.

Major Conduction Blockade

Blockade of neural impulses at the level of the spinal cord can be accomplished by two techniques: spinal or subarachnoid anesthesia, which involves injecting a small amount of local anesthetic agent into the intrathecal space, and epidural anesthesia, wherein a larger amount of drug is injected to surround the dura. While each has distinguishing features, for purposes of this discussion they will be considered together. The most feared complication of major conduction blockade is permanent paralysis following use of a spinal or epidural anesthetic.[2] Although rare in modern times, paralysis continues to be reported, most recently in obstetrical patients who inadvertently received a subarachnoid injection of 3% chloroprocaine (a drug intended for use only in the epidural space). Subsequent investigation implicated the solutions' pH and/or the presence of sodium bisulfate (an antioxidant) as the probable offensive elements.[31,73] Another cause of paralysis involves spinal cord compression secondary to epidural hematoma, which occurs principally in persons suffering from defects of coagulation. Thus the latter condition is one of the strongest contraindications to the use of epidural or spinal anesthesia.[1]

When spinal or epidural anesthesia is chosen for surgical procedures cephalad to the groin (T12 dermatome innervation), progressive blockade of the spinal sympathetic outflow occurs. The thoracolumbar sympathetic fibers exit the cord from T1 through L3 and are inhibited by anesthetic concentrations below those necessary to achieve sensory or motor blockade. As a result, the level of sympathetic involvement is usually estimated to be at least 2 dermatomes higher than the clinically determined sensory block. However, the effects of major conduction blockade on autonomic function are complex and have not been fully elucidated. A study of skin temperature changes during spinal anesthesia suggested that sympathetic inhibition may extend 6 levels higher than the somatic block.[22] Sympathetic inhibition causes vasodilatation of both resistance and capacitance vessels and could decrease systemic blood pressure. Indeed, hypotension is a frequent concomitant of spinal and epidural anesthesia, but it is not universal. Figure 9-1 shows the percent change in blood pressure as a function of sensory block level in a group of 60 patients.[78] The lack of correlation is striking. This finding may simply reflect differences in patient volume status, but could represent natural physiologic variability. It is well established but not widely appreciated that the body vasculature above the level of autonomic blockade reflexly constricts.[89] Figure 9-2 shows the results of a total body radionuclide study that illustrates this differential response.[4] An anomalous finding in this investigation is that the abdominal vasculature was seen to constrict rather than to dilate as would have been predicted by the level of blockade and the assumed innervation scheme. At a later point in this study the abdominal vasculature suddenly dilated in 25% (2 of 8) of the subjects, causing significant hypotension. No physiologic explanation for either the unexpected constriction or the sudden dilation of the visceral vasculature has been proposed.

The interplay of competing reflexes in partial sympathetic blockade is complex. Hypotension seen with

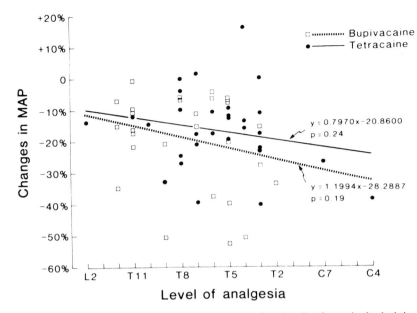

FIGURE 9-1. Maximum decrease in MAP versus level of analgesia after spinal administration of tetracaine (15 mg, with epinephrine) or bupivacaine (20 mg, without epinephrine). Patients had been prehydrated with 500 ml of crystalloid. No correlation was found between maximum decrease in MAP and level of analgesia for either drug.

Reproduced by permission from Phero JC et al: Hypotension in spinal anesthesia, Anesth Analg 66:549-552, 1987.

spinal and epidural anesthesia is rarely accompanied by an increase in heart rate. This unexpected absence of tachycardia is often attributed to blockade of cardiac accelerator fibers. However, baroreceptor-mediated increases in heart rate are only minimally blunted by ablation of myocardial sympathetics with a cervical epidural.[91] Alternately, the lack of heart rate response suggests that vagal stimulation may be triggered by decreased venous return and thereby attenuate normal accelerating impulses.[8]

The prophylaxis or treatment of hypotension is an important matter that awaits definitive evaluation. Generalizations are difficult because the occurrence of hypotension is unpredictable, and differences in underlying disease states alter the tolerance both to blood pressure decreases and to the various treatment options. To combat hypotension in obstetrical anesthesia, for example, it is common practice to give large amounts of crystalloid (1 or more liters) or colloid before and/or during the early stages of an epidural placed in parturients for cesarean section.[82] This technique is reasonably effective when combined with maneuvers to prevent uterine-caval

compression, but many individuals also require a vasopressor. Clearly, the administration of large amounts of crystalloid would be undesirable in patients with fluid retention syndromes including congestive heart failure and renal failure. A carefully balanced combination of small amounts of fluid, vasoconstriction, and inotropic support may be ideal,[15] an approach optimally undertaken using invasive hemodynamic monitoring.

The segmental vasodilatation accompanying major conduction blockade may be advantageous in certain patients. Some authorities suggest that spinal or epidural techniques are preferred in patients who have hypertension,[43] congestive heart failure,[45] or myocardial ischemia.[80] Their argument is that the afterload-reducing effect of the technique is specifically therapeutic in these conditions. Spinal anesthesia has been reported to acutely alleviate myocardial ischemia[95] and one echocardiographic study demonstrated improvement in baseline abnormalities of left ventricular wall-motion after epidural anesthesia in patients with myocardial disease.[7] However, when fluid was administered in the latter in-

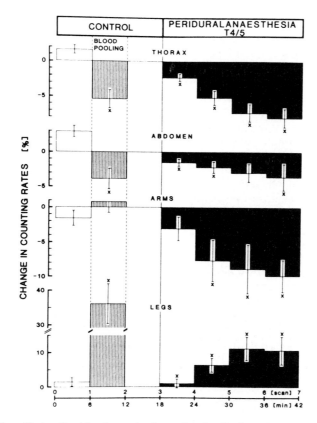

FIGURE 9-2. The effects of epidural anesthesia on the distribution of technicium-labeled erythrocytes in supine man (n = 8). Shown are seven sequential counting periods of 6 minutes each. Twenty ml of 2% lidocaine was injected at the start of period 4. Results are expressed as percent difference of time—period 3. During period 2 blood was pooled in the lower extremities by a tourniquet. Note that during epidural anesthesia lower body sequestration occurs in conjunction with volume depletion of upper extremity, thoracic, and surprisingly, the abdominal vasculature.

Reproduced by permission from Arndt J et al: Peridural anesthesia and the distribution of blood in supine humans, Anesthesiology 63:616-623, 1985.

vestigation (restoring venous return), the baseline abnormalities returned. This finding may temper the use of fluids as primary therapy for hypotension of neuraxis blockade in some patients. Another study has recently reported echocardiographic evidence of deterioration of myocardial function in patients with heart disease after epidural; this study does not mention volume loading.[85]

A practical objection to the use of spinal or epidural anesthesia to reduce preload and afterload is that the onset and intensity of effect cannot be modulated in a controlled fashion. Titration of short-acting agents, which more or less specifically alter different aspects of the cardiovascular system, and

assessment of the effects of therapy (through invasive monitoring) are usually considered central to anesthetic management of the critically ill. The lack of predictability, variable onset, and the fact that reversal must await block dissipation diminish most theoretical benefits of major conduction blockade in patients with heart disease.

With regard to regional anesthesia for the critically ill it is, of course, appropriate to use the full range of measurements and therapies outlined for general anesthesia.[38] The decision to use progressively extensive monitoring during anesthesia usually reflects the severity of systemic illness and the degree of surgical insult anticipated. Interestingly, the clinical perception that regional anesthesia is relatively safer appears to influence this decision. In a retrospective review of patients undergoing lower extremity vascular bypass procedures we found a significantly lower incidence of invasive monitoring in patients receiving regional anesthesia than in those having general anesthesia[9] in spite of some evidence that the former had more serious preoperative cardiovascular disease. The advisability of this practice is discussed in the Comparative Studies section.

Once an adequate block has been established and the surgery is underway, a smooth and stable intraoperative course is likely. In contrast to general anesthesia, regional anesthesia usually results in a virtually complete cessation of neural impulses from the operative site. Thus the fluctuations in vital signs seen during general anesthesia are blunted.[19] Exceptions to this occur during periods of blood loss, which may not be well tolerated and also at the time of block dissipation or redosing. Patients must be carefully monitored after redosing an epidural catheter, since cumulative effects can occasionally result in high blocks and precipitous drops in blood pressure. With high epidural or spinal levels, which are necessary to perform surgery on the upper abdomen, it is not uncommon to have virtually complete blockade of the thoracolumbar sympathetic chain. Since this includes the cardiac accelerator fibers (T1-T2) serious hypotension, with bradycardia, may occur. Several recent reports have emphasized the rapidity with which this combination can develop. Caplan et al[16] reviewed 14 cases of cardiac arrest during spinal anesthesia and noted that some individuals can develop a precipitous decrease in heart rate and blood pressure well after the time that the blockade level was assumed to be stabilized. Oversedation, with unrecognized hypoxia and/or hypercardia, was considered contributory in these cases. Frerichs et al[42] reported sudden asystole in an awake young healthy patient blocked to somatic level T3 when he received disturbing news that apparently initiated a vagal discharge. Another case report observed abrupt asystole in an individual with asymptomatic sick sinus syndrome undergoing epidural anesthesia to T8 somatic dermatome.[25]

It should be clear that regional anesthesia, especially major conduction blockade, is a serious undertaking that requires appropriate preoperative preparation, excellent patient rapport, and careful intraoperative monitoring and vigilance.[35]

We have discussed the effects of regional and general anesthesia with respect to the intraoperative period. However, most anesthesiologists today would consider antiquated the notion that their job is simply to "get the patient off the table." The complications of anesthesia are generally presumed to extend into the postoperative period and to include, for example, a myocardial infarction resulting from tachycardia caused by excessive incisional pain while the patient is in the recovery room. It is in the control of postoperative pain that epidural and spinal techniques may have their greatest use and desirability. (See Chapter 13.)

COMPARATIVE STUDIES

Many studies have appeared over the last 30 years that compare regional and general anesthesia using specific physiologic, biochemical, and metabolic end-points. The regional technique evaluated in virtually all of these investigations is major conduction blockade and most of this section will be concerned with a critique of these findings. First, however, we consider the status of more limited regional procedures.

Local Anesthesia

The safety of local anesthesia has been demonstrated in a large series of patients of mixed physiologic status undergoing ophthalmologic surgery.[5] This investigation did not directly compare local to general anesthesia but since it found such a low morbidity (virtually zero) associated with local anesthesia, even in patients with significant heart disease, it confirms a widely held clinical judgment and the results are generally accepted. This study also reported a much smaller number of patients who received general anesthesia, also without notable complications. The authors were unable to draw conclusions about this latter group because of the sample size.

There are no investigations of relative risk comparing general anesthesia with more extensive local procedures (such as surgeon-performed field block for inguinal hernia) or peripheral nerve techniques (such as an axillary block for upper extremity surgery). Although these methods are associated with some hazards as discussed previously, they enjoy considerable popularity, which varies between institutions and practitioners.

Also, there are no available data related to spinal anesthesia confined to low and/or one-sided dermatomes (thus minimizing autonomic involvement) although this technique is widely employed, with success, in extremely debilitated persons for lower extremity procedures such as amputations and debridements.

Major Conduction Blockade

The following is a review of studies that have compared epidural or spinal anesthesia with general anesthesia in respect to endocrine response, incidence of thromboembolic phenomena, intraoperative blood loss, measures of immune function, pulmonary effects, cardiovascular mortality, and morbidity. Since the two classes of anesthesia use such radically different methods it is not surprising that statistically significant variations are discovered. The clinical relevance of these findings, however, is often quite arguable. Results are difficult to interpret and compare because of problems of study design, patient selection, lack of randomization, and unspecified management guidelines. In spite of these drawbacks, conclusions of importance have been reported. This section discusses those findings that appear well documented and of clinical relevance.

Metabolic and endocrine surgical stress response. The physiologic response to accidental or surgical trauma results in alterations in hormonal levels and metabolic function. The majority of these changes are probably secondary to stimulation of high nervous centers by noxious input and subsequent efferent impulses to various endocrine organs.[55] Elevations of ACTH, ADH, prolactin, growth hormone, cortisol, aldosterone, epinephrine, and norepinephrine are seen during surgery under general anesthesia.[11,30] Regional blockade has been shown to inhibit these changes. Mechanisms by which epidural or spinal anesthesia accomplishes this inhibition include both blockade of afferent pain impulses from the surgical site and diminution of sympathetic efferent stimulation of the adrenal medulla.[30] These findings are most consistent for procedures performed on the lower abdomen and below.[77] For upper abdominal and thoracic procedures, epidural anesthesia fails to consistently block the endocrine metabolic stress response, even when the level of sensory loss suggests that noxious efferent impulses should not occur.[94] This finding is currently unexplained but may involve unblocked afferent autonomic pathways that do not follow somatosensory fibers.[39]

The techniques and conduct of general anesthesia used in these investigations deserve comment. The greatest endocrine response has been observed in studies that used nominal concentrations of volatile inhalational agents either alone or in combination with nitrous oxide.[39,59,77] Many clinicians feel that liberal use of opiates (in combination with other agents) are essential for patients where avoidance of the surgical stress response, or its hemodynamic sequelae, is of critical importance (for example, those with coronary artery disease).[88] Studies on endocrine response during high-dose narcotic and deep inhalation anesthesia have demonstrated smaller hormonal elevations.[26,44]

Finally, it should be noted that the implications of hormonal elevation in response to stress have not been explored (except for hemodynamic perturbations such as tachycardia that may be treated specifically). It has been suggested by some that the stress response to trauma or surgery could be conferring some physiologic benefit, thus making inhibition counterproductive.[17] In any event, the possible desirability of constant hormonal levels awaits further study.

Thrombosis and thromboembolism. Several prospective, randomized studies have investigated the incidence of perioperative thromboembolic phenomena after regional and general anesthesia.* For hip surgery and prostatectomy, a rather clear and consistent picture has emerged. The incidence of thrombotic complications as verified by phlebography or I-125 fibrinogen scan is 50% to 60% less under regional anesthesia than with general anesthesia. Probable explanations for this finding include increased blood flow to the lower extremities resulting from vasodilation and a regional anesthesia-induced antithrombotic state.[72] The antithrombotic effect may be caused by circulating epinephrine that is mixed with local anesthetics or by inhibition of platelet aggregation caused by circulating blood levels of the local anesthetic agent itself.[10] Whether the *intra*operative anesthetic technique is causally related to the findings is unknown, since all of these investigations have used the epidural to treat pain for hours to days postoperatively. It is thus possible that similar results would be obtained if a general anesthetic technique was used for the procedure and regional analgesia was administered only after the surgery. It is also quite possible that increased flow and antithrombosis could be reproduced with vasodilators and heparin or aspirin independent of the

*References 34, 48, 53, 68, 71, 72.

epidural technique. These possibilities in no way negate the value of the investigational results. They are mentioned only to caution the practitioner and consultant regarding recommendations made on the basis of these findings since other factors may be overriding and the same benefits obtained by other means.

Blood loss. Several investigations have concluded that blood loss is 30% to 40% less under regional anesthesia than with general anesthesia for elective hip replacement and during retropubic prostatectomy.[48,71,72] The lower rate of bleeding during regional anesthesia for these procedures is probably a result of lower arterial and venous pressures resulting from sympathetic blockade. In addition, perhaps, higher venous pressure in the general anesthesia group consequent to positive pressure ventilation causes more bleeding in those patients.[55] Deliberate hypotensive anesthesia with nitroprusside or nitroglycerin leads to similar reductions in blood loss.[81,93] The importance of vasodilatation in mediating blood loss is further suggested by investigations comparing thoracic epidurals with general anesthesia for upper abdominal procedures.[49,94] In these studies lower extremity vasodilation and decreased vascular pressures were not observed and blood loss was not different between the two groups. It is unlikely that the blood loss issue would be sufficiently overriding to determine the choice of regional anesthesia for a particular patient, especially since the same goal is accomplished reliably using general anesthesia in conjunction with other hypotensive techniques.

Immune function. Immunosuppression appears to be an acute sequela of the hormonal response to surgical stress. Since this stress response can be attenuated effectively (for certain procedures) by regional anesthesia, it seems probable that postoperative infections could also be reduced. Actually there is scant evidence for this potentially beneficial phenomenon. Studies evaluating the effect of different anesthetic regimens on immune function have not reported differences in outcome, and outcome studies have not concomitantly measured immune function. Yeager, et al[101] reported a 52% incidence of postoperative infections in patients receiving general anesthesia compared to 7% for those receiving a combined regional and general technique. Since postoperative treatment of infection was not controlled, immune function was not studied, and data collection was not conducted blindly, these findings

are inconclusive. If the results can be confirmed, then a truly compelling rationale for the use of regional analgesia—particularly in the postoperative period—will be established. Caution, however, should be used in the interpretation of positive correlations. A recent study of patients undergoing major upper abdominal surgery under general anesthesia showed that pulmonary complications, including infection, were reduced from 60% to 19% when postoperative respiratory therapy regimens were used.[84] Thus a difference in infection rates between regional and general anesthesia may be unrelated to direct effects on immune infection.

Pulmonary. Since ventilation is either assisted or controlled and oxygen supplementation is routine, serious difficulties with carbon dioxide and oxygen blood tensions are uncommon during general anesthesia, even in patients with advanced lung disease. The effects of regional anesthesia or intraoperative pulmonary function are variable. For low levels of blockade, lung function is minimally affected by the technique but at progressively higher thoracic levels the contribution of intercostal musculature to chest wall expansion will be reduced. Of no consequence in normal individuals, reduction of thoracic muscular activity can significantly compromise the pulmonary function of persons with advanced pulmonary disease.[28]

Bronchospasm may be triggered in susceptible individuals if endotracheal intubation is required under general anesthesia. Therefore, pulmonary reflexes must be grossly attenuated to avoid this hazard.[52] However, the volatile anesthetics are excellent bronchodilators and bronchospasm may actually be reversed with these agents.[51] Regional anesthesia is often chosen to prevent the intraoperative exacerbation of asthma.[58] The incidence of wheezing is certainly lower in patients undergoing regional anesthesia than in those having general anesthesia with intubation but not less than in patients having general anesthesia *without* intubation.[86]

Postoperative deterioration of pulmonary function is virtually universal but it appears to be more a function of the site of surgery than of the type of anesthesia. Upper abdominal and thoracic surgery results in a greater decline in lung function than lower abdominal cases while both are worse than limb procedures.[90] A theoretical advantage has been proposed for postoperative regional analgesia, because careful titration of drug concentration and amount can produce pain relief without significant

TABLE 9-1. Mortality following surgery, prospective randomized trials

Source		RA		GA		Time	P
Couderc et al	(1977)	7/50	(14%)	12/50	(24%)	(3 mo)	NS
McLaren et al	(1978)	4/51	(8%)	17/60	(28%)	(1 mo)	< 0.05
McKenzie et al	(1980)	5/49	(10%)	8/51	(16%)	(1 mo)	NS
White et al	(1980)	0/20	(0%)	0/20	(0%)	(1 mo)	NS
Davis et al	(1981)	3/64	(5%)	9/68	(13%)	(1 mo)	NS
Wickstrom et al	(1982)	3/73	(4%)	12/75	(16%)	(2 wk)	< 0.05
		14/73	(19%)	14/75	(19%)	(2 mo)	NS
Valentin et al	(1986)	15/253	(6%)	20/255	(8%)	(1 mo)	NS
		38/253	(15%)	38/255	(15%)	(6 mo)	NS
Yeager et al	(1987)	0/28	(0%)	4/25	(16%)	(1 mo)	< 0.04

muscle weakness.[76] Presumably the combination allows deep breathing, with diminution of atelectasis and possibly pneumonia, although studies to date have not confirmed this.[76,97]

Mortality. Studies relating anesthetic technique to perioperative mortality must be interpreted with caution for several important reasons: (1) Mortality is uncommon in healthy individuals undergoing routine procedures and sample sizes have to be extremely large to establish a difference between methods. (2) Anesthesia mortality in healthy patients is often caused by human error or clinical misjudgment. While error and misjudgment are important to considerations of risk management, any difference found between techniques caused by these factors may not be meaningful to the consultant or anesthesiologist trying to choose the best method of managing a particular patient. (3) Perioperative mortality in seriously ill high-risk patients may well be the result of disease severity or surgery-related factors independent of the anesthetic technique. Thus prospective, randomized trials require large numbers of individuals to ensure comparability of groups and treatments.

Table 9-1 lists the mortality results of several regional versus general studies in patients having hip surgery* as well as those of a recently published clinical trial of patients having high-risk surgery at a variety of sites.[101] Several features are noteworthy. Five of the hip surgery studies, including the largest study of 508 patients, reported no statistically significant difference in mortality between the two types of anesthesia. This is remarkable, since it is precisely

*References 29, 31, 64, 66, 96, 98, 99.

this group of patients in whom the only important, unequivocal difference in significant morbidity (thromboembolic phenomena) has been demonstrated. The only hip surgery studies showing a significant difference were those of McLaren et al[66] and Wickstom et al.[99] The McLaren study reports an extremely high mortality in general anesthesia group. In fact, most of the investigations in Table 9-1 show a mortality for the general anesthesia group that seems excessive. A recent randomized clinical trial of 152 patients undergoing general anesthesia for repair of fractured neck or femur reported death rates of 5.2% at 1 month and 15.1% at 6 months.[25] This is very comparable to the results of Valentin et al.[96] For both regional and general anesthesia may represent the realistic outcome of evenly-applied, high-quality clinical care.

Yeager et al[101] conducted a prospective randomized trial comparing general anesthesia with a combined epidural-general technique in patients undergoing either abdominal, major vascular, or intrathoracic surgery. Patients in the "combined" group received light general anesthesia (nitrous oxide plus intermittent narcotics) supplemented with epidural injection of a local agent. Postoperative analgesia in the latter group was mainly supplied by narcotics injected through the epidural catheter. Four of 25 (16%) in the general group and zero of 27 (0%) in the "combined" group died. This study has received wide attention, because the dramatic differences observed caused the investigators to abort the trial. Criticism has focused on many of the issues raised in this chapter.[23,54,57] The study patients had a wide variety of ancillary disease processes and most feel that the sample size was much too small to ensure comparability of groups and treatments. Further, the patients died on postoperative days 13, 17, 18, and 37, and it is difficult to imagine how the intraoperative anesthetic technique could be causally related to deaths so remote. It is possible that a cascade of debilitating events initiated during the perioperative period might culminate in death several days later. Alternately, postoperative use of epidural analgesia might diminish infectious or thromboembolic complications, the lethal effects of which would only manifest some time later. Of note is that a 16% death rate for elective (if major) surgery is high. Others have reported mortality rates of 1.7% to 8.5% for patients undergoing abdominal aneurysm repair,[14,27] one of the procedures heavily represented in the Yeager et al[101] study. In the absence of evidence to the contrary, it seems most probable that this small sample of patients had real differences in the severity of associated diseases and/or misadventures between the two study groups.

Cardiovascular morbidity. There have been virtually no recognized randomized prospective trials comparing the cardiovascular complications of regional and general anesthesia. The hip surgery investigations previously discussed failed to demonstrate differences in cardiovascular morbidity, although it is not at all clear that cardiovascular events were aggressively and systematically identified. Investigations of cardiovascular morbidity would require a study population known to be at risk for these complications, since the incidence of myocardial infarction and heart failure is very low overall. Regardless, these events constitute the major single category of serious perioperative morbidity.[88] Yeager et al[101] reported a cardiovascular failure (angina, myocardial infarction, new CHF, cardiogenic shock, and SVT) rate of 52% in their general group and 14% in the combined group. This remarkable finding must be closely examined. No management principles are given as part of the clinical protocol. Intraoperative anesthetic management and postoperative care are said to be "usual." No guidelines for invasive monitoring are presented. Anesthetic emergence problems in the general anesthesia group were largely side stepped because high dose narcotic techniques were used that shift several delicate clinical decisions to the intensive care unit staff. Time-to-extubation was much longer in the general anesthesia group as would be expected using this methodology. Finally, the report contains only lumped data. It would have been most instructive to have specific

patient/disease/surgery information on the study patients. While the complication rate is extremely high, perhaps the patients were at high risk for congestive morbidity. If they were, then it is even more important to know the criteria for use of invasive monitoring, proposed therapies, and the clinical algorithms that constitute the "usual" care at the authors' institution.

In a nonconcurrent study of 134 patients undergoing distal extremity vascular bypass grafting under regional (76) or general (56) anesthesia we found a greater incidence of perioperative myocardial ischemia or infarction in patients who received regional anesthesia.[9,62] Since this study was a chart review, it is subject to the possibility of dissimilarity between the groups and nonuniform data collection. Nonetheless, we could find no evidence that regional anesthesia was in any way superior. In a small subsequent prospective investigation using 24-hour Holter monitoring, serial ECGs, and creatine phosphokinase (CPK) isoenzymes in comparable groups, no difference was found in the rate of ischemia and infarction between regional and general anesthesia.[20,21] A prospective, randomized, clinical trial of regional anesthesia versus general anesthesia that uses clinical management protocols is needed to determine the relative risk in patients with heart disease.

The incidence of perioperative ischemia was not reported in the study by Yeager et al, but three myocardial infarctions occurred at unknown times in the general anesthesia group. It is noteworthy that most perioperative ischemia is probably silent[60] and is missed by standard 1-lead monitor systems employed in usual clinical care. Thus accurate assessment of the rate of ischemia would only come from more sophisticated technology such as 2-lead continuous Holter monitoring. As discussed above, both beneficial and detrimental effects on the determinants of myocardial oxygen consumption and demand will be observed with either regional or general anesthesia. At the same time general anesthesia, per se, is unlikely to have salutory effect on pump failure. Myocardial ischemia and failure can be prevented or managed using the monitoring and therapeutic modalities outlined above together with the direct and indirect effects of anesthesia, regardless of type.

SUMMARY

Both regional and general anesthetic techniques have advantages that recommend their use and complications or side effects that limit their appeal. Successful administration of either method depends on the physiologic status of the patient and on the skill and professional expertise of the practitioner. There is no consensus supporting absolute indications for the use of either regional or general anesthesia. However, from the data reviewed and broad clinical experience it seems reasonable to make the following recommendations:

1. Regional techniques that use modest doses of local anesthetics and do not involve systemic autonomic blockade may be preferable with the following strong provisions:
   a. No contraindication exists and the patient accepts
   b. The block can be initiated with alacrity and maintained with care
   c. The patient is appropriately monitored and vigilantly observed
   d. Everyone is prepared to progress to a general anesthetic or to abort the case, whichever is appropriate, should the blockade fail or side effects prove unacceptable.

2. In healthy patients epidural or spinal anesthesia, with or without sympathetic blockade, is an acceptable alternative to general anesthesia under exactly the same list of conditions. Individuals in this category having hip surgery or prostatectomy may actually benefit from receiving a regional technique.

3. Patients with cardiovascular, pulmonary, or other serious systemic illnesses who undergo major surgery are special cases in which either form of anesthesia may be acceptable or preferable. Careful monitoring and goal-directed control of physiologic variables throughout the entire perioperative period may be more important than the type of anesthesia. General anesthesia that is carefully prepared, monitored, and conducted cannot be ruled out in the seriously ill.

We have presented a point of view not heretofore stated explicitly in reviews discussing comparative risks of regional anesthesia and general anesthesia. Our thesis is that comparative studies addressing outcome must specify a management protocol to which the patient will be subjected throughout the investigational period, rather than simply outlining the treatments being compared. The wide disparity among morbidity and mortality rates for the same surgical procedure in different institutions implies either (1) end-points are variably defined or measured (mortality, however, seems unambiguous), (2) patient populations are quite divergent, or (3) the quality of perioperative care differs significantly. Resolution of these problems will not be easy. Clinicians are loath to specify, in print, their management principles, both because the matter seems too complex and because of a sense that clinical judgment may be restricted by adherence to a protocol. We feel the potential benefits justify an attempt to overcome these difficulties. The very activity of a group of clinicians mutually agreeing on a management scheme would serve to teach, communicate, and modify medical practice. The consequences of a particular methodology may then be evaluated and meaningful investigations conducted to resolve issues such as the relative safety of regional versus general anesthesia.

REFERENCES

1. Adriani J: Labat's regional anesthesia, ed 4, St Louis, 1985, Warren H Green Inc.
2. Adriani J and Naragi M: Paraplegia associated with epidural anesthesia, South Med J 79:1350-1355, 1986.
3. Albright GA: Cardiac arrest following regional anesthesia with etidocaine or bupivacaine, Anesthesiology 51:285-287, 1979.
4. Arndt J et al: Peridural anesthesia and the distribution of blood in supine humans, Anesthesiology 63:616-623, 1985.
5. Backer CL et al: Myocardial reinfarction following local anesthesia for ophthalmologic surgery, Anesth Analg 59:257-262, 1980.
6. Bailey PL and Stanley TH: Pharmacology of intravenous narcotic agents. In Miller RD (editor): Anesthesia, New York, 1986, Churchill Livingstone.
7. Baron JF et al: Left ventricular global and regional function during lumbar epidural anesthesia in patients with and without angina pectoris. Influence of volume loading, Anesthesiology 66:621-627, 1987.
8. Baron JF et al: Influence of venous return on baroreflex control of heart rate during lumbar epidural anesthesia in humans, Anesthesiology 64:188-193, 1986.
9. Beattie C et al: Myocardial ischemia may be more common with regional than with general anesthesia in high-risk patients, Anesthesiology 65:A518, 1986.
10. Borg T and Modig J: Potential anti-thrombotic effects of local anesthetics due to their inhibition of platelet aggregation, Acta Anaesthesiol Scand 29:739-742, 1985.

11. Brandt MR, Kehlet H, and Binder C: Effect of epidural analgesia on the glucoregulatory endocrine response to surgery, Clin Endocrinol 5:107-114, 1976.

12. Bromage PR: Epidural anesthesia, Philadelphia, 1978, WB Saunders Co.

13. Brown DL (editor): Risk and outcome in anesthesia, London, 1988, JB Lippincott Co.

14. Brown WO, Hollier LH, and Pairolero PC: Abdominal aortic aneurysm and coronary artery disease, Arch Surg 116:1484-1488, 1981.

15. Butterworth JF et al: Augmentation of venous return by adrenergic agonists during spinal anesthesia, Anesth Analg 65:612-616, 1986.

16. Caplan RA et al: Unexpected cardiac arrest during spinal anesthesia: a closed claims analysis of predisposing factors, Anesthesiology 86:5-11, 1988.

17. Carr DB: Commentary, Intell Rep Anesth 4(5):7, 1987.

18. Christensen P et al: Influence of extradural morphine on the adrenocortical and hyperglycemic response to surgery, Br J Anaesth 54:23-26, 1982.

19. Christopherson R et al: Hemodynamics lability and myocardial ischemia under general and regional anesthesia. Abstracts of the Eighth Annual Meeting of the Society of Cardiovascular Anesthesiologists, Montreal, 1986.

20. Christopherson R et al: Incidence of perioperative myocardial ischemia in patients having lower extremity vascular grafting. Abstracts of the 10th Annual Meeting of the Society of Cardiovascular Anesthesiologists, New Orleans, 1988.

21. Christopherson R et al: Perioperative myocardial ischemia and infarction occurs frequently in patients having peripheral vascular grafting under regional and general anesthesia, submitted 1989.

22. Chamberlin DP and Chamberlain BDL: Changes in skin temperature of the trunk and their relationship to sympathetic blockade during spinal anesthesia, Anesthesiology 65:139-143, 1986.

23. Clark JL: Epidural anesthesia and analgesia in high-risk surgical patients, Anesthesiology 67:1025-1026, 1987.

24. Cohen LI: Asystole during spinal anesthesia in a patient with sick sinus syndrome, Anesthesiology 68:787-788, 1988.

25. Coleman SA et al: Outcome after general anesthesia for repair of fractured neck of femur. A randomized trial of spontaneous vs. controlled ventilation, Br J Anaesth 60:43-47, 1988.

26. Cooper GM et al: Fentanyl and the metabolic response to gastric surgery, Anaesthesia 36:667-671, 1981.

27. Cooperman M, Pflug B, and Martin EW: Cardiovascular risk factors in patients with peripheral vascular disease, Surgery 84:505-509, 1978.

28. Cory PC and Mulroy MF: Postoperative respiratory failure following intercostal block, Anesthesiology 54:418-419, 1981.

29. Couderc E et al: Resultants comparatifs d l'anesthesia generale et peridural chez le grand viellard dans la chirurgie dela hanch, Anesth Analg (Paris) 34:987-997, 1977.

30. Covino BG: Reasons to preferentially select regional anesthesia. IARS Review Course Lectures, Anesth Analg 4(suppl):61-65, 1986.

31. Covino BG et al: Prolonged sensory motor deficit following inadvertent spinal anesthesia, Anesth Analg 59:390-400, 1980.

32. Crawford JS: Experiences with lumbar extradural analgesia for cesarean section, Br J Anaesth 52:821-825, 1980.

33. Damask AC et al: General vs. epidural which is the better anesthetic technique for femoral-popliteal bypass surgery? Anesth Analg 65:S39, 1986.

34. Davis FM and Laurenson VG: Spinal anesthesia or general anesthesia for emergency hip surgery in elderly patients, Anaesth Intensive Care 9:352, 1981.

35. Dawkins CJM: An analysis of the complications of extradural and caudal block, Anaesthesia 24:554-563, 1969.

35a. DeBakey ME and Lawrie GM: Combined coronary artery and peripheral vascular disease: recognition and treatment, J Vasc Surg 1:605-607, 1984.

36. De Jong RH, Ronfeld RA, and Derosa RA: Cardiovascular effects of convulsant and supraconvulsant doses of amide local anesthetics, Anesth Analg 61:3-9, 1982.

37. Derbyshire DR, Chmielewski A, and Fell D: Plasma catecholamine responses to tracheal intubation, Br J Anaesth 55:855-860, 1983.

38. DeWolf AM and Van Zundert AA: Spinal anesthesia and myocardial ischemia, Anesth Analg 66:582-583, 1987.

39. Engquist A et al: The blocking effect of epidural analgesia on the adrenocortical and hyperglycemic responses to surgery, Acta Anaesthesiol Scand 21:330-335, 1977.

40. FDA Drug Bulletin: Adverse reactions with bupivacaine, Rockville, Md, US Dept of Health and Human Services 13(3):23, 1983.

41. Freedman B et al: Fentanyl-halothane anesthesia maintains myocardial contractility, Anesthesiology 59:A35, 1983.

42. Frerichs RL, Campbell J, and Bassell GM: Psychogenic cardiac arrest during extensive sympathetic blockade, Anesthesiology 68:943-944, 1988.

43. Gal TJ and Cooperman LH: Hypertension in the immediate postoperative period, Br J Anaesth 47:70-74, 1975.

44. Gothert M and Wendt J: Inhibition of adrenal medullary catecholamine secretion by enflurane, Anesthesiology 46:400-403, 1977.

45. Greene NM: Physiology of spinal anesthesia, Baltimore, 1981, Williams & Wilkins.

46. Hamilton WK: Measures of outcome, Anesthesiology 65:419-425, 1986.

47. Hawkins WG: Medicolegal hazards of anesthesia, JAMA 163:746-748, 1957.

48. Hendolin H, Mattila MA, and Poikolainen E: The effect of lumbar epidural analgesia on the development of deep vein thrombosis of the legs after open prostatectomy, Acta Chir Scand 147:425-429, 1981.

49. Hendolin H, Tuppurainen T, and Lahtinen J: Thoracic epidural analgesia and deep vein thrombosis in cholecystectomized patients, Acta Chir Scand 148:405-409, 1982.

50. Hilgenburg JC: Intraoperative awareness during high-dose fentanyl oxygen anesthesia, Anesthesiology 54:341-343, 1981.

51. Hirschman CA and Bergman NA: Halothane and enflurane protect against bronchospasm in an asthma dog model, Anesth Analg 57:629-633, 1978.

52. Hirschman CA, Downes H, and Farbood A: Ketamine block of bronchospasm in experimental canine asthma, Br J Anaesth 51:713-718, 1979.

53. Hjorts NC et al: A controlled study on the effect of epidural analgesia with local anaesthetics and morphine on morbidity after abdominal surgery, Acta Anaesthesiol Scand 29:790-796, 1985.

54. Jenkins JG: Epidural anesthesia and analgesia in high-risk surgical patients, Anesthesiology 67:1024-1025, 1987.

55. Kehlet H: Epidural analgesia and the endocrine-metabolic response to surgery, update and perspectives, Acta Anaesthesiol Scand 28:125-127, 1984.

56. Kehlet H: Influence of regional anesthesia on postoperative morbidity, Ann Chir Gynaecol 73:171-176, 1984.

57. Kehlet H: Epidural anesthesia and analgesia in high-risk surgical patients, Anesthesiology 67:1022-1023, 1987.

58. Kehlet H et al: Effect of epidural analgesia on metabolic profiles during and after surgery, Br J Surg 66:543-546, 1979.

59. Kingston HG and Hirschman CA: Perioperative management of the patient with asthma, Anesth Analg 63:844-855, 1984.

60. Knight AA et al: Perioperative myocardial ischemia: importance of the preoperative ischemic pattern, Anesthesiology 68:681-688, 1988.

61. Levy JH et al: A retrospective study of the incidence and causes of failed spinal anesthetics in a university hospital, Anesth Analg 64:705-710, 1985.

62. Manolio TA et al: Regional versus general anesthesia in high-risk surgical patients: the need for a clinical trial, J Clin Anesth, accepted for publication, 1989.

63. Mark JB and Greenburg LM: Intraoperative awareness and hypertensive crisis during high-dose fentanyl-diazepam-oxygen anesthesia, Anesth Analg 62:698-703, 1983.

64. McKenzie PJ et al: Comparison of the effects of spinal anesthesia and general anesthesia on postoperative oxygenation and perioperative mortality, Br J Anaesth 52:49-54, 1980.

65. McLaren AD: Mortality studies. A review, Reg Anaesth 7:S172, 1982.

66. McLaren AD, Stockwell MC, and Reid VC: Anesthetic techniques for surgical correction of fractured neck of femur, Anaesthesia 33:10-14, 1978.

67. McPeck B: Inference, generalizability, and a major change in anesthetic practice, Anesthesiology 66:723-724, 1987.

68. Mellbring G et al: Thromboembolic complications after major abdominal surgery, Acta Chir Scand 149:263-268, 1983.

69. Merin RG: Is anesthesia beneficial for the ischemic heart? Anesthesiology 55:341-342, 1981.

70. Merin RG, Lowenstein E, and Gelman S: Is anesthesia beneficial for the ischemic heart? Anesthesiology 64:137-140, 1986.

71. Modig J et al: Comparative influences of epidural and general anesthesia on deep venous thrombosis and pulmonary embolism after total hip replacement, Acta Chir Scand 147:125-130, 1981.

72. Modig J et al: Thromboembolism after total hip replacement: role of epidural and general, Anaesthesia 62:174-180, 1983.

73. Moore DC et al: Chlorprocaine neurotoxicity: four additional cases, Anesth Analg 61:155-159, 1980.

74. Moore DC, Thompson GE, and Crawford RD: Long acting local anesthetic drugs and convulsions with hypoxia and acidosis, Anesthesiology 56:230-232, 1982.

75. Ngai SH: Action of general anesthetics in producing muscle relaxation. In Katz RL (editor): Muscle relaxants, Amsterdam, 1975, Exerpts Medica.

76. Pflug AE et al: The effects of postoperative peridural analgesia on pulmonary therapy and pulmonary complications, Anesthesiology 41:8-17, 1974.

77. Pflug AE and Halter JB: Effect of spinal anesthesia adrenergic tone and the neuroendocrine responses to surgical stress in humans, Anesthesiology 55:120-126, 1981.

78. Phero JC et al: Hypotension in spinal anesthesia, Anesth Analg 66:549-552, 1987.

79. Prys-Roberts C: Regulation of the circulation. In Prys-Roberts C (editor): The circulation in anesthesia, Oxford, Eng, 1980, Blackwell Publishing.

80. Prough DS et al: Myocardial infarction following regional anesthesia for carotid endarterectomy, Can Anaesth Soc J 31:192-196, 1984.

81. Qvist TF, Skovsted P, and Bredgaard-Sorensen M: Moderate hypotension anesthesia for reduction of blood loss during total hip replacement, Acta Anaesthesiol Scand 26:351-353, 1982.

82. Ramanathan S et al: Maternal and fetal effects of prophylactic hydration with crystalloids or colloids before epidural anesthesia, Anesth Analg 62:673-678, 1983.

83. Roberts SL and Tinker JH: Cardiovascular disease in risk and outcome. In Brown DL (editor): Anesthesia, London, 1988, Lippincott.

84. Roukema JA, Carol EJ, and Pring JG: The prevention of pulmonary complications after upper abdominal surgery in patients with non-compromised pulmonary status, Arch Surg 123:30-34, 1988.

85. Saada M et al: Segmental wall motion in coronary artery disease patients evaluated by two dimensional echocardiography after lumbar epidural anesthesia, Anesthesiology 67:A270, 1987.

86. Shnider SM and Papper EM: Anesthesia for the asthmatic patient, Anesthesiology 22:886-892, 1961.

87. Solazzi RW and Ward RJ: Analysis of anesthetic mishaps. The spectrum of medical liability cases, Int Anesthesiol Clin 22:43-59, 1984.

88. Stanley TH: Reasons to preferentially select general anesthesia. IARS Review Course Lectures, Anesth Analg 4(suppl):66-72, 1986.

89. Stanton-Hicks MD'A: Cardiovascular effects of extradural anesthesia, Br J Anaesth 47:253-261, 1975.

90. Tahir AH, George RB, and Weill H: Effects of abdominal surgery upon diaphragmatic function and regional ventilation, Int Surg 58:337-340, 1973.

91. Takeshima R and Dohi S: Circulatory responses to baroreflexes, valsalva maneuver, coughing, swallowing and nasal stimulation during acute cardiac sympathectomy by epidural blockade in awake humans, Anesthesiology 65:500-508, 1985.

92. Tarnow J, Markschies-Hornung A, and Schulte-Sasse U: Isoflurane improves the tolerance to pacing induced myocardial ischemia, Anesthesiology 64:147-156, 1986.

93. Thompson GE et al: Hypotensive anesthesia for total hip arthroplasty: a study of blood loss and organ function, Anesthesiology 48:91-96, 1978.

94. Traynor C et al: Effect of extradural analgesia and vagal blockade on the metabolic and endocrine response to upper abdominal surgery, Brit J Anaesth 54:319-323, 1982.

95. Urmey WF and Lambert DH: Spinal anesthesia associated with reversal of myocardial ischemia, Anesth Analg 65:908-910, 1986.

96. Valentin N et al: Spinal or general anesthesia for surgery of the fractured hip? A prospective study of mortality in 578 patients, Br J Anaesth 58:284-291, 1986.

97. Wahba WM, Don HF, and Craig DB: Postoperative epidural anesthesia: effects on lung volumes, Can Anaesth Soc J 22:519-527, 1975.

98. White IW and Chappel WA: Anesthesia for surgical correction of fractured femoral neck. A comparison of three techniques, Anaesthesia 35:1107-1110, 1980.

99. Wickstrom I, Holmberg I, and Stefansson T: Survival of female geriatric patients after hip fracture surgery. A comparison of five anesthetic methods, Acta Anaesthesiol Scand 26:607-614, 1982.

100. Wislon SL, Vaughan RW, and Stephen CR: Awareness, dreams, and hallucinations associated with general anesthesia, Anesth Analg 54:609-617, 1975.

101. Yeager M et al: Epidural anesthesia and analgesia in high risk surgical patients, Anesthesiology 66:729-736, 1987.

CHAPTER **10**

Intraoperative Complications

WILLIAM R. FURMAN

Unrecognized esophageal intubation
Aspiration of gastric contents
Neurologic injuries
    Peripheral nerve injuries caused by
      positioning
    Deficits after regional anesthetics

Air embolism
Intraoperative complications of massive
    transfusion
    Coagulopathies
    Metabolic
    Immunologic

Every aspect of anesthetic care can give rise to complications. These adverse effects range from minor and of short duration to devastating and permanent. This chapter discusses three important complications of operative anesthetic management: unrecognized esophageal intubation, aspiration of gastric contents, and neurologic injuries. It also covers two important complications of operative surgical management: air embolism and massive bleeding. Each of these problems can cause sequelae that may last beyond the perioperative period. In each case, the task of the anesthesiologist is either prevention or early detection and appropriate therapy.

UNRECOGNIZED ESOPHAGEAL INTUBATION

Intubation of the esophagus may occur when the larynx is difficult to visualize. If the error is not recognized and corrected properly, the resulting failure to oxygenate the patient can have catastrophic results. Because failure to successfully intubate the trachea is so important a cause of anesthetic mor-

bidity and mortality,[42] the management of such errors is an important aspect of the risk prevention program of almost all anesthesiology departments.

Adequate control of the airway, a fundamentally important aspect of anesthetic care, often requires intubation of the trachea. Most of the time, this is easily accomplished in the standard fashion with a laryngoscope. Among those patients who cannot be intubated in this manner are many in whom the potential difficulty is easily recognizable, such as those with craniofacial injuries, tumors, and deformities. In such cases, an alternative means of intubation, such as the use of a fiberoptic bronchoscope or other technique in which the patient remains awake, is often planned in advance, facilitating satisfactory management of the airway in these potentially difficult situations. A more serious problem concerns those patients who prove to be *unexpectedly* difficult to intubate, especially those in whom the anesthesiologist intubates the esophagus instead of the trachea and fails to recognize the error.

Prior to the widespread availability of devices capable of monitoring the concentration of carbon dioxide in exhaled gas, endotracheal tube placement could only be confirmed by visualization of the tube passing through the vocal cords, by auscultation over the chest and abdomen, and by observation of chest movement during inspiration. In some cases, attempts to verify placement by these methods may be inconclusive. Although no method is completely foolproof, monitoring of exhaled carbon dioxide is an objective means that provides confirmation instantaneously.[6] It is almost certain that CO_2 can only emanate from the lungs.[49,56,60] Because capnometers can reveal the presence of exhaled gas on a breath-by-breath basis, they are ideal as adjuncts to the physical methods described above and are also useful for early detection of inadvertent extubation during anesthesia.[65]

Esophageal intubations are not intrinsically harmful; it is the failure to identify the tube misplacement and remedy the situation that is potentially devastating. When an esophageal intubation is recognized, the tube should immediately be withdrawn and mask ventilation of the patient resumed to prevent hypoxia. The practice of having the patient breathe 100% oxygen prior to induction of anesthesia provides a high level of saturation of hemoglobin and affords safety during the time required for the intubation attempt,[28] but after a failed attempt, oxygenation must be resumed. After ventilation by mask is restored, the efforts to intubate the airway may continue.

If ventilation by mask is feasible, the technical difficulty involved in intubating the trachea is not life-threatening. However, if it is not possible to oxygenate and ventilate by mask after the induction of anesthesia, it is necessary to create a way for air to enter the trachea below the larynx. In truly emergent situations, a cricothyroid puncture may be performed with a large (10 to 15 gauge) catheter, and life support may be maintained while a more definitive tracheostomy is performed.[61]

ASPIRATION OF GASTRIC CONTENTS

Pulmonary aspiration of gastric contents is a complication of imperfect airway management that is an important cause of anesthetic morbidity and mortality. Hydrochloric acid is believed to be the most damaging chemical present in gastric contents. It has been suggested that when the gastric pH is below a critical value of 2.5, and a sufficiently large volume is as-

pirated, bronchopneumonia will result.[74] The critical volume of gastric contents that is required for significant lung injury has been theorized, but by no means proven, to be 25 ml, based on extrapolations from studies in animals such as rhesus monkeys.[37,58] The critical pH of 2.5 may be accurate, but many of the studies of the relationship between lung injury and the pH of the aspirate report average pH values, instead of average hydrogen ion concentrations.[70] This methodology may bias the results such that the critical pH is calculated as being higher than the data truly would support. Nonacid aspirates can also produce pulmonary damage, especially if the volumes are large, or particulate matter is present.[74]

In the operative setting, pulmonary aspiration occurs when an obtunded or unconscious patient actively vomits or passively regurgitates. Its prevention involves identification of patients at increased risk, reduction of the intragastric volume and gastric acidity, and successful protection of the airway.

The risk of regurgitation increases when the intragastric pressure is increased to the point where it can exceed the restraining ability of the gastroesophageal valve. The causes of increased intragastric pressure or decreased gastroesophageal valve function are many[34,70] (see the box below). When one of these factors is present and general anesthesia is required, regurgitation may be controlled by crico-

---

Causes of increased intragastric pressure

Decreased emptying

Pyloric or intestinal obstruction
Tense ascites
Pregnancy
Pain
Anxiety
Intraabdominal mass
Metabolic derangement
Increased intracranial pressure
Drug effects
    Narcotic
    Parasympathomimetic

Other causes of increased volume

Recent meal
Trauma
Obesity

esophageal pressure during the induction of unconsciousness,[62] or the airway may be secured under local or topical anesthesia first.

A decision must always be made regarding whether the indication for protection of the airway via rapid sequence induction is so strong as to justify the risk of failure of intubation once the patient is anesthetized and paralyzed. The strongest indications of risk of aspiration lie in patients who have had a recent meal, have gastrointestinal obstruction, are pregnant (especially at term), or have tense ascites. Trauma victims are almost always assumed to have recently eaten or drunk and therefore are considered most likely to be at high risk. There is great need to exercise discretion in the lower risk indications, however, as is emphasized by the fasting obese patient. Although there is some risk that the fasting gastric volume will be elevated and the pH reduced in such a patient, this risk must be weighed against the fact that many obese patients prove difficult to intubate.

Gastric acidity is temporarily reduced by antacids, although antacids can also damage the lungs.[26,34,74] Histamine (H-2) receptor antagonists and metoclopramide, alone and in combination, have been shown to reduce gastric acidity and diminish intragastric volume.[37,40] However, no controlled study has proven in humans that such a reduction in gastric volume or hydrogen ion concentration has a favorable effect on morbidity or mortality.[37] It is unlikely that such a study could be conducted in an ethical manner. Delaying nonemergent surgery for 8 or more hours to allow digestion of a recent meal can also be helpful, but none of these maneuvers ensures an empty stomach.

Protection of the airway in adults requires a cuffed endotracheal tube and may require positive-pressure ventilation, because aspiration around a low-pressure cuff may occur during spontaneous (negative-pressure) ventilation.[52]

When aspiration occurs, pulmonary injury may result from any of three separate factors (see the box above, right), depending on the nature of the inoculum.[3] In each case, ventilation-perfusion mismatching and intrapulmonary shunting occur rapidly, leading to hypoxia. Treatment is directed toward removal of any particulate material, followed by respiratory support.

The most commonly aspirated toxic fluid is hydrochloric acid. It produces a pulmonary burn,

The "triple threat" of aspiration		
Chemical	**Inert-airway obstruction**	**Bacterial infection**
Acid	Particulates	Primary
Hydrocarbons	Fluids	Superinfection
Mineral oil		
Bile		
Alcohol		
Fats		

which results in leakage of fluid into alveolar spaces, often causes bronchospasm, and characteristically leads to hypoxia.[3] Noncardiogenic pulmonary edema, pulmonary hemorrhage, and atelectasis occur early, and the adult respiratory distress syndrome may follow. These events may take place even in the absence of aspiration of particulate matter or a bacterial inoculum.

The management of witnessed aspiration is respiratory support.[2,3,11,12] Because oxygenation and ventilation are the initial concerns, clearing and intubating the airway must take place as soon as possible. Mechanical ventilatory support, sometimes including positive end-expiratory pressure (PEEP) is often required. Although studies have failed to demonstrate that the use of mechanical ventilation and PEEP improves survival in patients suffering from respiratory failure from a variety of causes including aspiration,[12,63,74] the standard approach to hypoxemia refractory to supplemental oxygen is to control ventilation and institute PEEP.

When particulate matter, such as solid gastric contents, are aspirated, the early management requires suctioning and removal of these particles to relieve atelectasis caused by obstruction of large airways.[34,74] Bronchoscopy may be required to achieve this, but pulmonary lavage is not indicated for the treatment of aspiration that is limited to gastric acid, because acid injures the lung almost instantly, and bronchial secretions effectively buffer the acid within minutes.[3,74]

Corticosteroids have been used in the treatment of acid aspiration, but most recent studies have failed to show any beneficial effect in either oxygenation or outcome.[11-13,20,74,75] Bacterially contaminated aspirates rarely occur in the operating room, although it is possible that histamine type 2 blocking agents can predispose the stomach to be colonized with gram-negative bacilli.[21] Usually, gastric acid that gains entry to the lung during induction of and emergence from anesthesia is sterile, therefore antibiotics are not indicated until an infection is actually documented by either a positive culture or a direct examination of purulent secretions. The lack of benefit of prophylactic antibiotics in terms of survival has been confirmed in several studies, and there is concern that antibiotics increase the risk that more resistant flora will cause subsequent infections.[3,12,74]

Symptomatic therapy of respiratory failure caused by aspiration of gastric contents is no different than that used for other causes of adult respiratory distress syndrome. Intensive nursing and medical support are required until recovery from the acute lung injury takes place. Reported mortality rates from aspiration range from 28% to 60%,[2,11,12] with little difference noted between surgical and nonsurgical occurrences.

NEUROLOGIC INJURIES

Injuries to the peripheral nervous system and prolonged deficits after regional anesthetics are complications of anesthetic management that typically are not evident during the course of the anesthetic. Rather, they are revealed in the postoperative period, either by incomplete resolution of a regional block or by the development of a neurologic deficit soon after surgery.

Peripheral Nerve Injuries Caused By Positioning

Peripheral nerves may be injured as a consequence of positioning for surgery. Anesthetized patients lack protective reflexes and are therefore unable to prevent being placed in positions that either stretch a nerve or nerve plexus or cause direct pressure to be applied to it. In either case, the common mechanism of injury is believed to involve the blood supply to the nerve; vasa nervorum are ruptured by stretching or are occluded by pressure, resulting in ischemia.[9,51]

The incidence of postoperative peripheral neuropathies has been reported in two large studies to be between 8 and 15 cases per 10,000 anesthetics.[19,51] Both surveys were retrospective, and therefore could have underestimated the true incidence of injury. In both studies, the most common injury was to the brachial plexus, followed by approximately equal frequencies of injury conforming to the distribution of the common peroneal, radial, and ulnar nerves (Table 10-1). These data suggest that this potentially preventable complication occurs once every few months in a hospital of average size.

The brachial plexus is susceptible to injury by stretching, if the upper extremity is malpositioned with respect to the head and torso, and by direct compression. In contrast, other peripheral nerve groups are injured by direct compression only, such as may occur when surgical instruments (retractors) or operating room personnel compress a nerve against a bony structure, or when the patient's weight causes a bony structure to entrap a nerve between it and an inadequately padded surface, such as an operating table.

Attention to details of operative positioning of the extremities prevents peripheral nerve injuries. Congenital anomalies, intraoperative hypotension and hypothermia, and the use of a tourniquet for hemostasis can all exacerbate the effects of adverse

TABLE 10-1. **Incidence of postoperative peripheral neuropathies**

	Source					
	Dhunér[19] 31 Injuries 30,000 cases 6 years		Parks[51] 72 Injuries 50,000 cases 13 years		Total 103 Injuries 80,000 cases	
Injury	#	#/10,000	#	#/10,000	#	#/10,000
Brachial plexus	11	3.6	28	5.6	39	4.9
Radial nerve	7	2.3	11	2.2	18	2.3
Ulnar nerve	8	2.7	9	1.8	17	2.1
Peroneal nerve	5	1.7	15	3.0	20	2.5
Other	0		9		9	

positioning. In addition, nerves affected by preexisting neurologic disorders such as diabetes mellitus, alcoholism, herpes zoster, and periarteritis nodosa are believed to be more susceptible to injury.[9,51]

Peripheral nerve injuries are often evident at the time of recovery from surgery, but they may not be reported by the patient until as long as 3 days later. Recovery time is variable and seems to correlate with the degree of injury. While some mild injuries resolve within 1 to 2 weeks, others may not begin to improve for 2 to 3 months and may continue to improve until 6 or more months after the injury. In less than 10% of cases, a residual neurologic deficit remains indefinitely. Treatment includes physiotherapy and protection from further injury, although there is no clear positive correlation between physiotherapy and improved extent or speed of recovery.[9,19,51]

Deficits After Regional Anesthetics

Most deficits following regional anesthetics are related to spinal or epidural anesthetics. Deficits occasionally occur after upper extremity nerve blocks, but there have been no large studies to determine the exact incidence or causes.[73] Although one incident of reflex sympathetic dystrophy 10 days after a 2-chloroprocaine brachial plexus block has been reported,[27] the local anesthetic agents are not generally believed to be directly toxic to peripheral nerves when administered in the recommended concentrations. However, the issue of inherent toxicity of 2-chloroprocaine remains open.[27,48]

Spinal and epidural anesthetics. Neurologic deficits following spinal and epidural anesthesia may be divided into major and minor sequelae. Prior to 1950, a significant number of patients suffered major deficits after spinal anesthesia. Three related syndromes of sensorimotor dysfunction were described: aseptic meningitis, cauda equina syndrome, and adhesive arachnoiditis (Table 10-2).[35] In addition, cases of transverse myelitis and intrathecal, epidural, and intervertebral disk space infections were reported.[10,22,68,77] During the past 3 decades, more rigorous attention to asepsis and to prevention of contamination of needles and ampoules by caustic disinfectants have reduced the risk of these major sequelae of spinal anesthesia to less than 1 per 10,000 cases.[35,55,68]

Although infectious complications of spinal and epidural anesthesia are still sporadically reported,[5,38] major deficits are most often ascribed to drug toxicity from the intrathecal injection of medications intended only for epidural use (2-chloroprocaine) or to the occurrence of epidural or subdural hematomas as complications of traumatic lumbar puncture (see the box below). In addition, spinal cord ischemia and infarction resulting from episodes of prolonged intraoperative hypotension have been implicated in some reports, although this matter has received little direct study.[35,68] Hypotension in other settings is rarely if ever causative of spinal cord infarction, making this mechanism an unlikely one. Finally, some cases of neurologic deficits that occur after spinal or epidural anesthesia are previously undiagnosed neurologic injuries or the coincidental worsening of preexisting neurologic pathology.[*]

Minor sensory neurologic defects that occur after spinal anesthesia (transient numbness or paresthesias in the perineum or lower extremities) are believed to result from a mild nonspecific toxic effect of local anesthetics in some cases and surgical positioning trauma in others. They are reported to occur in 3 to 8 cases per 1000, and they do not appear to be related to either trauma incurred during a technically difficult lumbar puncture or to the occurrence of paresthesias during needle insertion.[35,68,69]

*References 22, 35, 68, 69, 72, and 77.

> **Causes of major neurologic deficits occurring after epidural and spinal anesthesia**
>
> Unintended intrathecal injection
> Hematoma
> Local infection (abscess, meningitis)
> Severe hypotension (cord ischemia)
> Other (preexisting) pathology

TABLE 10-2. Neurologic deficits occurring after spinal anesthesia

Syndrome	Onset	Recovery
Aseptic meningitis	24 Hours	Days to 1 week
Cauda equina syndrome	Immediate	Weeks to months
Adhesive arachnoiditis	Months	Progressive

2-Chloroprocaine has been associated with prolonged neurologic deficits after epidural block. In some of these cases, inadvertent intrathecal injection is known to have taken place.[35] The question of whether 2-chloroprocaine is inherently neurotoxic or whether the preservative (bisulfite) is to be blamed remains unresolved. Several different experimental models have been employed to study this issue, and each has yielded conflicting results. Neurotoxicity can be produced when exposed nerves are bathed in 2-chloroprocaine. However, in vivo experiments in which the anesthetic is injected around the nerves in a manner approximating the clinical situation suggest that 2-chloroprocaine is not neurotoxic. These latter studies have shown that bisulfite can be toxic if the concentration is sufficiently high.[25] The current recommendation for prevention of prolonged block after epidural anesthesia is to meticulously test all epidural catheters for intrathecal placement before injection of anesthetic, especially when 2-chloroprocaine is used. If intrathecal injection of this agent occurs and leads to a persistent deficit, the only treatment available is supportive care.

AIR EMBOLISM

The clinical conditions that result when bubbles of undissolved gas gain entry to the vascular system are collectively called *air embolism*. When these bubbles are large enough, they can produce clinically noticeable obstructions to blood flow, either on the venous side in the pulmonary outflow tract (venous air embolization) or on the arterial side, such as in the coronary or cerebral circulation (systemic arterial air embolization). When the volumes of gas are small or enter the circulation slowly, no clinical signs or symptoms may result.[43]

Undissolved gas may gain entry to the circulation during surgery under a wide variety of circumstances. The most common situations involve surgical procedures that allow air entrainment through noncollapsible veins. In such cases, the surgical field is almost always above the level of the right atrium. Neurosurgical operations, especially those performed with the patient in the sitting position, are the most common. The reported incidence of detectable (although not necessarily clinically significant) embolization during neurosurgery varies from 6% to 66%, depending on the sensitivity of the method of detection.[32]

Air can also gain entry to the vascular system through vascular catheters of all kinds, including central venous lines and cannulae used for cardiopulmonary bypass or hemodialysis if a break in the integrity of the system occurs.[14,36,43] In addition, any procedure that involves the insufflation of gas into a body cavity, such as laparoscopy, hysteroscopy, or arthroscopy, can result in embolization of that gas.[43,59]

The minimum amount of air required to produce adverse clinical effects in man is postulated to be between 3 and 8 ml/kg injected rapidly, based on animal studies.[15,43] The mechanism by which venous air embolism becomes detrimental is believed to be obstruction of the pulmonary outflow tract, leading simultaneously to acute right heart failure and to impaired gas exchange. Subsequent events are generally attributable to the effects of hypoxia and hypercarbia, especially on the myocardium. There have also been reports of pulmonary edema following air embolism.[64]

When undissolved air gains entry to the systemic circulation (systemic arterial embolization) by passing through either the pulmonary circulation or the heart, localized ischemia and/or infarction can occur. Although the pulmonary circulation normally functions as a filter for air bubbles, this filtering capacity can be altered by a number of drugs, and recent animal studies suggest that the choice of anesthetic agents may exert an effect on the threshold for transpulmonary passage of venous air emboli.[76] Transcardiac passage probably occurs in the same way that paradoxical venous thromboemboli are believed to occur: an elevation of right-sided pressures favors intracardiac shunting through a patent foramen ovale, which may be present in up to 35% of the population.[30] The diagnosis of systemic air embolism is generally retrospective, posed as an explanation of a neurologic deficit or other localized injury incurred after an episode of venous air embolization; specific therapy is generally not feasible.[43]

Because of the high incidence of air embolism associated with certain surgical procedures, especially those performed with the patient in the sitting position, such procedures are generally performed with special attention to monitoring devices directed toward the early diagnosis and treatment of this problem. The diagnostic methods include auscultation for characteristic heart sounds via the esophageal stethoscope and via reflected ultrasound (Doppler device), end-tidal CO_2 monitoring, and the use of right atrial and pulmonary artery catheters.

Air emboli as small as 1 to 4 ml produce alterations in the heart sounds that may be heard through the esophageal stethoscope. Initially, the heart sounds develop a tympanic quality and the second heart sound may become louder. With increasing volumes of air, a coarse systolic murmur, and then a "mill-wheel" (systolic and diastolic) murmur develop. The Doppler device is considerably more sensitive and may respond to volumes as small as 0.25 ml if the probe is correctly positioned.[43,66] Capnometry, which is rapidly becoming standard anesthesia monitoring, rapidly indicates the presence of pulmonary outflow obstruction by undissolved gas. The sudden increase in the dead space to tidal volume ratio that results from a major pulmonary vascular obstruction by air is heralded by an equally sudden fall in the end-tidal CO_2.[8,65]

Right atrial and pulmonary artery catheters have also been used for the detection of air emboli. Both pulmonary artery pressures[41,47] and central venous pressures[54] rise after air embolization. In addition, any catheter placed in the right atrium represents a potential means of therapy. Multiport right atrial catheters appear to be most efficient in this regard[15]; however, entrained air can also be aspirated via the proximal lumen of a pulmonary artery catheter[41,47] or a special pulmonary artery catheter introducer sheath modified to have six 1-mm side holes near its distal end.[7]

When an air embolus is diagnosed, air can be aspirated from the right atrium if a catheter is in use. If N_2O is in use, it should be discontinued, for diffusion of N_2O into air bubbles will increase their size and clinical significance.[46,47] To prevent subsequent entrainment of air by the venous system, the surgical field should be flooded with irrigant, and the venous pressure should be elevated. Venous pressure may be increased by the infusion of intravenous fluids, by the use of continuous positive-pressure ventilation, or by direct compression of the jugular vein (during a sitting neurosurgical procedure).[67] The use of active lung inflation (manual compression of the anesthetic reservoir bag) or PEEP have been recommended, but the efficacy of these two latter maneuvers has recently been questioned.[53,67]

Although air embolism probably cannot be prevented, aggressive monitoring and therapy has led to early recognition and treatment and has reduced the morbidity and mortality associated with surgical procedures that have a high incidence of this complication. As a result, fatalities now tend to occur in settings where air emboli are so rare a complication that routine monitoring by Doppler probe and right atrial catheter is not indicated.[43] Perhaps the increased use of capnometry as a form of routine monitoring of all anesthetic administration will lead to earlier recognition of air emboli in these other settings and thus improve outcome.

INTRAOPERATIVE COMPLICATIONS OF MASSIVE TRANSFUSION

Massive transfusion is usually defined as the acute administration of more than 1.5 times the patient's estimated blood volume.[44,78] The infusion of such large volumes of blood is associated with a number of intraoperative coagulopathic, metabolic, and immunologic complications (see the box below). Because procedures that predictably result in massive blood loss (for example, trauma surgery and liver transplantation) are an important part of current surgical practice, an understanding of the management of complications of blood transfusion is particularly important.

Coagulopathies

Patients who receive large amounts of bank blood can develop significant clotting abnormalities. This can lead to an unfavorable cycle: they receive trans-

---

Intraoperative Complications of Massive Blood Transfusion

Coagulopathic
Dilutional thrombocytopenia
Factor V and VIII deficiency
Primary and secondary fibrinolysis

Metabolic
Citrate intoxication (hypocalcemia)
Acid-base imbalance
Potassium imbalance
Leftward shift of the oxyhemoglobin dissociation curve

Immunologic
Nonhemolytic (minor) reactions
Hemolytic (major) reactions

fusions of blood that does not clot properly, resulting in more bleeding, which requires more blood to be transfused, further exacerbating the coagulopathy. Evidence of a bleeding diathesis, such as hematuria, oozing from venipuncture sites or the surgical field, ecchymoses, or nasal or gingival bleeding may be observed during massive transfusion, and the diagnosis may be confirmed by laboratory testing of coagulation parameters. If possible, a specific diagnosis of the cause of bleeding should be made prior to therapy. However, this may be difficult during severe hemorrhage because many coagulation laboratories are unable to perform platelet counts, partial thromboplastin times (PTT), prothrombin times (PT), or to assess fibrinogen levels sufficiently quickly.[45] The principal causes of coagulation defects in massively transfused patients are dilutional thrombocytopenia, dilution of factors V and VIII, and fibrinolysis.[23,44,45]

Thrombocytopenia. Massive transfusions cause dilutional thrombocytopenia because the platelets contained in bank blood are deficient in both quantity and in viability. Forty percent of platelets stored in bank blood at 4° C for 3 hours and more than 85% of those stored for 24 hours are damaged and will be rapidly sequestered by the reticuloendothelial system once transfused. Abnormal bleeding in surgical patients is associated with platelet counts below about 65,000 per mm^3, therefore a previously normal individual must receive at least 12 to 15 units of blood before the platelet count falls to a clinically significant level.[44,45,57] Platelet transfusion may be required sooner if the initial counts were abnormally low, or if platelet function was initially abnormal. Otherwise, the administration of platelets is probably not indicated, and at least two studies have suggested that empiric platelet transfusions do not alter the incidence of nonsurgical bleeding.[31,57]

Factors V and VIII. Bank blood contains levels of factors V and VIII that are reduced to between 20% and 50% of normal; however, only 10% to 20% of the normal levels of these factors are required to prevent abnormal bleeding during surgery.[44,45] For this reason, no amount of transfusion of *whole* blood to a previously normal individual should adversely affect the coagulation cascade. Thus, there should be no need to administer fresh frozen plasma (FFP) for the purpose of reconstituting the levels of these factors during transfusion of whole blood, unless some other process, such as liver disease or a consumptive coagulopathy, is present.

When large amounts of *packed red blood cells* (greater than the patient's estimated blood volume) are transfused, FFP may be required because the packing process removes most of the plasma fraction. Until recently, the standard management of massive transfusion included the administration of two units of fresh frozen plasma after every six units of packed red blood cells infused.[23] Evidence for the utility of prophylactic administration of FFP has never been presented,[44,57] and a recent National Institutes of Health consensus conference concluded that "empiric use of FFP to reverse hemostatic disorders should be confined to those patients in whom factor deficiencies are presumed to be the sole or principle derangement."[17] As a volume expander or nutritional source, FFP is simply not justified. Safer, more effective alternatives exist.[17,24]

Fibrinolysis. Activation of the fibrinolytic system by endogenously released tissue thromboplastin may occur during massive transfusion of bank blood, or for reasons related to the need for the blood replacement (for example, portocaval, prostatic, uterine, or neurologic surgery or bacterial sepsis). The result is the formation of small fibrin thrombi in the bloodstream and consumption of and a decrease in factors I, II, V, and VIII, and platelets. The formation of small fibrin thrombi in the microvasculature is believed to diffusely activate the fibrinolytic system, resulting in the paradoxical combination of simultaneous clotting and bleeding (disseminated intravascular coagulation [DIC]).

When the activation of fibrinolysis occurs in association with DIC, the term *secondary fibrinolysis* is applied. It is speculated that primary fibrinolysis (fibrinolysis not associated with intravascular coagulation) may exist and that, when diagnosed, it should be treated with epsilon-aminocaproic acid after heparinization. Heparin therapy is also recommended for secondary fibrinolysis based on theory, but removal of the inciting cause of consumptive coagulopathy is always essential to its treatment. Transfusion of the consumed factors and platelets is controversial, but hard to abjure in the surgical patient who is bleeding.[23,45]

Metabolic

The potential metabolic consequences of massive transfusion include citrate toxicity, acidosis, hyperkalemia, and a leftward shift of the oxyhemoglobin dissociation curve. Although these abnormalities have been postulated to occur because of the composition of bank blood, in practice they rarely cause complications that require specific therapy. Most often, restoration of the intravascular volume in the bleeding patient is what is required to assure oxygen delivery to the tissues and proper metabolic balance.

Citrate intoxication. To ensure complete anticoagulation of bank blood, a planned excess of an anticoagulant containing citrate is added at the time of collection. Citrate prevents coagulation by chelating calcium ions; and rapid transfusion of bank blood (or fresh frozen plasma) reduces the recipient's serum ionized calcium concentration.[18] Earlier texts recommended routine administration of intravenous calcium salts to prevent the development of coagulopathy, myocardial depression, and rhythm disturbances.[44] Recent studies have shown that while ionized calcium levels do fall significantly during massive transfusion, they rebound rapidly on completion of the infusion, presumably because of hepatic metabolism of citrate and mobilization of calcium from tissue storage sites.[18,33,45,78] For these reasons, (1) citrate toxicity is not believed to be an important cause of coagulopathy, at least at rates of infusion up to 150 ml/min (20 units of whole blood per hour), and (2) routine calcium administration is not recommended unless evidence of clinically significant hypocalcemia, such as myocardial depression, develops. This may be more likely to occur in patients who are hyperventilated, hypothermic, or have liver disease.

Acid-base imbalance. Bank blood develops a number of biochemical and cellular changes, including hypercarbia, hypoxia, and acidemia. After 35 days, the P_{CO_2} rises to 200 mm Hg, the P_{O_2} falls to 20 mm Hg, and the pH averages 6.98, therefore rapid administration of stored blood has long been suspected capable of producing acidosis. For this reason, many authors have recommended routine administration of alkalinizing solutions during transfusion of more than 5 units. Studies carried out in trauma victims have not supported this approach; and the currently favored management is to aggressively restore the circulating volume and only treat metabolic acidosis that is confirmed by blood gas analysis.[31,44,78]

As a rule, the acid load will be well handled if tissue perfusion is maintained, and metabolism of the citrate included in the bank blood will provide a source of bicarbonate.[33] In addition, excessive alkalinization can theoretically be harmful because it may lead to impairment of oxygen delivery resulting from rightward shift of the oxyhemoglobin dissociation curve and from hyperosmolality.[16,44]

Potassium imbalance. During storage, the sodium-potassium pumping mechanism in the red blood cell membrane fails to function properly, and intracellular potassium leaks into the plasma fraction. After 35 days, the serum K^+ may be as high as 32 meq/L.[44,78] Nevertheless, routine administration of calcium in the absence of electrocardiographic evidence of significant hyperkalemia is not indicated. This is because the maximum total amount of potassium contained in one unit of blood is less than 10 meq, and only if a patient receives more than 10 units of 35-day-old-blood (an unlikely event) could 100 meq be administered. Even in that case, it would be expected that renal function and reuptake by the transfused cells would lower the serum potassium level, and that metabolism of citrate to bicarbonate would favor intracellular transfer of the ion as well. In the setting of renal failure and/or a persistent metabolic acidosis, hyperkalemia may be more likely, but laboratory or ECG evidence of potassium imbalance should be observed before treatment with calcium or glucose and insulin is initiated.

Alterations of the oxyhemoglobin dissociation curve. Oxygen delivery to the tissues may theoretically be adversely affected by three factors that increase the affinity of the hemoglobin molecule for oxygen: alkalosis, hypothermia, and reduced levels of 2,3-diphosphoglycerate (2,3-DPG).[1,44,78] Alkalosis is avoided by administering alkalinizing agents only when acidosis is documented. Hypothermia is not so much a specific complication of blood transfusion as a problem associated with all major surgical procedures. Its treatment and prevention require the use of all available modalities of heat conservation, including the warming of all blood through heat-exchanging devices, in an effort to prevent the cardiac arrhythmias that may occur when the core temperature falls below 32° C.

2,3-DPG levels are reduced in bank blood, and it is known that the infusion of large amounts of blood can reduce the recipient's levels transiently. The addition of adenine to bank blood results in higher levels of 2,3-DPG during storage, as well as longer red cell survival. Metabolically, frozen blood is more normal than other stored blood. While the alteration in the oxyhemoglobin relationship that attends a lower 2,3-DPG level has been shown to alter myocardial performance in isolated rabbit hearts with fixed coronary flow,[1] it is not yet known whether this effect is clinically significant in man.[39,45,78]

Immunologic

Intraoperative immunologic reactions to transfused blood may be classified as minor or major. The minor, non-life-threatening ones are usually leukoagglutinin reactions caused by antileukocyte antibodies possessed by the recipient. Major reactions occur when incompatible red blood cells are transfused.

Minor reactions. Minor transfusion reactions are characterized by fever, chills, and occasionally urticaria or other skin rashes. They are generally impossible to predict and therefore cannot be easily prevented. In the anesthetized patient, especially during an operative procedure characterized by significant blood loss, these symptoms may easily be overlooked if they are even recognizable at all.

The onset of a leukoagglutinin reaction is typically 30 to 120 minutes after the transfusion, and the episode may last as long as 48 hours.[4] In addition to fever and leukocytosis, tachycardia and hypotension may occur, and transient pulmonary infiltrates have also been reported.[71] If such a reaction is suspected during massive transfusion of a surgical patient, a reconfirmation of the correctness of the blood typing is necessary. Treatment with steroids may be beneficial; the utility of antihistamines is unclear.[4]

Hemolytic reactions. Hemolytic transfusion reactions occur when blood to which the recipient has antibodies or when plasma containing antibodies to the recipient's red blood cells is transfused. While reactions of the latter type are usually not severe, those of the former type may result in serious, life-threatening (40% to 60% mortality) hemolysis of the transfused blood. In the majority of such cases, the cause is a preventable break in the "chain of identity." The importance of conscientious positive identification at every step of the process by which a patient's blood type is determined and compatible units are selected and ultimately transfused cannot be overemphasized.[29,50]

The manifestations of a major hemolytic transfusion reaction in a conscious patient are listed in the box above, right. Many of these (back pain, dyspnea, angina, vomiting, diarrhea) are not recognizable in the anesthetized patient who is hemorrhaging. Others (circulatory collapse, oliguria, consumptive coagulopathy) may occur as a conse-

---

Signs and Symptoms of Major Transfusion Reactions
Urticaria
Circulatory collapse
Icterus
Hemoglobinuria
Oliguria
Severe back pain
Dyspnea
Angina
Vomiting
Diarrhea
Consumptive coagulopathy

---

quence of many other causes, and so are not specific indicators of a major blood incompatibility. A temporal relationship between the development of these symptoms and transfusion, especially if accompanied by the presence of hematuria, urticaria, or pigmented serum in a blood specimen should raise the suspicion of a potentially life-threatening transfusion reaction.

Treatment of such a reaction in a hemorrhaging surgical patient is especially difficult. It requires a halt to the transfusion while a reverification of the identification of the patient and of the units of blood takes place. In addition, a consumptive coagulopathy often ensues, compounding the problem. When such a reaction occurs, therapeutic measures intended to promote clearance of free hemoglobin and of antibody complexes, by alkalinizing the urine (sodium bicarbonate) and increasing urine output (crystalloid, mannitol, furosemide), are recommended despite the lack of theoretical or objective proof that they alter outcome. In addition, the development of DIC should be anticipated and a platelet count, PTT, and fibrinogen level determined. Guided by the results of these tests, treatment of DIC with heparin, FFP, and cryoprecipitate may be recommended, but have never been proven to alter outcome.[29,45]

REFERENCES

1. Apshein CS et al: Effect of erythrocyte storage and oxyhemoglobin affinity changes on cardiac function, Am J Physiol 248 (Heart Circ Physiol 17):H508-H515, 1985.
2. Arms RA, Dines DE, and Tinstman TC: Aspiration pneumonia, Chest 65:136-139, 1974.
3. Bartlett JG and Gorbach SL: The triple threat of aspiration pneumonia, Chest 68:560-566, 1975.

4. Barton JC: Nonhemolytic, noninfectious transfusion reactions, Semin Hematol 18:95-121, 1981.

5. Berman RS and Eisele JH: Bacteremia, spinal anesthesia, and development of meningitis, Anesthesiology 48:376-377, 1978.

6. Birmingham PK, Cheney FW, and Ward RJ: Esophageal intubation: a review of detection techniques, Anesth Analg 65:886-891, 1986.

7. Bowdle TA and Artru AA: Treatment of air embolism with a special pulmonary artery catheter introducer sheath in sitting dogs, Anesthesiology 68:107-110, 1988.

8. Brechner VL and Bethune RWM: Recent advances in monitoring pulmonary air embolism, Anesth Analg 51:255-261, 1971.

9. Britt BA, Joy N, and Mackay MB: Positioning trauma. In Orkin FK, and Cooperman LH, editors: Complications in anesthesiology, Philadelphia, 1983, JB Lippincott Co, pp 646-670.

10. Bromley LL, Craig JD, and Kessel AWL: Infected intervertebral disk after lumbar puncture, Br Med J 1:132-133, 1949.

11. Bynum LJ and Pierce AK: Pulmonary aspiration of gastric contents, Am Rev Resp Dis 114:1129-1136, 1976.

12. Cameron JL, Mitchell WH, and Zuidema GD. Aspiration pneumonia, Arch Surg 106:49-52, 1973.

13. Chapman RL et al: Effect of continuous positive-pressure ventilation and steroids on aspiration of hydrochloric acid (pH 1.8) in dogs, Anesth Analg 53:556-562, 1974.

14. Cohen MB et al: Introducer sheath malfunction producing insidious air embolism, Anesthesiology 67:573-575, 1987.

15. Colley PS and Artru AA: Bunegin-Albin catheter improves air retrieval and resuscitation from lethal venous air embolism in dogs, Anesth Analg 66:991-994, 1987.

16. Collins JA: Problems associated with the massive transfusion of stored blood, Surgery 75:274-195, 1974.

17. Consensus Conference: Fresh-frozen plasma, JAMA 253:551-553, 1985.

18. Cote CJ et al: Ionized hypocalcemia after fresh frozen plasma administration to thermally injured children, Anesth Analg 67:152-160, 1988.

19. Dhuner K-G: Nerve injuries following operations: a survey of cases occurring during a six-year period, Anesthesiology 11:289-293, 1948.

20. Downs JB et al: An evaluation of steroid therapy in aspiration pneumonitis, Anesthesiology 40:129-135, 1974.

21. Driks MR et al: Nosocomial pneumonia in intubated patients given sucralfate as compared with antacids or histamine type 2 blockers, N Engl J Med 317:1376-1382, 1987.

22. Dripps RD and Vandam LD: A long term follow-up of 10,098 spinal anesthetics. I. Failure to discover major sequelae, JAMA 156:1486-1491, 1954.

23. Ellison N: Hemostasis in the trauma patient, Semin Anesth 4:163-176, 1985.

24. Ewalenko P, Deloof T, and Peeters J: Composition of fresh frozen plasma, Crit Care Med 14:145-146, 1986.

25. Ford DJ and Raj PP: Peripheral neurotoxicity of 2-chloroprocaine and bisulfite in the cat, Anesth Analg 66:719-722, 1987.

26. Gibbs CP et al: Antacid pulmonary aspiration in the dog, Anesthesiology 51:380-385, 1979.

27. Gillespie JH, Menk EJ, and Middaugh RE: Reflex sympathetic dystrophy: a complication of interscalene block, Anesth Analg 66:1316-1317, 1987.

28. Gold MI, Duarte I, and Muravchick S: Arterial oxygenation in conscious patients after 5 minutes and after 30 seconds of oxygen breathing, Anesth Analg 60:313-315, 1981.

29. Greenwalt TJ: Pathogenesis and management of hemolytic transfusion reactions, Semin Hematol 18:84-94, 1981.

30. Gronert GA et al: Paradoxical air embolism from a patent foramen ovale, Anesthesiology 50:548-549, 1979.

31. Harrigan C et al: Serial changes in primary hemostasis after massive transfusion, Surgery 98:836-843, 1985.

32. Harris MM et al: Venous embolism during craniectomy in supine infants, Anesthesiology 67:816-819, 1987.

33. Kahn RC et al: Massive blood replacement: correlation of ionized calcium, citrate, and hydrogen ion concentration, Anesth Analg 58:274-278, 1979.

34. Kallos T, Lampe KF, and Orkin FK: Pulmonary aspiration of gastric contents. In Orkin FK, and Cooperman LH, editors: Complications in anesthesiology, Philadelphia, 1983, JB Lippincott Co, pp 152-164.

35. Kane RE: Neurologic deficits following epidural or spinal anesthesia, Anesth Analg 60:150-161, 1981.

36. Khoury GF et al: Air embolism associated with veno-venous bypass during orthotopic liver transplantation, Anesthesiology 67:848-851, 1987.

37. Kowalsky SF: Cimetidine in anesthesia: does it minimize the complications of acid aspiration? Drug Intell Clin Pharm 18:382-389, 1984.

38. Loarie DJ and Fairley HB: Epidural abscess following spinal anesthesia, Anesth Analg 57:351-353, 1978.

39. McConn R and Derrick JB: The respiratory function of blood, Anesthesiology 36:119-127, 1972.

40. Manchikanti L et al: Ranitidine and metoclopramide for prophylaxis of aspiration pneumonitis in elective surgery, Anesth Analg 63:903-910, 1984.

41. Marshall WK and Bedford RF: Use of a pulmonary-artery catheter for detection and treatment of venous air embolism, Anesthesiology 52:131-134, 1980.

42. Marx GF, Mateo CV, and Orkin LR: Computer analysis of postanesthetic deaths, Anesthesiology 39:54-58, 1973.

43. Michenfelder JD: Air embolism. In Orkin FK, and Cooperman LH, editors: Complications in anesthesiology, Philadelphia, 1983, JB Lippincott Co, pp 268-273.

44. Miller RD: Complications of massive blood transfusions, Anesthesiology 39:82-93, 1973.

45. Miller RD: Problems posed by transfusion. In Orkin FK, and Cooperman LH, editors: Complications in anesthesiology, Philadelphia, 1983, JB Lippincott Co, pp 461-475.

46. Munson ES and Merrick HC: Effect of nitrous oxide on venous air embolism, Anesthesiology 27:783-787, 1966.

47. Munson ES et al: Early detection of venous air embolism using a Swan-Ganz catheter, Anesthesiology 42:223-226, 1975.

48. Murphy TM: Complications of diagnostic and therapeutic nerve blocks. In Orkin FK, and Cooperman LH, editors: Complications of anesthesiology, Philadelphia, 1983, JB Lippincott Co, pp 106-116.

49. Murray IP and Modell JH: Early detection of endotracheal tube accidents by monitoring carbon dioxide concentration in respiratory gas, Anesthesiology 59:344-346, 1983.

50. Myhre BA, Bove JR, and Schmidt PJ: Wrong blood: a needless cause of surgical deaths, Anesth Analg 60:77-78, 1981.

51. Parks BJ: Postoperative peripheral neuropathies, Surgery 74:348-357, 1973.

52. Pavlin EG, VanNimwegan D, and Hornbein TF: Failure of high-compliance low-pressure cuff to prevent aspiration, Anesthesiology 42:216-219, 1975.

53. Pfitzner J and McLean AG: Venous air embolism and active lung inflation at high and low CVP, Anesth Analg 66:1127-1134, 1987.

54. Pfitzner J, McLean AG, and Crawshaw KM: Embolized air collection in the superior vena cava of "upright" sheep, Anesth Analg 66:1135-1140, 1987.

55. Phillips OC et al: Neurologic complications following spinal anesthesia with lidocaine: a prospective review of 10,440 cases, Anesthesiology 30:284-289, 1969.

56. Ping ST: Esophageal intubation, Anesth Analg 66:483, 1987.

57. Reed RL et al: Prophylactic platelet administration during massive transfusion, Ann Surg 203:40-48, 1986.

58. Roberts RB and Shirley MA: Reducing the risk of acid aspiration during cesarean section, Anesth Analg 53:859-868, 1974.

59. Saha AK: Air embolism during anaesthesia for arthrography in a child, Anaesthesia 31:1231-1233, 1976.

60. Salzarulo HH et al: Carbon dioxide detection and esophageal intubation, Anesth Analg 67:195-198, 1988.

61. Scuderi PE, McLeskey CH, and Comer PB: Emergency percutaneous transtracheal ventilation during anesthesia using readily available equipment, Anesth Analg 62:867-870, 1982.

62. Sellick BA: Cricoid pressure to control regurgitation of stomach contents during induction of anesthesia, Lancet 2:404-406, 1961.

63. Springer RR and Stevens PP: The influence of PEEP on survival of patients in respiratory failure, Am J Med 66:196-200, 1979.

64. Still JA, Lederman DS, and Renn WH: Pulmonary edema following air embolism, Anesthesiology 40:194-196, 1974.

65. Swedlow DB: Capnometry and capnography: the anesthesia disaster early warning system, Semin Anesth 5:194-205, 1986.

66. Tinker JH et al: Detection of air embolism: a test for positioning of right atrial catheter and doppler probe, Anesthesiology 43:104-106, 1975.

67. Toung TJK et al: Effect of PEEP and jugular venous compression on canine cerebral blood flow and oxygen consumption in the head elevated position, Anesthesiology 68:53-58, 1988.

68. Vandam LD: Complications of spinal and epidural anesthesia. In Orkin FK, and Cooperman LH, editors: Complications in anesthesiology, Philadelphia, 1983, JB Lippincott Co, pp. 75-105.

69. Vandam LD and Dripps RD: A long term follow-up of 10,098 spinal anesthetics. II. Incidence and analysis of minor sensory neurological defects, Surgery 38:463-469, 1955.

70. Vaughan RW, Bauer S, and Wise L: Volume and pH of gastric juice in obese patients, Anesthesiology 43:686-689, 1973.

71. Ward HN: Pulmonary infiltrates associated with leukoagglutinin transfusion reactions, Ann Intern Med 73:689-694, 1970.

72. Warner DO, Danielson DR, and Restall CJ: Temporary paraplegia following spinal anesthesia in a patient with a spinal cord arteriovenous malformation, Anesthesiology 66:236-237, 1987.

73. Winchell SW and Wolfe R: The incidence of neuropathy following upper extremity nerve blocks, Regional Anesth 10:12-15, 1985.

74. Wynne JW and Modell JH: Respiratory aspiration of stomach contents, Ann Intern Med 87:466-474, 1977.

75. Wynne JW et al: Steroid therapy for pneumonitis induced in rabbits by aspiration of foodstuff, Anesthesiology 51:11-19, 1979.

76. Yahagi N and Furuya H: The effects of halothane and pentobarbital on the threshold of transpulmonary passage of venous air emboli in dogs, Anesthesiology 67:905-909, 1987.

77. Yaskin HE and Alpers BJ: Neuropsychiatric complications following spinal anesthesia, Ann Intern Med 23:184-200, 1945.

78. Zauder HL: Massive transfusion, Int Anesthesiol Clin 30:157-170, 1982.

CHAPTER **11**

The Anesthetic Data Record

RICHARD M. SHAPIRO

The first anesthetic data record (ADR) appeared in 1895 containing pulse and respiratory rate changes associated with the administration of ether.[1] Since then anesthesia data recording has undergone vast changes. At present the ADR is considered to be the only definitive record of intraoperative events.[2] As such, it serves as medical-legal documentation of events that have occurred intraoperatively. In addition, anesthesiologists use the ADR as a teaching tool to evaluate the correctness of a given anesthetic, as a method to collect data for clinical research protocols, and as a method to determine if patients have had difficulties or complications associated with previously administered anesthetics.[2] Despite the obvious benefits afforded to anesthesiologists, the ADR can be of great value to consultants. Consultants can determine whether or not a relationship exists between intraoperative events and the postoperative complications they have been asked to evaluate and treat. Although the potential value of a well-documented ADR is obvious, the information contained in this document is often not readily recog-

nized by persons who are not anesthesiologists. Recognition of the information provided by the ADR requires an understanding of the general structure of the document, knowledge of commonly employed recording practices, and finally, insight into the value of the data recorded.

Despite every institution having its own ADR, all are similar in terms of their content and ability to meet the previously mentioned goals. This chapter will describe the general structure and the current recording practices used in completing the ADR at the Johns Hopkins Hospital. It is composed of two components, a preoperative evaluation section and the intraoperative data record section. I hope that the remainder of this textbook will provide the insight into the value of the data recorded.

PREOPERATIVE EVALUATION

Preoperative evaluation was incorporated into the ADR to standardize the preoperative assessment of patients coming to the hospital for surgery and to limit the variability found in residents' preoperative

138

PREOPERATIVE EVALUATION

DATE ______ TIME ______ AGE ______ SEX ______ RACE ______

PROCEDURE ______

DIAGNOSIS ______

MEDICATIONS ______

LAST P.O. ______ SOLIDS ______ LIQUIDS ______

USE BALLPOINT PEN

ALLERGIES ______

PATIENT DATA (1)

YES	NO	CARDIOVASCULAR DISEASE	YES	NO	HEPATIC DISEASE	YES	NO	HEMATOLOGIC DISEASE
		MI			HEPATITIS			SICKLE CELL
		HYPERTENSION			OTHER			COAGULOPATHY
		ARRHYTHMIA						OTHER
		ANGINA			**ENDOCRINE DISEASE**			**PEDIATRICS**
		CHF			DIABETES			PREMATURITY
		VALVULAR DISEASE			OTHER			CONGENITAL ABN
		PERIPHERAL VASC DISEASE						APNEA
		PAST CARDIAC SURGERY			**INFECTIOUS DISEASE**			OTHER
		OTHER			SEPSIS			**OBSTETRICS**
		PULMONARY			OTHER			PREECLAMPSIA ECLAMPSIA
		SMOKING Hx						PREMATURITY
		ASTHMA			**NEUROLOGIC DISEASE**			PLACENTA PREVIA ABRUPTIO
		COPD EMPHYSEMA BPD			SEIZURE			OTHER
		OTHER			ELEVATED ICP			**ANESTHETIC DIFFICULTIES**
		RENAL DISEASE			CEREBROVASC DISEASE			DIFFICULT INTUBATION
		RENAL FAILURE			NEUROMUSCULAR DISORDER			FAMILY HISTORY
		OTHER			OTHER			OTHER
								DRUG ABUSE
								ETOH
								OTHER

☐ HISTORY UNKNOWN EXCEPT AS NOTED ABOVE

EXPLANATION OF POSITIVE DATA ______

PHYSICAL EXAMINATION BP (RANGE) ______ P ______ R ______ T ______ WT ______ (Kg.)

☐ JVD ☐ PERIPHERAL EDEMA ☐ S3 GALLOP

(2)

LAB VALUES

NA ______ K ______ HCT ______

ABNL LAB: ______ (3)

ECG FINDINGS ☐ OFFICIAL ☐ UNOFFICIAL ☐ NORMAL ☐ ABNORMAL

☐ S-T ABNL ☐ CONDUCTION ABNL ☐ OTHER ☐ Q's ☐ ARRHYTHMIA ☐ LVH/RVH ☐ PVC's/MIN

IMPRESSION: (ASA STATUS) ______

PLANS: ______ (4)

COMPLETED BY: ______

CHART COPY JHH ANESTHESIA & CRITICAL CARE MEDICINE PREOP EVALUATION

FIGURE 11-1. Example of the preoperative evaluation record. *1*, patient data and medical review of systems; *2*, physical examination data; *3*, laboratory data; and *4*, assessment and anesthetic plan data.

notes. It was also done to permit computerized epidemiologic studies of the various patient populations admitted to the hospital for surgery. As can be seen from Figure 11-1, the preoperative evaluation sheet incorporates and highlights basic information every anesthesiologist should know before the administration of any anesthetic. It is divided into four parts: (1) patient and medical review of system data, (2) physical examination data, (3) laboratory data, and (4) assessment and anesthetic plan data.

Patient Data and Medical Review of Systems

Patient data and medical review of systems includes both patient and hospital information. Space is provided to record the patient's diagnosis, proposed surgical procedure, medications being taken, last oral intake, and allergies. The medical review of systems section consists of simple yes/no questions arranged by organ systems with space provided to elaborate on positive responses.

Physical Examination Data

Physical examination data provides space to record vital signs and to record significant positive and negative physical findings. Organ systems that need specific referencing include the neurologic, respiratory, and cardiovascular systems. Assessment of the patient's vascular access sites and airway is also mandatory before the administration of any anesthetic. Since lack of vascular access or a difficult airway can lead to major complications, plans can be altered in hopes of avoiding complications.

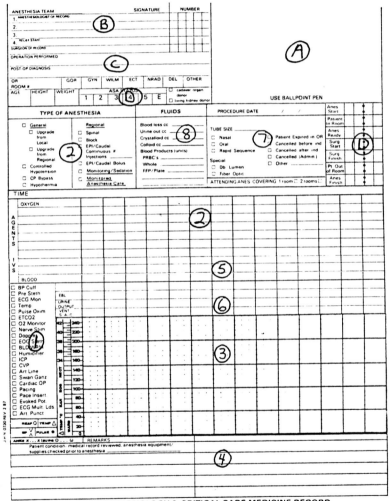

FIGURE 11-2. Example of the intraoperative data record. *A,* patient and hospital information; *B,* name of the anethesiologist and surgeon of record; *C,* type of procedure performed; *D,* operating room utilization data; *1,* monitors and equipment used; *2,* anesthetic agent section; *3,* hemodynamic and physiologic parameter section; *4,* remark (note) section; *5,* fluid section; *6,* urine output, estimated blood loss, and position section; *7,* endotracheal tube information section; and *8,* fluid summary section.

Laboratory Data

Laboratory data provides space to record basic laboratory studies, as well as space to enter studies obtained specific to each patient's disease process.

Assessment and Anesthetic Plan Data

Assessment and anesthetic plan data is where the patient's ASA status is assigned. As discussed in Chapter 3, the ASA status is a global indicator of disease severity that correlates with the risk of anesthesia. In addition, it allows the anesthesiologist to record the fact that these risks have been discussed with the patient, and that the patient either accepts or rejects them. Finally, space is provided to outline the anesthetic plan in terms of what monitoring will be required and what type of anesthesia is to be used.

INTRAOPERATIVE DATA RECORD

The intraoperative data record (Figure 11-2) frequently appears complicated and overwhelming to the novice or casual observer, primarily because of the large amount of data entered into each ADR. The ADR serves as a complete record of intraoperative events, providing anesthesiologists and consultants a means to reconstruct and identify events that could have contributed to or accounted for their patients immediate intraoperative or postoperative complications. If further clarification of intraoperative events is required, consultants should never hesitate to contact the anesthesiologist of record directly. In general, the information contained in the intraoperative data record can be classified into two types: administrative and clinical.

Administrative

Administrative space is provided to list the patient's name and hospital identification number, the names of the anesthesia team and surgeon of record, the patient's diagnosis and type of surgical procedure performed, and the operating room utilization data.

Clinical

The clinical section provides space for the accurate documentation of what occurs during any given anesthetic. It is composed of eight sections—each as important as the other. The first is used to document the type of monitors and equipment used during the anesthetic. Routine monitoring at our institution includes: a blood pressure cuff; a precordial or esophageal stethoscope—to permit auditory monitoring of respiration and heart sounds; a temperature probe to permit the detection of either hyperthermia or hypothermia; pulse oximetry to detect arterial oxygen desaturation; inspired oxygen monitoring to determine inspired oxygen concentrations to prevent the administration of hypoxic gas mixtures; end-tidal carbon dioxide monitoring to rapidly confirm the placement of endotracheal tubes, to monitor the adequacy of ventilation, and to monitor for pulmonary emboli, and ECG monitoring to detect arrhythmias and myocardial ischemia. Although this monitoring is routine at our institution, there is great interinstitution variability, ranging from just blood pressure and ECG monitoring to the aforementioned monitors plus mass spectrometry.

The second section is for the documentation of the type and dose of anesthetic administered. The specific agents employed to produce anesthesia are recorded in 6 to 9 lines. Since space is limited, this section is reserved for drugs given repeatedly or continuously, whereas drugs administered once or twice are recorded in the remark (note) section. Furthermore, consultants may find answers to the postoperative complications they have been called to evaluate and treat by noting what types of drugs were administered and when they were discontinued.

The patient's hemodynamic and physiologic responses to both the various anesthetic agents administered and to the various levels of surgical stimulation are documented in the third section. Routinely documented responses include heart rate, blood pressure, ECG rhythm, temperature, end-tidal carbon dioxide tension, oxygen saturation, and the inspired concentration of oxygen. Documentation of the patient's respiratory rate, tidal volume, minute ventilation, and peak airway pressures can also be included. Since the previously mentioned variables are plotted per time (5-minute intervals), anesthesiologists and consultants can determine whether a cause and effect relationship exists between complications and intraoperative events.

Space is provided in the fourth section to document specific aspects of the case's progress. Details of surgical and anesthetic complications, line insertion, and laryngoscopy are recorded.

The 1 to 3 lines of the fifth section are for running totals of administered colloid, blood products, and crystalloid.

The sixth section is where urine output, estimated blood loss, mode of ventilation (spontaneous, assisted, or controlled), and position of the patient are recorded.

Information concerning the endotracheal tube is described and recorded in the seventh section. In addition to listing the size and type of endotracheal tube used, space is provided to mention special equipment that might have been required for its placement (for example, fiberoptics).

Finally, space is provided in the eighth section to summarize the amount of crystalloid, colloid, and blood products administered, as well as the amount of urine recovered throughout the case.

COMPUTER-AIDED DATA RECORDS

Anesthetic data records are very labor intensive and are usually neglected in the name of patient care. To this end several groups have described the use of microcomputers to aid in the generation of the intraoperative data record.[3,4,5] At this time, several institutions are using such systems, while others are actively developing them. Proponents of computer aided data records argue that the complexity of modern anesthetics leave little time to chart physiologic

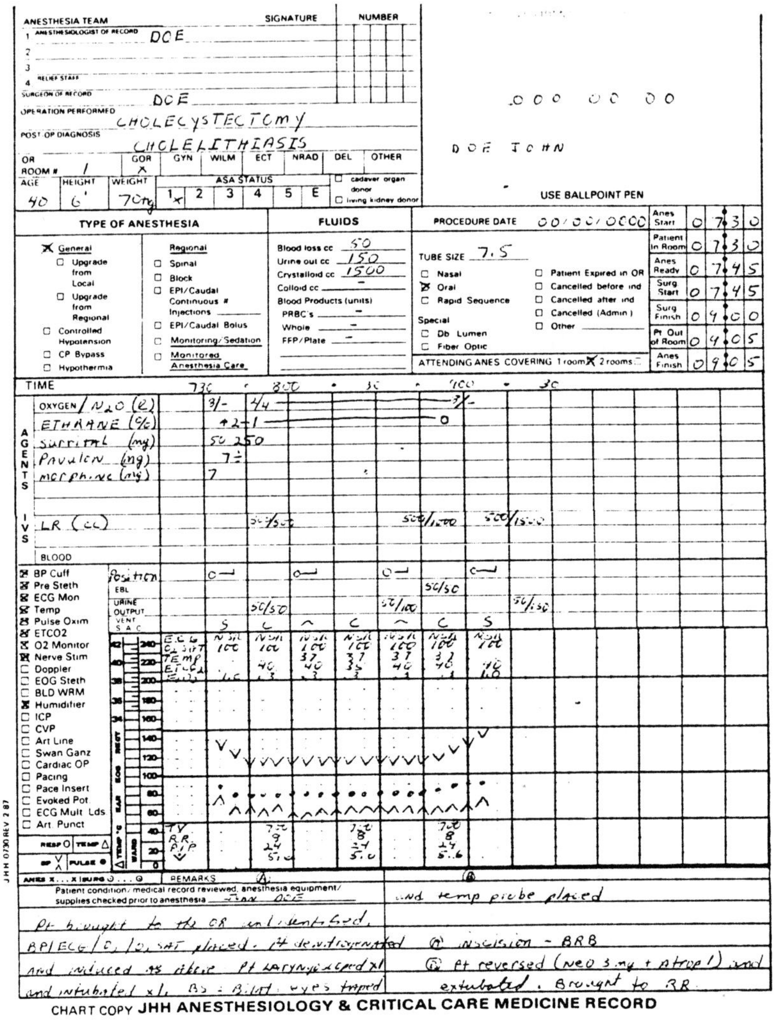

FIGURE 11-3. This example depicts the ADR of a 40-year-old male who undergoes an uncomplicated cholecystectomy.

variables as frequently as needed. To support this contention, studies comparing computerized ADRs to handwritten ADRs have shown that more information is captured with the computerized version, and that the data are recorded as they happen rather than later.[6] Controversy exists, however, as to what data should be collected, and at this time hardware to acquire all pertinent data is not yet available. Finally, opponents to computer-aided data records feel that automated data entry systems will decrease the vigilance of the anesthesiologist and lead to an increase in the number of complications.[7,8,9] Despite these problems and concerns, computerized data systems are coming of age, and once their size, cost, and reliability are improved their clinical use should become widespread.

EXAMPLES OF COMPLETED ADRS

What follows are examples of completed anesthetic data records and the information that can be obtained from them. Figure 11-3 describes a healthy 40-year-old male who has undergone an uncompli-

A

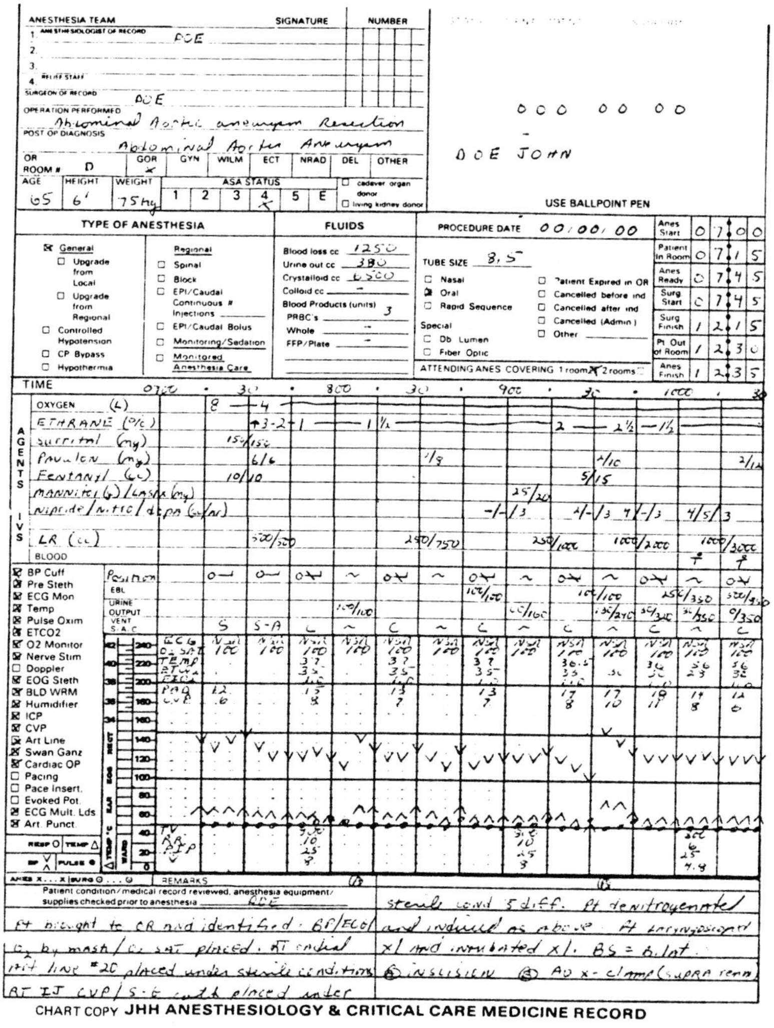

ANESTHESIA TEAM — SIGNATURE — NUMBER
1. ANESTHESIOLOGIST OF RECORD: DOE
SURGEON OF RECORD: DOE
OPERATION PERFORMED: Abdominal Aortic aneurysm Resection
POST OP DIAGNOSIS: Abdominal Aortic Aneurysm
OR ROOM #: D — GOR — GYN — WLM — ECT — NRAD — DEL — OTHER
AGE: 65 — HEIGHT: 6' — WEIGHT: 75 kg — ASA STATUS: 1 2 3 4 5 E (4)
000 00 00
DOE JOHN
USE BALLPOINT PEN

TYPE OF ANESTHESIA: General (checked); Upgrade from Local; Upgrade from Regional; Controlled Hypotension; CP Bypass; Hypothermia; Regional; Spinal; Block; EPI/Caudal Continuous # Injections; EPI/Caudal Bolus; Monitoring/Sedation; Monitored Anesthesia Care

FLUIDS: Blood loss cc 1250; Urine out cc 380; Crystalloid cc 6500; Colloid cc —; Blood Products (units) PRBC's 3; Whole —; FFP/Plate —

PROCEDURE DATE 00/00/00; TUBE SIZE 8.5; Nasal; Oral (checked); Rapid Sequence; Special: Db Lumen; Fiber Optic; Patient Expired in OR; Cancelled before ind; Cancelled after ind; Cancelled (Admin); Other
ATTENDING ANES COVERING 1 room / 2 rooms

Anes Start 0700; Patient In Room 0715; Anes Ready 0745; Surg Start 0745; Surg Finish 1215; Pt Out of Room 1230; Anes Finish 1235

TIME 0700 · 30 · 800 · 30 · 900 · 30 · 1000 · 30
AGENTS: OXYGEN (L); ETHRANE (%); Surital (mg); Pavulon (mg); Fentanyl (cc); Mannitol (g)/Lasix (mg); IVS: Nipride/Nitro/dopa; LR (cc); BLOOD

BP Cuff; Pre Steth; ECG Mon; Temp; Pulse Oxim; ETCO2; O2 Monitor; Nerve Stim; Doppler; EOG Steth; BLD WRM; Humidifier; ICP; CVP; Art Line; Swan Ganz; Cardiac OP; Pacing; Pace Insert.; Evoked Pot.; ECG Mult. Lds; Art. Punct.
Position; EBL; URINE OUTPUT; VENT; S.A.C.
RESP O — TEMP Δ — BP V Λ — PULSE ● — ANES X...X — SURG ⊙...⊙

REMARKS
Patient condition/medical record reviewed, anesthesia equipment/supplies checked prior to anesthesia DOE
Pt brought to OR and identified. BP/ECG/O2 SAT placed. RT radial art line #20 placed under sterile conditions. RT IJ CVP/S-G with placed under sterile cond. 5 diff. Pt denitrogenated and induced as above. Pt laryngoscoped x1 and intubated x1. BS = bilat. ① incision ② Ao x-clamp (supra renal)

CHART COPY JHH ANESTHESIOLOGY & CRITICAL CARE MEDICINE RECORD

FIGURE 11-4, A This example depicts the ADR of a 65-year-old patient who undergoes the repair of a suprarenal abdominal aortic aneurysm.

Continued.

cated cholecystectomy. The patient was monitored with a blood pressure cuff, precordial stethoscope, ECG, temperature probe, end-tidal carbon dioxide monitor, and an inspired-oxygen monitor. Equipment used included a nerve stimulator and a humidifier. The anesthetic consisted of oxygen, nitrous oxide, enflurane, surital (a short-acting thiobarbiturate used for induction), pancuronium bromide (a nondepolarizing muscle relaxant), and morphine sulfate. The hemodynamic and physiologic responses to both general anesthesia and surgery are seen. The ECG showed sinus rhythm throughout the case, and

the arterial oxygen saturation remained at 100%, while his temperature and end-tidal carbon dioxide levels remained stable. It can be seen that the anesthesiologist intubated the patient without difficulty and that on incision the blood was bright red. Other notes reveal the time of incision and the fact that the neuromuscular blockade was reversed with a combination of neostigmine and atropine. Finally, it can be noted that the patient received 1500 ml of lactated Ringer's solution with minimal blood loss. Figure 11-4, A and B describes a 65-year-old male who underwent the repair of a suprarenal abdominal aor-

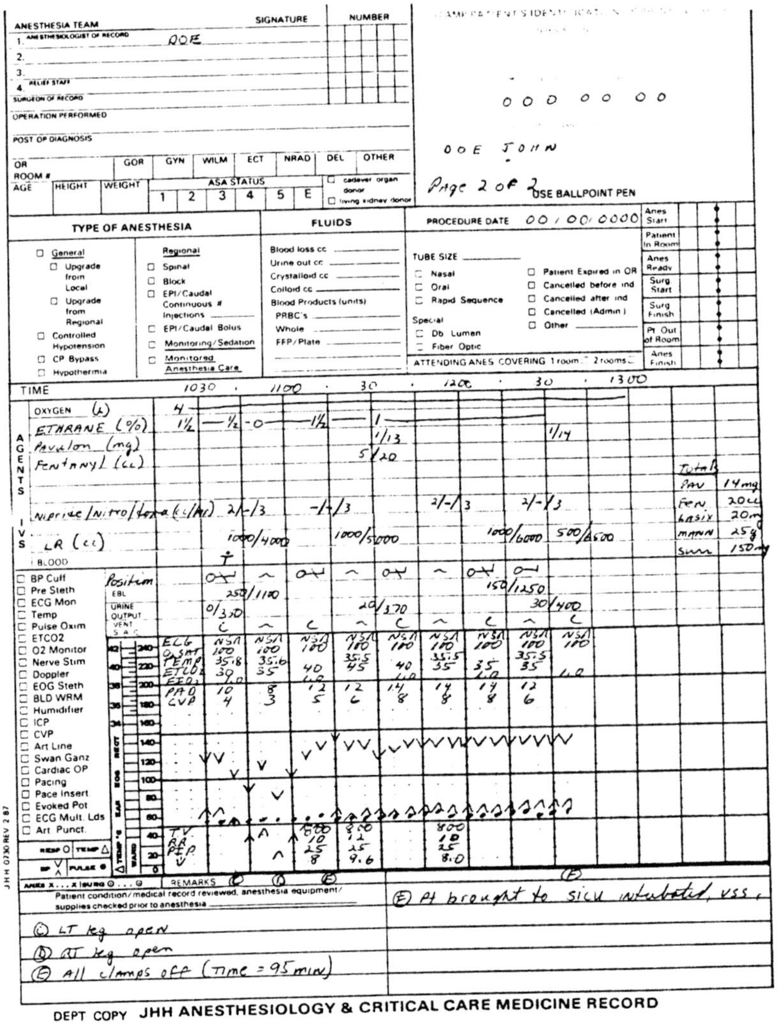

FIGURE 11-4, B

tic aneurysm. His preoperative medical history was positive for coronary artery disease, angina, and peripheral vascular disease. Preoperative medications included a beta-blocker and nitroglycerin. Postoperative consultation was required for the development of acute renal failure. Information obtained from the intraoperative data record is as follows. The patient was monitored with a blood pressure cuff, radial arterial line, precordial and esophageal stethoscopes, ECG, temperature probe, pulse oximeter, end-tidal carbon dioxide monitor, Foley cath-

eter, central venous pressure catheter, and a Swan-Ganz catheter. Equipment used included a nerve stimulator, a humidifier, and blood warmers. Agents used to produce anesthesia included oxygen, enflurane, thiamylal sodium (Surital), pancuronium, and fentanyl. He was also given mannitol, furosemide (Lasix), dopamine, nitroglycerin, and nitroprusside at various points during the procedure. His hemodynamic and physiologic responses to both the general anesthetic and to surgery are noted. As noted in the remarks section, placement of all intravascular

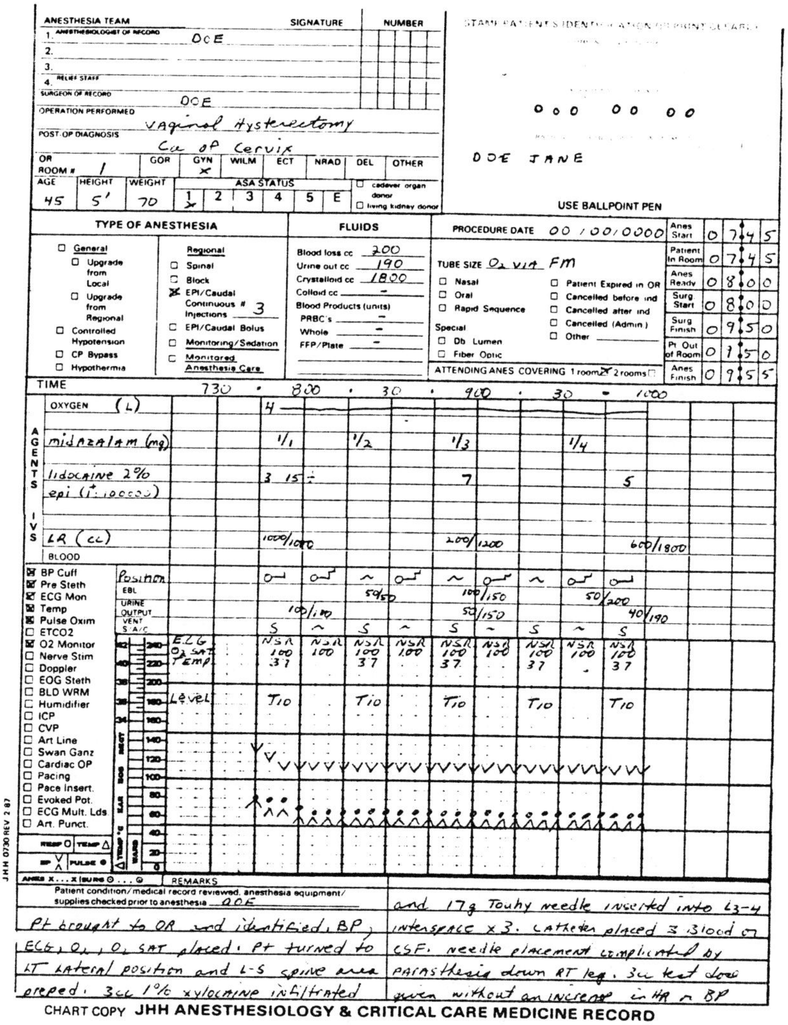

FIGURE 11-5. This example depicts the ADR of a 45-year-old female who undergoes a total vaginal hysterectomy.

monitors occurred without complications, and intubation occurred without problems. The total aortic cross-clamp time was reported to be 95 minutes with urine output being minimal during the case. In summary, the patient underwent repair of his suprarenal abdominal aortic aneurysm complicated by a prolonged aortic cross clamp time and by multiple episodes of hypotension. Thus this information explains the patient's postoperative renal failure and would not have been available if the intraoperative ADR was not consulted. Figure 11-5 describes a 45-year-old female who underwent a total vaginal hysterectomy for carcinoma of the cervix. Her past medical history is noncontributory and she takes no medications. Consultation was required postoperatively for the evaluation and treatment of a right foot drop. Information obtained from her intraoperative data record reveals that the patient was monitored with a blood pressure cuff, precordial stethoscope, ECG, and pulse oximeter. The anesthetic consisted of an epidural (2% xylocaine plus epinephrine) and a short-acting benzodiazepine for sedation. The patient's hemodynamic and physiologic response to both the anesthetic and surgery are noted. Of importance is the position the patient was placed in for the surgery (lithotomy), the anesthetic level achieved below T10, and the fact that paresthesias were noted during the placement of the epidural. Thus without referring to the intraoperative ADR one would assume that the neurologic deficit was secondary to

the epidural, and no consideration would be given to the possible occurrence of a peripheral neuropathy occurring secondary to positioning.

REFERENCES

1. Beecher HK: Texts and documents—the first anesthesia record, Surg Gynecol Obstet 71:689-693, 1940.
2. Dripps RD, Eckenhoff JE, and Vandam LD: The anesthesia data record. In Dripps RD (editor): Introduction to anesthesia—the principles of safe practice, ed 6, Philadelphia 1982, WB Saunders Co.
3. Apple HP, Schneider AJL, and Fadel J: Design and evaluation of a semiautomatic anesthesia record system, Med Instrum 16:69-71, 1982.
4. Mitchell MM: Automated anesthesia data management and recordkeeping, Med Instrum 16:279-282, 1982.
5. Prentice JW and Kenny GNC: Microcomputer based anesthetic record systems, Br J Anaesth 56:1433-1437, 1984.
6. Zollinger RM, Kreul JF, and Schneider AJL: Man-made versus computer generated anesthesia records, J Surg Res 22:419-424, 1977.
7. Lees DE: Computerized anesthesia records may have drawbacks, Anesthesiology 63:236-237, 1985.
8. Noel TA: Computerized anesthesia records may be dangerous, Anesthesiology 64:300, 1986.
9. Rosen AS and Rosenzweig W: Computerized anesthesia record, Anesthesiology 62:100-101, 1985.
10. Rosen AS and Rosenzweig W: On computerized anesthesia records, Anesthesiology 65:131-132, 1986.
11. Sarnat AJ: Do not fear computerized anesthesia records, Anesthesiology 65:132-133, 1986.

PART THREE

RECOVERY FROM SURGERY AND ANESTHESIA

CHAPTER 12

Commonly Encountered Recovery Room Problems

BRIAN A. ROSENFELD
CLAIR F. MILLER

Central nervous system
  Emergence phenomena
  Common neurologic findings
  Shivering and thermoregulation
Respiratory system
  Airway obstruction
  Hypoventilation
  Hypoxemia
Cardiovascular system
  Hypotension
  Hypertension

Myocardial ischemia and infarction
  Arrhythmias
Nausea and vomiting
Genitourinary system
  Oliguria
  Urinary retention
  Transurethral prostatectomy (TURP) syndrome

Successful completion of a procedure in the operating room does not ensure smooth and uneventful recovery from anesthesia and surgery. Postoperative complications severe enough to require treatment occur in 7% to 10% of general recovery room admissions.[16] Table 12-1 summarizes the incidence of problems encountered in a survey of 10,000 consecutive recovery room admissions at The Johns Hopkins Hospital. Surgical bleeding or exacerbation of preexisting medical conditions such as angina pectoris occasionally complicate early postoperative recovery. However, most recovery room problems are caused by adverse physiologic and pharmacologic effects of anesthetic drugs and techniques. Therefore, careful monitoring of anesthetized patients

must continue until the effects of anesthesia are completely reversed and protective reflexes are reestablished. Using an organ system format, this chapter discusses the problems that are most commonly encountered in the recovery room.

CENTRAL NERVOUS SYSTEM

Awakening from general anesthesia is often accompanied by neurologic signs and symptoms that would be considered pathologic in nonsurgical settings. Transient disorders of mentation, pathologic spinal reflexes, and movement disorders such as shivering are common central nervous system abnormalities observed in patients in the recovery room.

TABLE 12-1. Common recovery room problems

	Percent of patients
CENTRAL NERVOUS SYSTEM	2.4
Emergence phenomena	
Neurologic reflex changes	
Shivering and thermoregulation	
RESPIRATORY	5.5
Airway obstruction	
Hypoventilation	
Hypoxemia	
CARDIOVASCULAR	9.4
Hypotension	
Hypertension	
Myocardial ischemia	
Arrhythmias	
NAUSEA AND VOMITING	2.4
GENITOURINARY	NA
Oliguria	
Urinary retention	
TURP syndrome	

NA = Not available.

Emergence Phenomena

Emergence excitement occurs in 5% to 30% of recovery room admissions.[18,23] It is characterized by restlessness, disorientation, crying, moaning, and irrational talking during recovery from general anesthesia. In severe cases, patients may become delirious, shout, scream, and thrash aimlessly about; they may pose a danger to themselves and to recovery room staff. In a series of more than 12,000 surgical patients, Eckenhoff et al[18] observed emergence excitement in 5.3% of recovery room admissions. The incidence of excitement was higher after surgical procedures with emotional overtones such as breast surgery (fear of mutilation, cancer phobia) than after routine dental procedures, and was more common in the young than in the elderly patients. Anesthesia with either halogenated agents or ketamine, a dissociative agent, is associated with a higher incidence of emergence excitement than after spinal or narcotic-based general anesthetic techniques.[18,23] Scopolamine, an anticholinergic premedicant, also causes delirium, hallucinations, memory disturbances, and agitation in postoperative patients.[33]

Emergence excitement is a transient and self-limited phenomenon in most patients, and treatment is largely supportive. Abnormalities of arterial blood gases, electrolytes, or blood sugar can also cause mental status changes, and these physiologic abnormalities must be excluded in postoperative patients. Analgesic therapy often aborts or decreases the severity of excitement.[18] All restless patients require careful observation to prevent injury. Physostigmine, an anticholinesterase agent that penetrates the blood brain barrier, reverses the central anticholinergic effects of scopolamine within 5 to 10 minutes of administration and markedly improves mental status in patients who have received scopolamine.

Failure to regain consciousness promptly after discontinuation of anesthesia may be a result of the somnolent effects of intravenous agents, but more serious causes such as metabolic encephalopathy and acute neurologic injury must be investigated. The somnolent effects of narcotics and scopolamine can be reversed with naloxone and physostigmine, respectively.[33] Specific reversal agents for butyrophenones and benzodiazepines are not available, but physostigmine and other stimulants (theophylline, caffeine) have been reported to have general central nervous system arousal properties.[9,10,67] Persistent neuromuscular paralysis may mimic drug-induced coma, and evaluation of neuromuscular function with a nerve stimulator should be performed. If partial paralysis is found, treatment with anticholinesterase reversal agents should be attempted. The unconscious postoperative patient should also be evaluted and treated for metabolic causes of encephalopathy including hypoxia, hypercarbia, hypoglycemia, and electrolyte abnormalities. In the absence of drug or metabolic causes, it must be assumed that the comatose patient has suffered an acute neurologic injury from either ischemia or hemorrhage. Discovery of focal neurologic deficits on emergence from anesthesia reinforces the validity of this assumption.[46]

Common Neurologic Findings

Emergence from anesthesia in healthy patients is often accompanied by transient neurologic changes (sustained and nonsustained ankle clonus, bilateral hyperreflexia, the Babinski reflex, and decerebrate posturing) that are otherwise thought to be pathologic reflexes.[55] These changes can often be detected within minutes of discontinuation of anesthesia when

TABLE 12-2. Neurologic changes after 20 minutes in recovery room

	Percent of group		
	Halothane (n = 8)	Ethrane (n = 12)	N$_2$O—narcotic (n = 9)
Hyperreflexia	25	58	0
Clonus	75	83	44
Sustained clonus	0	50	0
Babinski	0	50	0

Adapted from Rosenberg et al: Anesthesiology 54:125, 1981.

the patient is still poorly responsive to verbal commands, but they may persist for more than 40 minutes into the postoperative period. These abnormalities occur more frequently after enflurane/N$_2$O anesthesia than after halothane or narcotic-based techniques (Table 12-2); their cause remains unexplained. Neurologic changes do not appear to be associated with adverse clinical consequences. However, the common presence of these transient abnormalities must be kept in mind when evaluating patients for possible acute central nervous system injury.

Shivering and Thermoregulation

Spontaneous shivering-like activity (postanesthetic tremor) is common during recovery from all types of general anesthesia. Uncontrolled motor activity may disrupt delicate surgical repairs and can result in dental damage. In addition, the subjective feeling of intense cold is often cited as being the most uncomfortable perioperative experience. Shivering increases metabolic rate and oxygen consumption by up to 400%, and it may not be tolerated in patients with compromised cardiovascular or respiratory function.[39,53] The causes and treatment of postanesthesia tremor have recently become areas of active, but unresolved, research.

Postanesthetic tremor is usually attributed to normal regulatory mechanisms that generate heat in response to interoperative hypothermia. Hypothermia during anesthesia results from decreased metabolic heat production (especially in patients with neuromuscular blockade), loss of heat to the environment, and decreased hypothalamic thermal regulation by anesthetic agents. Compensatory responses to hypothermia such as vasoconstriction, shivering, and

nonshivering thermogenesis are impaired. Postoperative shivering is usually thought to develop in response to decreased body temperature, but shivering may occur at normal body temperature after anesthesia, and mechanisms other than thermoregulation may also contribute to postanesthesia tremor.[24,55,58]

Recent evidence suggests that spontaneous tremor may be the result of increased spinal reflex activity during recovery from anesthesia. Electromyograms (EMG) of shivering muscle after isoflurane anesthesia reveal tonic and clonic activity similar to that produced by pathologic clonus in patients with spinal cord transection. Because EMG clonus is not observed during cold-induced shivering in unanesthetized volunteers, Sessler et al[58] suggest that a functional spinal cord transection (the brain is "asleep," the spinal cord is "awake") develops as the concentration of anesthetic decreases during recovery. The incidence of EMG clonus is highest at end-tidal concentrations of isoflurane between 0.1% and 0.19%; at higher concentrations, little muscular activity occurs and at lower concentrations, normal thermogenic shivering predominates.[58] While these conclusions have been questioned,[28] they offer a cogent explanation for development of postanesthesia tremor in normothermic patients and provide insight into potential mechanisms for other postoperative neurologic changes (clonus, Babinski reflex, hyperreflexia) that were previously discussed.

A variety of techniques are used to prevent or treat postanesthesia tremor. Hypothermic patients are rewarmed by increasing environmental temperature, warming and humidifying inspired air, and by using warming blankets and fluid warmers. To avoid increased cardiac work resulting from shivering-induced increases in metabolic rate and oxygen consumption, continuation of neuromuscular paralysis during rewarming is employed by some clinicians, particularly after cardiac surgical procedures. Meperidine (25 mg intravenously) successfully suppresses visible shivering in most patients and is associated with significant reductions in oxygen consumption and carbon dioxide production.[39] Other pharmacologic agents that may minimize shivering include methylphenidate (Ritalin), magnesium sulfate, calcium chloride, chlorpromazine, droperidol, and opiates. Stimulation of thermal receptors in blush areas of the skin appears to alter thermal signals reaching the central nervous system, because application of radiant heat to the face, neck, chest, and abdomen eliminates shivering within minutes in postoperative patients despite low core temperatures.[44,59] Flexion of the knees or elbows has been reported to minimize postanesthesia clonus in recovery room patients (clasp-knife responses).[5]

RESPIRATORY SYSTEM

Airway obstruction, hypoventilation, and hypoxemia are the major respiratory complications occurring in the recovery room.

Airway Obstruction

Airway obstruction in postoperative patients is common and can result in hypoxemia and hypercarbia. It may be caused by vomitus or secretions in the pharynx, the tongue falling back as a result of anesthetic related alterations of the genioglossus muscle, by laryngospasm, or by laryngeal edema secondary to operative trauma. Airway obstruction by the tongue is particularly common and can usually be alleviated by hyperextension of the neck and anterior displacement of the mandible. Occasionally placement of a nasal airway is required, these are usually better tolerated than oral airways, and are less likely to induce gagging, laryngospasm, or vomiting.

Laryngospasm, which occasionally occurs during emergence, is a protective reflex that is mediated by the superior laryngeal nerve that results in constriction of the extrinsic muscles of the larynx. Airflow obstruction occurs as a result of opposition of the true and false vocal cords in the midline. The diagnosis of laryngospasm is usually made when airway obstruction persists despite usual measures to relieve upper airway obstruction (proper head position, placement of an airway, and anterior displacement of the mandible). Treatment includes clearing secretions from the pharnyx and frequent, short positive pressure breaths using an ambu bag. Rarely, succinylcholine is required. Because respiratory muscle function is usually normal in patients with laryngospasm, marked negative intrathoracic pressures are generated that can occasionally result in hydrostatic pulmonary edema.[68] The mechanism responsible for the pulmonary edema is similar to a Mueller manuever (inspiration against a closed glottis) where increased venous return and decreased left ventricular function occur (Figure 12-1).[49] This form of pulmonary edema may occur at varying periods

of time after relief of laryngospasm, and an extended period of observation in the recovery room is required.

Upper airway obstruction caused by edema from surgical or anesthetic trauma is most common in patients with preexisting airway problems such as oropharyngeal tumors. Incomplete obstruction can often be treated with head-up positioning, humidified oxygen, and nebulized epinephrine; intravenous steroids have been shown to hasten the resolution of traumatic laryngeal edema.[11] Near complete or complete obstruction requires intubation with a small endotracheal tube or tracheostomy. Prolonged surgery in a head-down position can occasionally result in marked pharyngeal swelling. Such patients are at risk of airway obstruction and intubation until the swelling decreases is advised.

Vocal cord paralysis from damage to the recurrent laryngeal nerves particularly after surgery involving an enlarged thyroid can cause airway obstruction in the recovery room. This frequently requires tracheostomy but may resolve with time. Paradoxical vocal cord motion (PVCM) is a rare cause of airway obstruction that occurs in women with a history of functional disorders and paroxysms of upper airway obstruction.[29] Avoidance of endotracheal intubation, if possible, or extubation in a deep plane of anesthesia may prevent PVCM.

Hypoventilation

Hypoventilation is common in recovery room patients. Depressant effects of residual narcotics and inhalational agents on CO_2 responsiveness[36,66] account for most episodes of hypoventilation in the recovery room (Figure 12-2). The diagnosis of hypoventilation may be particularly difficult to make because inhalational agents also blunt the normal cardiovascular responses to hypercarbia (tachycardia, hypertension). Hypoventilation appears to be more common following intravenous narcotic than after general inhalation anesthesia, however inhalational agents depress the CO_2 response curve at subanesthetic concentrations.[45] Rarely narcotics can produce a biphasic respiratory depression pattern; depression that occurs on administration is followed several hours later by a second period of respiratory depression.[7] Epidural and intrathecal opiates can also produce respiratory depression that usually occurs 4 to 6 hours after administration.[17]

The only effective way to monitor alveolar ven-

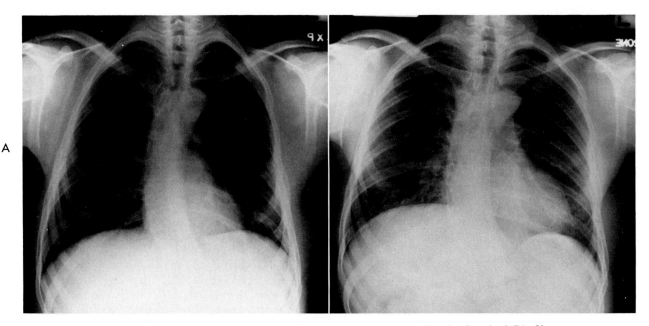

FIGURE 12-1. Chest x-rays taken in the same subject sequentially. **A,** Standard PA film at functional residual capacity. **B,** Film taken just before concluding a 10-second vigorous Mueller maneuver. There is a dramatic increase in pulmonary vascular markings, cardiomegaly, and dilation of the ascending aorta.

With permission from Montenegro HD (editor): Chronic obstructive pulmonary disease, New York, 1984, Churchill Livingstone.

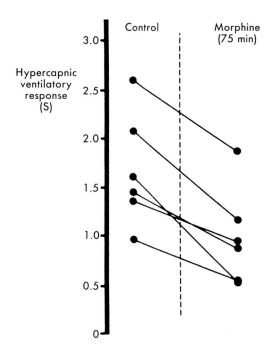

FIGURE 12-2. Ventilatory responses to hypercapnia as measured by the slope of the response S (in liters per minute per millimeter of mercury). Comparison of values before and at 75 minutes after the administration of 7.5 mg morphine subcutaneously shows a substantial and highly consistent depression of hypercapnic ventilatory drive in all subjects.

Reprinted with permission from Weil JV, McCullough RE, Kline JS, and Ingvar ES: N Engl J Med 292:1103-1106, 1975.

tilation in nonintubated patients is to directly measure PCO_2 in arterial blood. Alterations in respiratory frequency are unreliable. Pulse oximetry cannot be used to document hypoventilation, particularly when supplemental oxygen is being administered. As seen in the example below, when appropriate values are substituted into the alveolar gas equation, supplemental oxygen (40%) will result in a high alveolar PO_2 and normoxemia even when $PaCO_2$ is quite elevated. In the alveolar gas equation PaO_2 is the alveolar partial pressure of oxygen, FiO_2 is the inspired concentration of oxygen, (760-47) is the barometric pressure-water vapor pressure, $PaCO_2$ is the partial pressure of carbon dioxide in arterial blood, and R is the respiratory quotient.

$$PaO_2 = FiO_2(760\text{-}47) - PaCO_2/R$$

$$PaO_2 = .40(713) - 80/.8$$

$$PaO_2 = 285 - 90$$

$$PaO_2 = 189$$

Recently, nasal cannulae for monitoring end-tidal CO_2 have been introduced, however, their margin of error is so great as to make these devices unreliable.[2]

Narcotic-induced respiratory depression can be reversed by narcotic antagonists, and small doses (0.04 to 0.08 mg naloxone) can reverse the respiratory effects without precipitating severe pain.[51] It is most important to recognize that the duration of action of naloxone (1 to 4 hours) is shorter than some narcotics (methadone, CNS morphine) and repeat doses or a continuous infusion may be required.

Inadequate neuromuscular blocker reversal is another important cause of hypoventilation. Improper dosing of muscle relaxants or reversal agents or impaired excretion of the neuromuscular blocker as a result of renal failure while the reversal agent is being metabolized may lead to "recurarization."[41] Respiratory acidosis, metabolic alkalosis, hypokalemia, hypermagnesemia, and hypothermia impair return of adequate neuromuscular function.[42] Drugs such as antibiotics and diuretics can also adversely affect return of neuromuscular function.[4] Assisted ventilation may be required until neuromuscular function returns to normal.

Hypoxemia

Hypoxemia following anesthesia and surgery is common in patients not receiving supplemental oxygen.[63] Using continuous pulse oximetry during transfer of ASA class I and II patients breathing room air from the operating room to the recovery room, Tyler found that 30% of patients had O_2 saturations below 90% and 12% had O_2 saturations less than 85%. There was a significant correlation between development of hypoxemia and preoperative obesity or history of asthma. Accordingly, it is generally recommended that all patients receive supplemental oxygen during transport from the operating room to the recovery room and during their recovery room stay.

The cause of hypoxemia in the early postoperative period include anesthetic-induced hypoventilation, $\dot{V}/\dot{Q}$ mismatching, and intrapulmonary shunting. Inhalational agents alter respiratory muscle function and reduce functional residual capacity (FRC). The decrease in FRC is associated with diffuse microatelectasis in dependent lung regions that can be seen on intraoperative CT scans.[13] These changes may be more severe in patients with preoperative pulmonary dysfunction (elderly, obese, COPD, and pneumonia). Decreased FRC and hypoxemia rapidly reverse (1 to 3 hours) as inhalational anesthetic agents are eliminated from the body.[45] Pulmonary dysfunction after elimination of anesthetic agents is caused by pain-induced splinting and mechanical dysfunction of the diaphragm from upper abdominal and thoracic incisions (See chapter on perioperative changes in pulmonary function for a more detailed description). Additionally, the inhalational anesthetics and narcotics blunt the normal response to hypoxemia (Figure 12-3).[66] Monitoring arterial oxygenation in the recovery room with a pulse oximeter will help to detect hypoxemia early. Hypoxemia can be treated by increasing the inspired concentration of oxygen, upright positioning and lung expansion maneuvers such as incentive spirometry.[17] Less common causes of postoperative hypoxemia include cardiogenic and noncardiogenic pulmonary edema, pulmonary embolism, and acute bronchospasm, and are beyond the scope of this chapter.

CARDIOVASCULAR SYSTEM
Hypotension

Hypotension in the recovery room is usually caused by either residual effects of anesthesia or to hypovolemia. Hypotension is more common after regional than after general anesthesia because of the more pronounced and prolonged vasodilator effect of regional techinques. Local anesthetics in the epidural or subarachnoid space produce a "chemical sympathectomy" that results in arteriolar and ven-

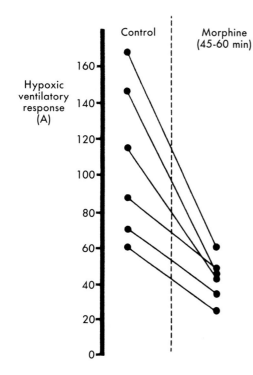

FIGURE 12-3. Ventilatory response to hypoxia as measured by the shape parameter A (high values of A denotes a vigorous ventilatory response) before and after the administration of morphine. The values after 7.5 mg morphine subcutaneously were obtained by averaging of the data at 45 and 60 minutes. It can be seen that the depression of hypoxic ventilatory drive observed was not only of considerable magnitude but also was highly consistent in that it occurred in every subject.

With permission from Weil JV, McCullough RE, Kline JS, and Ingvar ES: N Engl J Med 292:1103-1106, 1975.

odilation. Additionally, a high sympathetic block will involve the cardioaccelerator fibers T_1 to T_4 and the resulting vasodilation will not be accompanied by the usual reflex increases in heart rate. Elderly patients are particularly susceptible to regional anesthetic-induced hypotension that may be poorly tolerated because of underlying myocardial, renal, and cerebrovascular disease. The initial treatment of hypotension after spinal or epidural anesthesia is the Trendelenburg position to augment venous return. Judicious volume replacement and administration of alpha-adrenergic and beta-adrenergic agonists may be required if hypotension persists.[14] Fluid administration must be individualized because, as the sympathetic block recedes and the capacitance system regains tone, patients with marginal myocardial or renal function may be compromised by the increased pressures.

Hypovolemia causes hypotension in the normal awake state; additionally, residual effects of inhalation anesthetics (vasodilation, decreased myocardial contractility and blunting of baroreceptor reflex activity) will further exacerbate the effects of hypovolemia in recovery room patients. Patients may be hypovolemic from inadequate intraoperative blood and fluid replacement, or they may become hypovolemic in the recovery room from ongoing hemorrhage and third space losses. Determination of urine volume, osmolality and electrolytes, hematocrit and heart rate will frequently be sufficient to diagnose hypovolemia. Uncertainty about intravascular volume or fluid replacement should prompt measurement of central venous or pulmonary artery wedge pressure. Rarely, sepsis-induced hypotension can develop intraoperatively or in the immediate postoperative period in patients undergoing surgery for perforated abdominal viscera or abscess drainage. Management of these patients includes antibiotics, administration of fluids, and alpha agonists to increase systemic vascular resistance.

Hypertension

Transient arterial hypertension is common in recovery room patients. Gal and Cooperman observed postoperative hypertension (blood pressure greater than 190/100 mm Hg) in 60 (3.25%) of 1,844 patients.[22] Hypertension developed 10 to 30 minutes after completion of surgery and resolved without

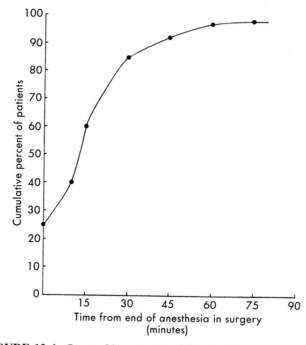

FIGURE 12-4. Onset of hypertension following the end of operation.

With permission from Gal TJ and Chapman LH: Br J Anaesth 47:70, 1975.

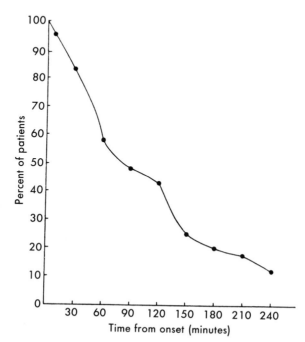

FIGURE 12-5. Duration of postoperative hypertension.

With permission from Gal TJ and Chapman LH: Br J Anaesth 47:70-74, 1975.

specific antihypertensive therapy within 3 hours in 47 (78%) patients (Figures 12-4 and 12-5). In the remaining 13 patients (22%), hypertension lasted beyond 3 hours and complications secondary to hypertension occurred in 6 of them. Preoperative hypertension was present in more than half the patients who developed postoperative hypertension.

Withdrawal of antihypertensive medications often contributes to development of postoperative hypertension in patients with preexisting hypertension. Rebound hypertension is most often caused by withdrawal of beta-blockers or clonidine.[40] Beta-blockers can be administered intravenously in the recovery room, but there is no intravenous clonidine preparation presently available. Clonidine can be administered transdermally, but requires 48 hours to reach therapeutic levels[60] and altered blood flow to the skin during the perioperative period may complicate absorption. If clonidine therapy is discontinued combined alpha-adrenergic and beta-adrenergic blockade should be used to prevent increased adrenergic responsiveness.

Hypertension can also reflect other problems such as hypoxemia, hypercarbia, and intracranial hypertension that should be treated immediately. Pain, intravascular volume overload, hypothermia, and bladder distension can also cause hypertension and should be corrected. If hypertension persists, specific antihypertensive medication should be administered according to the severity of the situation and the medical history of the patient. Systemic vasodilators frequently elicit reflex tachycardia that may be detrimental in patients with ischemic heart disease. A combined alpha-beta-blocker (labetalol) or a vasodilator in conjunction with a beta-blocker are preferred antihypertensive agents in this population of recovery room patients.

Myocardial Ischemia and Infarction

Myocardial ischemia and infarction (MI) occur with greater frequency and have a higher mortality in the perioperative period than in nonsurgical settings.[47,62] Events in the immediate postoperative period such as tachycardia, hypertension, hypotension, hypoxemia, hypercarbia, and hypothermia contribute to ischemia by disrupting the balance between myocardial oxygen supply and demand.

Intraoperative ischemia and infarction often go undetected[27] and recognition of postoperative myocardial ischemia or infarction may be more difficult. Patients with documented perioperative MIs fre-

quently do not complain of chest pain.[6,8] The incidence of clinically silent ischemia may be the highest in recovery room patients because of residual effects of anesthesia, narcotic analgesics, and patient difficulty differentiating ischemic pain from surgical pain. It is therefore important to recognize "anginal equivalents" (unexplained dyspnea, arrhythmias or hemodynamic changes) as markers of underlying ischemia in postoperative patients. Ischemia detection may be enhanced by continuous ECG monitoring of precordial leads V_4 to V_6 or a modified limb lead in the V_5 position.[34] However, the standard 12 lead ECG remains the best method for diagnosing ischemia and MI. Isolated T-wave changes (flattened or inverted) without other signs or symptoms of myocardial ischemia occur in 22% of postoperative patients with or without a preexisting history of CAD.[12] These isolated T-wave changes may not represent ischemia, and clinical judgement should guide management decisions.

Arrhythmias

Arrhythmias are extremely common in the recovery room, particularly sinus tachycardia. Other commonly encountered rhythm disturbances are sinus bradycardia, premature ectopic beats and accelerated ectopic rhythms. Sinus tachycardia in the recovery room is often caused by physiologic disturbances such as hypovolemia, fever, anemia, hypoxemia, and hypercarbia. These should be excluded before invoking pain or anxiety as the etiologic cause.

Causes of sinus bradycardia include (1) beta-blocker therapy, (2) neuromuscular blocker reversal agents, (3) local anesthetic effects on the cardioaccelerator fibers in patients wth regional anesthesia, (4) underlying heart disease, and (5) hypothermia. Bradycardia can also represent an ominous sign of severe hypoxemia that must always be ruled out. The neuromuscular blocker reversal agents (neostigmine, pyridostigmine, and edrophonium) cause bradycardia by increasing the available acetylcholine at all postganglionic receptors. To prevent profound cardiac effects, muscarinic blockers (atropine, glycopyrolate) are always given concomitantly; the net result is to increase acetylcholine only at the neuromuscular nicotinic receptor. However, the duration of action of acetylcholine esterase inhibitors is more prolonged than the muscarinic receptor antagonists. Theoretically, this can result in a period of unopposed muscarinic receptor stimulation, sinus bradycardia, and rarely, escape rhythms. These arrhythmias should only be treated if they are hemodynamically significant, because they will spontaneously revert in time.

Other causes of bradycardia in the recovery room include high spinal and epidural blocks that affect the cardioaccelerator sympathetic fibers (T_1 to T_4) and lead to unopposed vagal stimulation.

Mild hypothermia to 33°C decreases sinus node activity and also increases systemic vascular resistance that in turn reflexly slows heart rate.[56] Rewarming will reverse these changes. More severe hypothermia can result in atrial and ventricular arrhythmias.[57]

Ectopic rhythms (ventricular tachycardia, junctional tachycardia, atrial fibrillation, and atrial flutter) occur occasionally in recovery room patients. Recovery room patients often have electrolyte abnormalities, acid-base disturbances, residual inhalational anesthetic agents, central venous catheters, and particularly elevated catecholamines, which play an important role in generating and sustaining arrhythmias. Elevated postoperative catecholamines are probably the most important etiologic cause of postoperative tachyarrhythmias. Catecholamines accelerate impulse conduction velocity, shorten the refractory period, augment calcium influx into myocardial cells, and increase the amplitude of delayed after potentials enhancing the propensity for arrhthmias (Figure 12-6).[50] Additionally, catecholamines increase the slope of phase 4 spontaneous depolarization of the action potential that increases automaticity and the potential for ectopic beats and accelerated ectopic rhythms. Another cause of accelerated arrhythmias involves the inhalational anesthetics, particularly halothane, which sensitizes the myocardium to catecholamine stimulation.[31] The acute administration of theophylline compounds can also produce arrhythmias by this mechanism, and these agents should be used with caution in the immediate postoperative period.[38.54] Premature ventricular contractions (PVCs) and premature atrial contractions (PACs) are the most common ectopic rhythm disturbances in recovery room patients. These are rarely of clinical signficance unless associated with myocardial ischemia. The decision to treat these rhythm disturbances with an antiarrhythmic should be based on the clinical situation. Beta-blockers have been successful in terminating ventricular ectopy and some accelerated rhythms, felt to be secondary to catecholamines[30] while in other situations no therapy at all may be indicated. Obviously, accelerated arrhythmias, when associated with significant hemodynamic changes require treatment to slow and convert the rhythm disturbance.

NAUSEA AND VOMITING

Nausea and vomiting are often considered to be minor postoperative problems, but can result in significant discomfort and may prevent discharge of same day surgery patients. In addition, vomiting can result in tracheal aspiration when airway protective reflexes are depressed or when the jaw is wired after

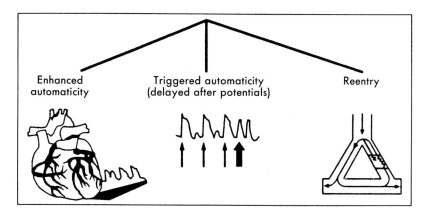

FIGURE 12-6. Mechanisms of arrhythmogenesis. The three proposed mechanisms for arrhythmia are enhanced automaticity, delayed after potential and reentry.

With permission from Podrid PJ, Venditti FJ, Levine PA, and Kline MD: Am J Cardiol 62:24H-33H, 1988.

oral surgery. Forceful muscular contractions that accompany retching and vomiting may also disrupt suture lines, cause bleeding, and can be extremely painful. Emesis results from stimulation of the vomiting center in the dorsal part of the lateral reticular formation, in the medulla, by autonomic afferents from the gastrointestinal tract and mediastinum, the vestibular component of the eighth cranial nerve, visual and cortical stimuli, and the chemoreceptor trigger zone (CRTZ) (Figure 12-7). Stimulation of the vomiting center causes reflex efferent activity resulting in emesis. Causes of vomiting in the postoperative period include drug effects, gastrointestinal (GI) distention, intraabdominal surgery, swallowed blood, pharyngeal stimulation, movement, and hypotension. The overall incidence of postoperative vomiting depends upon the criteria used for identification. Adrianni reported an incidence of 23%; while persistent vomiting occurred in 3.5%.[1] The incidence of postopertaive emesis appears to be highest after ophthalmic surgery, and is more common in women and in young patients.[64] There is also an increased incidence of vomiting in patients with previous postoperative emesis suggesting that some patients may be predisposed to the problem.[43]

The association of morphine premedication with postoperative nausea and vomiting is well known.[52] In a study of unpremedicated women undergoing uterine curettage, Riding observed a 22.4% incidence of nausea, retching, or vomiting. However, when morphine was added as a premedication, the incidence increased to 67%. When atropine was combined with morphine for premedication, emetic symptoms occurred in 37% of patients. The antiemetic effects of atropine were subsequently confirmed by preoperative administration of atropine alone, which reduced the incidence to 11.5%.[52] Narcotics are not always precipitants of emesis, and they may be antiemetic in the postoperative period. Over the first 12 to 24 postoperative hours, Andersen and Krohg noted that only 10% of patients had episodes of pain without nausea compared to 58.6% of patients who experienced pain with nausea.[3] These authors concluded that relief of pain decreases the severity of nausea and, when pain relief is inadequate, nausea often persists.

The association of postoperative emetic symptoms with inhalational agents such as ether and cyclopropane is well established. Similar data on halothane is conflicting, and studies to evaluate the effects of ethrane and forane on postoperative emesis are not available. Previous work has claimed that nitrous oxide causes emetic symptoms via central stimulation and gastrointestinal distention. A recent study by Muir et al isolated nitrous oxide as an etiologic agent, and in their study population found no increase in postoperative nausea and vomiting.[43] Relief of gastrointestinal distention by nasogastric suction-

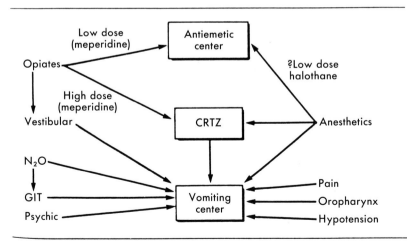

FIGURE 12-7. Sites of action of stimuli related to anaesthesia.

With permission from Palazzo MG et al: Can Anaesth Soc J 31:178-187, 1984.

TABLE 12-3. Activity of antiemetic drugs at neurotransmitter receptor sites

Drug	Dopamine (D$_2$)	Muscarinic cholinergic	Histamine (H$_2$)
ANTICHOLINERGICS			
Hyoscine	Negligible	+ + + + +	Negligible
Atropine	Negligible	+ + + + +	Negligible
Glycopyrrolate	Negligible	+ + + + +	Negligible
H$_1$ ANTIHISTAMINES			
Promethazine	+ + + +	+ + + + +	+ + + + +
Diphenhydramine	Negligible	+ + + +	+ + + + +
Cyclizine	+	+ + +	+ + + + +
PHENOTHIAZINES			
Fluphenazine	+ + + + +	+ + + +	+ + + + +
Prochlorperazine	+ + + + +	+ + + + +	+ + + +
Chlorpromazine	+ + + + +	+ + + +	+ + + + +
BUTYROPHENONES			
Droperidol	+ + + + +	Negligible	+
Haloperidol	+ + + + +	Negligible	+
MISCELLANEOUS			
Metoclopramide	+ + + +	Negligible	+
Domperidone	+ + + +	Negligible	Negligible

ing may decrease the incidence of vomiting after upper abdominal surgery, but may actually increase the incidence of nausea and retching. These data suggest that these latter symptoms may be caused by pharyngeal stimulation from the nasogastric tube.[32]

Management of postoperative emesis includes both preventive measures and pharmacologic strategies. Avoidance of gastric inflation during mask ventilation and gastric suctioning before extubation may decrese the incidence of postoperative emesis. Oropharyngeal packing will prevent blood from reaching the stomach during nasopharyngeal procedures. Because pharyngeal suctioning can provoke retching and vomiting, suctioning is best performed before reversal of muscle relaxation in the operating room. Excessive movement of the patient after regional anesthesia or opiate administration can also provoke nausea and should be avoided. Pain relief, hydration, and maintenance of normal blood pressure should contribute to prevention of postoperative emesis. Many pharmacologic agents such as anti-cholinergics, antihistamines, phenothiazines, sedatives, and antidopaminergics have antiemetic properties (Table 12-3). If antiemetics were innocuous, widespread prophylaxis would be acceptable. However, prophylaxis is probably indicated only for patients in whom vomiting would pose an excessive risk for aspiration or damage (oral surgery patients who have their jaws wired shut or patients undergoing eye and ear surgery).

The phenothiazines are effective antiemetic agents because of antidopaminergic, histaminic, and cholinergic properties, but their routine use is limited by a high incidence of side effects. The antidopaminergic qualities of the butyrophenones (haloperidol and droperidol) make this class of drugs especially effective against narcotic-induced vomiting. Droperidol is a highly effective antiemetic, with proven prophylatic efficacy at low doses (0.005 to 0.07 mg/kg).[48,34] Its duration of action (up to 24 hours) is longer than any other agent in common use, making it especially attractive for the postoperative period. Small doses of droperidol (up to 1.25

mg) in awake patients is associated with few neurologic side effects.[37] Metoclopramide and domperidone are specific antidopaminergic drugs that cause very little sedation in normal doses (domperidone does not cross the blood brain barrier). These agents increase lower esophageal sphincter pressure and promote gastric emptying. Prophylaxis with low dose metoclopramide (10 to 20 mg) appears to be effective only when administered at the end of surgery.[15] High dose metoclopramide (1 to 2 mg/kg) prophylaxis, similar to that used with cisplatinum chemotherapy, has not been evaluated in postoperative patients. These larger doses may be more effective and in cancer patients do not appear to increase the incidence of side effects.[25] Domperidone has not demonstrated efficacy as a prophylactic agent, but appears to be effective in treating active vomiting when given intravenously.[21,69]

The causes of postoperative emesis in any one patient are likely to be multifactorial. Prophylactic antiemetic measures should be used in all recovery room patients (avoidance of oral airways, excessive movement, treatment of pain). In addition, specific antiemetics should be used in patients with persistent nausea and vomiting. In the event of the first choice drug being ineffective, a second agent, preferably one with a different site of action, should be used.

GENITOURINARY SYSTEM

Postoperative oliguria, urinary retention, and the posttransurethral prostatic resection syndrome are the most common genitourinary problems encountered in recovery room patients.

Oliguria

As discussed in another chapter (Perioperative Management of Renal Disease), residual effects of anesthetic agents, perioperative activation of the sympathetic nervous system, and release of renin, angiotensin, and antidiuretic hormone contribute to transient reductions of urine volume in the postoperative period. Oliguria in the recovery room patient, however, is usually the result of either inadequate intravascular volume repletion or urinary retention in the absence of urinary tract obstruction.

Intraoperative fluid balance must be quickly assessed in the oliguric recovery room patient. Fluid requirements on the day of surgery include estimated preoperative losses (vomiting, diarrhea, ostomy drainage, and the dehydrating effects of bowel prep-

arations), maintenance requirements since discontinuation of oral intake, "third space" losses incurred in the operating room, operative blood loss, and loss of ascites, pleural fluid, or urine during the procedure. This volume of fluid may be quite high. Maintenance requirements are approximately 110 ml/hr for a 70 kg patient and operative third space losses during intraabdominal surgery may be as high as 8 to 10 ml/kg/hr. Third space losses may continue for many hours postoperatively. If intraoperative blood is replaced with crystalloid solutions, approximately 3 ml of crystalloid is required to compensate for each ml of blood lost to maintain normal intravascular volume. When estimated fluid requirements are compared to the volume of fluid and blood products actually administered intraoperatively, many oliguric postoperative patients are found to be volume depleted. Repletion of this deficit promptly restores urine flow in most cases. Failure to increase urine volume with a fluid challenge may indicate occult bleeding and continued intravascular contraction, or impaired myocardial function and decreased renal perfusion. Invasive measurements of cardiac output, central venous, and pulmonary capillary wedge pressures may be required to differentiate between these possibilities. Although some patients who are on chronic diuretic therapy occasionally require small doses of diuretics to maintain adequate urine flow (diuretic dependence), treatment of oliguria with diuretics in all other recovery room patients should be reserved for those with unequivocal evidence of intravascular fluid overload (pulmonary edema). Intravascular volume contraction can be exacerbated by injudicious use of diuretic agents. Inadequate left ventricular preload is a common cause of perioperatively-acquired renal failure. Excess volume administration can usually be easily treated in most patients. In contrast, development of postoperative renal failure severe enough to require dialysis therapy is associated with a 50% to 100% mortality rate (see chapter on Perioperative Management of Renal Disease).

Urinary Retention

Acute urinary retention is also a common postoperative complication. Surgical trauma to the detrusor muscle and damage to pelvic nerves may inhibit bladder emptying, and operations on genitourinary and on other pelvic structures are associated with the highest incidence of urinary retention.[19] Delayed recovery of autonomic and somatic nerve function after spinal or epidural anesthesia does not appear to be a common cause of postoperative oliguria; the incidence of urinary retention is similar after either general anesthesia or after regional techniques.[57] Heavily sedated postoperative patients are often unaware of acute bladder distention and may require urethral catheterization. Perioperative use of parasympatholytic agents such as atropine, scopolamine, and glycopyrrolate may partially inhibit bladder contraction and contribute to postoperative urinary retention. Administration of parasympathomimetic agents (pilocarpine or bethanechol) often increases detrusor muscle tone and promotes micturition, but these agents should be avoided in patients with obstructive urinary retention. Rather, bladder catheterization should always be used to treat retention in postoperative patients with known or suspected prostatic enlargement with obstruction.

Transurethral Prostatectomy (TURP) Syndrome

Exposure of large venous sinuses adjacent to the prostatic capsule during TURP provides a conduit for absorption (infusion under pressure) of large quantities of irrigation solution into the intravascular space. Absorption of a commonly used irrigant such as glycine results in the TURP syndrome, which is characterized by neurologic changes (dizziness, restlessness, confusion, visual disturbances, seizures, coma) and signs and symptoms of intravascular volume overload. This isotonic, solute-free solution is rarely associated with hemolysis, but it may cause acute water intoxication and severe hyponatremia when absorbed in large volume. Hahn[27] recently tagged glycine irrigant with ethanol and found that the concentration of ethanol in the exhaled breath in patients undergoing TURP correlated significantly with both the volume of glycine absorbed and with the level to which the serum sodium decreased. Signs and symptoms of absorption develop in up to 20% of patients having TURP procedures with glycine irrigation, but decreased serum sodium and increased serum levels of glycine and ammonia (a metabolic by-product of glycine) are observed in many asymptomatic patients postoperatively.[65] Wang et al[65] suggest that glycine acts as an inhibitory transmitter in the retina and may contribute to visual disturbances in the TURP syndrome. It remains a matter for speculation whether other neurologic aberrations are the result of hyperglycinemia, hyperammonemia, hyponatremia, or other unidentified factors.

Immediate treatment for the TURP syndrome is required because the fatality rate may exceed 1%.[61] The surgical procedure should be terminated as quickly as possible. Oxygen should probably be administered to all symptomatic patients with dyspnea or hypoxemia. Furosemide will aid in the excretion of excess free water and hasten the return of serum sodium levels to normal. Hypertonic saline should be administered if clinical signs of water intoxication are present (usually at serum sodium levels less than 120 meq/l). Anticonvulsant therapy with benzodiazepines, barbiturates, or dilantin are indicated if seizure activity develops. Effective treatment of pulmonary congestion or shock may require cardiac output determinations and pharmacologic therapy guided by invasive measurements of central venous and pulmonary capillary wedge pressures.

REFERENCES

1. Adriani J, Summers FW, and Antony SO: Is the prophylactic use of antiemetics in surgical patients justified? JAMA 175:666-671, 1961.
2. Andersen R and Krohg K: Pain as a major cause of postoperative nausea, Can Anaesth Soc J 23:366-369, 1976.
3. Anderson JA, Clark PJ, and Kafer ER: Use of capnography and transcutaneous oxygen monitoring during outpatient general anesthesia for oral surgery, J Oral Maxillofac Surg 45:3-10, 1987.
4. Argov Z and Mastaglia FL: Disorders of neuromuscular transmission caused by drugs, N Engl J Med 301:409-413, 1979.
5. Azzam FJ: A simple and effective method for stopping post-anesthesia clonus, Anesthesiology 66:98, 1987.
6. Baer S, NakhJavah F, and Kajani M: Postoperative myocardial infarction, Surg Gynecol Obstet 315-322, 1965.
7. Becker LD et al: Biphasic respiratory depression after fentanyl-droperidol or fentanyl alone used to supplement nitrous oxide anesthesia, Anesthesiology 44:291-296, 1976.
8. Becker RC and Underwood DA: Myocardial infarction in patients undergoing non-cardiac surgery, Cleveland Clin J Med 54:25-28, 1987.
9. Bidwai AV et al: Reversal of diazepam-induced post-anesthetic somnolence with physostigmine, Anesthesiology 51:256-259, 1979.
10. Bidwai AV et al: Reversal of innovar-induced post-anesthetic somnolence and disorientation with physostigmine, Anesthesiology 44:249-252, 1976.
11. Biller HF et al: Laryngeal edema an experimental

study, Annals Otol Rhinol Laryngol 79(6):1084-1087, 1976.

12. Breslow MJ et al: Changes in T-wave morphology following anesthesia and surgery: a common recovery room phenomenon, Anesthesiology 1986, 64: 398-402.

13. Brismar B et al: Pulmonary densities during anesthesia with muscular relaxation—a proposal of atelectasis, Anesthesiology 62:422-428, 1985.

14. Butterworth JF et al: Augmentation of venous return by adrenergic agonists during spinal anesthesia, Anesth Analg 65:612-616, 1986.

15. Clarke MM and Storrs JA: The prevention of postoperative vomiting after abortion; metoclopramide, Br J Anaesth 41:890-892, 1969.

16. Cooper JB et al: Effects of information feedback and pulse oximetry on the incidence of anesthesia complications, Anesthesiology 67:686-694, 1987.

17. Cousins MJ and Mather LE: Intrathecal and epidural administration of opioids, Anesthesiology 61:276-310, 1984.

18. Eckenhoff JE et al: The incidence and etiology of postanesthetic excitement. A clinical survey, Anesthesiology 22:667-673, 1961.

19. Egbert LD: Spinal anesthesia for anorectal surgery, Int Anesthesiol Clin 1:811, 1963.

20. Fairley HB: Oxygen therapy for surgical patients, Am Rev Respir Dis 122:37-44, 1980.

21. Fragen RJ and Caldwell N: A new benzimidazole antiemetic, domperidone, for the treatment of postoperative nausea and vomiting, Anesthesiology 49:289-290, 1978.

22. Gal TJ and Cooperman LH: Hypertension in the immediate postoperative period, Br J Anaesth 47:70-74, 1975.

23. Garfield JM et al: A comparison of psychologic responses to ketamine and thiopental-nitrous oxide-halothane anesthesia, Anesthesiology 36:329-338, 1972.

24. Goold JE: Postoperative spasticity and shivering: a review with personal observations of 500 patients, Anaesthesia 39:35-38, 1984.

25. Gralla RJ et al: Antiemetic efficacy of high-dose metoclopramide: randomized trials with placebo and prochlorperazine in patients with chemotherapy-induced nausea and vomiting, N Engl J Med 305:905-909, 1981.

26. Griffin RM and Kaplan JA: Myocardial ischaemia during non-cardiac surgery, Anaesthesia 42:155-159, 1987.

27. Hahn RG: Ethanol monitoring of irrigating fluid absorption in transurethral prostatic surgery, Anesthesiology 68:867-873, 1988.

28. Hamel HT: Anesthetics and body temperature regulation, Anesthesiology 68:833-835, 1988.

29. Hammer G, Schwinn D, and Wollman H: Postoper-ative complications due to paradoxical vocal cord motion, Anesthesiology 66:685-687, 1987.

30. Hanna MH, Heap DG, and Kimberley APS: Cardiac dysrhythmia associated with general anaesthesia for oral surgery, Anaesthesia 38:1192-1194, 1983.

31. Hashimoto K and Hashimoto K: The mechanism of sensitization of the ventricle to epinephrine by halothane, Am Heart J 83:652-658, 1972.

32. Holmes C: Postoperative vomiting after ether/air anaesthesia, Anaesthesia 20:199-206, 1965.

33. Holzgrafe RE et al: Reversal of postoperative reactions of scopolamine with physostigmine, Anesth Analg 52:921-925, 1973.

34. Iwamoto K and Schwartz H: Antiemetic effect of droperidol after ophthalmic surgery, Arch Ophthalmol 96:1378-1379, 1978.

35. Kaplan J (editor): Cardiac anesthesia, ed 2, New York, 1986, Grune & Stratton.

36. Knill RL and Gelb AW: Ventilatory responses to hypoxia and hypercapnia during halothane sedation and anesthesia in man, Anesthesiology 49:244-251, 1978.

37. Korttila K, Kauste A, and Auvinen J: Comparison of domperidone and metoclopramide in the prevention and treatment of nausea and vomiting after balanced general anaesthesia, Anesth Analg 58:396-400, 1979.

38. Levine JH, Michael JR, and Guarnieri TK: Multifocal atrial tachycardia: a toxic effect of theophylline, Lancet 12-14, 1985.

39. Macintyre PE et al: Effect of meperidine on oxygen consumption, carbon dioxide production, and respiratory gas exchange in post-anesthesia shivering, Anesth Analg 66:751-755, 1987.

40. Metz S, Klein C, and Morton N: Rebound hypertension after discontinuation of transdermal clonidine therapy, Am J of Med 82:17-19, 1987.

41. Miller RD and Cullen DJ: Renal failure and postoperative respiratory failure: recurarization? Br J Anaesth 48:253-256, 1976.

42. Miller RD and Savarese JJ: Pharmacology of muscle relaxants and their antagonists. In Miller RD (editor): Anesthesia, ed 2, New York, 1987, Churchill Livingstone.

43. Muir JJ et al: Role of nitrous oxide and other factors in postoperative nausea and vomiting: a randomized and blinded prospective study, Anesthesiology 66:513-518, 1987.

44. Murphy MT et al: Post-anesthetic shivering in primates: inhibition by peripheral heating and by taurine, Anesthesiology 63:161-165, 1985.

45. Nunn JF: Respiratory aspects of anesthesia. In Nunn JF (editor): Applied Respiratory Physiology, ed 3, London, 1987, Butterworths.

46. Oliver SB et al: Unexpected focal neurologic deficit on emergence from anesthesia: a report of three cases, Anesthesiology 67:823-826, 1987.

47. Pasternak RC and Braunwald JA: Acute myocardial

infarction. In Harrison's Principles of Internal Medicine, ed 11, New York, 1987, McGraw-Hill Book Co.

48. Patton CM, Moon MR, and Dannemiller FJ: The prophylactic antiemetic effect of droperidol, Anesth Analg 53:361-364, 1974.

49. Peters J, Kindred MK, and Robotham JL: Transient analysis of cardiopulmonary interactions. II. Systolic events, J Appl Physiol 64(4):1518-1526, 1988.

50. Podrid PJ et al: The role of exercise testing in evaluation of arrhythmias, Am J Cardiol 62:24H-33H, 1988.

51. Rawal N et al: Influence of naloxone infusion on analgesia and respiratory depression following epidural morphine, Anesthesiology 64:194-201, 1986.

52. Riding JE: Postoperative vomiting, Proc Roy Soc Med 53:671-677, 1960.

53. Rodriguez JL et al: Physiologic requirements during rewarming: suppression of the shivering response, Crit Care Med 11:490-497, 1983.

54. Roizen MF and Stevens WC: Multiform ventricular tachycardia due to the interaction of aminophylline and halothane, Anesth Analg 57:738-741, 1978.

55. Rosenberg H et al: Neurologic changes during awakening from anesthesia, Anesthesiology 54:125-130, 1981.

56. Rueler JB: Hypothermia: pathophysiology, clinical settings, and management, Ann Intern Med 89:519-527, 1978.

57. Scarborough RA: Spinal anesthesia from the surgeon's standpoint, JAMA 168:1324, 1958.

58. Sessler DI et al: Spontaneous post-anesthetic tremor does not resemble thermoregulatory shivering, Anesthesiology 68:843-850, 1988.

59. Sharkey A et al: Inhibition of post-anesthetic shiv-

ering with radiant heat, Anesthesiology 66:249-252, 1987.

60. Shaw JE: Pharmacokinetics of nitroglycerin and clonidine delivered by the transdermal route, Am Heart J 108:217-223, 1984.

61. Sunderrajan S et al: Post-transurethral prostatic resection hyponatremic syndrome: case report and review of the literature, Am J Kidney Dis 4:80-84, 1984.

62. Tarhan S et al: Myocardial infarction after general anesthesia, JAMA 220:1451-1454, 1972.

63. Tyler IL et al: Continuous monitoring of arterial oxygen saturation with pulse oximetry during transfer to the recovery room, Anesth Analg 64:1108-1112, 1985.

64. Vance JP, Neill RS, and Norris W: The incidence and aetiology of postoperative nausea and vomiting in a plastic surgical unit, Br J Plast Surg 26:336-339, 1973.

65. Wang JM et al: Transurethral resection of the prostate, serum glycine levels, and ocular evoked potentials, Anesthesiology 70:36-41, 1989.

66. Weil JV et al: Diminished ventilatory response to hypoxia and hypercapnia after morphine in normal man, New Engl J Med 292:1103-1106, 1975.

67. Weinstock M et al: Effect of physostigmine on morphine-induced postoperative pain and somnolence, Br J Anaesth 54:429-434, 1982.

68. Wilms D and Shure D: Pulmonary edema due to upper airway obstruction in adults, Chest 94:1090-1092, 1988.

69. Wilson DB and Dundee JW: Evaluation of the antiemetic action of domperidone, Anaesthesia 34:765-767, 1979.

CHAPTER **13**

Postoperative Pain Management

PATRICIA A. TEWES
DONALD R. TAYLOR
DENNIS L. BOURKE

Systemic opiates
Patient-controlled analgesia
Nonopioid analgesics
Regional anesthetic techniques
 Intrathecal and epidural analgesia

Intercostal nerve blocks
Intrapleural analgesia
Upper extremity analgesia
Transcutaneous electrical nerve stimulation
 (TENS)

A growing body of literature suggests that pain is inadequately treated in postoperative patients and that inadequate pain relief may have adverse physiologic and psychologic consequences. The now-classic study of Marks and Sachar[60] documented that 32% of medical inpatients who were treated with narcotic analgesics reported severe pain and that 41% had moderate pain. In a similar study, 75% of surgical patients reported moderate to severe pain during the postoperative period.[27] Despite increased awareness of pain undertreatment and development of many techniques to improve pain management, a recent study[30] found that 58% of medical-surgical inpatients reported excruciating pain during their hospitalization. Of patients with pain, only 45% recalled discussing their pain with a nurse, and this statistic was confirmed by review of nursing records.

Both a punitive attitude toward patients in pain and lack of knowledge concerning appropriate dosing and pharmacokinetics of analgesic drugs are listed as reasons for undertreatment of pain.[75] Bryan-Brown[23] reviewed 10,717 pages in surgical textbooks and noted that only 19 (0.2% of pages) were devoted to management of postoperative pain. These data suggest that pain management is not a high priority in surgical teaching and support the idea that lack of knowledge may be a major reason for undertreatment. In addition, pain medications are frequently prescribed in inadequate doses and at inappropriately long intervals.[29] Pain is also undertreated for fear of producing respiratory depression, but hypoxia is more often directly associated with untreated pain.

The physiologic consequences of undertreated postoperative pain may adversely influence perioperative outcome. Pain increases neuroendocrine activity and may increase the risk for myocardial ischemia in some patients. Stress-induced hypertension, cardiac arrhythmias, and metabolic changes may increase perioperative morbidity and mortality. Untreated pain may alter pulmonary function,[31,85,88] cause sleep disturbances,[59] impair ambulation, and increase the risk of deep venous thromboses.[77]

The complex relationship between psychologic factors and patient perceptions of pain was originally documented by Beecher,[8,9] who noted that 65% of severely wounded soldiers did not complain of pain. The authors suggested that pain perception may have been blunted by a sense of relief to be alive and leaving battle. Inadequate postoperative pain relief was characterized as a "cool and callous disgrace" by Colin MacInnes, an author who was dying of cancer.[23] Patients who have control over adverse stimuli such as pain appear to have less pain and fewer physiologic changes as a result.[6,18]

This chapter discusses many different methods for treatment of postoperative pain. Traditional routes for administration of systemic narcotics are considered first. A variation of continuous intravenous administration, patient-controlled analgesia, and the role of nonopioid analgesics in the perioperative period are then discussed. Finally, techniques of regional anesthesia appropriate for surgical patients are reviewed.

SYSTEMIC OPIATES

Although opioids have been used to relieve pain since the time of the ancient Greeks, there are still many misconceptions concerning their use. (See box above, right.) Ignorance of the pharmacokinetics of these drugs and inadequate dosing schedules resulting from concerns about respiratory depression and addiction have created a misconception among many physicians that narcotics do not relieve pain. However, when used with proper knowledge of pharmacokinetics (how the body handles the drug) and pharmacodynamics (the relationship between pharmacologic responses and drug concentrations), these drugs provide highly effective pain relief.[61]

Opiates are morphinelike analgesics with both spinal and central sites of action. They interact at specific opioid receptors and have properties similar to those of endogenous peptides including enkephalins, endorphins, and dynorphins.[48] There appear to be four distinct opioid receptors: (1) the mu receptor, which mediates analgesia, miosis, respiratory depression, and the opioid withdrawal syndrome; (2) the kappa receptor, which mediates spinal analgesia but not opioid withdrawal; (3) the sigma receptor, which mediates pupillary dilatation, tachypnea, and

Misconceptions about use of opioid drugs in acute pain
1. Doses should be as small and infrequent as possible to avoid development of addiction.
2. Doses larger than the standard do not increase pain relief and cause heavy sedation and respiratory depression.
3. Nursing and/or medical staff know when and how much pain relief each patient needs.
4. Patients requesting more pain relief than the standard are psychologically abnormal or are becoming addicted.
5. If nonopioid drugs are also ordered, these should be tried in preference to opioids.
6. What is needed is a powerful nonaddictive pain reliever.

Modified from Mather LE and Phillips GD: Opioids and adjuvants: principles of use. In Cousins MJ and Phillips GD (editors): Acute pain management, New York, 1986, Churchill Livingstone.

dysphoria; and (4) the delta receptor, which modulates the effects of the mu response. This last receptor is found mainly in periaqueductal gray matter and in the limbic system (Table 13-1). The symptoms produced by any particular opioid depend on the affinity of that drug for each of the different receptors.[48]

Morphine and all other opioids have many central nervous system effects, including analgesia, drowsiness, changes in mood, respiratory depression, and altered endocrine and autonomic nervous system function. Opioids are much more selective than other drugs that act on the CNS to produce analgesia. Inhalation of nitrous oxide, for example, produces more sedation and greater impairment of motor coordination for the same level of analgesia as an opiate. Currently, there is an attempt to find an opioid that specifically produces analgesia without the undesirable effects of respiratory depression, excessive sedation, and decreased gastrointestinal motility.

Of the opioid drugs currently available, morphinelike drugs (mu agonists) are the most widely used analgesics, and they all produce similar degrees of analgesia and side effects. They differ in duration of action and in the optimal route of administration.

TABLE 13-1.   Opiate receptors and the clinical properties of their agonists

Receptor type	Agonist	Effect of agonist on opiate withdrawl	Level of analgesia	Other effects
Mu (μ)	Morphine endorphins	Suppression	Supraspinal, dorsal horn	Miosis Respiratory depression Nausea Euphoria
Kappa (κ)	Ketocyclazocine dynorphin	No suppression	Spinal	Miosis Ataxia Sedation
Sigma (σ)	N-allylnormetazocine phencyclidine	No suppression	Suspraspinal, spinal	Pupillary Psychotomimetric Dysphoria Tachypnea
Delta (δ)	Enkephalins			

Fentanyl, for example, is minimally effective when given orally, but it is a potent analgesic intravenously. Many patients develop nausea with morphine, but not with meperidine. Thus the choice of drug for postoperative pain management depends on the individual patient, the duration of action, and the preferred route of administration. It has been suggested that visceral pain may be more responsive to kappa receptor agonists, whereas cutaneous electrical and thermal stimulation (somatic pain) respond best to mu and delta receptor agonists.[83] Use of mixed agonist-antagonist drugs such as pentazocine, nalbuphine, butorphanol, and buprenorphine is limited in the postoperative period because these drugs have a limited response (flat dose-response curve) on both analgesia and respiratory depression. A current area of active research is the search for a mixed agonist-antagonist with high analgesic properties but limited respiratory depression.

The route of administration of a narcotic is determined by the severity and location of pain. For major surgical procedures producing a high level of pain, parenteral or spinal axis administration is usually preferred, whereas oral administration may be sufficient in patients undergoing minor procedures (Table 13-2). Variability in the response to a given dose of opioid may be a result of individual differences in drug pharmacokinetics and to variable patient characteristics such as age, sex, and severity of pain. Pharmacokinetic studies in patients receiving 100 mg of intramuscular meperidine every 4

hours have shown a threefold difference in maximal blood concentrations and an eightfold difference at the time of occurrence of pain. Of these patients, 89% did not achieve adequate analgesia from the first dose, and over half still had severe pain after the second dose. Since duration of action of meperidine (Demerol) varies between 2 and 4 hours, the standard practice of administering a fixed dose of this drug every 3 to 4 hours is unlikely to produce satisfactory analgesia. Variability of intramuscular absorption may be decreased by using drugs that are more hydrophilic (morphine) than lipophilic (meperidine or fentanyl). Injection of lipophilic drugs into the deltoid rather than the gluteal muscle produces more consistent absorption because there is less fatty tissue near the deltoid muscle.

Intravenous boluses of narcotic drugs are effective more rapidly than intramuscular injections, and continuous infusions most effectively avoid the pain-sedation cycle seen with intermittent injections. Without a loading dose, continuous infusion will not achieve a steady state (the equilibrium of drug concentration between blood and tissues) until 4 to 6 times the half-life of the narcotic has elapsed. To avoid the side effects of a large bolus loading dose, a loading infusion may be given over 20 to 30 minutes. Transdermal administration of some drugs (fentanyl) provides consistent drug levels similar to continuous intravenous infusions; however, the times of onset and offset of drug effect is 6 to 12 hours because of slow penetration of the skin barrier. Epi-

TABLE 13-2. Characteristics of frequently used narcotic analgesics

Nonproprietary name	Trade name	Dose (mg) (sub-Q)	Duration of action (hours)	Withdrawal symptoms
Morphine		10	4-5	
Hydromorphone (dihydromorphinone)	Dilaudid	1.5	4-5	Like morphine
Oxymorphone (dihydrohydroxymorphinone)	Numorphan	1.0-1.5	4-5	Like morphine
Metopon (methyldihydromorphinone		3.5	4-5	Like morphine
Codeine		120 (10-20)	(4-6)	
Hydrocodone (dihydrocodeinone)	Hycodan	(5-10)	(4-8)	Between morphine and codeine
Drocode (dihydrocodeine)	Synalgos-DC	60	4-5	Between morphine and codeine
Oxycodone (dihydrohydroxycodeinone)		10-15 (3-5)	4-5 (4-5)	Close to morphine
Pholcodine (β-morpholinylethylmorphine)		(5-15)	4-5	Much less than codeine
Levorphanol	Levo-Dromoran	2	4-5	Like morphine
Methadone	Dolophine	8-10	3-5	
Dextromoramide		5-7.5	4-5	Like methadone
Dipipanone		20-25	4-5	Like methadone
Phenadoxone		10-20	1-3	Less than morphine
Meperidine	Demerol	75-100	2-4	
Alphaprodine	Nisentil	40	1-2	Like meperidine

Modified from Jaffe JH and Martin WR: Opioid analgesics and narcotics. In Gilman AJ et al: Goodman and Gilman's the pharmacological basis of therapeutics, New York, 1985, Macmillan Publishing Co.

dural and intrathecal administration of narcotics is discussed in a later section.

Use of "prn" fixed doses of drugs often leads to erratic fluctuation in drug levels and unsatisfactory analgesia in postoperative patients. Patient requests for analgesic therapy are often followed by a time delay before the nursing staff is able to administer the drug, and a cycle of severe pain alternating with excessive sedation after drug administration is established. A system of patient-administered medication at the time that pain is first perceived provides one solution to this common problem.

PATIENT-CONTROLLED ANALGESIA

Patient-controlled analgesia (PCA) is now widely accepted as a safe and effective method of postoperative pain management. It allows patients to titrate narcotic drug dose to need in a timely and practical fashion to eliminate the cycle of pain alternating with sedation (Figure 13-1) that is associated with parenteral injections.[71] Small, self-administered boluses of drug achieve constant blood levels that approximate those obtained with continuous intravenous infusions (Figure 13-2) but provide patient comfort and safety by administering only enough drug to control pain. Initial attempts to deliver intravenous narcotics to patients on demand consisted of having a nurse-observer administer small intravenous doses of narcotic at the patient's request.[84] This technique produced superior pain relief with smaller total drug dosage than parenteral bolus injections, but it was an impractical system because of the demands placed

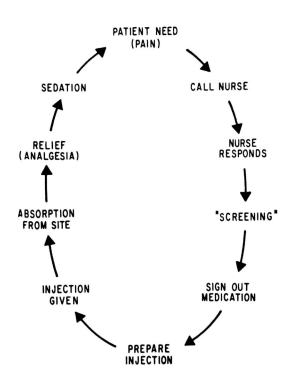

FIGURE 13-1. The cyclic character of conventional analgesic therapy.

From Graves DA et al: Patient-controlled analgesia, Ann Int Med 99:360-366, 1983.

on the nursing staff.[93] Therefore, researchers developed specialized patient-controlled analgesia devices to deliver analgesic drugs on demand.

Several features of modern PCA systems minimize the risk of drug overdose and increase analgesic efficacy. First, as narcotic blood levels rise, analgesia is normally achieved before sedation, and sedation precedes respiratory depression.[12,39] Thus inappropriate triggering of the system produces sedation that subsequently limits further dosing. Small bolus doses of 1 to 3 mg of morphine or its equivalent are commonly used to take advantage of this graded response. Second, all PCA devices have a lockout period during which requests by the patient for further bolus doses are ignored by the machine. The lockout interval forces the patient to experience the maximal analgesic effect of a bolus dose before a subsequent dose can be delivered. Maximal respiratory depression normally occurs within 7 minutes after administration of morphine, and a minimal lockout interval of 5 to 6 minutes is commonly used. Finally, a continuous background infusion (0.5 to 2.0 mg of morphine per hour) is possible with most PCA devices to maintain constant serum levels and to increase the efficacy of small PCA boluses in regaining pain control. Use of the basal infusion mode requires periodic assessment of patient demands for bolus doses to appropriately adjust the rate of infusion for safe and maximal benefit.

Whereas almost every available intravenous analgesic has been evaluated for PCA therapy (see box on p. 168), no drug has been found to be superior to morphine.[106] The usual PCA doses for morphine and meperidine are given in Table 13-3. However, individual patient variability to the pharmacologic effects of narcotic agents precludes standardized recommendations for dose based on age, sex, or body weight.[4,54,95,96] Thus the typical morphine PCA bolus dose is empirically started at 1 mg with a lockout interval of 6 minutes. Initial studies demonstrated that the pharmacologic and mechanical safety features of PCA devices achieved analgesia without oversedation.[14,95] While many patients forgo complete pain relief to minimize sedation,[4,14] the level

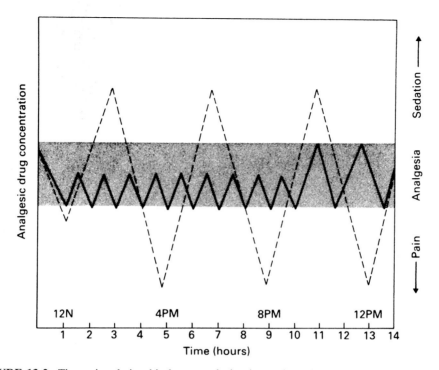

FIGURE 13-2. Theoretic relationship between dosing interval, analgesic drug concentration and clinical effects when comparing a patient-controlled analgesia system (*solid line*) to conventional intramuscular therapy (*broken line*).

From White PF: Use of a patient-controlled analgesia infuser for the management of postoperative pain. In Harmer M, Rosen M, and Vickens MD: Patient-controlled analgesia, Boston, 1985, Blackwell Scientific Publications.

Analgesics used with PCA therapy

Alfentanil	Methadone
Buprenorphine	Morphine
Fentanyl	Nalbuphine*
Hydromorphone	Oxymorphone
Ketamine**	Pentazocine*
Meperidine	Sufentanil

*Agonist-antagonist
**Phencyclidine derivative

---

of sedation with PCA is probably equivalent to that observed postoperatively with intramuscular analgesia.[32,46,54,103]

Studies of the efficacy of PCA compared to intramuscular narcotics for postoperative analgesia are conflicting. Some authors have found PCA superior to intramuscular narcotics,[16,46,53,104] whereas others have shown the two methods to be equally effective in relieving postoperative pain.[44,54,103] Comparisons between epidural narcotics, PCA, and intramuscular injections[32,44] in cesarean section patients found that epidural narcotics provided pain relief superior to that of either PCA or intramuscular narcotics, but patients preferred PCA. Other studies have also confirmed this favorable patient response to PCA.[44,54,57,89,96] In one questionnaire, 26 of 27 PCA patients liked having control over their postoperative pain management and were pleased that they did not have to wait for a nurse to administer an analgesic injection.[89] Although not specifically studied, it is generally accepted that ablation of the pain cycle with PCA reduces patient anxiety in the postopera-

TABLE 13-3. Usual PCA doses for meperidine and morphine*

Drug	Bolus dose (mg)		Lockout interval (min)		Basal infusion (mg/hr)	
	Average	Range	Average	Range	Average	Range
Meperidine	10	5-30	6	5-15	5	5-20
Morphine	1	0.5-3	6	5-15	0.5	0.5-2

*These are suggested as starting doses only. After initiating therapy titrate dose to analgesia versus sedation.

tive period,[106] and this effect may be caused in part by decreased dependence on nursing staff for analgesic therapy.[12]

Kleiman et al[54] reported that PCA patients tolerated early postoperative mobilization better than patients treated with intramuscular analgesics despite pain scores that were similar in both groups. One study demonstrated a 22% reduction in hospital stay in thoracotomy patients treated with PCA,[35] but this study has not been repeated by others. PCA decreases the amount of time nurses spend administering analgesics and may reduce labor costs; however, overall analgesic cost to the patient may increase because of equipment and drug preparation costs.[45,57] Nighttime sleep patterns are improved with PCA therapy.[32]

Patients should be maintained on PCA therapy until oral pain medications are begun. Daily narcotic requirements normally decrease approximately 50% every 12 to 24 hours over the first 3 postoperative days (except for intraabdominal procedures when narcotic consumption remains constant during the first 3 days and then decreases).[24] As the number of PCA bolus doses decreases, downward adjustment of the basal infusion rate may be required to prevent sedation. When patients are able to take liquids, oral analgesics should be started and the basal infusion stopped. If the PCA bolus is being avidly used during this time, the dosage of oral analgesic drugs should be increased.

Complications are rare in patients who are appropriately selected for PCA therapy. Mental alertness and ability to understand the concept of PCA and instructions on how to use the device are required. Elderly patients who become confused at night and patients who are unwilling to self-administer narcotics are not good candidates for PCA. Patients with significant liver, renal, or pulmonary disease should be approached with caution. Hypovolemic patients

are at increased risk of narcotic-induced respiratory depression.[96] Narcotic addiction is considered by some to be a contraindication,[79] whereas other practitioners consider these patients on a case-by-case basis.[42] Finally, a trained nursing staff is essential because nursing error is perhaps the greatest source for mishaps with PCA therapy.

Pharmacologic side effects of PCA therapy are the same as those observed after narcotic administration by any other route. Clinically important respiratory depression occurs in less than 1% of hospitalized medical patients after parenteral narcotics,[65,66] and the risk of respiratory depression with PCA is similarly low.[43,106] Jensen et al[49] reported three cases of respiratory arrest during PCA: (1) a cracked PCA syringe siphoned its full contents into a patient; (2) a microprocessor malfunction allowed a patient to use the drug at an excessive rate, and the nurse replaced the syringes as quickly as the patient used them; and (3) a physician ordered combined PCA and intramuscular therapy that resulted in narcotic overdose. All three patients were successfully resuscitated with naloxone and recovered uneventfully. Respiratory depression resulting from programming errors and accidental intravenous bolus administration during changing of a drug cartridge have been reported.[105] One case of respiratory depression during PCA therapy in a hypovolemic patient was successfully treated with fluid resuscitation alone, and another patient required naloxone and volume replacement.[96] A well-trained and vigilant nursing staff is the most important factor in minimizing complications. PCA devices that program the drug dose in mass units rather than volume units, automatic nursing intervention standards, and physician availability for immediate evaluation and treatment of patients are also important to decrease the risk of respiratory depression.[49]

The incidence of nausea and vomiting with PCA

is equal to or less than that observed with intramuscular narcotics.[32,44,46,54] Most patients with nausea obtain symptomatic relief with metoclopramide, and PCA is rarely discontinued for intractable nausea. Pruritus may be more common with PCA therapy than with intramuscular injections, but it is significantly less frequent than with epidural narcotics.[32,44] Pruritus associated with PCA or intramuscular injections responds to antihistamines, but that produced by epidural narcotics may require naloxone for reversal.[44]

PCA therapy is evolving. Studies are underway to further evaluate the role of PCA in postoperative pain management, and the method is being used to administer analgesics by epidural,[26,33,87] subcutaneous,[99] and oral[102] routes. Patient-controlled anxiolysis with midazolam has been reported in intensive care units.[58] PCA is being used in the management of cancer pain[47,101] and during sickle cell crisis.[82] While PCA has gained relatively rapid acceptance for postoperative analgesia, the complete scope of its role in pain management remains undefined.

NONOPIOID ANALGESICS

Nonopioid drugs such as sedatives, antipsychotics, antidepressants, stimulants, and antiinflammatory agents have been used to supplement narcotic action in the postoperative period, but the role of these drugs in this setting is not well defined. Although sedatives (benzodiazepines, barbiturates) may actually increase nociception, their effects to enhance sedation and sleep may be desirable in some patients. Sedation should not, however, be considered a substitute for adequate analgesia. Hydroxyzine, an antihistamine with sedative properties, is frequently used to supplement narcotic analgesia, but studies of the efficacy of this drug in postoperative patients yield conflicting results.[3] Antipsychotic drugs such as the phenothiazines (chlorpromazine, promethazine) and the butyrophenones (haloperidol) have little analgesic efficacy, and each agent may adversely enhance narcotic-induced bradycardia and respiratory depression.[7] Use of phenothiazines and butyrophenones as narcotic adjuvants is probably not indicated, but they are used effectively in small doses to treat postoperative nausea and vomiting. Although antidepressants such as amitriptyline or imipramine are useful in treatment of chronic pain, they have not been evaluated for use in the treatment of acute postoperative pain. Similarly, psychomotor stimulants such as *d*-amphetamine are sometimes used in patients with chronic cancer pain to counteract the sedative effects of narcotics, but these agents probably have no role in acute postoperative pain management.

Aspirin-like drugs inhibit production of prostaglandins from damaged cells and are particularly useful in the treatment of pain associated with inflammation. Prostaglandins sensitize pain receptors to mechanical and chemical stimulation.[37] Antiinflammatory drugs are useful in the treatment of low-to-moderate intensity pain and also appear to have some synergism with narcotics. Since these drugs may interfere with platelet function, they should be used with caution in patients on anticoagulants or with bleeding disorders.

Other analgesic agents such as nitrous oxide and ketamine have been used for postoperative pain management. However, each of these agents have powerful sedative effects with comparatively low-level analgesic effects, and their use in surgical patients should be restricted to intraoperative management supervised by anesthesiologists.

REGIONAL ANESTHETIC TECHNIQUES

Despite many advantages over conventional systemic analgesic methods, use of regional anesthetic techniques to provide postoperative analgesia has not gained widespread acceptance. This reluctance may be caused by generalized resistance to change and unfamiliarity of people who are not anesthesiologists with the technical skills and specific knowledge required.

The many advantages of regional analgesic techniques, however, are causing practice patterns to change. Many regional analgesic techniques have the unique ability to completely block afferent pain stimuli. This effect not only provides analgesia, but it also prevents activation of various neurohumoral responses to pain such as catecholamine release and increased sympathetic nervous system activity. Stress-induced hyperglycemia and glucose intolerance are attenuated and perioperative changes in metabolic rate, oxygen demand, and myocardial work are minimized. Regional techniques achieve analgesia without sedation. Compared to parenteral narcotics, epidural analgesia has been associated with earlier postoperative ambulation, more rapid return of bowel function, shorter postoperative hospital stay, and decreased incidence of both pulmonary and thromboembolic complications.[28,55,76,77,85] Regional analgesic techniques can be divided into peripheral, regional, or axial (spinal and epidural) blocks.

Intrathecal and Epidural Analgesia

Before the analgesic effectiveness of spinal opiates was demonstrated, intrathecal or epidural routes for postoperative pain control were seldom used. The only effective drugs were local anesthetics that not only alleviated pain, but also caused sympathetic and motor blockade. For these reasons, postoperative analgesia by the intrathecal or epidural routes was usually limited to special circumstances and required specialized nursing care. However, the finding that epidural and intrathecal narcotics produced profound analgesia without these undesirable side effects has stimulated interest in their use.

Discovery of highly specific opiate receptors in the central nervous system in 1973 spurred the search for endogenous opiate-like substances. In 1975, two pentapeptides (Met-Enkephalin and Leuenkephlin) with analgesic activity indistinguishable from that produced by morphine and other narcotic analgesics were discovered. Other investigations revealed the existence of specific opioid receptors in the spinal cord with high concentrations of both Mu and Kappa receptors in the lamina I and II of the substantia gelatinosa. The lamina II location coincides with termination areas for polymodal nociceptive C fibers. Most opioids act at these receptor sites to inhibit release of substance P, a neurotransmitter of nociceptive stimuli. Subsequent research culminated in 1979 with the use of intrathecal morphine to control pain in humans. Since that time, numerous studies have demonstrated the efficacy of both epidural and intrathecal narcotic administration in the control of pain. By either route, narcotics ultimately act on opioid receptors in the substantia gelatinosa to interrupt afferent nociceptive transmission.

Intrathecal analgesia. Although a number of options are available, single dose morphine is the most common method of intrathecal analgesia. Intrathecal morphine produces analgesia that is usually superior to conventional analgesic administration methods.[11,62] Surprisingly, the site of injection does not have to coincide with the affected segments to be effective. Lumbar administration of intrathecal morphine can provide adequate analgesia after either hemorrhoid, thoracic, or head and neck surgery. Intrathecal morphine doses range from 0.2 to 1.0 mg, depending on age, body size, and the location of pain. Onset of analgesia requires 45 to 60 minutes after injection, and it is common practice to administer intrathecal morphine several hours before the end of surgery to achieve good postoperative pain control. Duration of action is 12 to 24 hours. Nearly all of an intrathecal dose of morphine acts at the spinal level, although some fraction of the dose may be transported in the CSF to supraspinal receptors. Since morphine is not lipophilic, very little crosses membranes to enter the systemic circulation. After typical intrathecal doses, peak plasma concentrations may reach 1 to 2 ng/ml as compared with therapeutic plasma levels of 14 to 18 ng/ml following parenteral administration of standard analgesic doses of 0.5 to 1.5 mg/kg.

Side effects and complications are related to systemic and supraspinal effects. The most common side effects are pruritus, urinary retention, nausea, and vomiting.[19,20] These undesirable effects all respond to low doses of intravenous naloxone that do not antagonize analgesia (0.5 μg/kg/hr).[78] Pruritis can often be effectively treated with antihistamines. The most serious side effect, respiratory depression caused by narcotic action on supraspinal opioid receptors, can occur as long as 18 hours after intrathecal narcotic administration. The incidence of respiratory depression following intrathecal narcotics (less than 1%) is slightly higher than after epidural (less than 0.2%) or conventional parenteral methods of administration.[22,40] Respiratory depression responds immediately to intravenous naloxone. Concern about respiratory depression has been exaggerated, probably because of the long latency and the unpredictability of onset.

Epidural analgesia. Although the mechanism of action and quality of analgesia are similar, epidural analgesia offers more options and several practical advantages over intrathecal analgesia. Both techniques work by attenuating noxious afferent input at the spinal level. However, epidural administration permits more precise control of drug concentration and limits systemic effects, since the drug is not immediately mixed with the cerebrospinal fluid. Further, because catheters are commonly placed in the epidural space and only rarely in the intrathecal space, epidural analgesia is more amenable to long-term, continuous therapy.

Local anesthetics administered into the epidural space completely block afferent nociceptive impulses and attenuate neurohumoral reflex responses to pain. However, local anesthetics invariably block sympathetic fibers and often block other sensory modalities and motor efferents as well. Consequently, patients receiving epidural local anesthetics for postoperative analgesia require extensive, labor-intensive monitoring in an ICU. For these reasons, use of local anesthetics for postoperative pain control is limited to special instances where it is essential to avoid the deleterious effects of narcotics or to patients who require blockade of only a very few spinal segments.

Epidural narcotics, on the other hand, have a potentially much wider range of uses and do not require intensive monitoring. Epidural narcotics can provide extensive and profound analgesia without blocking other sensory modalities, motor efferents, or the sympathetic nervous system.

The route by which narcotics injected into the epidural space reach the substantia gelatinosa is not precisely known, however, it is believed that the arachnoid granulations located in the dural cuffs are the major pathway of diffusion. Some additional narcotic may penetrate the dura directly, and some may diffuse into the spinal reticular arteries and then to the substantia gelatinosa. The longer path from epidural injection sites to the spinal opioid receptors requires approximately a tenfold increase of epidural narcotic dose (2 to 10 mg) compared to intrathecal morphine (0.1 to 1.0 mg).[67] Larger dose requirements and epidural site of deposition result in considerable plasma uptake. After epidural injection of morphine, plasma profiles are very similar to those with intramuscular injection of a similar dose; however, the local CSF-to-plasma concentration ratio is typically 50 to 150:1 after 1 to 2 hours.

The onset, duration, and extent of action of epidural narcotics are primarily a function of lipophilicity.[97] Morphine, which is relatively hydrophilic, has an onset of 45 to 90 minutes and a duration of 12 to 24 hours. In contrast, the more lipophilic fentanyl has an onset of 10 to 20 minutes and a duration of about 1 hour. The longer duration of morphine makes it more suitable for postoperative analgesia

as a single injection. Continuous postoperative infusion through a catheter may be most effectively accomplished with lipophilic drugs such as fentanyl. Because the duration of action is shorter, fentanyl infusions can be adjusted hourly to obtain the optimal infusion rate. The greater lipid solubility of fentanyl may lower the incidence of respiratory depression and other complications because there is less cephalad spread of the drug to supraspinal receptors.

Analgesia from epidural and intrathecal narcotics does not appear to be intensified by the addition of vasoconstrictors, as it is with local anesthetics.[73] There is some evidence that epidural narcotic analgesia is enhanced when the narcotic infusion is mixed with dilute concentrations of local anesthetics; however the mechanism is not known.[25,36]

Complications from epidural narcotics are similar to those seen with intrathecal narcotics; minor complications include pruritus (14%), urinary retention (12%), and nausea and vomiting (11%).[19,20] Because these side effects all result from low doses of systemically absorbed narcotics acting at supraspinal opioid receptor sites,[40] they are effectively reversed by low-dose infusions of naloxone without substantially reversing analgesia. The incidence of delayed respiratory depression associated with epidural narcotics is less than 0.2%, and this incidence compares favorably with that observed after parenteral narcotic administration.[21,22,38] It should be noted that the incidence of all complications from epidural narcotics is highest in volunteers, lower in patients with acute pain, and seldom seen in chronic-pain patients.

Intercostal Nerve Blocks

Intercostal nerve blocks with local anesthetics have been effectively used to treat acute pain from thoracotomy incision, fractured ribs, and abdominal incisions. In the past, the use of intercostal nerve block was limited by several factors: (1) duration of analgesia was typically less than four hours despite using long-acting agents with epinephrine, (2) adequate analgesia often required blocks at several different levels and resulted in high serum drug concentration levels, and (3) multiple-level intercostal blocks increased the incidence of pneumothorax. For these reasons, intercostal blocks have been reserved for patients with fractured ribs or patients with chest tubes in whom pain prevented adequate pulmonary toilet.

As early as 1981, there were reports of multiple levels of analgesia from a single intercostal nerve block.[74] Subsequent radiographic studies confirmed that injection of sufficiently large volumes of drug caused the local anesthetic to diffuse centrally and then vertically to provide analgesia over multiple dermatome levels. Since that time, the technique has evolved to include placement of a catheter in the subcostal neurovascular space to provide prolonged analgesia either by intermittent injection or by continuous infusion of local anesthetic.[70] Continuous intercostal nerve block has been particularly valuable in patients with fractured ribs, but has also been useful in both thoracotomy patients and in obese patients after cholecystectomy.[34,68,69] Pain is relieved with minimal systemic effects. Pulmonary complications are reduced because coughing and deep breathing are promoted, narcotic respiratory depression is absent, and early ambulation is facilitated. Normal bowel function is regained early postoperatively because of reduced narcotic dosage and early ambulation. Because of these advantages, it seems likely that continuous intercostal nerve block will be used more extensively to treat postoperative pain as experience with this technique grows.

Intrapleural Analgesia

In 1986, Reiestad and Stromskag[80] introduced a technique involving placement of a catheter into the intrapleural space. Local anesthetics injected through this catheter provided postoperative analgesia for cholecystectomy, breast surgery, and renal surgery. Subsequent papers have advocated intrapleural analgesia for a variety of acute pain conditions, including postoperative thoracotomy and abdominal incisions. An epidural catheter is usually placed in the intrapleural space at the eighth rib through an epidural needle with loss of resistance technique. Local anesthetic solutions can be given through the catheter either by intermittent injections (5 to 20 ml) or by continuous infusion. Bupivacaine (0.25% to 0.5%) with epinephrine has been the preferred local anesthetic agent. Although experience with intrapleural catheters is limited, reports of pneumothorax are rare.

It is believed that drugs spread through the ipsilateral intrapleural space and diffuse into intercostal nerves to produce analgesia over a wide area of the thorax. Like continuous intercostal block, the intrapleural technique provides analgesia with minimal sedation, respiratory depression, or sympathetic blockade. In contrast to epidural or intercostal catheters, intrapleural catheters have little chance of migrating into vascular structures. Intrapleural analgesia offers much promise, but extended clinical trials are lacking, and currently available information consists of isolated studies and occasional case reports.

Upper Extremity Analgesia

Postoperative analgesia for surgery of the upper extremity can be provided with the subclavian or axillary perivascular regional techniques described by Winnie.[107] Either technique is amenable to intermittent injection or continuous infusion of local anesthetics. Although seldom required for adequate postoperative pain control, these special techniques produce sympathetic blockade that may improve blood flow when circulation is compromised by vasospasm. Trauma patients or patients with severe pulmonary disease may benefit from these approaches by avoiding the sedative and/or respiratory depressant effects of systemic analgesics. Intolerance to conventional analgesics may also be an indication for the use of these regional anesthetic techniques. Since these techniques are time consuming and require technical expertise, patients require closer observation and more intensive care than patients treated with conventional analgesic methods. To avoid repeating these efforts every few hours, catheters can be placed either in the axillary or interscalene perivascular space.

The axillary approach is ideal for analgesia and/or sympathetic blockade below the elbow, but it may occasionally be contraindicated because of proximity to axillary lymph nodes in patients with infection or metastatic disease. Axillary catheters are difficult to secure in place if treatment is required for more than 48 hours.

The subclavian approach to the interscalene space is the preferred block for analgesia of the upper arm and/or shoulder. It could also be used for sympathetic block of the forearm and hand, but blocking the C7 and T1 dermatomes is difficult. The major advantage of subclavian block is ease of securing a continuous infusion catheter for long periods of time.

When intermittent injections are used, the concentration and volume of drug should be the lowest that will block the distribution and modality desired. Since little information is available in the current literature, it is probably best to estimate infusion rates after a period of experience with intermittent injections.

Transcutaneous Electrical Nerve Stimulation (TENS)

Use of electricity to produce analgesia may date to Greek and Roman times. The electric ray, which can emit as much as 200 V, was used in the first century AD to treat a variety of painful disorders.[50,52] Electrical analgesia has been used only sporadically since ancient times, but recent advances have stimulated new interest in electroanalgesia, TENS.

Gate-control theory forms the theoretic basis for afferent stimulation techniques of analgesia. Electrical stimulation of large afferent fibers effectively closes a gate at the spinal level to painful stimuli traveling in smaller fibers. A central mechanism may also modulate the gating system via descending pathways.[64] Evidence for an alternative theory suggests that electrostimulation releases endorphins in the substantia gelatinosa and thereby inhibits transmission of pain stimuli. This latter theory attractively explains the fact that only a brief period of stimulation often produces prolonged analgesia.[1] However, naloxone has not been effective in antagonizing analgesia produced by TENS.[86]

TENS is usually delivered as a balanced, biphasic, asymmetric spiked wave pulse. This form prevents electrolysis and annoying muscular contractions and provides a pleasant, tingling sensation to the patient. Useful pulse widths range from 60 to 150 msec. Pulse frequencies range from 10 to 100 Hz, but 80 to 100 Hz appear to be the most effective frequencies for acute pain. Current amplitude is determined by trial and error; the maximum current that causes neither pain nor twitching is usually between 12 to 20 mAmp.

Numerous studies have demonstrated the usefulness of TENS in treating a variety of chronic pain syndromes, and TENS is often a first line of treatment for chronic pain of unknown etiology. TENS has many advantages that would make it an ideal postoperative analgesic. It is nontoxic, noninvasive, simple to use, and does not require high levels of nursing care. It does not cause addiction, respiratory depression, or sedation. Other complications associated with narcotics such as pruritus, nausea, vomiting, urinary retention, and orthostatic hypotension do not occur with TENS. Unfortunately, studies of the effectiveness of TENS in the postoperative period are inconclusive.

While TENS relieves musculoskeletal pain, permits early range of motion exercises, and improves outcome after knee surgery, it is not effective in treating visceral pain during the first 24 hours postoperatively. TENS does not improve spirometric pulmonary function or arterial blood gases postoperatively despite reduced narcotic analgesic requirements. Postoperative ileus may resolve more rapidly in the presence of TENS; this effect may be caused by reduced narcotic doses. Only one study in the literature suggests an association of TENS with a shorter postoperative hospital stay.[50] These variable responses may result from lack of manufacturing standards for TENS devices and lack of standardized user-controlled parameters such as lead placement.

While TENS is virtually free of undesirable side effects, it is not presently capable of providing reliable analgesia in the immediate postoperative period. It may be a useful adjunct to conventional methods in selected cases, such as peripheral musculoskeletal procedures. At the current state of development, TENS is neither cost effective nor therapeutically effective in the majority of postoperative patients. Continued research and development of standardized treatment schedules may eventually demonstrate benefit to postoperative patients.

SUMMARY

Recent evidence indicates that effective perioperative pain control not only provides physical comfort to patients, but also attenuates many adverse physiologic and psychologic effects of anesthesia and surgery. A few studies suggest that pain ablation improves outcome and decreases length of postoperative hospital stay.* These findings indicate that postoperative analgesia is more important than is generally appreciated, and emphasizes the fact that uninformed and punitive approaches to pain management are detrimental.

Many available drugs and techniques effectively blunt painful stimuli, but comparative studies of analgesic efficacy do not unequivocally support use of one strategy over another. Analgesic efficacy of standard methods of parenteral narcotic administration appear to be less than that of most of the specialized techniques discussed in this chapter. Whether the effectiveness of parenteral agents is limited by development of serious complications before equianalgesic levels are achieved is unclear; many comparative studies use conventional narcotic dosing schedules that are inadequate by standard pharmacokinetic principles. Theoretic and practical considerations suggest that continuous epidural infusions of short-acting, lipophilic agents such as fentanyl may provide superior analgesia. However, some patients prefer PCA over epidural narcotics despite decreased analgesic efficacy of PCA. Thus, management techniques that allow patient control over administration of analgesic medications may be preferable to ones that place control in the hands of hospital staff. More studies to evaluate the effects of analgesic techniques on perioperative outcome are needed.

Choice of analgesic technique must account for overall medical status of the patient, history of untoward drug reactions, availability of appropriate equipment and trained staff, location and type of surgery, and patient preference. Many ongoing investigations of both new methods for pain control and refinement of existing ones may improve analgesic therapy and decrease perioperative morbidity and mortality in the future.

*References 28, 35, 55, 76, 77, 85.

REFERENCES

1. Anderson SA: Pain control by sensory stimulation. In Bonica JJ, Liebeskind JL, and Albe-Fessard DG (editors): Advances in pain research and therapy, vol 3, New York, 1979, Raven Press.
2. Armitage EN: Local anesthetic techniques for prevention of postoperative pain, Br J Anaesth 58:790–800, 1986.
3. Atkinson JH, Kremes EF, and Garfin SR: Psychopharmacological agents in the treatment of pain, J Bone Joint Surg 67A(2):337–342, 1985.
4. Atwell JR et al: The efficacy of patient controlled analgesia in patients recovering from flank incisions, J Urol 132:701–703, 1984.
5. Austin KL, Stapleton JW, and Mather LE: Multiple intramuscular injections: a major source of variability in analgesic response to meperidine, Pain 47-62, 1980.
6. Averill JR: Personal control over aversive stimuli and its relationship to stress, Psychol Bull 80:286, 1973.
7. Baldessarini RJ: Drugs and the treatment of psychiatric disorders. In: Gilman AG et al: Goodman and Gilman's the pharmacological basis of therapeutics, New York, 1985, McMillan Publishing Co.
8. Beecher HK: Pain in men wounded in battle, Ann Surg 123:96–105, 1946.
9. Beecher HK: The powerful placebo, Am Med Assoc J 159:1602–1606, 1955.
10. Benedetti C, Bonica JJ, and Bellucci G: Psychophysiology and therapy of postoperative pain: a review. In: Benedetti C (editor): Advances in pain research and therapy, New York, 1984, Raven Press.
11. Bengtsson M, Lofstrom J, and Merits H: Postoperative pain relief with intrathecal morphine after major hip surgery, Reg Anaesth 8:138–141, 1983.
12. Bennett RL and Griffen WO: Patient-controlled analgesia, Contemp Surg 23(12):76–86, 1982.
13. Bennett RL and Griffen WO: Effect of patient-controlled analgesia in nocturnal sleep and spontaneous activity following laparotomy, Anesthesiology 61:205, 1984.
14. Bennett R et al: Morphine titration in postoperative laparotomy patients using patient-controlled analgesia, Curr Ther Res 32:45–52, 1982.
15. Bennett RL et al: Patient-controlled analgesia: a new concept of postoperative pain relief, Ann Surg 195:700–705, 1982.
16. Bennett RL et al: Postoperative pulmonary function with patient-controlled analgesia (abstract), Anesth Analg 61:171, 1982.
17. Bennett RL et al: Patient-controlled analgesia and analgesic outcome, nocturnal sleep, and spontaneous activity, Surg Forum 35:57–59, 1984.
18. Bowers KS: Pain, anxiety and perceived control, J Consult Clin Psychol 32:596, 1968.
19. Bromage PR, Camporesi E, and Chestnut D: Epidural narcotics in postoperative analgesia, Anesth Analg 59:473–480, 1980.
20. Bromage P et al: Nonrespiratory side effects of epidural morphine, Anesth Analg 61:490–495, 1982.
21. Brownridge P: Epidural and intrathecal opiates for pain relief, Anaesthesia 38:74–79, 1983.
22. Brownridge P, Wrobel J, and Watt-Smith J: Respiratory depression following accidental subarachnoid pthedine, Anaesth Intensive Care 11:237–241, 1983.
23. Bryan-Brown CW: Development of pain management in critical care. In Cousins MJ and Phillips GD: Acute pain management, New York, 1986, Churchill Livingstone.
24. Bullingham Res: Postoperative pain, Postgrad Med J 60:847–851, 1984.
25. Chestnut DH et al: Continuous infusion during labor: a randomized, double-blind comparison of 0.0625% bupivicaine/0.0002% fentanyl versus 0.125% bupivicaine, Anesthesiology 68:754–759, 1988.
26. Chrubasik J and Wiemeas K: Continuous-plus-on-demand epidural infusion of morphine for postoperative pain relief by means of a small externally worn infusion device, Anesthesiology 64:263–267, 1985.
27. Cohen F: Postsurgical pain relief: patients' status and nurses' medication choices, Pain 9:265–274, 1980.
28. Cohen SE and Woods WA: The role of epidural mor-

phine in the postcesarean patient: efficacy and effects on bonding, Anesthesiology 58:500–504, 1983.

29. Cronin M, Redfern PA, and Utting JE: Psychometry and postoperative complaints in surgical patients, Br J Anaesth 45:879–886, 1973.

30. Donovan M, Dillon P, and McGuire L: Incidence and characteristics of pain in a sample of medical surgical inpatients, Pain 30:69–78, 1987.

31. Drummond GB and Littlewood DG: Respiratory effects of extradural analgesia after lower abdominal surgery, Br J Anaesth 49:999–1004, 1977.

32. Eisenach JC, Grice SC, and Dewan DM: Patient-controlled analgesia following cesarean section: a comparison with epidural and intramuscular narcotics, Anesthesiology 68:444–448, 1988.

33. Estok PM et al: Use of patient controlled analgesia to compare intravenous to epidural administration of fentanyl in the postoperative patient, Anesthesiology 67:A230, 1987.

34. Eugberg G: Respiratory performance after upper abdominal surgery. A comparison of pain relief with intercostal blocks and centrally acting analgesia, Acta Anaesthesiol Scand 29:427–433, 1985.

35. Finley RJ, Kerri-Szanto M, and Boyd D: New analgesic agents and techniques shorten postoperative hospital stay, Pain 2:S397, 1984.

36. Fischer R et al: Comparison of continuous epidural infusion of fentanyl-bupivacaine and morphine-bupivacaine in management of postoperative pain, Anesth Analg 67:559–563, 1988.

37. Flower (1985)

38. Glurel A et al: Epidural morphine for postoperative pain relief in anorectal surgery, Anesth Analg 65:499–502, 1986.

39. Graves DA et al: Patient-controlled analgesia, Ann Int Med 99:360–366, 1983.

40. Gueneron J et al: Effect of naloxone infusion on analgesia and respiratory depression after epidural fentanyl, Anesth Analg 67:35–38, 1988.

41. Gustafsson L, Schildt B, and Jacobsen KJ: Adverse effects of extradural and intrathecal opiates. Report of a nationwide survey in Sweden, Br J Anaesth 54:479–483, 1982.

42. Hammonds WD and Hord AH: Additional comments regarding an anesthesiology-based postoperative pain service (letter), Anesthesiology 69:139–140, 1988.

43. Harmer M: Respiratory effects of patient-controlled analgesia. In Harmer M, Rosen M, and Vickers MD: Patient-controlled analgesia, Boston, 1985, Blackwell Scientific Publications, Inc.

44. Harrison DM et al: Epidural narcotic and patient-controlled analgesia for post-cesarean section pain relief, Anesthesiology 68:454–457, 1988.

45. Harvie KW: A major advance in the control of postoperative knee pain, Orthopedics 2:26–27, 1979.

46. Hecker BR and Albert L: Patient-controlled analgesia: a randomized, prospective comparison between two commercially available PCA pumps and conventional analgesic therapy for postoperative pain, Pain (35):115–120, 1988.

47. Hill HF, Saeger LC, and Chapman RC: Patient-controlled analgesia after bone marrow transplantation for cancer. Postgraduate Medicine A special Report: Patient Controlled Analgesia, A More Rational Approach to Pain Management, 1986, McGraw-Hill Book Co.

48. Jaffee JH: Opioid analgesics and antagonists. In Gilman AJ et al: Goodman and Gilman's the pharmacological basis of therapeutics, New York, 1985, Macmillan Publishing Co.

49. Jensen JR: Patient-controlled analgesia pump problems and solutions, Perspect Healthcare Risk Management Fall:8–10, 1987.

50. Kane K and Taub A: A history of local electrical analgesia, Pain 1:125–140, 1975.

51. Kehlet H: The modifying effect of general and regional anesthesia on the endocrine-metabolic response to surgery, Reg Anaesth 7(Suppl):538, 1982.

52. Kellawaye P: The part played by electrical fish in the early history of bioelectricity and electrotherapy, Bull Hist Med 20:112–137, 1946.

53. Kerri-Szanto M and Heaman S: Postoperative demand analgesia, Surg Gyn Obstet 134:647–651, 1972.

54. Kleiman RL et al: A comparison of morphine administered by patient-controlled analgesia and regularly scheduled intramuscular injection in severe postoperative pain, J Pain Symp Management 3:15–22, 1988.

55. Lane E et al: Epidural morphine for postoperative analgesia: a double blind study, Anesth Analg 61:236–240, 1982.

56. Lee A et al: Postoperative analgesia by continuous extradural infusion of bupivacaine and diamorphine, Br J Anaesth 60:845–850, 1988.

57. Levi P: Patient controlled analgesia: traditional versus mechanical, JONA 16:18–32, 1986.

58. Loper KA, Ready LB, and Brody M: Patient-controlled anxiolysis with midazolam, Anesthesiology 67:1118–1119, 1988.

59. Marks RA and Sachar EJ: Undertreatment of medical inpatients with narcotic analgesia, Ann Int Med (2):173–181, 1978.

60. Marks RA and Sachar EJ: Undertreatment of medical inpatients with narcotic analgesia, Ann Int Med (2):173–181, 1978.

61. Mather LE and Phillips GD: Opioids and adjuvants: principles of use. In Cousins MJ and Phillips GD: Acute pain management, New York, 1986, Churchill Livingstone.

62. Mathews E and Abrams L: Intrathecal morphine in

open heart surgery, Lancet 1:543, 1980.

63. Melzak R: The McGill pain questionnaire: major properties and strong methods, Pain 1:277–279, 1975.

64. Melzak R and Wall P: Pain mechanisms: a new theory, Science 150:971–979, 1965.

65. Miller RR and Jack H: Clinical effects of meperidine in hospitalized medical patients, J Clin Pharmacol 4: 180–189, 1978.

66. Miller RR and Jack H: Clinical effects of parenteral narcotics in hospitalized medical patients, J Clin Pharmacol 4:165–171, 1980.

67. Moore R et al: Dural permeability to narcotics: in vitro determination and application to extradural administration, Br J Anaesth 54:1117–1122, 1982.

68. Murphy D: Continuous intercostal nerve blockade for pain relief following cholecystectomy, Br J Anaesth 55:521–524, 1983.

69. Murphy D: Intercostal nerve blockade for fractured ribs and postoperative analgesia. Description of a new technique, Regional Anaesth 8:151–153, 1983.

70. Murphy D: Continuous intercostal nerve blockade. An anatomical study to elucidate its mode of action, Br J Anaesth 56:627–630, 1984.

71. Nayman J: Measurement and control of postoperative pain, Ann Royal Coll Surgeons Eng 61:419–426, 1979.

72. Nordberg G et al: Pharmokinetic aspects of epidural morphine analgesia, Anesthesiology 58:545–551, 1983.

73. Nordberg G et al: Epidural morphine: influence of adrenalin admixture, Br J Anaesth 58:598–604, 1986.

74. O'Kelly E and Gary B: Continuous pain relief for multiple fracture ribs, Br J Anaesth 53:989–991, 1981.

75. Peck CL: Psychological factors in acute pain management. In Cousins MJ and Phillips GD: Acute pain management, New York, 1986, Churchill Livingstone.

76. Rawal N et al: Epidural morphine for postoperative pain relief: a comparative study with intramuscular narcotic and intercostal nerve block, Anesth Analg 61:93–98, 1982.

77. Rawal N et al: Comparison of intramuscular and epidural morphine for postoperative analgesia in the grossly obese: influence on postoperative ambulation and pulmonary function, Anesth Analg 63:583–592, 1984.

78. Rawal N et al: Influence of naloxone on analgesia and respiratory depression following epidural morphine, Anesthesiology 64:191–194, 1986.

79. Ready LB et al: Development of an anesthesiology based postoperative pain management service, Anesthesiology 68:100–106, 1988.

80. Reiestad R and Stromskag K: Interplural catheter in the management of postoperative pain: a preliminary report, Reg Anaesth 11:89–91, 1986.

81. Riebrel LN: Cardiopulmonary complications after major surgery: a role for epidural analgesia, Surg 102:660–666, 1987.

82. Schechter NL, Berien FB, and Katz SM: The use of patient controlled analgesia in adolescents with sickle cell pain crisis: a preliminary report, J Pain and Symp Management 3:109–113, 1988.

83. Schmauss C and Yaks TL: In vitro studies on spinal opiate receptor systems mediating aminoception. II. Pharmacological profiles suggesting a differential association of mu, delta, and kappa receptors with visceral chemical and cutaneous thermal stimuli in the rat, J Pharmacol Exp Ther 228:1–12, 1983.

84. Sechzer PH: Objective measurement of pain, Anesthesiology 29:209–210, 1968.

85. Shulman M et al: Postthoracotomy pain and pulmonary function following epidural and systemic morphine, Anesthesiology 61:569–575, 1984.

86. Sjolund BH and Erikson MBE: The influence of naloxone on analgesia produced by peripheral conditioning stimulation, Brain Res 173:295–302, 1979.

87. Sjostrom S, Tamsen A, and Hartvig P: Patient-controlled analgesia with epidural opiates: a preliminary report. In Harmer M, Rosen M, and Vickers MD: Patient-controlled analgesia, Boston, 1985, Blackwell Scientific Publications, Inc.

88. Spencer AA and Smith G: Post-operative analgesia in lung function: a comparison of morphine with extradural block, Br J Anaesth 43:144–148, 1971.

89. Spetzler B and Anderson L: Patient-controlled analgesia in the total joint arthroplasty patient, Clin Orthop 215:122–125, 1987.

90. Sriwatanakul K et al: Analyses of narcotic analgesic usage in the treatment of postoperative pain, JAMA 250:926–929, 1983.

91. Stapleton JV, Austin KL, and Malher LE: A pharmocokinetic approach to postoperative pain: continuous infusion of pethidine, Anaesth Intensive Care 7:25–32, 1979.

92. Szyfelbein SK, Osgood PF, and Carr DB: The assessment of pain and plasma B-endorphin immunoactivity in burned children, Pain 22:173–182, 1985.

93. Tammisto T: Analgesics in postoperative pain relief, Acta Anaesthesiol Scand 70(suppl):47–50, 1978.

94. Tammisto T and Tigerstedt I: Narcotic analgesics in postoperative pain relief in adults, Acta Anaesthesiol Scand 74(suppl):161–164, 1982.

95. Tamsen A et al: Patient controlled analgesic therapy in the early postoperative period, Acta Anaesthesiol Scand 23:462–470, 1979.

96. Tamsen A et al: Patient-controlled analgesic therapy: clinical experience, Acta Anaesthesiol Scand 74 (suppl):157–160, 1982.

97. Tan S, Cohen S, and White P: Sufentanyl for analgesia after cesarean section: intravenous versus epidural administration, Anesth Analg 65(suppl):1, 1986.

98. Towsen A et al: CSF and plasma kinetics of morphine and meperidine after epidural administration, Anesthesiology 59:A196, 1983.

99. Urquhart ML, Klapp K, and White PF: Patient-controlled analgesia: a comparison of intravenous versus subcutaneous hydromorphine, Anesthesiology 69:428–432, 1988.

100. Utting JE and Smith JM: Postoperative analgesia, Anaesthesia 34:320-332, 1979.

101. Vinik HR et al: Patient-controlled analgesia in hospitalized patients a multicenter evaluation. Postgraduate Medicine A Special Report: Patient Controlled Analgesia A More Rational Approach to Pain Management, New York, 1986, McGraw-Hill Book Co.

102. Wall R: Oral patient controlled analgesia for postoperative pain control. Presented at the Acute Pain Service Conference Washington, DC, 1988, Georgetown University.

103. Welchew EA: On-demand analgesia: a double blind comparison of on demand intravenous fentanyl with regular intramuscular morphine, Anaesthesia 38:19–25, 1983.

104. White PF: Use of a patient-controlled analgesia infuser for the management of postoperative pain. In Harmer M, Rosen M, and Vickers MD: Patient-controlled analgesia, Boston, 1985, Blackwell Scientific Publications Inc.

105. White PF: Mishaps with patient-controlled analgesia, Anesthesiology 66:81–83, 1987.

106. White PF: Use of patient-controlled analgesia for management of acute pain, JAMA 259:243–247, 1988.

107. Winnie AP: Plexus anesthesia, vol 1. Perivascular techniques of brachial plexus block, Philadelphia, 1983, WB Saunders Co.

CHAPTER 14

Neuroendocrine Responses to Surgery

MICHAEL J. BRESLOW

Effects of anesthetics on sympathoadrenal and
neuroendocrine function
Effects of surgical stimulation on endocrine and
sympathoadrenal function
Mechanisms responsible for perioperative
neuroendocrine changes

Potential adverse effects of the stress response to
surgery
Pharmacologic modulation of the "stress
response"
Recommendations and conclusions

In 1929 Cannon described the "fight or flight"
reaction and proposed that secretion of catecholamines during stress is an important compensatory
response.[12] Selye in 1950, expanding on the observations of Cannon, advanced his theory of the "adaptation response" to injury.[65] In this classic treatise,
Selye proposed that the body responds to "threats to
survival" by increasing sympathetic nervous system
activity and adrenal epinephrine secretion, which act
to maintain blood pressure and cardiac output, and
by secreting cortisol and antidiuretic hormone (arginine vasopressin), which alter fuel homeostasis,
immune function, and fluid balance. Studies by
Sandberg et al[63] and Hammond and Moore[32] in the
1950s showed that surgical trauma is associated with
increased plasma levels of cortisol and catecholamines. These neuroendocrine changes following
surgery were widely believed to be necessary for
survival, a conclusion supported by the salutary effect of glucocorticoid replacement therapy on perioperative mortality in patients with Addison's disease.[28] Introduction of new assay techniques in the

30 years following these initial reports has greatly
added to our knowledge of perioperative sympathoadrenal and endocrine changes. Unfortunately,
our understanding of why endocrine changes occur
is still incomplete. More importantly, our understanding of end-organ effects of surgically induced
sympathoadrenal and neuroendocrine changes are incomplete. An emerging body of knowledge suggests
that the adaptation response of Selye, while clearly
adaptive when injury occurs in nonmedical settings,
may be harmful when it occurs following controlled
surgical trauma in patients with underlying medical
problems. This chapter reviews the diffuse changes
in endocrine and sympathetic nervous system activity that occur in the perioperative period. Rather than
focusing on phenomenological studies, however, I
will emphasize studies investigating mechanisms
and end-organ effects. It is my belief that the neuroendocrine response to surgery is responsible for
the majority of physiologic changes that occur in the
perioperative period and that modulating this response may be of significant therapeutic benefit in
selected patients.

EFFECTS OF ANESTHETICS ON SYMPATHOADRENAL AND NEUROENDOCRINE FUNCTION

Induction of anesthesia is usually associated with a decrease in sympathetic tone, particularly when sympathetic tone is increased before administration of anesthetic agents because of anxiety, hypovolemia, or pain. This effect on sympathetic tone, which occurs with almost all anesthetic agents in use today, can result in precipitous declines in arterial blood pressure when blood pressure is dependent on increased sympathetic tone (that is, low cardiac output states caused by marked hypovolemia or severe cardiac dysfunction). In most instances, however, induction of anesthesia is associated with only small decreases in plasma epinephrine and norepinephrine levels[40,49] and is well tolerated hemodynamically. Ketamine, an arocyclohexalamine related to phencyclidine, differs from almost all other anesthetic agents in current use in that it increases circulating catecholamine levels.[2] This effect on plasma catecholamine levels occurs as a result of direct central nervous system stimulation of sympathetic activity and also via inhibition of neuronal catecholamine reuptake.[54] Because of this effect on plasma catecholamine levels, ketamine is often used for induction of anesthesia in hemodynamically unstable patients.

The effects of anesthetic agents on endocrine function appear to be fairly minimal, with the following two exceptions. Halter et al[31] have shown that the insulin response to an intravenous glucose load is attenuated in anesthetized patients (Figure 14-1). The mechanism responsible for this action is not known, nor is it known if it occurs with all anesthetic regimens. Etomidate, a recently introduced sedative used for induction and maintenance of anesthesia, alters endocrine function by specifically interfering with the biosynthesis of cortisol.[76] Etomidate lowers plasma cortisol and aldosterone levels and blocks the usual ACTH-mediated increase in these adrenal steroids that normally occurs during surgical stimulation.[23,75] This effect of etomidate appears to last several hours following administration of a single dose. Despite concern that inhibition of cortisol synthesis might be poorly tolerated in selected high-risk patients, there have been no reports of adverse effects when etomidate is used for induction of anesthesia. However, prolonged use of etomidate for sedation has been associated with increased mortality.[45]

EFFECTS OF SURGICAL STIMULATION ON ENDOCRINE AND SYMPATHOADRENAL FUNCTION

Surgical incision is promptly followed by increases in plasma epinephrine,[32,62] norepinephrine,[32,62] arginine vasopressin,[7,16] ACTH,[55] cortisol,[63] growth hormone,[55] beta endorphin,[17] prolactin,[3] and prostaglandin metabolite[71] levels. The magnitude

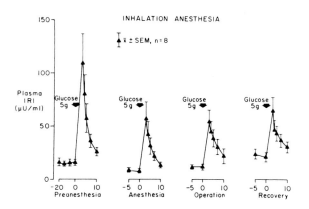

FIGURE 14-1. Arterial plasma immunoreactive insulin *(IRI)* levels before and after administration of glucose (5 g IV) measured before and after induction of inhalation anesthesia, during surgery, and 90 minutes after discontinuation of anesthesia. Data are mean of 8 patients ± SE.

From Halter JB and Pflug AE: Relationship of impaired insulin secretion during surgical stress to anesthesia and catecholamine release, J Clin Endocrinol Metab 51:1093–1098, 1980.

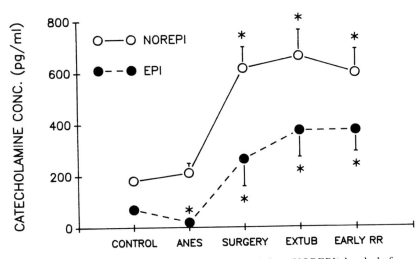

FIGURE 14-2. Plasma epinephrine *(EPI)* and norepinephrine *(NOREPI)* levels before, during, and immediately following abdominal surgery. ANES, induction of anesthesia; EXTUB, extubation; EARLY RR, 30 minutes after admission of the recovery room. * = p ≤ 0.05 compared with control. Data are mean of 8 patients ± SE.

From Halter JB, Pflug AE, and Porte D: Mechanisms of plasma catecholamine increases during surgical stress in man, J Clin Endocrinol Metab 45:936–944, 1977.

and duration of this diffuse response appears to vary with the extent of surgical trauma,[15] with larger operations resulting in greater and more prolonged elevations. Recent data also suggest that younger patients may have a more pronounced response than older patients.[3] A detailed review of selected changes follows:

Epinephrine and norepinephrine. Plasma epinephrine and norepinephrine levels increase twofold to sixfold intraoperatively[30] (Figure 14-2). The magnitude of the change in plasma catecholamine levels varies considerably from patient to patient. In general, more extensive surgical procedures are associated with larger rises.[15] Both epinephrine and norepinephrine levels are significantly elevated in the early postoperative period.[62] Most studies, however, suggest that epinephrine levels return to baseline values within 12 to 24 hours following surgery,[62] while plasma norepinephrine levels remain elevated for up to 5 days postoperatively[15] (Figure 14-3). Using ³H-norepinephrine turnover techniques, Hilsted et al showed that elevated norepinephrine levels following surgery are a result of increased release from sympathetic nerves and do not reflect alterations in catecholamine clearance.[36] The relatively transient adrenal medullary response to surgery contrasts with

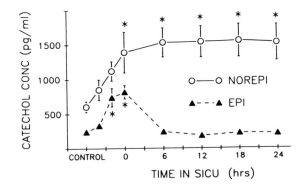

FIGURE 14-3. Plasma epinephrine *(EPI)* and norepinephrine *(NOREPI)* levels before induction of anesthesia (control), at two points during surgery, and 0, 6, 12, 18, and 24 hours following aortic surgery. SICU, surgical intensive care unit; OR, operating room. Data are mean of 12 patients ± SE. * p < 0.05 compared to preinduction value.

the more prolonged increase in sympathetic nervous system activity. Similar divergent responses have been reported in experimental animals subjected to various physiologic stimuli.[81] The physiologic significance of this divergent response is not known.

Arginine vasopressin (AVP). Plasma levels of AVP increase markedly with surgery, reaching approximately 20 pM/L (25 pg/ml) during cholecystectomy and 50 pM/L (65 pg/ml) during thoracic surgical procedures.[7,16] Plasma AVP levels usually range from 0 to 8 pM/L, and change in response to plasma osmolarity. The increase in plasma AVP levels with surgery, therefore, more closely approximates those encountered during major physiologic stresses such as hemorrhagic hypotension[11] and hypoxia.[57] Plasma AVP levels have been reported to remain elevated for up to 5 days following major surgery.[7] Other investigators, however, have found a more transient response following cholecystectomy.[16]

Renin angiotensin system. In contrast to the fairly substantial data available concerning changes in plasma norepinephrine, epinephrine, and AVP levels during surgery, there are little data on the renin angiotensin system. Although renin and angiotensin II levels rise in some patients intraoperatively,[33,61,77] this is not a consistent finding, nor does it appear to follow a predictable pattern. Data from Robertson and McKalis suggest the changes in plasma renin activity are correlated with intravascular volume, and increases are only noted when hypovolemia occurs.[61] Plasma renin levels have been reported to be normal in the postoperative period.[61]

ACTH/cortisol. Increases in glucocorticoid secretion following surgery have been recognized for many years.[63] Based on the consistency of this hypercortisolemia in surgical patients and the high perioperative mortality in patients with Addison's disease before the introduction of glucocorticoid replacement therapy, it has become commonplace for clinicians to replicate this glucocorticoid response in patients with possible adrenal insufficiency by intraoperative and postoperative administration of glucocorticoids in supraphysiologic doses. Recent data indicate that during surgery there is constant secretion of ACTH, which contrasts with the pulsatile secretion that occurs normally.[70] In addition, adrenal sensitivity to ACTH is increased twofold intraoperatively.[70] The mechanism responsible for this increased sensitivity, however, is not known.

Beta endorphin. Plasma levels of beta endorphins are elevated during surgery to approximately three times basal levels.[17,18] This increase in endorphins is not observed with induction of anesthesia, but only after incision.[17,18] In one study, use of a narcotic-based anesthetic prevented intraoperative increases in plasma beta endorphin levels; however, with emergence from general anesthesia, endorphin levels increased markedly.[18] Postoperative morphine administration appears to lower plasma endorphin levels.[17]

Thyroid hormone. Surgery is associated with transient increases in total and free T4 and in free T3.[14] Pituitary TSH secretion has also been reported to increase intraoperatively.[1] In the postoperative period, however, marked reductions in free T3 and T4 occur that persist for approximately 1 week.[14] Associated with this decrease in free T3, significant increases in levels of reverse T3 are noted postoperatively.[14] This pattern of altered deiodination of thyroxine following surgery is analogous to that described in patients with severe nonthyroidal illness (sick euthyroid syndrome).[78] The metabolic implications of these changes are not well understood.

MECHANISMS RESPONSIBLE FOR PERIOPERATIVE NEUROENDOCRINE CHANGES

As recognized by Selye, physiologic stressors result in increased sympathetic nervous system activity and diffuse hormonal activation. Studies in experimental animals have confirmed that physiologic stressors, such as hemorrhage and hypoxia, result in marked stimulation of these systems.[10,29,57] Although both hypoxia and hypotension can occur intraoperatively, they are uncommon and cannot be implicated in the postoperative stress response in most patients. Hypothermia, which is a more common perioperative physiologic alteration, can also increase sympathetic nervous system activity. However, the transient nature of postoperative hypothermia cannot account for increases in sympathoadrenal and endocrine secretion that persist for days following major surgical procedures. The most likely cause of these changes, therefore, is pain. Painful stimuli in animals have been shown to reproduce these changes.[37] Denervation before limb scald injury blocks this response in experimental animals,[37] indicating that humoral factors are not involved. Studies in paraplegic humans have confirmed that intact neural pathways to the central nervous system are required for expression of the stress response.[38] In a similar vein, interruption of afferent neural input by use of spinal and epidural local anesthetics can prevent intraoperative and postoperative increases in

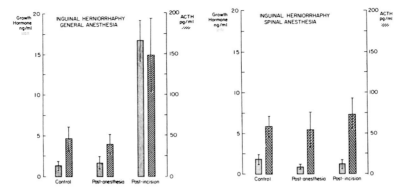

FIGURE 14-4. Plasma growth hormone and ACTH levels before surgery, after induction of anesthesia, and 1 hour after skin incision. Left panel shows data from 9 patients undergoing inguinal herniorrhaphy with general anesthesia and right panel shows data from 7 patients undergoing the same procedure with spinal anesthesia. Data shown are means ± SE.

From Newsome HH and Rose JC: The response of human adrenocorticotrophic hormone and growth hormone to surgical stress, J Clin Endocrinol 33:481–487, 1971.

ACTH,[55] growth hormone,[55] cortisol,[48] and plasma catecholamines.[62] Demonstration of this effect is shown in Figure 14-4. While some of these changes following conduction blockade may reflect interruption of efferent nerve impulses to sympathetic nerves and to the adrenal medulla, prevention of pituitary secretory responses (growth hormone, ACTH) strongly suggests that the predominant explanation is elimination of afferent stimuli. Supporting this conclusion are data demonstrating attenuation of the rise in norepinephrine and AVP when epidural narcotics are used for postoperative analgesia[7,62] (Figure 14-5). These data, when taken together, strongly suggest that pain is the afferent impulse that elicits the stress response in surgical patients.

Potential Adverse Effects Of The Stress Response To Surgery

The generalized adaptation response is clearly beneficial when injury occurs in nonmedical settings. Survival of experimental hemorrhagic shock and hypoxia are both adversely affected by adrenalectomy.[6,53] The box on p.185, left, lists several beneficial effects of this response. With controlled surgical trauma and careful anesthetic management, however, hypovolemia, hypotension, and hypoxia should not occur, and it is less clear that the "adaptation response" is adaptive. More importantly,

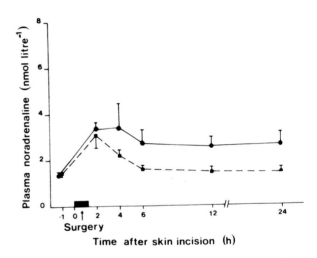

FIGURE 14-5. Plasma noradrenaline concentrations before and after cholecystectomy with general anesthesia plus postoperative parenteral morphine (———); and general anesthesia plus extradural morphine (------). Data are mean of 8 patients ± SE.

From Rutberg H et al: Effects of the extradural administration of morphine, or bupivacaine, on the endocrine response to upper abdominal surgery, Br J Anaesth 56:233–238, 1984.

Potential beneficial effects of the stress response to injury and probable mediators

I. Maintenance of central blood pressure
   A. Peripheral vasoconstriction
      Sympathetic nervous system
      Epinephrine
      Vasopressin
      Angiotensin
   B. Increased cardiac performance
      Sympathetic nervous system
      Epinephrine
II. Maintenance of intravascular volume
   A. Decreased urinary losses
      Sympathetic nervous system
      Vasopressin
      Aldosterone
   B. Transfer of intracellular volume to extracellular space
      Adrenocortical hormones
III. Increased production of fuel substrates
      Epinephrine
      Cortisol
      Glucagon

Potential adverse effects of the stress response to injury

   I. Hypertension
  II. Myocardial ischemia
 III. Arrhythmias
 IV. Hyperglycemia
  V. Hypermetabolism and nitrogen loss
 VI. Hypokalemia
VII. Hyponatremia
VIII. Fluid retention

---

the physiologic changes elicited by these mediators can have significant adverse effects in patients with underlying medical problems. The complications (see box above, right) that can result from these physiologic changes account for considerable perioperative morbidity and mortality and will be discussed in some detail.

Hypertension. Intraoperative increases in arterial blood pressure usually occur either in response to painful and/or stressful stimuli, such as laryngoscopy, incision, or visceral traction, or near the completion of the surgical procedure when anesthetic depth is decreasing before the patient's awakening. In both settings, anesthetic depth is presumably inadequate to prevent either the sympathetic nervous system response to pain or the end-organ vascular and cardiac changes elicited by this response. Consistent with this hypothesis, circulating catecholamine levels have been shown to increase during these intraoperative events,[34] and rises in arterial blood pressure can be prevented by pretreatment with adrenergic receptor antagonists.[47] The observation that increases in arterial blood pressure correlate with

increases in plasma catecholamine levels[30,77] also implicates sympathetic hyperactivity in intraoperative hypertension. Management of intraoperative hypertension, however, is usually not problematic, since most anesthetic agents diminish sympathetic outflow and blunt end-organ responses to sympathetic stimulation. However, since all anesthetics must eventually end, hypertension is a frequent and occasionally problematic postoperative occurrence.

The incidence of postoperative hypertension is approximately 5% following routine surgical procedures.[21,24] Following more extensive and traumatic operations, in particular operations on the abdominal aorta,[27] extracranial cerebral vessels,[4,46] and coronary vessels[22,77], the incidence of hypertension approaches 50%. Potential adverse effects of hypertension include (1) myocardial ischemia (secondary to increased myocardial oxygen consumption), (2) low cardiac output (secondary to increased afterload), (3) leakage from fresh vascular anastomoses, and (4) neurologic deficits following carotid endarterectomy. In addition, postoperative hypertension frequently requires close monitoring of therapy, thus adding to the cost of hospitalization. While postoperative hypertension may have many different etiologies, there are considerable data implicating sympathetic nervous system hyperactivity. Several studies have demonstrated correlations between perioperative increases in blood pressure and increases in plasma catecholamine levels[30,77] (Figure 14-6). In addition, data from a recently completed double-blind, placebo-controlled trial in our institution to evaluate the contribution of sympathetic nervous system hyperactivity to postoperative increases in blood pressure support this conclusion.[8a] In this

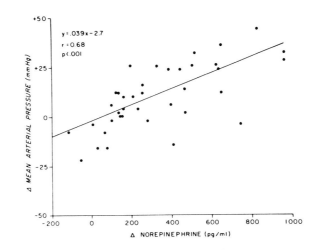

FIGURE 14-6. Regression analysis of changes in mean arterial blood pressure from baseline versus changes in plasma norepinephrine levels for 8 patients having abdominal surgery. Data obtained after induction of anesthesia, during surgery, at extubation, and 30 and 120 minutes postoperatively.

From Halter JB, Pflug AE, and Porte D: Mechanisms of plasma catecholamine increases during surgical stress in man, J Clin Endocrinol Metab 45:936–944, 1977.

study, epidural morphine was used to attenuate the sympathetic nervous system response to abdominal aortic surgery, and the incidence of hypertension in this experimental group was compared to the incidence in a control group who received epidural saline and parenteral narcotics for postoperative pain relief. Patients receiving epidural morphine required less parenteral morphine and had lower pain scores, lower plasma norepinephrine levels, and a reduced incidence of postoperative hypertension (4 of 12 versus 9 of 12). Plasma epinephrine and arginine vasopressin levels were similar in both groups, suggesting that sympathetic nervous system activity is the predominant mediator of postoperative hypertension. Sympathetic nervous system hyperactivity may not, however, account for hypertension following coronary artery bypass grafting (CABG). Suppression of sympathetic nervous system activity with clonidine does not prevent post-CABG hypertension,[34] and stellate ganglion blockade attenuates post-CABG hypertension without diminishing sympathetic nervous system activity.[22] These data suggest that factors other than sympathetic nervous system activity, such as cardiopulmonary bypass, hypothermia, or afferent cardiac reflexes, contribute to postoperative hypertension in this setting. Sympa-

thetic nervous system hyperactivity, however, appears to be the major mediator of hypertension following surgical procedures other than open heart surgery.

Myocardial ischemia. Despite improvements in anesthetic technique, myocardial infarction continues to account for a significant percentage of perioperative deaths. Myocardial infarction occurred in approximately 2% of 1001 consecutive elective surgical patients over 40 years of age followed by Goldman et al and accounted for approximately one third of all deaths in this series.[25] The incidence of myocardial infarction is higher following extensive surgical procedures, such as operations involving the abdominal aorta, and when coronary artery disease is more prevalent in the study population (for example, in patients having vascular operations).[39,74] Despite considerable intraoperative hemodynamic turbulence, the majority of perioperative infarctions occur not during surgery but 1 to 3 days postoperatively.[59,74] Although many hypotheses have been advanced to account for this delayed peak incidence of myocardial infarction, the pathogenesis of postoperative myocardial infarction is not known. A possible etiologic role of sympathetic nervous system hyperactivity is suggested by data correlating postoperative increases in arterial blood pressure and heart rate with increases in plasma catecholamines and the demonstration that increased sympathetic tone can cause coronary vasoconstriction and myocardial ischemia in experimental animals.[35] Both hypertension and tachycardia increase myocardial oxygen consumption and can adversely affect the balance between oxygen supply and consumption. In contrast, coronary vasoconstriction can precipitate ischemia by reducing coronary blood flow. While the role of sympathetic nervous system hyperactivity in postoperative myocardial infarction is unproven, standard therapy includes maneuvers to minimize pain-induced sympathetic nervous system activation and aggressive use of adrenergic receptor antagonists to control heart rate and blood pressure. While more work in this area is required to clarify the mechanisms responsible for postoperative myocardial infarction, it is important to appreciate the hemodynamic consequences of sympathetic nervous system hyperactivity and the potential consequence of these changes in patients with coronary artery disease.

Arrhythmias. Ventricular ectopy and supraventricular tachycardias are common in the perioperative period, particularly following major surgical procedures and in patients with underlying medical illnesses.[26,42,43] While certainly multifactorial in origin, sympathetic nervous system hyperactivity appears to contribute to the high incidence of these rhythm disturbances. Although seldom fatal, postoperative tachyarrhythmias can precipitate myocardial ischemia and/or lower cardiac output, and often they necessitate overnight monitoring in a critical care setting. Because of the known effects of sympathomimetic agents on automaticity, beta-adrenergic receptor antagonists are often used to treat ectopy and control heart rate in these patients.

Hyperglycemia. Blood sugar routinely rises intraoperatively and remains elevated in the postoperative period.[8] While rarely problematic in healthy patients, this glycemic response to surgery can result in significant hyperglycemia in diabetic patients, complicating management and potentially increasing morbidity. In an elegant series of studies, Eigler et al showed in dogs that replication of plasma levels of glucagon, cortisol, and epinephrine encountered during stress, by infusion of exogenous hormones, results in similar elevations in blood sugar.[20] Using radiotracer techniques, they demonstrated that these mediators act synergistically to increase blood sugar

levels by increasing glucose production and decreasing glucose use. Similar glycemic responses to triple hormone infusion have recently been reported in humans.[66] Further confirmation of the role of stress hormones comes from the work of Tsuji,[67] who demonstrated that preoperative administration of the beta-adrenergic receptor antagonist propranolol attenuated the glycemic response to surgery. More impressive still are the data of Brandt et al, which show that attenuation of the hormonal response to surgery by use of epidural local anesthetics completely prevents intraoperative hyperglycemia.[8]

Hypermetabolism and nitrogen loss. Following injury, metabolic rate and protein breakdown increase. This posttraumatic hypermetabolism is proportional to the extent of injury and can increase to twice basal levels. The accompanying accelerated protein breakdown, which can result in malnutrition, has been proposed as a possible contributor to organ failure following extensive trauma.[13] Similar metabolic changes have been described following elective surgery, with nitrogen loss increasing more than twofold.[67,68] Bessey et al have shown that infusion of cortisol, glucagon, and epinephrine into normal volunteers for 72 hours, at rates sufficient to increase plasma levels of these hormones to those encountered following mild to moderate injury, results in 20% to 30% increases in oxygen consumption, metabolic rate, and nitrogen excretion.[5] Recently Tsuji et al demonstrated that increased urinary nitrogen excretion following gastrectomy is associated with increases in plasma epinephrine, glucagon, and cortisol.[68] These authors found that epidural local anesthetics and epidural narcotics, when used for intraoperative and postoperative analgesia, can attenuate excessive nitrogen excretion following gastrectomy (Figure 14-7). Use of epidural local anesthetics and opiates was also associated with smaller increases in catecholamines, cortisol, and glucagon, suggesting that pain-induced increases in these stress hormones are responsible for the observed metabolic changes.

Hypokalemia. Intravascular infusion of catecholamines results in cellular uptake of potassium.[9] This translocation of potassium appears to be mediated by beta$_2$ adrenoreceptors.[9] Catecholamine-mediated extracellular to intracellular shift of potassium has been suggested as a possible cause of otherwise unexplained hypokalemia in postoperative patients.[52] In addition, increased plasma levels of

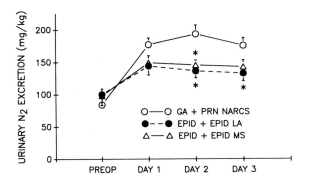

EFFECT OF DIFFERENT ANALGESIC REGIMENS
ON POSTOP NITROGEN LOSS

FIGURE 14-7. Daily urinary nitrogen excretion obtained before upper abdominal surgery and on the first 3 postoperative days. Thirty patients had the procedure performed under general anesthesia and received parenteral narcotics for postoperative analgesia (*GA + PRN NARCS*). The remaining patients had the procedure performed using a continuous epidural anesthetic (0.5% bupivicaine) for intraoperative analgesia, and either had an epidural bupivicaine infusion continued postoperatively (*EPID + EPID LA*, n = 20) or had morphine 4 mg every 12 hours administered through the epidural catheter (*EPID + EPID MS*, n = 20). * = p < 0.05 compared to general anesthesia group.

From Tsuji H et al: Effects of epidural administration of local anaesthetics or morphine on postoperative nitrogen loss and catabolic hormones, Br J Surg 74:421–425, 1987.

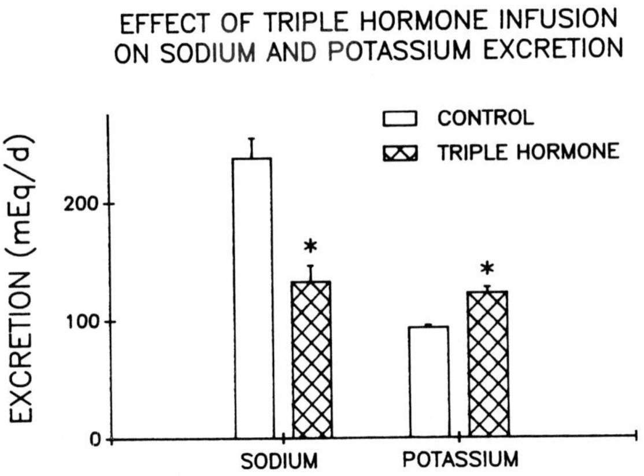

EFFECT OF TRIPLE HORMONE INFUSION
ON SODIUM AND POTASSIUM EXCRETION

FIGURE 14-8. Twenty-four hour sodium and potassium excretion before *(control)* and during combined infusion of cortisol, glucagon, and epinephrine *(triple hormone)*. Data are mean of 9 male volunteers ± SE. * = p ≤ 0.05 compared to control.

From Bessey PQ et al: Combined hormonal infusion simulates the metabolic response to injury, Ann Surg 200:264–281, 1984.

mineralocorticoids postoperatively probably result in increased renal loss of potassium. While the clinical implications of transient decreases in extracellular potassium concentration are probably negligible, treatment of this laboratory abnormality is common and results in considerable effort and expense.

Hyponatremia. Moore and colleagues, in an elegant series of papers in the 1950s,[19] demonstrated impaired free water excretion in surgical patients and correctly attributed this defect to elevated levels of antidiuretic hormone (AVP). Subsequent introduction of radioimmunoassay techniques for measurement of AVP have confirmed that marked increases in AVP occur postoperatively and can persist for several days.[7,16] Thus, all surgical patients essentially have a "syndrome of inappropriate ADH" in which AVP levels are elevated without regard for plasma osmolality. Consistent with this, administration of excessive quantities of hypotonic fluids to postoperative patients can result in hyponatremia, and seizures and death have been reported in this setting.[82]

Fluid retention. Postoperative weight gain is extremely common and often exceeds 10% of body weight. Most of this weight gain is caused by accumulation of fluid in the interstitial space. This fluid accumulation, often referred to as "third space losses," varies with the type of surgery, extent of tissue trauma, and nature of replacement fluid composition. In most instances, intraoperative fluid replacement is titrated to maintain normal intravascular volume, and thus weight gain does not reflect hypervolemia. Most patients excrete this excess fluid without problem as it is reabsorbed from the interstitial space during recovery. Balance studies, however, suggest that sodium and water retention occur in all patients postoperatively, and this state persists for several days.[56] Possible mechanisms responsible for this sodium avidity include hypercortisolemia and increased renal sympathetic nerve activity. Sodium and water retention have been demonstrated in normal volunteers during prolonged administration of cortisol, glucagon, and epinephrine[5] (Figure 14-8). This effect of triple hormone infusion occurs with cortisol infusion alone, and is presumably a result of mineralocorticoid actions. In postoperative patients, elevated plasma AVP levels may also contribute to water retention and hypervolemia. These postoperative abnormalities of salt and water balance can result in significant hypervolemia and pulmonary edema in patients with underlying cardiac and/or

renal disease, necessitating close attention to volume status in these patients. While routine use of diuretics is not necessary, selected patients will require diuretic therapy postoperatively.

Pharmacologic Modulation of the "Stress Response"

High-dose narcotic anesthetic regimens can attenuate intraoperative increases in ACTH, cortisol, growth hormone, AVP, and catecholamines. With emergence from anesthesia, however, plasma levels of these compounds promptly increase to levels encountered in other postoperative patients. Since maintaining high-dose narcotic anesthesia for several days is not practical, this technique cannot be used to modulate the postoperative stress response. Regional anesthetic techniques, in which local anesthetics are used to provide nerve conduction blockade, result in complete analgesia—assuming the block is successful. As discussed earlier, these techniques prevent intraoperative rises in all hormone systems studied, including ACTH, cortisol, growth hormone, and catecholamines. Continuation of conduction blockade postoperatively is also possible and has been shown to significantly attenuate the sympathetic nervous system and endocrine response to surgery, as well as several sequelae of this response. Local anesthetics, however, are not specific for sensory fibers and, in addition to analgesia, can produce motor blockade and sympathectomy. As a result patients frequently must be confined to bed, which represents a significant disadvantage of these techniques when used postoperatively in awake patients. The relatively recent identification of spinal cord opiate receptors and the recognition of their role in modulating afferent pain impulses has led to the use of epidural and subarachnoid opiates for postoperative pain relief (see Chapter 13 for a more complete discussion of this subject). These techniques provide prolonged analgesia (4 to 24 hours per dose, depending on which opiate is employed) that is superior to analgesia routinely achieved with parenteral narcotics,[44,60] and significant side effects (principally respiratory depression) appear to occur only infrequently ($\leq 1\%$). As mentioned earlier in this chapter, epidural opiates have been shown to attenuate postoperative norepinephrine and AVP increases. While presumably this effect on sympathetic nervous system and posterier pituitary secretory activity results from superior analgesia, direct central nervous sys-

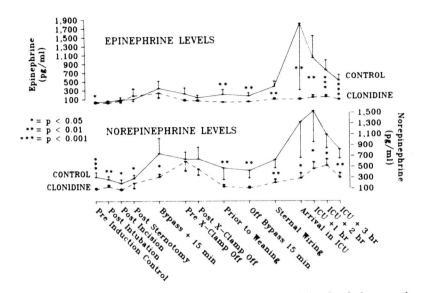

FIGURE 14-9. Comparison of plasma epinephrine and norepinephrine levels in control patients (n = 10) and in patients receiving clonidine before and during coronary artery bypass grafting (n = 10).

From Flacke JW et al: Reduced narcotic requirement by clonidine with improved hemodynamic and adrenergic stability in patients undergoing coronary bypass surgery, Anesthesiology 67:11–19, 1987.

tem effects on sympathetic outflow cannot be excluded. The effect of epidural and/or spinal opiates on other hormone systems is not known. A small but real incidence of significant respiratory depression with these techniques, however, has resulted in many hospitals limiting their use to closely monitored nursing units (intensive care units, overnight recovery rooms, or special postoperative wards).

Recently intraoperative administration of the alpha$_2$-adrenergic agonist clonidine has been shown to significantly attenuate intraoperative increases in norepinephrine, epinephrine, and cortisol[34,64] (Figure 14-9). This effect of clonidine is presumably caused by central nervous system effects of the drug. The nonspecific alpha-adrenergic receptor antagonist phentolamine has also been shown to modulate the stress response to surgery, completely preventing intraoperative increases in growth hormone.[73] These effects of alpha$_2$ agonists and antagonists are interesting, and these agents may provide a useful means of pharmacologically manipulating the stress response to surgery. At this time, however, the implications of such manipulation are unknown, and their use is strictly investigational. For example, it is not known whether intraoperative use of alpha$_2$

agonists might blunt the sympathetic nervous system response to hemorrhage, and thus eliminate an important compensatory response to potentially life-threatening intraoperative hemorrhage.

Recommendations and Conclusions

The preceding section describes several methods to attenuate the sympathetic nervous system and endocrine response to surgery. The question that remains to be answered is whether we should attempt to prevent this diffuse neuroendocrine response, and in which patients. An important and as yet incompletely answered aspect of this question concerns the potential benefit of the stress response in the perioperative period. As previously mentioned, it is standard practice to administer supraphysiologic doses of glucocorticoids to all surgical patients with possible adrenal insufficiency. Whereas this replicates the hypercortisolemia that occurs in normal patients, recent data suggest this may be unnecessary. Udelsman et al randomized adrenalectomized monkeys undergoing cholecystectomy to receive no glucocorticoid replacement, normal replacement doses of glucocorticoids, or supraphysiologic doses such as are routinely administered clinically.[69] They observed hypotension and excess mortality in animals not receiving any glucocorticoids. However, the other two groups did equally well, suggesting that normal physiologic levels of glucocorticoids are adequate to tolerate the stress of surgery. In addition, regional anesthetic techniques, which are associated with an absent intraoperative stress response, are not associated with excess mortality and/or morbidity. In fact, a recent paper suggests that the converse may be true.[80] However, many questions remain. Does the stress response improve immune function? Recent data suggest it may do just the opposite.[41] Are interventions that eliminate pain superior to direct central nervous system suppression of the stress response? Until these questions are answered, widespread changes in clinical practice cannot be justified. However, there do seem to be sufficient data establishing the safety of aggressive analgesic regimens to attenuate the stress response to justify their use in high-risk patients. In our institution, high-risk patients, especially those with coronary artery disease who are undergoing extensive surgical procedures, usually receive epidural or spinal opiates for postoperative analgesia. In addition, they are closely monitored in the intensive care unit for 24 to 96 hours, during which time heart rate and blood pressure are aggressively maintained near normal levels. Whether more aggressive therapy with alpha$_2$ agonists is indicated in larger numbers of patients is unknown at this time and warrants further investigation.

REFERENCES

1. Adashi EY et al: Impact of acute surgical stress on anterior pituitary function in female subjects, Am J Obstet Gynecol 138:609-614, 1980.
2. Appel R et al: Sympathoneuronal and sympathoadrenal activation during ketamine anesthesia, Clin Pharmacol Ther 16:91-95, 1979.
3. Arnetz BB et al: Age-related differences in the serum prolactin response during standardized surgery, Life Sci 35:2675-2680, 1984.
4. Asiddao CB et al: Factors associated with perioperative complications during carotid endarterectomy, Anesth Analg 61:631-637, 1982.
5. Bessey PQ et al: Combined hormonal infusion simulates the metabolic response to injury, Ann Surg 200:264-281, 1984.
6. Bond RF and Johnson III G: Cardiovascular adrenoreceptor function during compensatory and decompensatory hemorrhagic shock, Circ Shock 12:9-24, 1984.
7. Bormann BV et al: Influence of epidural fentanyl on stress-induced elevation of plasma vosopressin (ADH) after surgery, Anesth Analg 62:727-732, 1983.
8. Brandt MR et al: Rapid decrease in plasma-triiodothyronine during surgery and epidural analgesia independent of afferent neurogenic stimuli and of cortisol, Lancet 2:1333-1336, 1976.
8a. Breslow MJ et al: Epidural morphine decreases postoperative hypertension by attenuating sympathetic nervous system hyperactivity, JAMA 261: in press, 1989.
9. Brown MJ, Brown DC, and Murphy MB: Hypothalemia from beta$_2$-receptor stimulation by circulating epinephrine, N Engl J Med 309:1414-1419, 1983.
10. Cameron V et al: Stress hormones in blood and cerebrospinal fluid of conscious sheep: effect of hemorrhage, Endocrinology 116:1460-1465, 1985.
11. Cameron V et al: Effect of central naloxone on hormone and blood pressure responses to hemorrhage in conscious sheep, Life Sci 41:571-577, 1987.
12. Cannon WB: Bodily changes in pain, hunger, fear, and rage, ed 2, New York, 1934, D Appleton & Co.
13. Cerra FB: Hypermetabolism, organ failure, and metabolic support, Surgery 101:4-14, 1987.
14. Chan V, Wang C, and Yeung RTT: Pituitary-thyroid responses to surgical stress, Acta Endocrinol 88:490-498, 1978.
15. Chernow B: Hormonal responses to graded surgical stress, Arch Intern Med 147:1273-1278, 1987.
16. Cochrane JPS et al: Arginine vasopressin release following surgical operations, Br J Surg 68:209-213, 1981.
17. Dubois M et al: Surgical stress in humans is accompanied by an increase in plasma beta-endorphin immunoreactivity, Life Sci 29:1249-1254, 1981.
18. Dubois M et al: Effects of fentanyl on the response of plasma beta-endorphin immunoreactivity to surgery, Anesthesiology 57:468-472, 1982.
19. Dudley HF et al: Studies on antidiuresis in surgery: effects of anesthesia, surgery and posterior pituitary antidiuretic hormone on water metabolism in man, Ann Surg 140:354-364, 1954.
20. Eigler N, Sacca L, and Sherwin RS: Glucagon, epinephrine, and cortisol in the dog: a model for stress-induced hyperglycemia, J Clin Invest 63:114-123, 1979.
21. Eltringham RJ: Complications in the recovery room, J Royal Soc Med 72:278-280, 1979.
22. Fouad FM et al: Possible role of cardioaortic reflexes in postcoronary bypass hypertension, Am J Cardiol 44:866-872, 1979.
23. Fragen RJ et al: Effects of etomidate on hormonal responses to surgical stress, Anesthesiology 61:652-656, 1984.
24. Gal TJ and Cooperman LH: Hypertension in the immediate postoperative period, Br J Anaesth 47:70-74, 1975.

25. Goldman L et al: Cardiac risk factors and complications in non-cardiac surgery, Medicine 57:357-370, 1978.

26. Goldman L: Supraventricular tachyarrhythmias in hospitalized adults after surgery, Chest 73:450-454, 1978.

27. Goldman L and Caldera DL: Risks of general anesthesia and elective operation in the hypertensive patient, Anesthesiology 50:785-792, 1979.

28. Greene CH, Walters W, and Rowntree LG: Surgical operations in Addison's disease, Ann Surg 98: 1013-1017, 1933.

29. Hall RC and Hodge RL: Changes in catecholamine and angiotensin levels in the cat and dog during hemorrhage, Am J Physiol 221:1305-1309, 1971.

30. Halter JB, Pflug AE, and Porte D: Mechanisms of plasma catecholamine increases during surgical stress in man, J Clin Endocrinol Metab 45:936-944, 1977.

31. Halter JB and Pflug AE: Relationship of impaired insulin secretion during surgical stress to anesthesia and catecholamine release, J Clin Endocrinol Metab 51:1093-1098, 1980.

32. Hammond WG, Aronow L, and Moore FD: Studies in surgical endocrinology. III. Plasma concentrations of epinephrine and norepinephrine in anesthesia, trauma and surgery, as measured by a modification of the method of Weil-Malherbe and Bone, Ann Surg 144:715-731, 1956.

33. Hawkins S et al: Changes in pressor hormone concentrations in association with coronary artery surgery, Br J Anaesth 58:1267-1272, 1986.

34. Helbo-Hansen R et al: Clonidine and the sympatico-adrenal response to coronary artery by-pass surgery, Acta Anaesthesiol Scand 30:235-242, 1986.

35. Heusch G and Deussen A: The effects of cardiac sympathetic nerve stimulation on the perfusion of stenotic coronary arteries in the dog, Circ Res 53:8-15, 1983.

36. Hilsted J, Christensen NJ, and Madsbad S: Whole body clearance of norepinephrine, J Clin Invest 71:500-505, 1983.

37. Hume DM and Egdahl RH: The importance of the brain in the endocrine response to injury, Ann Surg 150:697-712, 1959.

38. Hume DM, Bell CC, and Bartter F: Direct measurement of adrenal secretion during operative trauma and convalescence, Surg 52:174-186, 1962.

39. Jeffrey CC et al: A prospective evaluation of cardiac risk index, Anesthesiology 58:462-464, 1983.

40. Joyce JT, Roizen MF, and Eger II EI: Effect of thiopental induction on sympathetic activity, Anesthesiology 59:19-22, 1985.

41. Keller SE et al: Stress-induced suppression of immunity in adrenalectomized rats, Science 221:1301-1304, 1983.

42. Krowka MJ et al: Cardiac dysrhythmia following pneumonectomy: clinical correlates and prognostic significance, Chest 91:490-495, 1987.

43. Kuner J et al: Cardiac arrhythmias during anesthesia, Dis Chest 52:580-587, 1967.

44. Lanz E et al: Epidural morphine for postoperative analgesia: a double-blind study, Anesth Analg 61:236-240, 1982.

45. Ledingham I and Watt I: Influence of sedation on mortality in critically ill multiple trauma patients, Lancet 1:1270, 1983.

46. Lehv MS, Salzman EW, and Silen W: Hypertension complicating carotid endarterectomy, Stroke 1:307-313, 1970.

47. Leslie JB et al: Ablation of the hemodynamic responses to tracheal intubation with preinduction intravenous labetalol, Anesthesiology 67: A30, 1987.

48. Loughran PG, Moore J, and Dundee JW: Maternal stress response associated with caesarean delivery under general and epidural anaesthesia, Br J Obstet Gynaecol 93:943-949, 1986.

49. Mannelli M et al: A study of human adrenal secretion. Measurement of epinephrine, norepinephrine, dopamine and cortisol in peripheral and adrenal venous blood under surgical stress, J Endocrinol Invest 5:91-95, 1982.

50. Masala A et al: Effect of clonidine on stress-induced cortisol release in man during surgery, Pharmacol Res Commun 17:293-298, 1985.

51. Matsubara Y et al: Plasma glucagon changes in surgical patients, Jpn J Surg 9:327-334, 1979.

52. Morgan DB and Young RM: Acute transient hypokalemia: new interpretation of a common event, Lancet 2:751-752, 1982.

53. Nahas GG et al: Influence of acute hypoxia on sympathectomized and adrenalectomized dogs, Am J Physiol 177:13-15, 1954.

54. Nedergaard OA: Cocaine-like effect of ketamine on vascular adrenergic neurones, Eur J Pharmacol 23:153-161, 1973.

55. Newsome HH and Rose JC: The response of human adrenocorticotrophic hormone and growth hormone to surgical stress, J Clin Endocrinol 33:481-487, 1971.

56. Quesne LP and Lewis AAG: Postoperative water and sodium retention, Lancet 1:153-158, 1953.

57. Raff H, Tzankoff SP, and Fitzgerald RS: ACTH and cortisol responses to hypoxia in dogs, J Appl Physiol 51:1257-1260, 1981.

58. Raff H et al: Vasopressin, ACTH, and corticosteroids during hypercapnia and graded hypoxia in dogs, Am J Physiol 244:E453-E458, 1983.

59. Rao TLK, Jacobs KH, and El-Etr AA: Reinfarction following anesthesia in patients with myocardial infarction, Anesthesiology 59:499-505, 1983.

60. Rawal N et al: Epidural morphine for postoperative pain relief: a comparative study with intramuscular narcotic and intercostal nerve block, Anesth Analg 61:93-98, 1982.

61. Robertson D and Michelakis AM: Effect of anesthesia and surgery on plasma renin activity in man, J Clin Endocrinol 34:831-836, 1972.

62. Rutberg H et al: Effects of the extradural administration of morphine, or bupivacaine, on the endocrine response to upper abdominal surgery, Br J Anaesth 56:233-238, 1984.

63. Sandberg AA et al: The effects of surgery on the blood levels and metabolism of 17-hydroxycorticosteroids, J Clin Invest 33: 1509-1516, 1954.

64. Satta G et al: Effect of clonidine on stress-induced cortisol release in man during surgery, Pharmacol Res Comm 17:293-298, 1985.

65. Selye H: Stress and the general adaptation syndrome, Br Med J 1:1383-1390, 1950.

66. Shamoon H et al: Synergistic interactions among antiinsulin hormones in the pathogenesis of stress hyperglycemia in humans, J Clin Endocrinol Metab 52:1235-1241, 1981.

67. Tsuji H et al: Inhibition of metabolic responses to surgery with B-adrenergic blockade, Br J Surg 67:503-505, 1980.

68. Tsuji H et al: Effects of epidural administration of local anaesthetics or morphine on postoperative nitrogen loss and catabolic hormones, Br J Surg 74:421-425, 1987.

69. Udelsman R et al: Adaptation during surgical stress: a reevaluation of the role of glucocorticoids, J Clin Invest 77:1377-1381, 1986.

70. Udelsman R et al: Responses of the hypothalamic-pituitary-adrenal and renin-angiotensin axes and the sympathetic system during controlled surgical and anesthetic stress, J Clin Endocrinol Metab 64:986-994, 1987.

71. Utsunomiya T et al: Maintenance of cardiodynamics with aspirin during abdominal aortic aneurysmectomy (AAA), Ann Surg 194:602-608, 1981.

72. Vandam LD and Moore FD: Adrenocortical mechanisms related to anesthesia, Anesthesiology 21:531-551, 1960.

73. Vigas M et al: Alpha-adrenergic control of growth hormone release during surgical stress in man, Metabolism 26:399-402, 1977.

74. von Knorring J: Postoperative myocardial infarction: a prospective study in a risk group of surgical patients, Surg 90:55-60, 1981.

75. Wagner RL and White PF: Etomidate inhibits adrenocortical function in surgical patients, Anesthesiology 61:647-651, 1984.

76. Wagner RL et al: Inhibition of adrenal steroidogenesis by the anesthetic etomidate, N Engl J Med 310:1415-1421, 1984.

77. Wallach R et al: Pathogenesis of paroxysmal hypertension developing during and after coronary bypass surgery: a study of hemodynamic and humoral factors, Am J Cardiol 46:559-565, 1980.

78. Wartofsky L and Burman KD: Alterations in thyroid function in patients with systemic illness: the euthyroid-sick syndrome, Endocrine Rev 3:164-218, 1982.

79. Weinstein GS et al: The renin-angiotensin system is not responsible for hypertension following coronary artery bypass grafting, Ann Thorac Surg 43:74-77, 1987.

80. Yeager MP et al: Epidural anesthesia and analgesia in high-risk surgical patients, Anesthesiology 66:729-736, 1987.

81. Young JB, Rosa RM, and Landsberg L: Dissociation of sympathetic nervous system and adrenal medullary responses, Am J Physiol 247:E35-E40, 1984.

82. Zimmerman B and Wangensteen OH: Observations of water intoxication in surgical patients, Surg 31:654-669, 1952.

CHAPTER 15

Changes in Lung Function Following Anesthesia and Surgery

CLAIR F. MILLER
JACKIE L. MARTIN

Alterations of pulmonary function commonly develop during and after anesthesia and surgery, and all surgical patients are at risk for postoperative pulmonary complications. Although many pulmonary changes that occur intraoperatively resemble postoperative changes, they probably depend on different factors, but the transition from intraoperative to postoperative mechanisms is poorly understood. Decreased lung volumes caused by general anesthesia, for example, rapidly return to preoperative values in the early postoperative hours. However, pulmonary restrictive defects that last up to 2 weeks postoperatively depend on the site of surgical incision rather than the anesthetic technique employed. This chapter reviews (1) intraoperative changes in respiratory function, (2) postoperative pulmonary dysfunction, and (3) prevention and treatment of postoperative pulmonary complications.

INTRAOPERATIVE RESPIRATORY FUNCTION: EFFECTS OF ANESTHESIA
Airway Patency and Protection

Induction of general anesthesia predisposes to upper airway obstruction, impairs protective reflexes that normally guard against pulmonary aspiration, and depresses ciliary clearance of mucous and foreign material from the tracheobronchial tree. Hypoglossal nerve activity is depressed by halogenated anesthetics, barbiturates, and benzodiazepines, and even sedative concentrations of these agents may cause the tongue to fall against the posterior pharyngeal wall and obstruct the upper airway.[62,83] Air

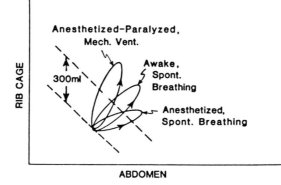

FIGURE 15-1. Diagram of relative contribution of tidal volume from the rib cage and abdomen in awake, anesthetized, and anesthetized-paralyzed states. The relative contribution from the rib cage to tidal volume is smaller during anesthesia with spontaneous breathing than in awake state.

From Rehder K and Marsh HM: Respiratory mechanics during anesthesia and mechanical ventilation. In Machlem PT and Meed J (editors): Handbook of Physiology, Baltimore, 1986, Waverly Press, Inc.

flow during inspiration may draw the epiglottis over the tracheal entrance in anesthetized patients who are breathing spontaneously without endotracheal intubation.[16] Sedation with 50% nitrous oxide in oxygen in healthy young volunteers decreases the number of swallows and prolongs the latent period of initiation of the swallowing reflex in response to injections of water into the pharynx.[85] Increasing the concentration of inhaled nitrous oxide progressively depresses the swallowing reflex in cats and predisposes to tracheal aspiration.[84] Clearance of mucous and inhaled particulate matter by airway cilia is markedly reduced at anesthetic concentrations of halogenated agents.[89] Tracheal mucous flow is similarly impaired during inhalation of either cold air[61] or air at relative humidity less than 75%.[43] Cuffed endotracheal tubes also reduce tracheal mucous velocity, but they may prevent tracheal aspiration.[107]

Lung Volumes

Administration of general anesthesia regularly and predictably decreases functional residual capacity (FRC) 15% to 25% below awake, supine values.[34,58,59,135] FRC decreases immediately on induction of anesthesia and remains stable at this new level throughout the anesthetic course.[59] All general anesthetic agents decrease FRC during spontaneous and mechanical ventilation whether or not neuromuscular blocking drugs are used.

Compression of lung tissue caused by anesthesia-induced changes in the shape and motion of the chest wall appear to be responsible for decreased FRC in anesthetized humans.[17,31,108] The rib cage appears to collapse on induction of general anesthesia as anteroposterior thoracic diameter decreases and lateral diameter increases.[129] These changes are not proportional because decreases occur in both thoracic cross-sectional area and volume.[56] The rib cage contribution to the tidal volume decreases and paradoxical (abdominal-diaphragmatic) breathing develops despite upper airway patency during spontaneous ventilation (Figure 15-1).[66,126,129] Whether anesthetic agents directly depress rib cage musculature, depress monosynaptic spinal reflex arcs, or alter supraspinal neural input to intercostal muscles is not known. Anesthetics directly decrease diaphragm muscle tone at end-expiration, and tonic relaxation causes cephalad displacement of the diaphragm that further decreases thoracic volume.[47,82] Hedenstierna et al[56] confirmed by computed tomography (CT) of the chest that the combined effects of decreased cross-sectional area of the chest and cranial displacement of the diaphragm account for reduced thoracic volume associated with decreased FRC after induction of general anesthesia (Figure 15-2).

Acute reduction of FRC is associated with pulmonary parenchymal collapse during both spontaneous and mechanical ventilation. Atelectasis (de-

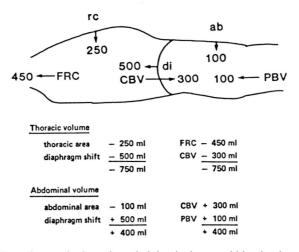

FIGURE 15-2. Mean changes in thoracic and abdominal gas and blood volumes (milliliters) after induction of anesthesia with mechanical ventilation. rc, rib cage; di, diaphragm; ab, abdomen; CBV, central blood volume; PBV, peripheral blood volume.

From Hedenstierna G et al: Functional residual capacity, thoracoabdominal dimensions, and central blood volume during general anesthesia with muscle paralysis and mechanical ventilation, Anesth 62:247–254, 1985.

termined by CT) develops in dependent lung regions within 10 to 15 minutes after anesthesia induction.[17,123] Alveolar collapse may be a result of the reduction of end-expiratory lung volume below closing capacity (CC) in some patients.[34] However, Juno et al[68] and Bergman et al[13] suggest that both CC and FRC decrease in parallel after induction of general anesthesia, and other unidentified mechanisms may contribute to airspace collapse. The extent of atelectasis may be greater in obese patients and in patients who have low anteroposterior and wide lateral chest wall diameters, presumably because these patients have low FRC before induction of anesthesia.[118] Breathing at low volumes increases elastic recoil of the lung and decreases lung compliance.[10,135] The role of surfactant in mediating these changes is not clear.[100] Despite decreased lung volume and compliance, anesthetized patients are able to increase their work of breathing in response to resistance and elastance loading.[81,87] Ability to increase work may preserve minute ventilation during partial airway obstruction intraoperatively and in the early postoperative period.

Gas Exchange

While minute ventilation must be increased after induction of anesthesia to compensate for increased alveolar dead space and wasted ventilation in apparatus dead space,[88] impaired oxygenation is the major consequence of decreased FRC and air space collapse after induction of general anesthesia. Before development of the Clarke electrode for direct measurement of partial pressure of oxygen in arterial blood (PaO_2), perioperative arterial desaturation was thought to be restricted to patients undergoing thoracotomy with lung resection. However, Nunn et al[86] observed mean PaO_2 values of 58 mm Hg (room air breathing) in young healthy patients immediately after minor procedures under general anesthesia. Bendixen et al[10] reported that both PaO_2 and total pulmonary compliance decreased (22% and 15%, respectively) intraoperatively after 30 minutes of anesthesia administration at constant FiO_2 and normal $PaCO_2$. Both authors suggested that the decrease in PaO_2 resulted from either anesthesia-induced intrapulmonary shunt or development of ventilation-to-perfusion (VA/Q) inequality, because PaO_2 remained low despite normal $PaCO_2$ values.[10,86] Later studies by Hewlett et al[59] and Hickey et al[60] showed that the alveolar to arterial oxygen difference ($P(A-a)O_2$) increases after anesthesia induction, and that $P(A-a)O_2$ increases in direct proportion to the amount that FRC decreases.[59]

In the absence of direct right-to-left anatomic

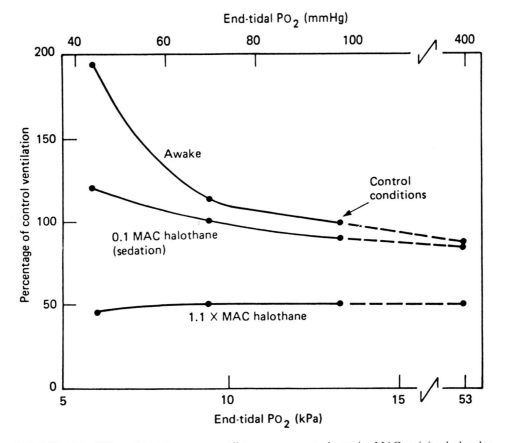

FIGURE 15-3. Effect of halothane on ventilatory response to hypoxia. MAC, minimal alveolar concentration required for anesthesia.

From Nunn JF: Control of breathing. In Applied Respiratory Physiology, ed 3, London, 1987, Butterworth Publishers.

shunts, increased $P(A-a)O_2$ must result from either intrapulmonary shunt, perfusion of lung regions with low VA/Q ratios, or both. Recent assessments of VA/Q ratios by multiple inert gas elimination techniques reveal that both abnormalities develop after anesthesia induction in association with decreased FRC. The pattern of abnormality that develops may depend on patient age and underlying pulmonary disease. In young (24 to 33 years) healthy volunteers, Rehder et al[101] reported a wide range of VA/Q ratios after anesthesia induction, but intrapulmonary shunt values remained less than 1%. In older surgical patients (37 to 61 years) without lung disease, Bindslev et al[15] found that intrapulmonary shunt increased on induction of anesthesia, but shunt did not entirely account for increases in $P(A-a)O_2$.

Dueck et al[35] found large increases in both shunt and areas of low VA/Q ratios in elderly patients (52 to 75 years) with chronic pulmonary disease. These studies suggest a tendency for increased shunting in older patients and in patients with preexisting lung disease.

Tokics et al,[123] using chest CT, related VA/Q ratios to atelectasis before and after induction of anesthesia in patients (mean age 42 years) without lung disease. Intrapulmonary mean shunt values increased from 1.2% to 6.5% and dependent atelectasis developed after 15 minutes of halothane anesthesia. The magnitude of the shunt correlated directly to the extent of atelectasis (r = 0.84). Positive end-expiratory pressure (PEEP) reduced the amount of atelectasis, but did not alter shunt fraction. These authors con-

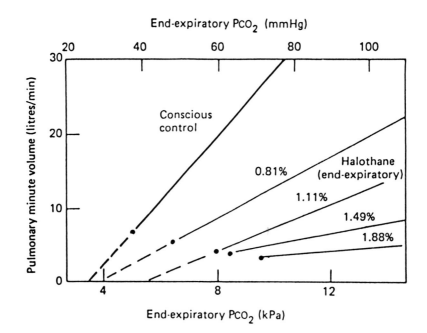

FIGURE 15-4. Effect of ventilatory response to $PaCO_2$ at different concentrations of halothane.

From Nunn JF: Control of breathing. In Applied Respiratory Physiology, ed 3, London, 1987, Butterworth Publishers.

cluded that development of atelectasis and shunt in dependent lung areas is the major cause of impaired oxygenation during anesthesia.[123] However, in another series of young healthy patients (mean age 28 years), shunt fraction increased only in patients in whom FRC under anesthesia decreased below awake CC.[34] The shunt effect directly correlated with body mass index (weight/height²) and was greater in smokers than in nonsmokers. Perfusion of lung regions with low (but not zero) VA/Q ratios accounted for increases in $P(A-a)O_2$ in patients in whom FRC under anesthesia remained above awake CC.[34]

Pulmonary blood flow normally decreases in atelectatic regions of lung to maintain equality of VA/Q ratios. Decreased alveolar oxygen concentration mediates vasoconstriction of the pulmonary arterial tree locally (hypoxic pulmonary vasoconstriction) to limit blood flow.[11] Inhalational, but not intravenous, anesthetic agents inhibit hypoxic pulmonary vasoconstriction, and this effect appears to be a major determinant of maldistribution of pulmonary blood flow under anesthesia.[12,78,119]

Lung volume reduction invariably accompanies induction of anesthesia, and decreased FRC is associated with impaired oxygenation. Oxygenation abnormalities develop as a result of either intrapulmonary shunt or perfusion of lung units with low VA/Q ratios. The magnitude of shunt appears to depend on the amount of atelectasis that develops, and atelectasis is greater in smokers and in obese patients.

Respiratory Drive

All halogenated anesthetic agents markedly impair normal ventilatory responses to hypoxia and hypercarbia. Figure 15-3 illustrates the hypoxic ventilatory response to both sedative and anesthetic alveolar concentrations of halothane in man.[72] Impaired hypoxic drive appears to result from depression of chemoreceptors at the carotid bodies by anesthetic agents.[30,70] Figure 15-4 shows that halothane decreases ventilatory response to increased $PaCO_2$ in dose-dependent fashion. Halothane also markedly reduces the peripheral chemoreceptor-mediated ven-

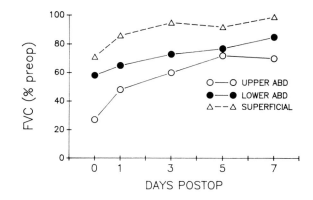

FIGURE 15-5. Influence of site of surgical incision on postoperative changes in forced vital capacity (FVC).

From Alexander JI et al: Br J Anaesth 45:34–40, 1973; Ali J et al: Am J Surg 128:376–382, 1974; and Meyers JR et al: Arch Surg 110:576–583, 1975.

tilatory response to acute metabolic acidemia in humans.[71]

POSTOPERATIVE RESPIRATORY FUNCTION

Decreased FRC, atelectasis, and increased P(A-a)O$_2$ are regular and expected consequences of general anesthesia in all patients. However, these abnormalities are observed postoperatively only in patients in whom the chest or abdominal cavity has been opened. The magnitude and duration of late postoperative pulmonary abnormalities vary markedly according to the site of surgical incision.

Influence of Surgical Incision Site

FRC decreases more after abdominal or thoracic incisions than after lower abdominal procedures. Superficial (nonabdominal, nonthoracic) procedures are not associated with postoperative FRC reduction (Table 15-1).[2,4,80,115] P(A-a)O$_2$ increases postoperatively in direct proportion to the amount that FRC decreases.[2,26] Forced vital capacity (FVC) and forced expiratory volume in one second (FEV$_1$) also decrease more after upper abdominal than after lower abdominal or superficial incisions, but the ratio of FEV$_1$/FVC remains normal (Figure 15-5).[2,3,80] FRC and FVC slowly return to preoperative values over 12 to 14 days after abdominal or thoracic procedures.[7,21] Thus postoperative patients develop acute

TABLE 15-1. Postoperative FRC changes by site of incision (percent of preoperative values)

Site	Postoperative days			
	1	**3**	**5**	**7**
Upper abdomen	71	81	90	90
Lower abdomen	88	115	101	102
Peripheral	97	103	108	86
Thoracic	83	85	93	88
Sternotomy	59	58	65	NA

NA, not available.
From Alexander JI et al: Br J Anaesth 45:34-40, 1973; Ali J et al: Am J Surg 128:376-382, 1974; Meyers JR et al: Arch Surg 110:576-583, 1975; Stock MC et al: Crit Care Med 12:969-972, 1984.

restrictive pulmonary defects that vary in duration and severity according to the site of surgical incision.

Proposed Causes of Prolonged Postoperative Pulmonary Abnormalities

The reasons for prolonged postoperative pulmonary restrictive abnormalities are not well understood. The following explanations, which are discussed below, are often proposed: (1) persistent effects of anesthetic agents, (2) restrictive effects of pain and muscle splinting, and (3) diaphragm dysfunction.

Persistent effects of anesthesia. At least three studies suggest that FRC rapidly returns to preoperative values after surgery, and that mechanisms other than anesthesia are responsible for low FRC throughout the late postoperative course.[3,24,38] Although FRC was not measured intraoperatively, Ali et al[3] observed a 16-hour delay before FRC decreased below preoperative values after upper abdominal surgery. Dureuil et al[38] and Colgan et al[24] also found FRC to be unchanged from preoperative values at 4 hours after upper abdominal surgery, but neither author made subsequent FRC determinations. Although other investigators have reported decreased FRC at 4 hours after abdominal and cardiac surgical procedures,[115,116] serial measurements of FRC beginning intraoperatively and continuing throughout the postoperative hours have not been reported.

Indirect evidence suggests that mechanisms other than anesthesia are responsible for late postoperative pulmonary abnormalities. First, serial determinations of atelectasis by chest CT throughout the perioperative period suggest that postoperative atelectasis occurs more commonly and more extensively after upper abdominal than after lower abdominal surgery.[117] This differential effect is unlikely to be the result of anesthetic agents alone. Second, although metabolites of halogenated anesthetic agents are present in body stores at low concentration for many postoperative days,[25,114] atelectasis and pneumonia occur as frequently with epidural as with general anesthesia techniques for abdominal procedures.[57,120] Ravin et al[97] found that both spinal and general anesthesia techniques were associated with identical reductions in FVC, FEV_1, and PaO_2 at 24 and 48 hours after lower abdominal surgery. Thus, anesthetic metabolites do not appear to mediate postoperative pulmonary abnormalities. A third argument against anesthesia as a primary mediator of late postoperative pulmonary restrictive dysfunction is the rapid return of lung volume, mechanical function, and gas exchange to preoperative values after superficial procedures.

Pain and muscle splinting. Pain and muscle splinting have also been thought to cause postoperative pulmonary restrictive dysfunction, but little evidence supports this hypothesis. In patients who received no analgesic therapy after upper abdominal surgery, Wahba et al[131] found that although administration of epidural lidocaine eliminated pain and

increased FVC from 37% to 55% of preoperative values, FRC did not increase. Jakobson et al[63] also found unchanged FRC when pain was relieved by intercostal nerve blocks with etidocaine at 24 hours after cholecystectomy. Bromage et al[18] gave parenteral morphine to postoperative patients who had pain and noted that FEV_1 increased from 37% to 45% of preoperative values. Subsequent administration of either epidural local anesthetic or epidural narcotic further increased FEV_1 from 45% to 67% of preoperative values after upper abdominal or thoracic procedures; FRC was not measured.[18] These studies suggest that pain relief may decrease postoperative splinting and partially correct spirographic abnormalities, but pulmonary restriction (decreased FRC) remains unchanged. It seems unlikely that pulmonary restriction results from the effects of epidural or intercostal neural blockade, because neither technique decreases FRC in volunteers who have not had surgical interventions.[55,132]

Diaphragm dysfunction. Similarities between pulmonary abnormalities that accompany abdominal surgery and those observed in patients with neuromuscular disease and diaphragm failure have stimulated interest in postoperative respiratory muscle activity. Indices of diaphragm dysfunction (decreased volume displacement, decreased transdiaphragmatic pressure swings during tidal breathing, paradoxical motion of the diaphragm, and increased rib cage and decreased diaphragm contribution to tidal volume) occur as early as 1 hour postoperatively and may persist for 7 to 10 days after upper abdominal and thoracic surgery.[38,45,77,111] Ford et al[45] suggest that postoperative failure of the diaphragm to contract effectively during inhalation, combined with increased expiratory muscle effort, may be responsible for FRC reduction after upper abdominal surgery.

Causes of postoperative diaphragm dysfunction remain a matter of speculation. Residual anesthetic agents are unlikely to be mediators for the reasons discussed before, and analgesic therapy with epidural fentanyl does not improve diaphragm function after upper abdominal surgery.[111] Contractility appears to be normal during bilateral electrical phrenic nerve stimulation.[38] Mechanical irritation of the diaphragm during abdominal surgery[103] or as a result of postoperative pneumoperitoneum[14] may alter diaphragm function either directly or via chest wall or peritoneal reflexes that inhibit phrenic nerve activity.[38] Intraoperative phrenic nerve injury does not account for diaphragm dysfunction after pulmonary resection.[77] Despite transient phrenic nerve paresis from cold cardioplegia solution during cardiopulmonary bypass, Wilcox et al[137] were unable to establish a relationship between postoperative atelectasis and phrenic nerve conduction abnormalities after cardiac surgery. Aminophylline partially improves diaphragm function after cholecystectomy, but whether aminophylline acts as a diaphragmatic inotrope or as a central nervous system stimulant is not clear.[37] Both Ford et al[44] and Dureuil et al[37] noted anecdotally that some postoperative patients, when asked, are able to reverse their pattern of breathing from predominantly thoracic to abdominal breathing. Volitional control over breathing pattern suggests that diaphragmatic abnormalities may be partially mediated by central neural mechanisms that control respiratory drive, and this response may partially explain the beneficial effects that doxapram is reported to have on postoperative pulmonary function.[52,139]

Consequences of Intraoperative and Postoperative Changes

Induction of general anesthesia decreases FRC and impairs oxygenation in all surgical patients, but these changes rapidly return to preoperative values in the early postoperative hours. Other pulmonary effects of anesthetic agents including decreased ventilatory drive, impaired airway protective reflexes, and tendency for upper airway obstruction also resolve rapidly as anesthetic gases are eliminated from the body. When these transient pulmonary abnormalities persist into the immediate postoperative hours, they are often identified as early postoperative pulmonary complications. (Respiratory complications in the recovery room are reviewed in Chapter 12.)

However, decreases in FRC that persist for many postoperative days result from either diaphragm dysfunction or from other unidentified pathophysiologic abnormalities that reduce lung volumes after abdominal or thoracic procedures. Prolonged postoperative FRC and FVC reductions are associated with atelectasis, decreased pulmonary compliance, increased work of breathing,[130] and rapid respiratory rate at low tidal volume without sighs.[8,39] Poor cough effort increases susceptibility of postoperative patients to retained secretions, bacterial contamination of the airway, and pneumonia. Thus acute reduction of lung volume is probably the major cause of late postoperative pulmonary complications. Identification of FRC reduction as the central abnormality establishes a focus for prevention and treatment of postoperative pulmonary complications.

POSTOPERATIVE PULMONARY COMPLICATIONS

Late postoperative pulmonary complications are leading causes of morbidity and mortality in surgical patients.[22,36,75] While decreased FRC, FVC, and increased P(A-a)O$_2$ are expected consequences of upper abdominal and thoracic procedures, accentuation of these effects may result in pneumonia, respiratory failure, and death. Although deaths occur rarely after anesthesia and surgery (1.5% to 2.0% of all cases),[9,46] Lunn et al[75] found that respiratory complications accounted for 24% of clinical causes of death in 197 patients who died within 6 days of operation. In a series of 10,000 major operative procedures, Martin et al[79] found that 10% of all operative deaths occurred in patients with pneumonia, and development of pneumonia was associated with a 46% mortality.

Incidence

Diagnostic criteria for postoperative pulmonary complications usually include radiographic abnormalities (atelectasis, lobar collapse, or infiltrate) and clinical signs or symptoms that reflect newly acquired pulmonary pathology (fever, leukocytosis, rales, tubular breath sounds, cough, sputum production, or dyspnea). Although postoperative complication rates vary widely depending on the specific radiographic and/or clinical criteria used for detection, pulmonary complications after upper abdominal surgery are as common today as they were 20 years ago (Table 15-2). Unfortunately, the diagnostic criteria used in these studies do not differentiate between complications with clinically important sequelae such as pneumonia and those that may be considered normal consequences of surgical intervention. Atelectasis, for example, is a noninfectious complication that develops in up to 90% of patients after cardiac surgery and resolves without adverse effects in most patients.[115] However, atelectasis is often the first clinically apparent postoperative abnormality in a pathophysiologic sequence that results in bacterial contamination and development of pneumonia in 1.3% of all surgical procedures.[79] Risk factors for pulmonary complications must be iden-

TABLE 15-2. Incidence of pulmonary complications after upper abdominal surgery

Author and reference number	Number of patients	Criteria		Incidence of PPC (percent)
		PE	CXR	
1968-1980				
Wightman[136]	118	+	+	20
Latimer[74]	46	+	+	76
Van De Water[127]	30	+	+	30
Bartlett[6]	150	+	+	17
Craven[27]	70	+	+	59
Lyager[76]	103	+	+	37
Jung[67]	126	+	+	41
1981-1988				
Alexander[1]	134		+	35
Celli[20]	174	+		46
Stock[116]	65	+	+	37
Ricksten[102]	43		+	16
Schwieger[109]	40	+	+	35
O'Connor[90]	40	+		35
Roukema[106]	153	+	+	41

PPC, postoperative pulmonary complications; PE, physical examination; CXR, chest radiography.

tified to guide preventive and treatment techniques and thus decrease postoperative pulmonary morbidity and mortality.

Risk Factors

Risk factors for development of life-threatening postoperative complications such as pneumonia also identify patients who are likely to develop less severe pulmonary abnormalities. A prospective study of 520 surgical patients found significant associations by linear discriminant analysis between postoperative pneumonia and (1) upper abdominal or thoracic sites of surgery, (2) prolonged operative procedure, (3) increased severity of underlying diseases, (4) history of smoking, and (5) poor preoperative nutrition.[50] The incidence of pneumonia increased as age and body weight increased, but the association of these variables with pneumonia lost significance after other variables were controlled for separately.[50] Large clinical surveys that assess the overall incidence of postoperative radiographic and clinical pulmonary abnormalities document increased complication rates in the presence of the risk factors listed in the box above, right.[73,74,136]

Risk factors for postoperative pulmonary complications

Abdominal or thoracic incision
Prolonged operative procedure
Patient characteristics
    Preexisting pulmonary disease
    Smoking history
    Increased age
    Obesity
    Poor nutritional status

Site of incision. The incidence of pulmonary complications appears to increase in direct proportion to the amount that FRC and FVC decrease postoperatively, and the site of surgical incision is probably the primary determinant for these changes. Latimer et al[74] summarized the results of 19 surgical series from 1922 to 1969 and found the highest incidence of postoperative pulmonary complications after upper abdominal or thoracic procedures; the lowest rates occurred after operations at peripheral body sites. Incidence rates are higher after upper abdominal than after lower abdominal incisions.[1,73,74,136] Subcostal incisions for cholecystectomy have been associated with fewer pulmonary complications and better pulmonary mechanical function (FVC, FEV_1) than midline incisions.[49]

Length of procedure. Operative procedures lasting more than 2 to 3 hours are consistently associated with increased rates of postoperative pulmonary complications,* but this association remains unexplained. Caplan et al[19] found that after 47 hours of anesthesia for reimplantation of eight severed fingers, a 21-year-old man had a prolonged and stormy emergence from general anesthesia. Tracheal extubation was delayed for 36 hours for fear of upper airway incompetence; full cognitive function did not return until the third postoperative day. Although other pulmonary complications did not develop in this patient, prolonged emergence after several hours of anesthesia in older patients with other risk factors may predispose to postoperative airway obstruction, aspiration, and pneumonia.

Patient characteristics. Postoperative death rates are sevenfold to tenfold higher in patients with

*References 33, 50, 74, 106, 136.

chronic bronchitis or chronic obstructive pulmonary disease (COPD) than in patients without these diseases.[46,120] Preexisting lung disease may be a leading risk factor for development of postoperative pulmonary complications. Wightman et al[136] found that complications developed in 26% of patients with chronic respiratory disease compared to 8.2% in those with normal lung function preoperatively. Similar observations have been made by other investigators.[74,113] Cigarette smoking, a major cause of chronic lung disease, increases airway mucous production, decreases mucociliary clearance, promotes small airway closure, and increases the incidence of postoperative pulmonary complications whether or not the patient has a history of preexisting bronchitis or COPD.[73,93]

Postoperative pulmonary complications are less clearly associated with either old age or obesity than with other risk factors. While most studies report higher complication rates with increased age (greater than 70 years of age), old age may simply be a marker for underlying pulmonary dysfunction. In nonsurgical settings, obesity is often associated with VA/Q inequality, intrapulmonary shunt, and impaired oxygenation,[5,92] but Ray et al[99] report that FRC and FVC do not decrease significantly until body weight exceeds 250% of predicted body weight. These findings may explain why some investigators observe increased complication rates in obese patients[20] and others do not.[136] Increased gastric volume and decreased gastric pH in obese patients predispose to extensive lung injury if aspiration occurs perioperatively.[128]

Protein-energy malnutrition is associated with decreased FVC and FEV_1 preoperatively,[138] and postoperative pulmonary complications occur more frequently in malnourished than in normal patients.[50,138] The finding of Windsor et al[138] that pneumonia developed in 21% of protein-depleted versus 7% of non-protein-depleted patients after abdominal surgery suggests that malnutrition also impairs normal host defenses against airway colonization and invasion by bacteria in the postoperative time.

In a series of 136 patients who developed postoperative pneumonia, Martin et al[79] found that 69% of cases were caused by gram-negative organisms, and gram-negative pneumonitis was a major determinant of death in these patients. Evidence is rapidly accumulating that retrograde airway colonization from the stomach by gram-negative intestinal bacteria is a major mechanism for nosocomial pneumonia in both postoperative and intensive care unit patients.[32,91] Parr et al[91] found gastric colonization by gram-negative intestinal bacteria in 23% of patients after cholecystectomy, and gastric colonization was significantly associated with culture of the same organisms in sputum and with development of postoperative radiographic abnormalities. Maintenance of gastric acidity throughout the postoperative period appears to prevent gastric colonization and to decrease the incidence of gram-negative pneumonias.[32] Gram-negative intestinal bacteria may be important opportunistic pathogens in patients with protein-energy malnutrition.

Postoperative pulmonary complications contribute significantly to surgical morbidity and mortality. The incidence of radiographic and clinical signs of pulmonary pathology varies directly with the amount that FRC and FVC decrease postoperatively, and complications are most common after upper abdominal or thoracic incisions. Duration of surgical procedure and factors related to preoperative medical condition of the patient also influence complication rates, but the interactive effect of each variable with the other remains a matter of speculation because few studies employ multivariate analysis. Noninfectious complications occasionally evolve into bacterial bronchitis or pneumonia that are associated with high mortality rates, but risk factors and mediators of this transition are poorly defined. Methods to decrease the incidence of postoperative pulmonary complications and improve outcome have logically focused on techniques to minimize postoperative FRC reduction.

Prevention and Treatment of Pulmonary Complications

Preoperative identification of high risk patients should guide the use of chest physiotherapy maneuvers, lung expansion techniques, and analgesic strategies to augment lung function, reduce complication rates, and improve outcome.

General considerations. The incidence of pulmonary complications in patients with abnormal preoperative spirometry and/or arterial blood gas analysis in 40% to 60% compared to 0% to 10% in normal patients.[74,113] On the basis of comprehensive review of the literature, Tisi[121,122] recommends preoperative spirographic and arterial blood gas analyses for patients in the following categories: (1) those scheduled for upper abdominal or thoracic surgery, (2) cigarette smokers with cough, (3) obese patients, (4) patients older than 70 years of age, and (5) patients with chronic pulmonary disease (defined as presence of any bedside physical finding suggestive of lung disease). If pulmonary resection is planned, such patients should also have radioisotopic lung scanning to evaluate regional lung function. All other surgical candidates with abnormal spirographic or blood gas analyses should receive preoperative and postoperative chest physiotherapy.[121,122]

It has been shown that high-risk patients who receive standardized preoperative and postoperative chest physiotherapy have fewer postoperative complications than untreated controls.[20,53,106,113] Nevertheless, Fogh et al[42] observed in patients undergoing abdominal procedures that even the combined predictive power of spirometry, radioisotopic scintigraphy, and standard chest radiography did not identify those patients who developed postoperative complications severe enough to require treatment. No single spirographic abnormality is unequivocally predictive of postoperative pulmonary complications,[51,53] and the specificity of any measurement may be insufficient to justify the cost of routinely applied preoperative and postoperative respiratory therapy programs.[95,125] Chest physiotherapy maneuvers (percussion, postural drainage, vibration, and deep breathing and coughing exercises) appear to be most beneficial in patients who have lobar atelectasis or large volumes of secretions, and they may precipitate bronchospasm in acutely ill patients without preexisting reactive airways disease.[69] Thus preoperative spirographic and arterial blood gas testing appear to be helpful in identifying high-risk patients who may benefit from perioperative chest physiotherapy, but predictive tests and specific therapeutic recommendations for individual patients have not been definitively established.

Prophylactic measures should be used throughout the perioperative time to decrease pulmonary morbidity and mortality. When indicated, bronchodilator therapy should be optimized preoperatively and continued throughout the perioperative course. Preoperative smoking cessation should be encouraged in all patients. Short term abstinence decreases carboxyhemoglobin levels within hours, but postoperative complication rates decrease only in patients who have abstained from smoking for more than 8 weeks before surgery.[93,133] No particular anesthetic

technique has been found to eliminate or decrease the incidence of postoperative pulmonary complications, and anesthetic management is based on the desires and physiologic requirements of the patient. Careful intraoperative and postoperative airway management is required to prevent bronchospasm, maintain airway patency, and prevent pulmonary aspiration of foreign material. Early extubation of the trachea and maintenance of gastric acidity in the postoperative time may reduce the likelihood of bacterial colonization of the airway and decrease the incidence of enteric bacterial pneumonias.[32,65] Patients should receive supervised instruction on the use of specialized respiratory therapy and analgesic devices to improve compliance with and enhance the effectiveness of these important therapeutic modalities.

Lung expansion techniques. Lung inflation strategies that are commonly used postoperatively include cough and deep breathing exercises (CDE, a major component of chest physiotherapy programs) and use of mechanical devices such as incentive spirometry (IS), intermittent positive pressure breathing (IPPB), and continuous positive airway pressure (CPAP). Each technique is based on sound physiologic principles and should promote periodic lung expansion, increase FRC, and decrease the incidence of postoperative pulmonary complications.[6,96] To compare the effectiveness of lung expansion techniques in decreasing postoperative pulmonary complications, Table 15-3 lists complication rates reported in a number of prospective, randomized studies of patients having upper abdominal or thoracic procedures (high-risk patients who should receive perioperative chest physiotherapy[122]). Complication rates in these patients are markedly less than in untreated control groups with either CDE, IS, or IPPB (upper panel, Table 15-3). Celli et al[20] found "absence of respiratory treatment" to be a major risk factor by discriminant function analysis for development of postoperative complications.

Among the treatment techniques, mask CPAP appears to be marginally more effective than either CDE, IS, or IPPB in decreasing postoperative pulmonary complications (Table 15-3). The low complication rate in the CPAP group of Ricksten et al[102] may reflect the combined effects of CPAP and CDE, since all patients in this study received perioperative chest physiotherapy with CDE. While the mean postoperative FRC values among the CDE, IS, and CPAP

TABLE 15-3. Effects of lung expansion techniques on the incidence of pulmonary complications after abdominal or thoracic surgery

Author and reference numbers	Number of patients	Incidence of PPC (percent of group)				
		No RX	Treatment			
			CDE	IS	IPPB	CPAP
STUDIES WITH UNTREATED CONTROLS						
Stein[113]	48	60	22			
Craven[27]	70	71		46		
Celli[20]	81	88	33	30	32	
Schwieger[109]	40	30		40		
Roukema[106]	153	60	19			
STUDIES WITH CDE CONTROLS						
Bartlett[6]	150		25	9		
Lyager[76]	94		33	51		
Stock[116]	65	POD 1	33	50		44
		POD 3	42	41		23
Rickstein[102]	43	POD 1	33			11
		POD 3	40			4
O'Connor[90]	40		45	25		
UNCONTROLLED COMPARATIVE STUDIES						
Van De Water[127]	30			20	40	
Jung[67]	81			49	36	

No RX, no respiratory therapy; CDE, cough and deep breathing exercises; IS, incentive spirometry; IPPB, intermittent positive pressure breathing; CPAP, continuous positive airway pressure.

groups were similar, Stock et al[116] found more rapid recovery of FRC with CPAP than with CDE. Recovery of FRC with IS was similar to that of CPAP.[116] The benefits of any frequently administered, well-supervised postoperative respiratory therapy modality may derive partly from early ambulation and resumption of the upright position that is associated with greater FRC and FVC after upper abdominal surgery than the supine position.[57]

Postoperative pulmonary complications can be reduced by lung inflation maneuvers, but choice of technique appears to depend on factors other than the relative improvement in pulmonary function deriving from various techniques. Untoward effects of lung expansion techniques are rare, but bloating and abdominal distension may limit the usefulness of IPPB.[20] CPAP may be preferred over IS in some cases because it is painless and requires no effort from the patient. Perhaps the most remarkable observation to be made from Table 15-3 is that 20% to 30% of all postoperative patients develop pulmonary complications despite treatment with lung inflation techniques.

Analgesic therapy. As previously discussed, postoperative FRC reduction does not appear to be the result of pain and muscle splinting, because postoperative measurements of FRC before and after analgesic therapy are identical. However, effort-dependent tests of pulmonary function (FVC, FEV_1) improve with pain relief.[18,63,131] Changes in FVC, FEV_1, and peak expiratory flow rates (PEF) after analgesic therapy with a variety of specialized techniques at 24 hours after abdominal or thoracic surgery are compared in Table 15-4 to controls who received only parenteral narcotics for pain relief. These studies show that postoperative spirographic abnormalities are often improved by analgesic therapy. Hendolin et al[57] showed that FVC is significantly lower in patients after upper abdominal surgery who subsequently develop complications than in those without postoperative pulmonary pathology. This link between spirographic abnormalities and

TABLE 15-4. Effects of analgesic techniques on postoperative spirographic abnormalities

Author and reference numbers	Number of patients	Site		FVC		FEV$_1$		PEF	
		TH	AB	C	RX	C	RX	C	RX
EPIDURAL LOCAL ANESTHETICS									
Spence[112]	21		+	32	27	31	30		
Pflug[94]	20		+	54	75			57	69
Hendolin[57]	70		+	57	64	64	68	63	72
EPIDURAL NARCOTICS									
Bromage[18]	66		+			45	67		
Rawal[98]	60		+					57	90
Shulman[110]	30	+		44	65	44	67	45	67
Jayr[64]	146		+	53	52	50	52		
Rosenberg[105]	40		+					58	55
TENS									
Ali[3]	40		+	39	65				
Galloway[48]	40		+					40	41
Rooney[104]	50	+		38	51	42	52		
PCA									
Welchew[134]	20		+	47	42	50	46	55	57
Rosenberg[105]	40		+					58	54

All control groups received parenteral narcotics.
TH, thoracic incision; AB, abdominal incision; C, control; RX, treatment; TENS, transcutaneous electric nerve stimulation; PCA, patient-controlled analgesia; FVC, forced vital capacity; FEV$_1$, forced expiratory volume in one second; PEF, peak expiratory flow rate.

development of complications suggests that analgesic therapy may decrease the incidence of postoperative pulmonary complications.

Pulmonary complication rates after specialized analgesic techniques are compared in Table 15-5 to matched controls who received parenteral narcotics. Complications are clearly fewer with a number of analgesic strategies. Until definitive comparative studies are done, however, choice of technique appears to depend more on available anesthetic skill and expertise than on improvement in pulmonary function.[23]

The beneficial effects of analgesic therapy on FVC, FEV$_1$, and PEF apparently enhance coughing ability, facilitate early ambulation, improve patient cooperation with respiratory therapy maneuvers, and decrease the incidence of postoperative pulmonary complications. Ricksten et al[102] combined effective analgesic therapy (epidural morphine) with aggressive perioperative respiratory therapy (CDE and CPAP) and noted that the incidence of postoperative pulmonary complications decreased markedly in high-risk surgical patients (Table 15-3). While pulmonary restrictive defects probably persisted unaltered, the combined benefits of analgesic and respiratory therapy maneuvers appear to be greater than with either technique alone.

SUMMARY

Alterations of pulmonary function are regular and predictable consequences of anesthesia and surgery. Accentuation of these changes occasionally result in serious pulmonary complications and death. General anesthetic agents are responsible for complications in the early postoperative hours; abnormalities of diaphragm function appear to mediate late pulmonary complications after abdominal or thoracic procedures. Late complications are rare in patients after procedures at peripheral body sites.

Induction of general anesthesia predisposes to airway obstruction, blunts airway protective reflexes, decreases FRC, impairs oxygenation, and inhibits ventilatory drive mechanisms in all patients. While these changes are completely reversible as anesthetic

TABLE 15-5. Effects of analgesic techniques on the incidence of pulmonary complications after upper abdominal surgery

Author and reference number	Number of patients	Incidence of PPC (percent in each group)					
			Treatment				
		CON	EPI LA	EPI NARC	ICNB	TENS	PCA
Spence[112]	21	70	18				
Pflug[94]	20	82	46				
Rosenberg[105]	80	40		55	47		45
Cuschieri[28]	106	30				23	
Cuschieri[29]	50	64	24				
Hasenbros[54]	129	38		12			
Hendolin[57]	70	50	27				
Engberg[40]	417	16			12		
Jayr[64]	146	50		64			

Control groups received parenteral narcotics.

CON, control; EPI LA, epidural local anesthetics; EPI NARC, epidural narcotics; ICNB, intercostal nerve block; TENS, transcutaneous electrical stimulation; PCA, patient controlled analgesia; PPC, postoperative pulmonary complications.

agents are eliminated from the body, careful intraoperative and early postoperative anesthetic management is required to prevent arterial hypoxemia, tracheal aspiration of foreign material, and respiratory arrest.

After abdominal or thoracic procedures, decreases in FRC and oxygenation are greatest in patients with preexisting lung disease, obese patients, smokers, and elderly patients, whether or not general anesthesia is used. Aggressive management of these patients with chest physiotherapy, lung expansion techniques, and effective analgesic therapy decreases the incidence of postoperative atelectasis, lobar collapse, pneumonia, and death. Future recommendations for prevention and treatment of postoperative pulmonary complications may include strategies to increase postoperative diaphragm function, specific directions for preoperative and postoperative nutritional support, and definitive techniques to prevent bacterial contamination of the airway.

REFERENCES

1. Alexander GD et al: Maximal inspiratory volume and postoperative pulmonary complications, Surg Gyn Obstet 152:601-603, 1981.
2. Alexander JI et al: The role of airway closure in postoperative hypoxaemia, Br J Anaesth 45:34-40, 1973.
3. Ali J, Yaffe CS, and Serrette C: The effect of transcutaneous electric nerve stimulation on postoperative pain and pulmonary function, Surgery 89:507-512, 1981.
4. Ali J et al: Consequences of postoperative alterations in respiratory mechanics, Am J Surg 128:376-382, 1974.
5. Barrera F et al: The distribution of ventilation, diffusion, and blood flow in obese patients with normal and abnormal blood gases, Am Rev Resp Dis 108:819-830, 1973.
6. Bartlett RH et al: Studies on the pathogenesis and prevention of postoperative pulmonary complications, Surg Gyn Obstet 137:926-933, 1973.
7. Beecher HK: Effect of laparotomy on lung volume, demonstration of a new type of pulmonary collapse, J Clin Invest 12:651-658, 1933.
8. Beecher HK: The measured effect of laparotomy on the respiration, J Clin Invest 12:639-650, 1933.
9. Beecher HK and Todd DT: A study of the deaths associated with anesthesia and surgery: based on a study of 599,548 anesthesias in ten institutions 1948-1952, inclusive, Ann Surg 140:2-34, 1954.
10. Bendixin HH, Hedley-Whyte J, and Laver MB: Impaired oxygenation in surgical patients during general anesthesia with controlled ventilation. A concept of atelectasis, N Engl J Med 269:991-996, 1963.
11. Benumof JL: Mechanism of decreased blod flow to atelectatic lung, J Appl Physiol 46:1047-1048, 1979.
12. Benumof JL and Wahrenbrock EA: Local effects of anesthetics on regional hypoxic pulmonary vasoconstriction, Anesthesiology 43:525-532, 1975.
13. Bergman NA and Tien YK: Contribution of the closure of pulmonary units to impaired oxygenation

during anesthesia, Anesthesiology 59:395-401, 1983.

14. Bevan PG: Post-operative pneumoperitoneum and pulmonary collapse, Br Med J 2:609-613, 1961.

15. Bindslev L et al: Ventilation-perfusion distribution during inhalation anesthesia. Effects of spontaneous breathing, mechanical ventilation and positive end-respiratory pressure, Acta Anaesthesiol Scand 25:360-371, 1981.

16. Boiden MP: Airway patency in the unconscious patient, Br J Anaesth 57:306-310, 1985.

17. Brismar B et al: Pulmonary densities during anesthesia with muscular relaxation—a proposal of atelectasis, Anesthesiology 62:422-428, 1985.

18. Bromage PR, Camporesi E, and Chestnut D: Epidural narcotics for postoperative analgesia, Anesth Analg 59:473-480, 1980.

19. Caplan RA and Long MC: Prolonged anesthesia—management and sequelae of a two-day general anesthetic, Anesth Analg 63:353-358, 1984.

20. Celli BR, Rodriguez KS, and Snider GL: A controlled trial of intermittent positive pressure breathing, incentive spirometry, and deep breathing exercises in preventing pulmonary complications after abdominal surgery, Am Rev Resp Dis 130:12-15, 1984.

21. Churchill ED and McNeil D: The reduction in vital capacity following operation, Surg Gyn Obstet 44:483-488, 1927.

22. Cohen MM et al: A survey of 112,000 anaesthetics at one teaching hospital (1975-1983), Can Anaesth Soc J 33:22-31, 1986.

23. Coleman DL: Control of postoperative pain. Nonnarcotic and narcotic alternatives and their effect on pulmonary function, Chest 92:520-528, 1987.

24. Colgan FJ and Mahoney PD: The effects of major surgery on cardiac output and shunting, Anesthesiology 31:213-221, 1969.

25. Cousins MJ et al: Metabolism and renal effects of enflurane in man, Anesthesiology 44:44-53, 1976.

26. Craig DB: Postoperative recovery of pulmonary function, Anesth Analg 60:46-52, 1981.

27. Craven JL et al: The evaluation of the incentive spirometer in the management of postoperative pulmonary complications, Br J Surg 61:793-797, 1974.

28. Cuschieri RJ, Morran CG, and McArdle CS: Transcutaneous electrical stimulation for postoperative pain, Ann R Coll Surg Engl 67:127-129, 1985.

29. Cuschieri RJ et al: Postoperative pain and pulmonary complications: comparison of three analgesic regimens, Br J Surg 72:495-498, 1985.

30. Davies RO, Edwards MW, and Lahiri S: Halothane depresses the response of carotid body chemoreceptors to hypoxia and hypercapnia in the cat, Anesthesiology 57:153-159, 1982.

31. Don HF, Wahba M, and Cuadrado L: The effects of anesthesia and 100 per cent oxygen on the functional residual capacity of the lungs, Anesthesiology 32:521-529, 1970.

32. Driks MR et al: Nosocomial pneumonia in intubated patients given sucralfate as compared with antacids or histamine type 2 blockers. The role of gastric colonization, N Engl J Med 317:1376-1382, 1987.

33. Dripps RD and Deming MV: Postoperative atelectasis and pneumonia: diagnosis, etiology and management based upon 1240 cases of upper abdominal surgery, Ann Surg 124:94-110, 1946.

34. Dueck R et al: The lung volume at which shunting occurs with inhalation anesthesia, Anesthesiology 69:854-861, 1988.

35. Dueck R et al: Altered distribution of pulmonary ventilation and blood flow following induction of inhalational anesthesia, Anesthesiology 52:113-125, 1980.

36. Duncan PG and Cohen MM: Postoperative complications: factors of significance to anaesthetic practice, Can J Anaesth 34:2-8, 1987.

37. Dureuil B et al: Effects of aminophylline on diaphragmatic dysfunction after upper abdominal surgery, Anesthesiology 62:242-256, 1985.

38. Dureuil B et al: Diaphragmatic contractility after upper abdominal surgery, J Appl Physiol 61:1775-1780, 1986.

39. Egbert LD and Bendixen HH: Effect of morphine on breathing pattern: a possible factor in atelectasis, J Am Med Assoc 188:485-488, 1964.

40. Engberg G and Wiklund L: Pulmonary complications after upper abdominal surgery: their prevention with intercostal blocks, Acta Anaesthesiol Scand 32:1-9, 1988.

41. Faust RJ and Nauss LA: Post-thoracotomy intercostal block: comparison of its effects on pulmonary function with those of intramuscular meperidine, Anesth Analg 55:542-546, 1976.

42. Fogh J et al: The predictive value of preoperative perfusion/ventilation scintigraphy, spirometry and x-ray of the lungs on postoperative pulmonary complications. A prospective study, Acta Anaesthesiol Scand 31:717-721, 1987.

43. Forbes AR: Humidification and mucus flow in the intubated trachea, Br J Anaesth 45:874-878, 1973.

44. Ford GT and Guenter CA: Toward prevention of postoperative pulmonary complications, Am Rev Resp Dis 130:4-5, 1984.

45. Ford GT et al: Diaphragm function after upper abdominal surgery in humans, Am Rev Resp Dis 127:431-436, 1983.

46. Fowkes FGR et al: Epidemiology in anaesthesia. III: Mortality risk in patients with coexisting physical disease, Br J Anaesth 54:819-824, 1982.

47. Froese AB and Bryan AC: Effects of anesthesia and paralysis on diaphragmatic mechanics in man, Anesthesiology 41:242-255, 1974.

48. Galloway DJ et al: A clinical assessment of electroanalgesia following abdominal operations, Surg Gyn Obstet 159:453-456, 1984.

49. Garcia-Valdecasas JC et al: Subcostal incision versus midline laparotomy in gallstone surgery: a prospective and randomized trial, Br J Surg 75:473-475, 1988.

50. Garibaldi RA et al: Risk factors for postoperative pneumonia, Am J Med 70:677-680, 1981.

51. Gass GD and Olsen GN: Preoperative pulmonary function testing to predict postoperative morbidity and mortality, Chest 89:127-135, 1986.

52. Gawley TH et al: Role of doxapram in reducing pulmonary complications after major surgery, Br Med J 1:122-124, 1976.

53. Gracey DR, Divertie MB, and Didier EP: Preoperative pulmonary preparation of patients with chronic obstructive pulmonary disease. A prospective study, Chest 76:123-129, 1979.

54. Hasenbos M et al: Post-operative analgesia by high thoracic epidural versus intramuscular nicomorphine after thoracotomy. Part III. The effects of per- and post-operative analgesia on morbidity, Acta Anaesthesiol Scand 31:608-615, 1987.

55. Hecker BR, Bjurstrom R, and Schoene RB: Effect of intercostal nerve blockade on respiratory mechanics and CO_2 chemosensitivity at rest and exercise, Anesthesiology 70:13-18, 1989.

56. Hedenstierna G et al: Functional residual capacity, thoracoabdominal dimensions, and central blood volume during general anesthesia with muscle paralysis and mechanical ventilation, Anesthesiology 62:247-254, 1985.

57. Hendolin H et al: The effect of thoracic epidural analgesia on respiratory function after cholecystectomy, Acta Anaesthesiol Scand 31:645-651, 1987.

58. Hewlett AM et al: Functional residual capacity during anaesthesia. II. Spontaneous respiration, Br J Anaesth 46:486-494, 1974.

59. Hewlett AM et al: Functional residual capacity during anaesthesia. III. Artificial ventilation, Br J Anaesth 46:495-503, 1974.

60. Hickey RF et al: Effects of halothane anesthesia on functional residual capacity and alveolar-arterial oxygen tension difference, Anesthesiology 38:20-24, 1973.

61. Hill L: The ciliary movement of the trachea studied in vitro: a measure of toxicity, Lancet 2:802-805, 1928.

62. Hwang J, St John WM, and Bartlett D: Respiratory-related hypoglossal nerve activity: influence of anesthetics, J Appl Physiol 55:785-792, 1983.

63. Jakobson S and Ivarsson I: Effects of intercostal nerve blocks (etidocaine 0.5%) on chest wall mechanics in cholecystectomized patients, Acta Anaesthesiol Scand 21:497-503, 1977.

64. Jayr C et al: Postoperative pulmonary complications: general anesthesia with postoperative parenteral morphine compared with epidural analgesia, Surgery 104:57-63, 1988.

65. Johanson WG et al: Nosocomial respiratory infections with gram negative bacilli: the significance of colonization of the respiratory tract, Ann Intern Med 77:701, 1972.

66. Jones JG et al: Rib cage movement during halothane anaesthesia in man, Br J Anaesth 51:399-407, 1979.

67. Jung R et al: Comparison of three methods of respiratory care following upper abdominal surgery, Chest 78:31-35, 1980.

68. Juno P et al: Closing capacity in awake and anesthetized-paralyzed man, J Appl Physiol 44:238-244, 1978.

69. Kirilloff LH et al: Does chest physical therapy work? Chest 88:436-444, 1985.

70. Knill RL and Clement JL: Site of selective action of halothane on the peripheral chemoreflex pathway in humans, Anesthesiology 61:121-126, 1984.

71. Knill RL and Clement JL: Ventilatory responses to acute metabolic acidemia in humans awake, sedated, and anesthetized with halothane, Anesthesiology 62:745-753, 1985.

72. Knill RL and Gelb AW: Ventilatory responses to hypoxia and hypercapnia during halothane sedation and anesthesia in man, Anesthesiology 49:244-251, 1978.

73. Laszlo G et al: The diagnosis and prophylaxis of pulmonary complications of surgical operations, Br J Surg 60:129-134, 1973.

74. Latimer RG et al: Ventilatory patterns and pulmonary complications after upper abdominal surgery determined by preoperative and postoperative computerized spirometry and blood gas analysis, Am J Surg 122:622-632, 1971.

75. Lunn JN, Hunter AR, and Scott DB: Anaesthesia-related surgical mortality, Anesthesiology 38:1090-1096, 1983.

76. Lyager S et al: Can postoperative pulmonary conditions be improved by treatment with the Bartlett-Edwards incentive spirometer after upper abdominal surgery? Acta Anaesthesiol Scand 23:312-319, 1979.

77. Maeda H et al: Diaphragm function after pulmonary resection: relationship to postoperative respiratory function, Am Rev Resp Dis 137:678-681, 1988.

78. Marshall BE and Marshall C: Anesthesia and pulmonary circulation. In Covino BG et al: Effects of Anesthesia, Baltimore, 1985, Waverly Press, Inc.

79. Martin LF et al: Postoperative pneumonia: determinants of mortality, Arch Surg 119:379-383, 1984.

80. Meyers JR et al: Changes in functional residual capacity of the lung after operation, Arch Surg 110:576-583, 1975.

81. Moote CA, Knill RL, and Clement J: Ventilatory compensation for continuous inspiratory resistive and elastic loads during halothane anesthesia in humans, Anesthesiology 64:582-589, 1986.

82. Muller N et al: Diaphragmatic muscle tone, J Appl Physiol 47:279-284, 1979.

83. Nishino T et al: Comparison of changes in the hypoglossal and the phrenic nerve activity in response to increasing depth of anesthesia in cats, Anesthesiology 60:19-24, 1984.

84. Nishino T et al: Effects of increasing depth of anaesthesia on phrenic nerve and hypoglossal nerve activity during the swallowing reflex in cats, Br J Anaesth 57:208-213, 1985.

85. Nishino T et al: Depression of the swallowing reflex during sedation and/or relative analgesia produced by inhalation of 50% nitrous oxide in oxygen, Anesthesiology 67:995-998, 1987.

86. Nunn JF: Hypoxaemia after general anaesthesia, Lancet 2:631-632, 1962.

87. Nunn JF and Ezi-Ashi TI: The respiratory effects of resistance to breathing in anesthetized man, Anesthesiology 22:174-185, 1961.

88. Nunn JF and Hill DW: Respiratory dead space and arterial to end-tidal CO_2 tension difference in anesthetized man, J Appl Physiol 15:383-389, 1960.

89. Nunn JF et al: The effect of inhalational anaesthetics on the swimming velocity of tetrahyemia pyriformis, J Cell Sci 15:537-554, 1974.

90. O'Connor M, Tattersall MP, and Carter JA: An evaluation of the incentive spirometer to improve lung function after cholecystectomy, Anaesthesia 43:785-787, 1988.

91. Parr NJ et al: Gram-negative intestinal bacteria, gastric colonization and postoperative pulmonary complications, J R Coll Surg Edinb 33:9-12, 1988.

92. Pasulka PS et al: The risks of surgery in obese patients, Ann Intern Med 104:540-546, 1986.

93. Pearce AC and Jones RM: Smoking and anesthesia: preoperative abstinence and perioperative morbidity, Anesthesiology 61:576-584, 1984.

94. Pflug AE et al: The effects of postoperative peridural analgesia on pulmonary therapy and pulmonary complications, Anesthesiology 41:8-17, 1974.

95. Poe RH et al: Can postoperative pulmonary complications after elective cholecystectomy be predicted? Am J Med Sci 295:29-34, 1988.

96. Pontoppidan H: Mechanical aids to lung expansion in nonintubated surgical patients, Am Rev Resp Dis 122:109-119, 1980.

97. Ravin MB: Comparison of spinal and general anesthesia for lower abdominal surgery in patients with chronic obstructive pulmonary disease, Anesthesiology 35:319-322, 1971.

98. Rawal N et al: Epidural morphine for postoperative pain relief: a comparative study with intramuscular narcotic and intercostal nerve block, Anesth Analg 61:93-98, 1982.

99. Ray S et al: Effects of obesity on respiratory function, Am Rev Resp Dis 128:501-506, 1983.

100. Rehder K, Sessler AD, and Marsh HM: General anesthesia and the lung, Am Rev Resp Dis 112:541-563, 1975.

101. Rehder K et al: Ventilation-perfusion relationship in young healthy awake and anesthetized-paralyzed man, J Appl Physiol 47:745-753, 1979.

102. Ricksten S et al: Effects of periodic airway pressure by mask on postoperative pulmonary function, Chest 89:774-781, 1986.

103. Road JD et al: Diaphragm function and respiratory response after upper abdominal surgery in dogs, J Appl Physiol 57:576-582, 1984.

104. Rooney S et al: A comparison of pulmonary function tests for postthoracotomy pain using cryoanalgesia and transcutaneous nerve stimulation, Ann Thorac Surg 41:204-207, 1986.

105. Rosenberg PH, Heino A, and Scheinin B: Comparison of intramuscular analgesia, intercostal block, epidural morphine and on-demand-i.v.-fentanyl in the control of pain after upper abdominal surgery, Acta Anaesthesiol Scand 28:603-607, 1984.

106. Roukema JA, Carol EJ, and Prins JG: The prevention of pulmonary complications after upper abdominal surgery in patients with noncompromised pulmonary status, Arch Surg 123:30-34, 1988.

107. Sackner M et al: Effects of oxygen breathing and tracheal intubation on tracheal mucous velocity of anesthetized dogs, Bull Eur Physiopathol Respir 9:403, 1973.

108. Schmid ER and Rehder K: General anesthesia and the chest wall, Anesthesiology 55:668-675, 1981.

109. Schwieger I et al: Absence of benefit of incentive spirometry in low-risk patients undergoing elective cholecystectomy, Chest 89:652-656, 1986.

110. Shulman M et al: Postthoracotomy pain and pulmonary function following epidural and systemic morphine, Anesthesiology 61:569-575, 1984.

111. Simonneau G et al: Diaphragm dysfunction induced by upper abdominal surgery: role of postoperative pain, Am Rev Resp Dis 128:899-903, 1983.

112. Spence AA and Smith G: Postoperative analgesia and lung function: a comparison of morphine with extradural block, Br J Anaesth 43:144-148, 1971.

113. Stein M and Cassara EL: Preoperative pulmonary function and therapy for surgery patients, J Am Med Assoc 211:787-790, 1970.

114. Stier A et al: Urinary excretion of bromide in halothane anesthesia, Anesth Analg 43:723-728, 1964.

115. Stock MC et al: Comparison of continuous positive airway pressure, incentive spirometry, and conservative therapy after cardiac operations, Crit Care Med 12:969-972, 1984.

116. Stock MC et al: Prevention of postoperative pulmonary complications with CPAP, incentive spirometry, and conservative therapy, Chest 87:151-157, 1985.

117. Strandberg A et al: Atelectasis during anaesthesia and in the postoperative period, Acta Anaesthesiol Scand 30:154-158, 1986.

118. Strandberg A et al: Constitutional factors promoting development of atelectasis during anaesthesia, Acta Anaesthesiol Scand 31:21-24, 1987.

119. Sykes MK et al: The effect of inhalational anaesthetics on hypoxic pulmonary vasocontriction and pulmonary vascular resistance in the perfused lungs of the dog and cat, Br J Anaesth 44:776-787, 1972.

120. Tarhan S et al: Risk of anesthesia and surgery in patients with chronic bronchitis and chronic obstructive pulmonary disease, Surgery 74:720-726, 1973.

121. Tisi GM: Preoperative evaluation of pulmonary function: validity, indications, and benefits, Am Rev Resp Dis 119:293-310, 1979.

122. Tisi GM: Preoperative identification and evaluation of the patient with lung disease, Med Clin North Am 71:399-412, 1987.

123. Tokics L et al: Lung collapse and gas exchange during general anesthesia: effects of spontaneous breathing, muscle paralysis, and positive end-expiratory pressure, Anesthesiology 66:157-167, 1987.

124. Toledo-Pereyra LH and Demeester TR: Prospective randomized evaluation of intrathoracic intercostal nerve block with bupivacaine on postoperative ventilatory function, Ann Thorac Surg 27:203-205, 1979.

125. Torrington KG and Henderson CJ: Perioperative respiratory therapy (PORT): program of preoperative risk assessment and individualized postoperative care, Chest 93:946-951, 1988.

126. Tusiewicz K, Bryan AC, and Froese AB: Contributions of changing rib cage-diaphragm interactions

127. Van De Water JM et al: Prevention of postoperative pulmonary complications, Surg Gyn Obstet 135: 229-233, 1972.

128. Vaughan RW, Bauer S, and Wise L: Volume and pH of gastric juice in obese patients, Anesthesiology 43:686-689, 1975.

129. Vellody VPS et al: Compliances of human rib cage and diaphragm-abdomen pathways in relaxed versus paralyzed states, Am Rev Resp Dis 118:479-491, 1978.

130. Viale JP et al: Oxygen cost of breathing in postoperative patients: pressure support ventilation vs continuous positive airway pressure, Chest 93:506-509, 1988.

131. Wahba WM, Don HF, and Craig DB: Post-operative epidural analgesia: effects on lung volumes, Can Anaesth Soc J 22:519-527, 1975.

132. Wahba WM et al: The cardio-respiratory effects of thoracic epidural anaesthesia, Can Anaesth Soc J 19:8-19, 1972.

133. Warner MA, Divertie MB, and Tinker JH: Preoperative cessation of smoking and pulmonary complications in coronary artery bypass patients, Anesthesiology 60:380-383, 1984.

134. Welchew EA: On-demand analgesia. A double-blind comparison of on-demand intravenous fentanyl with regular intramuscular morphine, Anaesthesia 38:19-25, 1983.

135. Westbrook PR et al: Effects of anesthesia and muscle paralysis on respiratory mechanics in normal man, J Appl Physiol 34:81-86, 1973.

136. Wightman JAK: A prospective survey of the incidence of postoperative pulmonary complications, Br J Surg 55:85-91, 1968.

137. Wilcox P et al: Phrenic nerve function and its relationship to atelectasis after coronary artery bypass surgery, Chest 93:693-698, 1988.

138. Windsor JA and Hill GL: Risk factors for postoperative pneumonia: the importance of protein depletion, Ann Surg 208:209-214, 1988.

139. Winnie AP et al: Chemical respirogenesis. II. Reversal of postoperative hypoxemia with the "pharmacologic sigh," Anesth Analg 50:1043-1055, 1971.

to the ventilatory depression of halothane anesthesia, Anesthesiology 47:327-337, 1977.

CHAPTER **16**

Prevention of Perioperative Infectious Complications

MARIA D. ALLO

Patient factors predisposing to infection
  Skin
  Eyes and ears
  Mouth
  Nose and nasopharynx
  Gastrointestinal tract
  Small intestine/biliary tract

Colon
Genitourinary tract
Epidemiologic factors
Prophylactic antibiotics
  Systemic prophylaxis
  Bowel preparation
  Intraperitoneal antibiotics

Infection accounts for much of the morbidity and mortality associated with surgical procedures and has significant economic impact as well. It has been estimated in one study[5] that the indirect and direct costs for nosocomial infections in 1967 was about $9.8 billion in the aggregate and about $6000 to $10,000 per patient. Needless to say, these costs have only increased with time.

The first two sections of this chapter discuss the causes of preventible surgical infections, which include patient, environmental, and technical factors. Understanding and awareness of these issues may in some cases prevent these untoward complications.

The last section deals with the indications and limitations of prophylactic antibiotics.

PATIENT FACTORS PREDISPOSING TO INFECTION

Prevention of infection in the surgical patient ideally begins with the preoperative visit. At that time evidence of conditions known to alter host defenses

in the surgical patient should be sought, and if possible modified. Attention must also be paid to the infection status of the patient before the operation. The presence of chronic or subacute infection preoperatively is a relative contraindication to the performance of an elective operation, and an absolute contraindication if prosthetic grafts or devices are to be inserted, except in those instances when the operation is being performed as part of the treatment for the infection. During the preoperative visit, assessment is made regarding special precautions or modifications of technique to reduce infectious risk, for example, avoidance of nasotracheal intubation and nasogastric tubes, when possible, in patients with a history of chronic or recurrent sinus infection.

Any underlying process or surgical procedure that disrupts the usual barriers to contamination within the body increase perioperative infection risk. A brief review of systems will focus on the local factors that provide natural barriers to infection and, when violated, constitute increased risk for infection.

212

Skin

Intact skin, though sometimes heavily colonized by bacteria on its external surface, will not permit absorption of microorganisms internally. The skin flora has both resident and transient bacteria. The transient bacteria generally come from the environment and remain on the skin surfaces. In intact skin they do not compete with the resident flora for niches in the microecosystem of the skin surface. Cleansing of the skin surface usually eliminates them. The resident flora, in contrast, occupy specific niches and actually facilitate the barrier function of the skin. For example, diphtheroids grow adjacent to sebaceous glands and break down sebum into free fatty acids that inhibit many nonresident bacteria. In general, large inocula are needed to infect intact tissue. In studies in which live organisms are injected into the soft tissue of guinea pigs, more than 10^9 *Staphylococcus aureus* are required to produce consistent infection, and this is independent of the site inoculated.[22] Factors that increase susceptibility to soft tissue infections include breaks in the skin, decreases in blood supply or tissue perfusion,[8] alterations in lymphatic drainage caused by lymphedema or venous stasis,[7] trauma, even in the absence of a break in the skin,[11] and some occupational exposures.[20] A diverse lot including animal handlers, bakers, hairdressers, dock workers, janitors, upholsterers, and physicians have occupational exposures demonstrated to increase risk for skin infection.

The preoperative appearance of the skin should be carefully noted. The presence of folliculitis, furuncles, or carbuncles suggests infection with *S. aureus* until proved otherwise. Since most healthy patients are rarely affected by those conditions, a history of severe or recurrent infection should prompt investigation for diabetes mellitus, hypogammaglobulinemia, Job syndrome, or neutrophil defect. Not uncommonly, poor hygiene, skin zoonoses (lice, scabies), seborrhea, poor nutrition, hyperhidrosis, and obesity are associated. Preoperative management should include frequent soap and water showers to reduce overall colonization and sterile dressings to any open or draining lesions. Elective procedures should be postponed until draining lesions resolve.

Decubitus ulcers are another potential source of sepsis in the postoperative period, and are sometimes present in elderly or debilitated patients coming to the hospital for surgery to correct other conditions.

Care to reduce local pressure and maintain local hygiene should be instituted before sepsis ensues. Early mobilization, if possible, and frequent turning with inspection of pressure points should be done perioperatively.

Eyes and Ears

The production of tears and the ability to blink provide very effective local defense against infection in the eye. Disruption of these activities eliminates the mechanical, chemical, and immunologic factors that make eye infections relatively infrequent.[16]

A history of chronic "ear infections" should prompt investigation preoperatively for causes of eustachian tube obstruction, especially chronic sinusitis, allergies, or chronic nasopharyngitis. If infection is found, treatment with decongestants and antibiotics should precede elective surgery, particularly operations in which endotracheal, nasotracheal, or nasogastric intubation is planned. Intraoperatively, inadvertent instillation of fluid or betadine into the ear canal can produce a situation akin to "swimmer's ear" or cause local skin irritation and breakdown that can progress to external otitis. Postoperatively, prolonged nasotracheal or nasogastric intubation may be associated with acute sinusitis or otitis.

Mouth

Poor oral hygiene profoundly affects the mouth flora with respect to both types and numbers of organisms found. The presence of dental plaque and/or caries has been associated with significantly increased numbers of anaerobic bacteria. Patients with such an altered flora are at increased risk for anaerobic pulmonary infections associated with aspiration or altered host defenses secondary to general anesthesia.[25] Removal of carious teeth when indicated, and aggressive oral hygiene to treat gingivitis and/or periodontitis should be initiated before elective surgery, especially when insertion of a vascular graft or prosthetic heart valve or other device is contemplated. Bacteremia with seeding of metastatic sites including prostheses commonly occurs from dental sources and is a major source of endocarditis. Because correction of dental problems is associated with bacteremia, even when prophylactic antibiotics are used (for example, in patients with vascular grafts), failure to correct known dental problems before surgery puts the patient at unnecessary risk once the prosthesis is in place.

Other mouth infections are of concern perioperatively. Sialadenitis is associated with decreased salivary flow, increased viscosity of salivary secretion, and mechanical obstruction of the salivary ducts. In patients with a history of sialadenitis preoperatively, one should try to elicit factors that cause chronic irritation to the salivary glands such as cigarette smoking and factors that cause chronic infection such as poor dental hygiene or use of drugs that diminish salivary flow (for example, digitalis, or sympathomimetic drugs). Systemic diseases that affect salivary flow include cystic fibrosis, cirrhosis, gout, diabetes, and adrenal cortical disease.

Postoperative dehydration can precipitate acute suppurative parotitis, which is caused by ascending infection along the parotid duct, usually with *S. aureus* (90%) or *Streptococcus pyogenes*. The clinical picture is one of a large tender parotid with erythema of the overlying facial skin. Patients should be rehydrated and treated with antibiotics directed against *S. aureus*. Rarely this condition requires treatment with radiation, or surgical drainage.

Nose and Nasopharynx

In a patient without clinically apparent infection, nasal organisms play little role in increasing infection risk associated with surgery.

Gastrointestinal Tract

Normally the low pH of the stomach effectively prevents heavy colonization of the stomach with bacteria. Distal obstruction, H_2 blockers or other conditions that raise gastric pH are associated with significant increases in the number of bacteria recovered from the stomach. In general, however, prophylactic antibiotics are not used in gastric surgery unless the patient is obstructed or achlorhydric.

Small Intestine / Biliary Tract

The upper gastrointestinal tract is sparsely colonized with bacteria, and the biliary tract is sterile in the absence of biliary tract disease or surgical intervention that alters communication between the biliary tract and the GI tract, for example, choledochoenterostomy. The jejunum has a predominant gram-positive flora consisting of small numbers (<100,000) of enterococci, lactobacilli, and diphtheroids. Gram-negative bacilli and strict anaerobes are not usually present. Enterobacteriaceae are not present proximal to the ileum but are found in increasing numbers as one samples distally. In the distal ileum about half of normal people are colonized with *Candida albicans*.

Small bowel injury is rarely a cause of significant peritonitis. In patients with inflammatory bowel disease, however, abscess is a problem. Nagler[15] estimated that between 12% and 28% of patients with Crohn's disease develop enteroparietal, intramesenteric, or interloop abscesses. There is no similar incidence of abscess formation with ulcerative colitis. The usefulness of bowel preps for small bowel operations to prevent wound infections is debatable. There are no studies looking at wound infection rates after parenteral antibiotics, and the largest study of bowel prep for small bowel operations had its lowest wound infection rate in the untreated control group who received neither mechanical prep nor antibiotics.[18] Probably in the absence of a bacterial overgrowth syndrome special bowel prep is unnecessary for small bowel operations.

Colon

No part of the body packs as many bacteria per unit volume as the colon (10^{11} to 10^{12} CFU/CC). It has been estimated that bacteria comprise one third of the dry weight of human feces.[13] Leakage of colon contents is virtually always associated with inoculation of large numbers of bacteria, and for this reason reduction of the colonic bacterial load has become an important goal in the prevention of infectious complications of colon operations. Most bowel preps in use today involve both mechanical cleansing and intraluminal or systemic antibiotics.

Genitourinary Tract

Nosocomial bacteriuria, and subsequent urinary infection is the most common hospital acquired infection.[14] Preoperative urinalysis should indicate presence of urinary tract infection. In addition, history of burning, frequency, nocturia, or urgency should be sought as part of the preoperative evaluation. Active urinary tract infection should be treated before performance of elective operation. Patients at risk for urinary tract infection include those with urologic conditions associated with obstruction or with communication between the gastrointestinal and genitourinary tracts, and men with chronic prostatitis. A history of recurrent nephrolithiasis and persistently high urinary pH suggest infection with urea-splitting bacteria such as *Morganella* or *Proteus*.

Instrumentation and indwelling catheters predispose to bacteriuria and increase risk of infection. In males condom catheters should be used when incontinence (rather than urinary retention) is the indication for a urinary drainage device.

EPIDEMIOLOGIC FACTORS

The largest and most frequently quoted study looking at technical factors predisposing to wound infections was done at Foothills Hospital by Cruse and Foord.[6] They studied 23,649 wounds and cited an overall infection rate of about 4.7%. Factor analysis was done to determine what factors were contributory. It was found that there was no decrease in infection rate with showering; the infection rate was about 2% in patients showering with ordinary bath soap and in patients who did not shower. However, the rate was cut roughly in half if an antiseptic detergent was used. Skin preparation has also been an area of investigation. The ideal disinfectant should have a high germicidal potential, a broad antimicrobial spectrum, and should be able to penetrate well into the spaces in which disinfection is desirable. Among commonly used agents, hexachlorophene is probably the most commonly used phenol-type disinfectant. On contact it is bacteriostatic but requires prolonged contact to exert its bacteriocidal potential. In addition to killing bacteria it is also effective against most pathogenic fungi. Furthermore, it does not lose its potency in the presence of soap. The major disadvantage of hexachlorophene is its ability to be absorbed through the skin. It has been reported to cause neurologic symptoms in some patients. Consequently the FDA has restricted over-the-counter sales of some hexachlorophene-containing products and strongly warns against its use on burned or denuded skin, on mucous membranes or on newborns because of its ability to accumulate with repeated use. Many hospitals have substituted other agents for hexachlorophene for scrubbing. Because prolonged contact is required for maximal efficacy it is not used very frequently as an antiseptic for the operative site.

Alcohol was the principal topical disinfectant until relatively recently. It has the advantage of being bacteriocidal, cheap, colorless, and able to exert a cleansing action. The main disadvantage of alcohol is that it has no effect on spores, although it is effective against bacteria and many viruses and fungi. When used as a skin preparation, solutions of greater than 70% isopropyl alcohol are probably most effective.

Iodine has been used as an antiseptic since the nineteenth century and is extremely effective as a bacteriocidal and a sporicidal agent. It is also effective against fungi, viruses, and protozoans. Acidic solutions increase its efficiency although it is effective over a wide pH range. Free iodine is used as 2% iodine tincture or as iodine in an aqueous solution. In general, strong iodine solutions (greater than 5% iodine) are not used as skin preparations because they may cause burns to the skin. Iodophors are iodines combined with stabilizing agents that will free iodine once it is in solution. The most common combination is that of iodine and polyvinylpyrrolidone (povidone iodine), which releases free iodine when it is dissolved in water. There is no evidence that definitively shows that this form of iodine is more effective and/or less toxic than using aqueous or alcohol solutions or free iodine. Iodophors need to be in contact with the skin for at least 5 minutes to provide reliable degerming whereas elemental iodine solutions work much more quickly when applied topically.

Chlorhexidine is a biguanidine substance that is used for skin degerming and is effective against gram-positive bacteria and most gram-negative bacteria. It seems to work well even in the presence of organic matter including pus or blood and is not absorbed through intact skin. One of its major advantages is that 15 to 30 seconds are required to give about a 99% reduction in skin bacterial counts and it remains on the skin for several hours after contact and retains its activity there. The major drawback to its use is that it is irritating to the eyes and can cause deafness if instilled into the ear of a person with a perforated tympanic membrane.

Finally the use of quaternary ammonium compounds such as benzalkonium chloride has fallen out of favor, despite the fact that they are relatively harmless and inexpensive, because they are fairly inactive against gram-negative bacteria and are rapidly inactivated by soap or other foreign bodies on the skin. Consequently, they are used primarily for degerming of denuded skin or mucous membranes, for bladder irrigation, or for retention lavage, and are very rarely used as a primary skin degerming agent.

At the present time, the procedure recommended most commonly consists of cleansing the area to be prepared with soap or nonirritating detergent followed by an application of a degerming agent. The skin wash can be done as a preoperative shower or cleansing before coming to the operating room followed by painting of the skin in the operating room, or the entire procedure can be carried out as part of the preoperative preparation in the operating room.

Studies by Seropian et al[23] have suggested that shaving immediately before operation is an effective way to remove body hair and that doing so in the operating room prevented bacterial growth in razor nicks. Seropian's study found that shaved patients had a higher infection rate than those who were not shaved and that use of a depilatory also produced a very low infection rate. Clipping of the body hair rather than shaving decreases the infection rate (compared to patients who are shaved). Present recommendations are (1) if the patient is to be shaved it should be done at the time of operation and not the night before, ideally less than two hours before operation, (2) clipping of the hair is better than shaving because it leaves no razor nicks, which are sites for bacterial growth, and (3) not shaving does not in any way add to the risk of infection and in fact may result in a lower operative infection rate than shaving.

Paskin and Lerner[19] published a study that found that the incidence of wound infection doubled with the use of adherent plastic drapes and this may be attributed to the occlusive dressing allowing bacteria to proliferate underneath the drape or to the use of a nonsterile solution to get the drapes to stick. The major advantage of these drapes is that they demarcate the area designated for operation, and prepped by cleansing and degerming, as described above. Cloth drapes and plastic drapes serve the same purpose, and one has no major advantage over the other as long as the drapes are not soaked, (soaking causes bacteria to strike through the barrier), and the draping does not become dislodged and therefore expose areas that have not been topically prepared.

Just as preparing the patient's skin is important, so is it helpful to cleanse and disinfect the hands of personnel coming into contact with the surgical wound. Gloves protect the surgeon from contact with the patient's secretions but are less important than skin cleansing as protection for the patient against contamination from the surgeon's hand. The cleansing solutions mentioned previously for patient skin preparation have also been used for surgical handwashing. Of those cited, chlorhexidine is probably

the agent of choice since it requires brief contact with the skin to be effective, leaves a residual film on the skin, and has a broad antibacterial spectrum.

Studies have been done to look at factors in the hospital environment that affect infection rate. The most important factor identified was the individual surgeon. Intraoperative breaks in technique appear to have the greatest influence on postoperative wound infection rates. Surgical wards and postoperative dressing techniques did not affect clean wound infection rates. Cruse and Foord's study[6] showed a twofold increase in infection rate when preoperative hospital stay increased from 1 day to 1 week. It did not, however, address differences in severity of illness, which would prompt longer preoperative hospital stay. In a similar vein, length of operating time has been correlated with increased infection risk. Again, the reasons for the procedure taking a long time may, in fact, be more important than the time itself.

The introduction of foreign bodies or other contaminants at the time of operation has been shown to increase the likelihood of infection. Foreign bodies in the wound include hemostatic agents, suture material, glove powder, lint, drains, and coagulum. When drains are used, closed suction drainage is preferable to open drains, such as Penrose drains.[1]

The impact of good surgical technique in the prevention of infection has been addressed in many studies. The importance of gentle handling of tissue, meticulous hemostasis, and adherence to principles of asepsis are obvious.

PROPHYLACTIC ANTIBIOTICS

The use of antibiotics as prophylaxis against wound infection was controversial until relatively recently. Even though the literature is replete with studies whose conclusions conflict, a sound body of literature and experience defines the indications and techniques of antibiotic prophylaxis.

Systemic Prophylaxis

Experimental studies by Burke and colleagues[2,12] established that perioperative inhibition of host defenses occurs within a limited time frame, and that administration of antibiotics must correspond to this critical period to be effective. It was shown that antibiotics given *after* contamination with staphylococci were ineffective. Therefore, to be effective, prophylactic antibiotics directed against the most likely contaminating pathogens must be present in appropriate levels before the contamination. There was no advantage to continuing antibiotics beyond the immediate perioperative period, and in fact there are disadvantages to doing so. The disadvantages include selection of resistant organisms, drug reactions, and superinfection.

Subsequently, many clnical studies have confirmed the observations of Burke and shown that in select cases antibiotics appropriately chosen and timed decreased the incidence of postoperative wound sepsis when compared to no antibiotics or placebo. The presentation of a specific advantage of one antibiotic over another for prophylaxis has been much harder to demonstrate. A review by Solomkin et al[24] evaluated studies comparing efficacy of antibiotics used empirically in intraabdominal sepsis and indicated several flaws common to studies of antibiotic prophylaxis including small sample size and poor patient stratification. Nevertheless, randomized prospective studies have established the efficacy of antibiotic prophylaxis for several specific indications. These include potentially contaminated abdominal operations,[9] and gastric and duodenal procedures, in patients who are achlorhydric or who have low bacterial counts in their gastric aspirate.[17]

The usefulness of prophylactic antibiotics in patients undergoing biliary operations is more controversial. Most authors consider them of value in so-called "high-risk" patients. These include patients presenting with biliary obstruction and elderly (over 70 years of age) patients. Patients undergoing routine cholecystectomy may not benefit from antibiotic administration preoperatively and studies can be found that support and refute their use. Chetlin and Elliott[3] define criteria to determine risk of postoperative infection in patients undergoing biliary operations that have proved helpful. Another area of controversy is the need for antibiotic prophylaxis for acute appendectomy. There is currently no consensus as to whether or which antibiotics are appropriate in this setting.

Although most authors concede that prophylaxis is indicated for elective operations on the colon, there is some controversy as to whether intraluminal bowel preparation precludes the need for concomitant systemic antibiotic prophylaxis. This issue is discussed later in the section on bowel preparation.

Systemic antibiotics are not generally recommended for clean procedures. Clean procedures are defined as operations that do not violate a colonized area of the body and whose risk of infection is less than 1%. Examples include inguinal herniorrhaphy, thyroidectomy, or mastectomy. There are no studies showing a difference in infection rate for patients undergoing clean procedures who have received antibiotics as compared to those who were not treated. The exception is patients with prosthetic grafts in place, or being inserted as part of the procedure. In such patients the risk of infection remains less than 1% but the consequences of infection, should it occur, are potentially disastrous. Thus prophylactic antibiotics are generally used in patients undergoing arterial reconstruction, joint replacement, or cardiac valve replacements.

Patients operated upon following penetrating trauma to the abdomen probably benefit from antibiotic administration preoperatively. The patients at greatest risk for infection are those who have sustained colon injuries. Since these patients frequently cannot be identified preoperatively, and since the risks associated with single dose antibiotic administration are few, preoperative antibiotics administered before surgery in doses adequate to provide good tissue and blood levels are probably indicated. Studies comparing specific antibiotics or combinations have failed to show a consistent difference in efficacy. Therefore, choice of drug should be predicated on cost and safety criteria.

Among obstetrical patients Ledger[10] has shown that there was a decrease in infectious complications in premenopausal women undergoing hysterectomy when a cephalosporin was administered preoperatively.

In summary, prophylactic antibiotics are useful when there is a high probability of postoperative wound infection. To be effective, the drug should be administered before surgery and discontinued shortly thereafter. Finally, the choice of antibiotic is flexible. Consideration should include low toxicity, ease of administration, coverage of the expected potential pathogens, and low cost.

Bowel Preparation

Operations on the colon have been associated with a high incidence of wound infection, and as early as the 1940s attention was directed toward decreasing septic complications. Poth is credited with defining the characteristics of the "ideal intestinal antiseptic," which would have rapid action, be minimally absorbed systemically, minimally toxic, active intraluminally in the intestine, and cover a broad antibacterial spectrum.[21] Subsequently, several prospective, randomized, double blind studies established the efficacy of several bowel preparation regimens that used both mechanical cleansing and oral, relatively nonabsorbable antibiotics.[4,26] These studies clearly demonstrated a reduced incidence of wound sepsis in the antibiotic treated group as compared to the control group who had mechanical preparation only. More recent studies have used various oral antibiotic combinations with no substantive differences in outcome as long as both aerobic and anaerobic components of the gut flora were covered. The issue of systemic prophylaxis in addition to oral antibiotics plus mechanical cleansing is unresolved.

Intraperitoneal Antibiotics

There are no definitive experimental data to support the use of intraperitoneal antimicrobial agents, nor is there any published work to suggest that topical agents are better prophylaxis than either systemic or intraluminal regimens. Unfortuantely most of the studies done have not excluded patients who received systemic or intestinal antibiotics.

REFERENCES

1. Alexander JW, Korelitz J, and Alexander NS: Prevention of wound infections. A case for closed suction drainage to remove wound fluids deficient in opsonic proteins, Am J Surg 132:59-63, 1976.
2. Burke JF: The effective period of preventive antibiotic action in experimental incisions and dermal lesions, Surgery 50:161-168, 1961.
3. Chetlin SH and Elliott DW: Preoperative antibiotics in biliary surgery, Arch Surg 107:319-323, 1973.
4. Clarke JS et al: Preoperative oral antibiotics reduce septic complications of colon operations: results of prospective randomized, double blind clinical study, Ann Surg 186:251-259, 1977.
5. Cruse PJE: Wound infections: epidemiology and clinical characteristics. In Howard RJ and Simmons RL (editors): *Surgical Infectious Diseases*, ed 2, East Norwalk, Conn, 1988, Appleton & Lange.
6. Cruse PJE and Foord R: A five year prospective study of 23,649 surgical wounds, Arch Surg 107:206, 1973.
7. Delong TG and Simmons RL: Role of lymphatics in bacterial clearance from early soft tissue infection, Arch Surg 117:123-128, 1982.
8. Duncan WC, McBride ME, and Knox JM: Experimental production of infections in human, J Invest Dermatol 54:319-323, 1970.
9. Gugliemo BJ et al: Antibiotic prophylaxis in surgical procedures—a critical analysis of the literature, Arch Surg 118:943-955, 1983.
10. Ledger WJ, Sweet RL, and Headington JT: Prophylactic cephaloridine in the prevention of postoperative pelvic infections in premenopausal women undergoing vaginal hysterectomy, Am J Obstet Gynecol 115:766-774, 1973.
11. Madden JE et al: Studies in the management of the contaminated wound: IV resistance to infection of surgical wounds made by knife, electrosurgery and laser, Am J Surg 119:222-224, 1970.
12. Miles AA, Miles EM, and Burke J: The value and duration of defense reactions of the skin to the primary lodgement of bacteria, Br J Exp Pathol 38:79-96, 1957.
13. Moore WEC and Haldeman LV: Human fecal flora: the normal flora of 20 Japanese-Hawaiians, Appl Microbiol 27:961-979, 1974.
14. Mulholland SG and Bruun JA: A study of urinary tract infections, J Urol 110:245-248, 1973.
15. Nagler SM and Poticha SM: Intraabdominal abscess in regional enteritis, Am J Surg 137:350-354, 1979.
16. Newell FW: Physiology and biochemistry of the eye. In Newell FW: Ophthalmology principles and concepts, ed 4, St. Louis, 1978, The CV Mosby Co.
17. Nichols RL et al: Efficacy of antibiotic prophylaxis in gastroduodenal surgery, Ann Surg 182:557-561, 1975.
18. Parker TH and O'Leary JP: Effect of preparation of the small bowel on microflora and postoperative wound infections, SGO 146:379-382, 1978.
19. Paskin DL and Lerner HJ: A prospective study of wound infections, Am J Surg 35:627-629, 1969.
20. Pittelkon R: Occupational dermatoses. In Zenz C (editor): Occupations medicine, Chicago, 1975, Year Book Medical Publishers, Inc.
21. Poth EJ: Intestinal antisepsis in surgery, JAMA 153:1516-1521, 1953.
22. Roettinger W et al: Role of inoculation site as a determinant of infection in soft tissue wounds, Am J Surg 126:354-358, 1973.
23. Seropian R and Reynolds BM: Wound infections after preoperative depilatory versus razor preparation, Am J Surg 121:251-254, 1971.
24. Solomkin J et al: Antibiotic trials in intraabdominal infections: a critical evaluation of study design and outcome reporting, Ann Surg 200:29-39, 1984.
25. Sommers HM: Indigenous microbiota in humans. In Howard RJ and Simmons RL (editors): Surgical infectious diseases, ed 2, Norwalk, Conn, 1988, Appleton & Lange.
26. Washington JA et al: Effect of preoperative antibiotic regimen on development of infection after intestinal surgery: prospective randomized, double blind study, Ann Surg 180:567-572, 1974.

PART FOUR

SPECIFIC PROBLEMS

CHAPTER **17**

Coronary Artery Disease

BRIAN A. ROSENFELD

Myocardial infarction (MI) is a frequent cause of mortality within the perioperative period. In addition, complications from myocardial ischemia (pulmonary edema and cardiac arrhythmias) together with MI, are major causes of morbidity and lengthened hospital stay.

Successful perioperative management requires preoperative identification of those patients with coronary artery disease (CAD) who are likely to develop perioperative ischemia. Careful clinical assessment may need to be supplemented by noninvasive and invasive testing. Results of such an evaluation are then used to determine whether to proceed with the planned surgery, a more limited surgical procedure,

or myocardial revascularization. These studies will also serve to guide perioperative management strategies.

In this chapter, I examine (1) preoperative risk assessment, including both routine and specialized testing, (2) criteria for altering plans for surgery, (3) determinants of perioperative ischemia, (4) modalities for monitoring and diagnosing ischemia, and (5) the management of patients at risk before, during, and after surgery.

PREOPERATIVE RISK ASSESSMENT

The risk to all surgical patients of suffering a perioperative MI is approximately 0.13% to

TABLE 17-1. Computation of multifactorial index score to estimate cardiac risk in noncardiac surgery

	Points
S_3 gallop or jugular venous distention on preoperative physical examination	11
Transmural or subendocardial myocardial infarction in the previous 6 months	10
Premature ventricular beats, more than 5/min documented at any time	7
Rhythm other than sinus or presence of premature atrial contractions on last preoperative electrocardiogram	7
Age over 70 years	5
Emergency operation	4
Intrathoracic, intraperitoneal, or aortic site of surgery	3
Evidence of important valvular aortic stenosis*	3
Poor general medical condition†	3

From Goldman L: Cardiac risks and complications of noncardiac surgery, Ann Intern Med 98:504-513, 1983.
*Findings of a cardiologist's examination, noninvasive testing, or cardiac catheterization.
†As evidenced by electrolyte abnormalities (potassium, < 3.0 mEq/L; HCO_3, < 20 mEq/L), renal insufficiency (blood urea nitrogen, > 50 mg/dl; creatinine, > 3.0 mg/dl), abnormal blood gases (PO_2, < 60 mm Hg; PCO_2, > 50 mm Hg), abnormal liver status (elevated aspartate transaminase or signs at physical examination of chronic liver disease), or any condition that has caused the patient to be chronically bedridden.

TABLE 17-2. Goldman multifactorial risk assessment

Class	Points	Risk	
I	0-5	0.7%	Complication
		0.2%	Death
II	6-12	5.0%	Complication
		2.0%	Death
III	13-25	11%	Complication
		2.0%	Death
IV	≥ 26	22%	Complication
		56%	Death

From Goldman L: Cardiac risks and complications of noncardiac surgery, Ann Intern Med 98:504-513, 1983.
Complications were defined as myocardial infarction, pulmonary edema or ventricular tachycardia.

0.66%.[100,104] Patients who have previously sustained an MI have a greater risk, typically between 4% and 8%, and the risk increases substantially if the infarction has been within 6 months.[96,100] The perioperative mortality associated with reinfarction has been reported to be 23% to 70%.[2,104] However, many of these studies were retrospective and conducted at a time when invasive hemodynamic monitoring and postoperative intensive care unit (ICU) observation were not common. In contrast, two more recent studies, one by Wells and Kaplan and the other by Rao et al, have reported less than 2% incidence of reinfarction with a previous MI.[83,109] In patients with a recent MI (0 to 6 months), they found a reinfarction rate of less than 6%. In both studies, patients were fully evaluated and their physiologic status was optimized preoperatively. Most patients underwent intraoperative monitoring with pulmonary artery and systemic arterial catheters. Blood pressure, heart rate, cardiac rhythm, and hematocrit levels were kept within a narrow range. In addition, most patients were monitored for up to 96 hours postoperatively in an ICU, where these hemodynamic and physiologic parameters were kept from fluctuating widely. Some authors have questioned the conclusions of Rao et al, because they used historical controls and because of the type of surgery their patients underwent (10% ophthalmologic).[60] Nevertheless, it seems clear that optimal perioperative management can reduce mortality in surgical patients with CAD. In spite of the improved outcome in the studies of Wells and Rao, patients with a recent MI continue to be at increased risk, and whenever possible surgery should be delayed at least 3 months after the infarction.

Risk Indices

Attempts to preoperatively assess operative risk began with Dripps and the development of the ASA classification.[25] In 1978, Goldman published a cardiac risk index (CRI) for prospectively determining the cardiac morbidity and mortality on the basis of history, physical exam, resting ECG, and routine laboratory studies (Table 17-1).[35] This index, which is described in detail in Chapter 3, stratifies patients into four groups, assigning each group a relative risk of cardiac complications (Table 17-2). While the CRI has proved reliable in a general surgical population, its reliability in predicting risk in certain patient groups is limited. For example, in patients over 65 years of age the CRI had a low sensitivity (31%) in predicting cardiac complications,[34] and in elective abdominal aortic surgery, patients' cardiac complications consistently exceeded those predicted by the CRI.[12,45]

Attempting to improve on this low sensitivity in high-risk patients, Detsky and colleagues specifically evaluated a high-risk population, using additional variables.[24] These included a history of MI (longer than 6 months ago), angina class 3 or 4 (Canadian Cardiovascular Society), unstable angina within 3 months of surgery, and a history of pulmonary edema. Using a pretest probability and adjusting it with their "variable index," they derived a post-test probability of sustaining a cardiac complication. While this index is more cumbersome, it incorporates important additional information into risk assessment and may be more reliable than the CRI in high-risk patients.

Use of a risk index is valid for most surgical patients; however, the risk for an asymptomatic patient with significant CAD may go undetected. This limitation is particularly important in patients with peripheral vascular disease (PVD). These patients have an extremely high incidence of concomitant CAD but are frequently asymptomatic because of limitations in their activity caused by claudication or prior amputation. The high incidence of CAD in patients with peripheral vascular disease was demonstrated by Hertzer et al.[42] In this study coronary angiograms were performed on 1000 consecutive patients scheduled for elective peripheral vascular surgery. The study population included 263 patients with abdominal aortic aneurysms, 295 patients with cerebrovascular disease, and 381 patients with lower extremity ischemia. Before the angiograms, patients were classified on the basis of their history and resting ECG as having CAD or not; 446 patients had no indication of CAD, while 554 patients were suspected of having CAD. Results of this study, presented in Table 17-3, clearly demonstrate the high incidence of CAD in both groups of PVD patients. Tomatis, in a similar study, confirms this apparent lack of correlation between history, resting ECG, and CAD. In his group of patients with PVD 16%, with normal ECGs and no history of angina, previous MI, or congestive heart failure, had severe CAD as determined by coronary angiogram.[103]

In spite of the results of the studies by Hertzer and Tomatis, routine preoperative coronary angiography in all patients with PVD is not justified. The morbidity and expense of the procedure outweigh its yield as a preoperative screening test. These studies do demonstrate, however, that many patients with PVD may have low risk-index scores but clinically significant CAD, and they would benefit from further preoperative cardiac evaluation.

In a general surgical population, the CRI remains

TABLE 17-3.   Angiographic classification of coronary artery disease, according to clinical indications

	Clinical coronary disease			
	No indication		Suspected	
	Number	%	Number	%
Normal coronary arteries	64	14	21	4
Mild to moderate CAD*	218	49	99	18
Advanced but compensated CAD†	97	22	192	34
Severe, correctable CAD‡	63	14	188	34
Severe, inoperable CAD§	4	1	54	10

From Hertzer NR: Coronary artery disease in peripheral vascular patients, Ann Surg 199:223-233, 1984.

*Mild to moderate CAD, with measurable disease of one or more coronary arteries but no lesion exceeding 70% stenosis.

†Advanced but compensated CAD, with greater than 70% stenosis of one or more coronary arteries but no immediate indication for myocardial revascularization using coronary artery bypass grafting (CABG) because of adequate intercoronary collateral circulation or because the involved vessel supplied myocardium already replaced by scar.

‡Severe, correctable CAD, with greater than 70% stenosis of one or more coronary arteries serving unimpaired myocardium and representing immediate or foreseeable risk for myocardial infarction.

§Severe, inoperable CAD, with greater than 70% stenosis of multiple coronary arteries representing inadequate targets for CABG because of diffuse, distal disease or generalized ventricular impairment.

the most easily determined and useful risk index overall for preoperative evaluation.[111] In certain patient groups, particularly the elderly and those with vascular disease, it will underestimate the cardiac risk of surgery. In these groups the Detsky index may prove more sensitive, but even it will overlook most patients with clinically silent CAD.

Preoperative Testing

The goal of preoperative testing is to identify patients with CAD who would benefit from (1) myocardial revascularization (CABG) surgery before their noncardiac surgery, (2) intensive intraoperative and postoperative measures to reduce the operative risk, (3) a more limited surgical approach, or (4) avoidance of surgery altogether.

The need for further coronary artery testing in all surgical patients should be determined by the routine preoperative assessment (history, physical exam, ECG, and chest x-ray examination) and the magnitude of surgery planned. Risk indices can serve as a relative guide for deciding which patients require further evaluation. For patients with known or suspected CAD, further preoperative testing can delineate the extent of disease.

Exercise stress testing. Exercise stress testing (EST) provides valuable information about suspected coronary disease.[36] Because of the ease and minimal expense of EST, it has been suggested as a preoperative screening test for many patients. One study evaluated this use in patients over 40 years of age and found such a low yield that they concluded EST has no place as a routine preoperative screening test.[15] This conclusion suggests that EST should be used only in patients with suspected CAD.

In spite of the exercise requirement, EST is informative in patients with claudication symptoms, and studies have shown that 29% to 38% of patients with PVD will develop ECG evidence of ischemia.[21,66] These same studies demonstrated that 27% of patients with PVD who had neither a history of angina or MI, nor an abnormal ECG had ischemia with exercise. This group subsequently experienced a 26% perioperative MI rate, again pointing out the insensitivity of the standard preoperative assessment of patients with PVD. EST is frequently limited by the patient's physical endurance and obscured by baseline ECG changes. Moreover, the overall sensitivity of the test is questionable, as demonstrated by Gage in a comparison of EST to coronary angiography.[32]

MUGA scan. The resting gated blood pool (MUGA) study does not provide direct evidence of coronary disease but yields important information on left ventricular function. A study done on 100 patients in the hospital for peripheral vascular surgery found a significantly higher incidence of perioperative MI in those with ejection fractions (EF) less than 35%.[76] Myocardial revascularization has been shown to improve survival in patients with triple-vessel CAD and poor left-ventricular function (EF < 30%).[81] The MUGA scan can therefore be useful in identifying these patients at increased risk of perioperative MI who might also benefit from coronary angiography and CABG.

Dipyridamole thallium scan (DTS). Dipyridamole administered orally or intravenously in conjunction with thallium scanning is a sensitive and specific test for CAD.[46,57] Dipyridamole is a potent dilator of normal coronary arteries, with attenuated effects on stenotic coronary vessels. Thallium-201 is absorbed by myocardial cells based on their perfusion but not by scar from infarcted tissue. Scans performed at 5 minutes and at 3 hours will differentiate myocardium perfused normally from myocardium with "relative hypoperfusion" (Figure 17-1). The test is performed on patients at rest without increasing myocardial oxygen requirements and is not limited by ECG abnormalities or concomitant medications. The cost is one sixth that of coronary angiography, making it appealing as a screening test.

This technique was used by Boucher et al to estimate the cardiac risk in patients with suspected CAD who were to undergo peripheral vascular surgery.[9] In this study, a positive scan was associated with a 50% incidence of perioperative cardiac events, whereas normal scans or those showing persistent defects (old MI) had none. Six of the patients with abnormal scans underwent coronary angiography before surgery, and all had severe multivessel CAD. Two subsequent studies evaluated DTS as a screening test for patients with PVD. One study demonstrated a good correlation with perioperative MI when two of nine myocardial segments showed hypoperfusion.[22] The other study used clinical information from the patients to determine low-risk and high-risk groups.[27] They then demonstrated such a strong correlation between perioperative cardiac events and the high-risk positive-scan group that they recommend coronary angiography in this group.

These results demonstrate that DTS alone may not be sufficiently sensitive as a general screening test

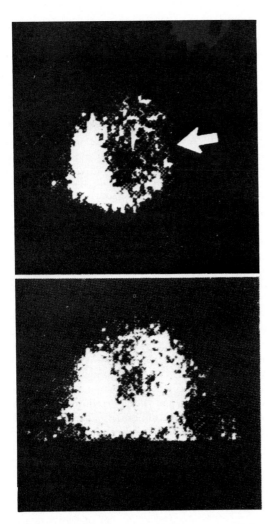

FIGURE 17-1. Dipyridamole thallium myocardial perfusion scintigrams in the left anterior oblique (LAO) position in a patient with a reversible perfusion defect. The scan done at 5 minutes demonstrates a lateral wall perfusion defect *(arrow)* that is not present on the scan done at 3 hours consistent with transient myocardial ischemia.

in patients with PVD. Adding clinical criteria increases the sensitivity of the test, but as we have learned from other studies, 15% to 20% of PVD patients who might qualify for myocardial revascularization are classified as low-risk by clinical criteria. Most surprising from this study is the incidence of perioperative MI in the high-risk group, considering that this information was known preoperatively

by the surgeon, anesthesiologist, and intensivist.

Ambulatory ECG monitoring. Ambulatory monitoring for myocardial ischemia has recently shown promise in providing important prognostic information. Silent ischemia during ambulatory monitoring appears to select a subset of patients whose CAD is associated with an increased morbidity and mortality.[86] This is also true of patients with unstable angina.[38] Perioperative cardiac morbidity and mortality also increases in patients with silent ischemia documented by preoperative Holter monitoring.[82] This association may have been previously demonstrated in 1985 by Slogoff and Keats, whose patients with "ischemia on arrival" were predominantly asymptomatic and associated with increased perioperative MI.[91] Further study using ambulatory monitoring should define its precise role in preoperative evaluation.

The decision to proceed with further testing should be based not only on the perioperative risk to the patient, but on the long-term benefits of identifying and quantitating the extent of their CAD. At present, there is no single test, short of coronary angiography, that will reliably identify patients with CAD, and even angiography cannot predict perioperative events. Some newer modalities appear promising and should also establish a role in preoperative testing.

Criteria for Altering Plans for Surgery

Once patients with significant CAD have been identified, a decision must be made whether to proceed immediately with the planned surgery. The alternatives to doing the planned surgery with intensive intraoperative and postoperative management are canceling the surgery, doing a more limited procedure, or doing coronary artery bypass grafting (CABG) first. Some surgical problems are not amenable to limited approaches, and in ones that are there is very little data on whether risk is actually reduced. In one group of 135 patients who had positive ESTs, the use of an axillo-femoral approach was compared to an intraabdominal aortic cross clamp procedure and found to be associated with less risk of both perioperative MI (17% to 27%) and mortality (13% to 20%), but neither of these differences was statistically significant.[3] Percutaneous angioplasty of peripheral vascular lesions is also felt to be safer, but a recent retrospective study showed no statistical difference in perioperative angina and MI when patients having angioplasty were compared to those having surgery.[71]

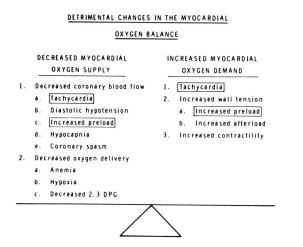

DETRIMENTAL CHANGES IN THE MYOCARDIAL
OXYGEN BALANCE

DECREASED MYOCARDIAL
OXYGEN SUPPLY

1. Decreased coronary blood flow
   a. Tachycardia
   b. Diastolic hypotension
   c. Increased preload
   d. Hypocapnia
   e. Coronary spasm
2. Decreased oxygen delivery
   a. Anemia
   b. Hypoxia
   c. Decreased 2,3 DPG

INCREASED MYOCARDIAL
OXYGEN DEMAND

1. Tachycardia
2. Increased wall tension
   a. Increased preload
   b. Increased afterload
3. Increased contractility

FIGURE 17-2. Detrimental changes in the myocardial oxygen balance. Note that tachycardia and increased preload affect both sides of the balance.

From Kaplan J: Cardiovascular physiology. In Kaplan J (editor): Cardiac Anesthesia, ed 2, New York, 1987, Grune & Stratton, Inc.

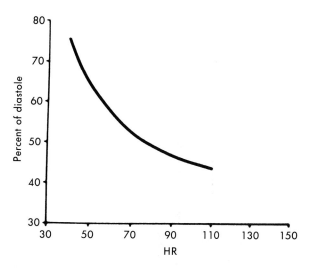

FIGURE 17-3. Relationship between heart rate (HR) and percent diastole. Small changes in HR produce dramatic changes in the percent diastole at slower HRs.

From Boudoulas H et al: Changes in diastolic time with various pharmacologic agents, Circulation 60:164-169, 1979.

The use of CABG before or concomitantly with noncardiac surgery is advocated by some surgical centers.[6,19,67] Large uncontrolled, nonrandomized studies report an improved outcome in patients undergoing noncardiac surgery after coronary revascularization (including the mortality associated with the CABG procedure).[6,19,67] These centers, however, have tremendous expertise in this area and their results may not be representative. While the results of these studies look promising, we await a large multicenter, randomized trial for an answer to this question. At present, the decision to proceed with CABG before noncardiac surgery should be based on (1) the patients' wishes, (2) severity of CAD, (3) the CABG experience at the institution, and (4) the experience of the anesthesiologists and intensivists dealing with high-risk patients at the institution.

PERIOPERATIVE CAUSES OF MYOCARDIAL ISCHEMIA
Supply and Demand

The balance between myocardial oxygen supply and demand governs the development of myocardial ischemia (Figure 17-2). Factors causing either an increase in myocardial oxygen consumption or a decrease in supply can lead to ischemia and infarction. Myocardial oxygen consumption (MVO_2) is deter-

mined by heart rate, preload, afterload, and contractility. The effect that each of these parameters has on the development of ischemia has been examined, and it is apparent that tachycardia is the single most important hemodynamic variable causing ischemia.[99] Tachycardia increases MVO_2 and decreases myocardial blood supply at the same time. It decreases blood supply by shortening diastole, which is when most coronary blood flow occurs. For example, when heart rate is increased from 60 to 150 beats per minute, diastolic time per minute falls from 40 seconds to 20 to 25 seconds.[47] This relationship between heart rate and percent diastole is nonlinear, and greater decreases in diastole occur with heart rate changes at the lower range (Figure 17-3). Increasing preload has been shown to be the next most important hemodynamic cause of myocardial ischemia. Higher preload pressures increase MVO_2 by increasing myocardial wall tension. At the same time, myocardial oxygen supply decreases as a result of the elevated transmural pressure on intramyocardial arterioles. This effect on supply can be seen by the following formula:

Coronary perfusion pressure (CPP) =
    Aortic diastolic pressure −
        Left ventricular end-diastolic pressure

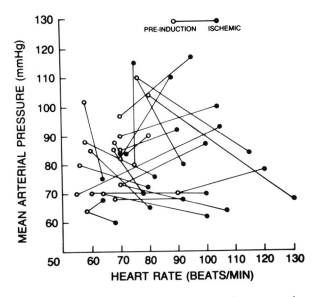

FIGURE 17-4. Mean arterial pressure and heart rate values at preinduction and at the time ischemic ECG changes were observed. In this study ischemic ECG changes were associated with significant increases in the heart rate with no consistent relationship between ischemia and either the systolic or mean arterial pressure.

From Kotter GS et al: Myocardial ischemia during cardiovascular surgery as detected by an ST segment trend monitoring system, J Cardiothorac Anesth l:190-199, 1987.

Afterload is felt to exert the least effect on myocardial ischemia because any increase in myocardial wall tension from increased afterload is partially counterbalanced by an increase in coronary perfusion pressure. The significance of tachycardia-induced ischemia has been validated clinically in many studies (Figure 17-4).[53,59,91,92]

Myocardial blood supply was previously felt to be determined, in patients with CAD, by the degree of obstruction present in the coronary arteries. This led to the assumption that controlling heart rate, blood pressure, and preload would preclude the development of ischemia. It is now known that the epicardial vessels and intramyocardial arterioles have intrinsic dynamic vasomotor tone.[13,28] This tone may be affected by factors demonstrating circadian rhythm, and be responsible for the increase in ischemia and MI found between 6 AM and 12 PM daily.[16] Much of the evidence supporting changes in myocardial supply as the cause of ischemia comes from Deanfield's data. In this study ambulatory patients had

frequent ischemic events as indicated by Holter monitor without any increase in heart rate.[23]

Intraoperative studies support the fact that hemodynamic parameters and myocardial ischemia do not always go hand-in-hand. Three studies evaluating the use of prophylactic nitroglycerin on ischemia during continuous ECG monitoring were unable to demonstrate a correlation between ECG ischemia and changes in heart rate and/or blood pressure.[18,33,102] In another study, myocardial lactate production was measured in anesthetized patients and there was no correlation between the rate-pressure product (heart rate × blood pressure) and lactate production.[94] Further evidence to suggest that a relative decrease in coronary flow is the cause of some ischemia comes from the work of Kleinman et al.[51] These authors used thallium-201 perfusion scans during induction of anesthesia to qualitatively assess regional myocardial flow. In their study, 45% of patients (10 of 22) developed positive scans (defect on scan compared to preoperative scan) during intubation in spite of insignificant changes in their baseline hemodynamics (HR 66 ± 3 to 71 ± 4, SBP 133 ± 6 to 128 ± 8). Two of these 10 patients had persistently positive scans postoperatively. One of the two had a perioperative MI, and the significance of the defect in the other patient was unknown.

The conclusion to be drawn from these studies is that there is a spectrum of clinical presentation of patients with CAD. On one end is classic fixed obstruction, where controlling myocardial oxygen supply and demand by altering heart rate, preload, afterload, and contractility should control ischemia. On the other end are pure supply-side alterations in myocardial oxygen delivery caused by changes in vascular tone. Somewhere in the middle will be most patients, with variable components of both processes. The implications this has for perioperative management are (1) controlling hemodynamic variables alone may not preclude the development of ischemia, (2) close observation of the ECG will reveal ischemia otherwise unsuspected from the patient's heart rate or blood pressure, and (3) anesthetic agents and other yet-to-be determined factors probably contribute to alterations in local myocardial blood flow.

Physiologic Changes

In the perioperative period there are neural, hormonal, hemodynamic, and hematologic changes capable of inducing myocardial ischemia and infarction. The neurohormonal changes in the perioperative period reflect catecholamine stimulation of the cardiovascular system. Through the sympathetic nervous system and adrenal medulla, catecholamines increase heart rate, contractility, and blood pressure, which is detrimental to patients with CAD. Certain events surrounding the operative period lead to sympathetic stimulation. It is at these times when appropriate therapy can attenuate the release of catecholamines and also block the cardiovascular response.

Preoperative anxiety, preinduction intravascular line placement, laryngoscopy and intubation, surgical stress, emergence, and postoperative pain are events usually associated with cardiovascular stimulation.[17]

Anxiety

Preoperative anxiety related to the impending surgery may be responsible for elevated epinephrine levels measured in patients before anesthetic induction.[40] Surprisingly, there are no studies in the literature assessing whether analgesics and/or sedative hypnotics in the immediate preoperative period (a common practice of anesthesiologists) cause any change in the elevated catecholamines. One study measuring beta-endorphins and ACTH as humoral markers of stress, showed that diazepam, meperidine, and diphenhydramine individually caused a significant attenuation of the stress response compared with control and placebo.[108] A preoperative visit by the anesthesiologist has also been shown to be beneficial in reducing anxiety levels in patients.[56]

Line Placement

Two studies have examined the hemodynamic changes and ischemia associated with placement of arterial and pulmonary artery (SGC) catheters. Lunn et al showed a significant increase in heart rate and blood pressure associated with line placement.[61] In this study, patients were premedicated with diazepam (10 mg orally), morphine sulfate (0.1 mg/kg), and scopolamine (0.5 mg intramuscularly 90 minutes before arrival in the operating room [OR]). The subgroup that was not on beta-blockers had greater increases in heart rate and blood pressure than the treated group, but both groups demonstrated statistically significant increases. A case report by Kotrly (using the ST segment trend monitor) graphically depicts the onset of ischemia with cannulation of the internal jugular vein and the subsequent resolution

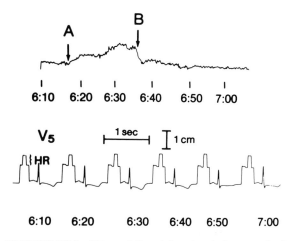

FIGURE 17-5. ST trend line *(above)* and the record of electronically stored V₅ complexes *(below)*. Although the trend line reflects ST segment changes in all three leads that compose the orthogonal set (V5, AVF, −V1), only the stored V₅ complexes are shown because depression is most obvious in this lead. The generally upward direction of the ST trend line from points *A* to *B* indicates the increasing deviation of the ST segment (J point + 60 msec) from the isoelectric line. Point *A* denotes the time when the patient was put in the head-down position for cannulation of the internal jugular vein. Point *B* denotes the time when the patient's head was elevated and intravenous nitroglycerin infusion started.

To improve clarity, 1 sec and 1 cm (1 millivolt) calibration lines have been substituted for the standard ECG grid lines. Because the electronic markers between stored complexes represent 10 min of elapsed time, the 1 sec scale may only be used to measure interval times between points on any single ECG complex. The height of the narrow pulse on top of each separating markers preceding the V5 complexes corresponds to the heart rate (HR) with each millimeter being equal to 10 beats/min. By measuring these pulses, it can be seen that the heart rate increased from approximately 50 to 67 beats/min between 6:10 and 6:30.

From Kotrly KJ et al: Intraoperative detection of myocardial ischemia with an ST segment trend monitoring system, Anesth Analg 63:343-345, 1984.

with administration of nitroglycerin (Fig. 17-5).[52] Contrary to these reports, Waller was unable to demonstrate statistically significant increases in hemodynamic variables or ischemia with intravascular line placement.[107] This study was similar to Lunn's in the dose of diazepam, morphine, and scopolamine. The differences were that these patients received an additional 1 to 2 inches of nitropaste with their routine cardiac medications and, on their arrival in the OR, their level of sedation was evaluated and supplemental sedation administered as needed.

Placement of vascular cannulae is associated with pain and anxiety in patients who are not appropriately medicated. When cannulation is not proceeding smoothly because of anatomic or technical problems, the patient's hemodynamics and anxiety cannot be overlooked. Waller's study has clearly shown that when patients with CAD are adequately premedicated and receive supplemental sedation as needed, they can easily tolerate these procedures.

Intubation

Laryngoscopy and intubation is associated with marked sympathetic stimulation, causing tachycardia and hypertension. Russell et al documented a significant rise in plasma norepinephrine (NE) levels with laryngoscopy and intubation that correlated with a rise in mean arterial pressure from 77 ± 6.6 to 122 ± 5.9 mm Hg.[88] Attempts to control this stimulation have included local and intravenous lidocaine, narcotics, beta-blockers, and vasodilators. Treatment with beta-blockers (especially esmolol, the new short-acting agent) appears to provide the best protection.[20]

Emergence

Emergence from anesthesia and the immediate postoperative period (0 to 2 hours) represents a time when neurohormonal and physiologic stresses can induce myocardial ischemia. Awareness of pain, the discomfort of an endotracheal tube, hypothermia, changes in vascular tone, and muscle paralysis are all factors that can lead to myocardial ischemia.

The severity of the underlying CAD and the extent of the operative procedure should dictate whether patients are allowed to emerge (awaken) in the operating room at the end of the operation. Many anesthetics are planned to keep the patient anesthetized and paralyzed until transferred to the ICU to make the transition from anesthesia to consciousness as smooth as possible. The reasons for delaying emergence are (1) titrating analgesic drugs (to insure adequate pain relief) against residual anesthetic agents is difficult and can be associated with sympathetic stimulation from either inadequate pain relief or hypercarbia from respiratory depression, (2) reversing muscle paralysis enables the emerging semistuporous patient to thrash about, increasing myocardial

oxygen requirements and potentially pulling out necessary catheters, and (3) reversing paralysis in a hypothermic patient can lead to shivering.

The phenomenon of postoperative shivering is felt to represent either a neuromuscular response to lowered body temperature or a recovery of spinal activity before recovery of inhibitory upper motor neurons.[14] Shivering markedly increases systemic metabolic demands, and measurements of total body oxygen consumption have shown increases of up to 700% during shivering.[87] In this situation, ventilation and cardiac output must increase proportionately to meet these demands. If patients are mechanically ventilated at a fixed rate, the increase of CO_2 production can lead to hypercarbia. In patients with CAD the increase in myocardial demand can precipitate ischemia, and failure to meet systemic oxygen requirements can lead to acidosis and hypoxemia. Subclinical shivering has recently been demonstrated with a strain gauge and electronic recorder; whether subclinical shivering leads to increases in systemic metabolism is not known. The pharmacologic therapies for controlling patients who are actively shivering are paralysis or meperidine.[63]

In response to surgery and/or pain, postoperative cathecholamine levels show a persistent elevation of both norepinephrine (NE) and epinephrine (E).[64] These levels will vary depending upon the magnitude of the operation, with most E levels returning to near baseline within 24 hours and NE levels remaining elevated for up to 5 days.[64] Efforts to block the catecholamines or the cardiovascular response to adrenergic stimulation include the use of systemic and epidural narcotics, beta-blockers, and vasodilators. Adequate analgesia and sedation, sufficient to attenuate the sympathetic response to pain, are beneficial for the patients sense of well-being and their CAD. However, overzealous use of these drugs can lead to hypotension, respiratory depression, and disorientation, particularly in elderly patients. Postoperative use of regional anesthetic techniques (that is, epidural narcotics, plexus blocks, and local nerve blocks), when applicable, provides excellent analgesia and decreases the problem of systemic narcotic administration.

Hemodynamic Changes

In hypothermic patients, rewarming is associated with peripheral vasodilation and a fall in systemic vascular resistance (SVR) and central venous pres-

TIMING OF POSTOPERATIVE MI

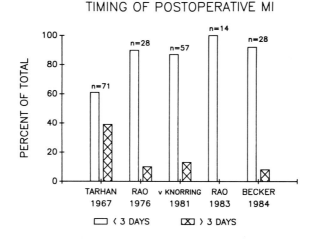

FIGURE 17-6. Timing of postoperative myocardial infarction from studies looking at noncardiac surgery patients.

From Tarhan S et al: JAMA 220:1451-1454, 1972; Rao TLK, Jacobs KH, and El-Etr AA: Anesthesiology 59:499-505, 1983; von Knorring J: Surgery 90:55-60, 1981; and Becker RC and Underwood DA: Cleve Clin J Med 54:25-28, 1987.

sure (CVP). Transvascular escape and third spacing of fluid (into areas of tissue disruption and intraabdominal viscera) is another factor requiring administration of large amounts of fluid in the postoperative period. Failure to keep up with the fluid requirements during this time can lead to hypotension and tachycardia. After 24 to 48 hours, patients usually begin to reaccumulate this extravascular fluid into the intravascular space (assuming that no pathologic process has intervened). During this reaccumulation phase, patients continue to require careful hemodynamic monitoring and drug therapy to avoid tachycardia and hypertension from volume overload. Patients with poor left-ventricular function and/or renal insufficiency are particularly at risk during this period.

Hematologic Changes

Alterations in clotting and fibrinolysis occur in patients postoperatively, inducing a hypercoagulable state.[10] While this reaction is teleologically beneficial for overall hemostasis, patients with stenotic coronary artery lesions may be at risk for the development of coronary thrombosis. Recent studies have also documented elevated levels of fibrinogen and fibrin degradation products in patients with unstable angina and MI.[41,54] Over time some clotting parameters in

postoperative patients increase (fibrinogen and factor VIII) and some decrease (antithrombin III).[10] These levels appear to peak on postoperative days 2 and 3, coincidental with the peak development of postoperative MI (Figure 17-6).[70] It is not known yet whether there is a link between postoperative clotting abnormalities and MI, but this is an area of active research.

MONITORING FOR MYOCARDIAL ISCHEMIA

Modalities for monitoring myocardial ischemia include the standard surface electrocardiogram (ECG), computer-assisted scanning of ST segments, pulmonary artery catheters (SGC), and two-dimensional transesophageal echocardiography (2D-TE). Although these techniques are not available in all hospitals, it is important to understand their advantages and disadvantages and their relative sensitivity for identifying ischemia.

ECG

The surface ECG is the most commonly used technique for detecting myocardial ischemia. Either ST segment elevation or 1 mm or more of horizontal or downsloping ST depression is indicative of myocardial ischemia (Figure 17-7).[36] Precordial lead V5

ECG Patterns indicative of Myocardial Ischemia

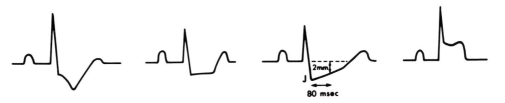

ECG Patterns not indicative of Myocardial Ischemia

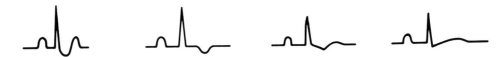

FIGURE 17-7. Electrocardiographic criteria for myocardial ischemia.

From Goldschlager N: Use of the treadmill test in the diagnosis of coronary artery disease in patients with chest pain, Ann Intern Med 97:383-388, 1982.

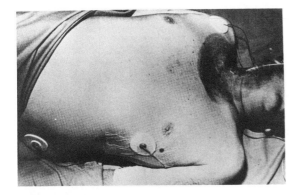

FIGURE 17-8. The CS5 lead arrangement is demonstrated. Standard lead I should be selected to monitor a modified V5 lead. From Kaplan J: Cardiovascular physiology.

In Kaplan J (editor): Cardiac Anesthesia, ed 2, New York, 1986, Grune & Stratton, Inc.

is the most informative lead for monitoring and diagnosing ischemia; data from EST indicate that 89% of ST segment information contained in the conventional 12-lead ECG is found in this lead.[48] When using a 3-lead ECG system, a modified V5 lead can be obtained by moving lead I to the V5 position and monitoring lead I (Figure 17-8).

Patients with high-grade obstruction of the right coronary artery (RCA), or right ventricular (RV) hypertrophy and an RCA lesion should also be monitored for RV ischemia. Recent studies suggest that leads II and V5 may not provide a sufficiently sensitive means for diagnosing RV ischemia. Alternative surface ECG leads, particularly V4R and CR4R (fifth intercostal space at the right midclavicular line), have been shown to be most effective in this situation.[50] The esophageal electrocardiogram has also been used to detect for RV ischemia. Using this technique, Trager and Kaplan were able to detect ST segment changes when no changes were evident in lead II.[105]

Computer Assisted ST Segment Scanning

Modifications to improve the sensitivity of the ECG include reviewing periodically run ECG strips, intraoperative Holter monitor recordings, continuous ECG hardcopy printout, and a recent innovation, microcomputer scanning of the ECG.[53] This technique uses a microprocessor to measure and trend each ST segment. Changes above (ST segment elevation) or below (ST segment depression) the baseline are transformed into a positive value and displayed on a trend monitor (see Figure 17-5). This technique is felt to improve the ability to detect ischemia.

For some patients, any monitoring modality using

ECG ST segments is of limited value. Baseline ECG abnormalities demonstrating either bundle branch block or pacemaker-induced depolarization render ST segment interpretation impossible, and patients with LVH or digoxin repolarization changes are difficult to assess. If these abnormalities are present, another monitoring tool should be employed for detecting ischemia.

Pulmonary Artery Catheter

Use of the pulmonary artery (PA) catheter to diagnose myocardial ischemia was first demonstrated by Kaplan and Wells in 1981.[49] This technique is based on the observation that during cardiac catheterization patients developing angina had an associated increase in left-ventricular end-diastolic pressure (LVEDP) or pulmonary capillary wedge pressure (PCWP) that preceded ECG changes. In their study during CABG, these authors considered patients developing a new AC wave greater than 15 mm Hg or a V-wave greater than 20 mm Hg to have ischemia. Eighteen of 40 patients (45%) developed signs of myocardial ischemia before cardiopulmonary bypass. In these 18 patients, 10 had ischemia detected by PCWP tracings alone, 5 had both ST depression and abnormal PCWP tracings, and 3 developed ST segment depression without PCWP abnormalities. Subsequent studies comparing this method to continuous ECG monitoring, continuous Holter monitoring, and myocardial lactate production have been unable to consistently demonstrate a correlation between elevated PCWP and myocardial ischemia.[93,101] These authors and others hypothesize that increases in LVEDP or PCWP are secondary to global decreases in left-ventricular compliance (from impaired diastolic relaxation) and may not occur during focal ischemia. Though relatively insensitive to focal ischemia, PCWP monitoring still represents an indirect method for detecting myocardial ischemia when the ECG cannot be used because of baseline abnormalities. Kaplan and Well's study suggests that the ECG and PCWP monitoring, when used together, have greater sensitivity for detecting myocardial ischemia than either one alone.

Two-dimensional Transesophageal Echocardiography

Limitations in the sensitivity and specificity of ECG and PCWP monitoring have led to the intraoperative use of two-dimensional transesophageal echocardiography (2D-TE). This method reveals focal changes in systolic wall dimensions and motion abnormalities thought to be caused by ischemia, which frequently precede ECG changes.[93] Comparing surface echocardiography to ECG, Wohlgelernter studied patients undergoing coronary angioplasty of the LAD artery.[110] After 20 seconds of balloon inflation (total coronary occlusion) all patients had profound regional dysfunction by echocardiogram, but only 64% developed ECG changes, which increased to 80% of patients at 60 seconds of total ischemia. Two patients with profound abnormalities by echocardiogram had no ECG changes. The authors concluded from this study that the surface ECG does lag behind the two-dimensional echocardiogram in documenting ischemia, but the ECG still provides a highly sensitive technique for detecting myocardial ischemia.

The improved sensitivity of these other monitoring modalities over the standard ECG must be weighed against the increased morbidity, cost, and manpower required for their use. In high-risk patients the use of alternative monitoring techniques may be warranted; however, their use in all patients with CAD is not advocated and cannot supplant the surface ECG and vigilence.

DIAGNOSING ISCHEMIA AND INFARCTION

The diagnosis of myocardial ischemia and infarction in the postoperative period can be problematic. Patients with postoperative MI have a very high incidence of silent (painless) infarction, ranging from 20% to 80% (Table 17-4).[4,5,26] Painless infarction is felt to be secondary to the coexisting pain of surgery and the use of analgesics, which mask the myocardial pain symptoms. Clinically silent ischemia places a greater burden on the physician, who must be aware of changes that may be manifestations of underlying myocardial ischemia (anginal equivalents). Unexplained arrhythmias, hypotension, a sudden increase in pulmonary capillary wedge pressure, or right-sided heart pressure may all represent ongoing ischemia. If these events occur, an ECG should be obtained immediately to document any changes.

The postoperative ECG is the least expensive and most easily obtained marker of myocardial ischemia and infarction. However, the postoperative ECG will frequently contain T-wave changes that may not be

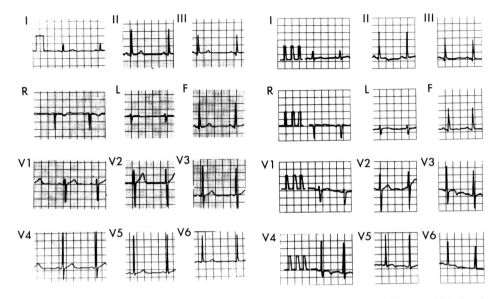

FIGURE 17-9. Preoperative **(A)** and postoperative **(B)** ECGs of a 31-year-old man, ASA 1, who underwent parotid gland resection under morphine—N$_2$O—ethrane anesthesia. Note flattened-T-waves in the inferior leads and inverted or biphasic T-waves in the anterolateral leads on the postoperative ECG.

From Breslow MJ et al: Changes in T-wave morphology following anesthesia and surgery: a common recovery room phenomenon, Anesthesiology 64:398-402, 1986.

TABLE 17-4.   Silent perioperative myocardial infarction

Study	Year	Number of patients	Incidence of silent infarction
Driscoll[26]	1961	12	83%
Baer[4]	1965	41	39%
Tarhan[100]	1972	28	21%
Goldman[35]	1978	18	50%
Steen[96]	1978	28	61%
von Knorring[106]	1981	35	37%
Rao[83]	1983	42	53%

indicative of myocardial ischemia (Figure 17-9). Breslow et al evaluated 394 random noncardiac surgical patients for postoperative ECG changes.[11] Of this group 71 (19%) had new T-wave abnormalities, 46 had new T-wave flattening, and 25 had new T-wave inversions. The incidence of postoperative T-wave changes was no different in patients with preexisting CAD than in those without (23% versus 18%). Intraabdominal pathologic conditions and autonomic nervous system imbalance were thought to

be responsible for these nonishemic repolarization changes. This same phenomenon was probably demonstrated in 1959 by Driscoll et al.[26] These authors, looking at the incidence of postoperative MI, had a subgroup of 30 patients with inverted T-waves that resolved over 7 days without apparent complications. Postoperative ECG changes involving T-waves alone appear to be relatively common, nonspecific, and clinical judgment should dictate further work-up.

Measurement of creatine phosphokinase (CPK) MB isoenzyme levels is extremely helpful in diagnosing postoperative MI. Postoperative patients will routinely have elevations of total CPK levels because of surgical tissue trauma, however, the MB isoenzyme level should be negligible, and when elevated, it has been found to be a reliable marker of myocardial damage.[85]

MANAGEMENT STRATEGIES
Pharmacologic Therapy

The perioperative period, as we have shown, is associated with elevated catecholamines and hemodynamic fluctuations. These changes require ther-

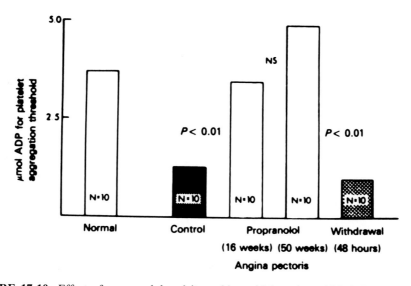

FIGURE 17-10. Effect of propranolol and its sudden withdrawal on APD-induced platelet aggregability in patients with angina pectoris. After propanolol, platelets of treated patients are less sensitive to ADP (geometric mean) than they were before treatment, and they are not significantly different from normal. Forty-eight hours following abrupt propranolol withdrawal, platelets of patients have returned to their pretreatment hyperresponsiveness to ADP. From Frishman WH and Weksler BB: Effects of B-adrenoceptor blocking agents on platelet function in normal subjects and patients with angina pectoris.

In Roskamm H and Graefe KH (editors): Advances in β-blocker therapy, Amsterdam, 1980, Excerpta Medica.

apy with beta-blockers and vasoactive agents in most patients with CAD, and in rare instances mechanical devices can be employed. Proper usage of these agents is important during this particularly vulnerable period.

Beta-blockers

There is substantial published evidence that acute withdrawal of beta-blockers will induce a hyperadrenergic state that can exacerbate angina and cause infarction.[31] This effect is thought to result from an increased number and sensitivity of beta receptors (up regulation) in the myocardium, and also on platelets. Failure to maintain adequate beta-blockade leads to increases in heart rate, state of myocardial contractility, and platelet aggregation (Figure 17-10). Consistent with this mechanism of "up regulation" is the attenuated hyperadrenergic response seen when beta-blockers with partial agonist activity (for example, pindolol) are withdrawn.[98] This increase in adrenergic activity normally develops over 24 to 72 hours; however, studies have demonstrated that patients withdrawn from beta-blockers 10 hours

before surgery are not protected from increases in heart rate and blood pressure during endotracheal intubation[74] (Figure 17-11). Consequently, it is recommended that patients receive their beta-blockers the morning of surgery and throughout the perioperative period. For patients with CAD who were previously not receiving beta-blockers, there still exists the need to blunt the elevated perioperative catecholamines. This need was demonstrated in a study on patients undergoing AAA repair, which revealed a significant reduction in heart rate, blood pressure, perioperative arrhythmias and MI in the group that received beta-blockade.[77]

In certain patients the use of beta-blockers has been questioned, and in others it is considered relatively contraindicated. Patients with rest angina were previously thought to be at increased risk if they took beta-blockers because these agents could potentiate vasoconstriction (unopposed alpha stimulation) in epicardial coronary vessels. Gottlieb et al, however, demonstrated that patients with rest angina who were already receiving nitrates and calcium channel blockers could receive propanolol safely,

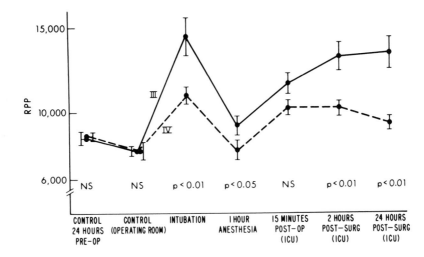

FIGURE 17-11. Mean rate-pressure product (RPP) of group III patients (propranolol discontinued 10 hours before surgery) and group IV patients (propranolol maintained until 2 hours before surgery, restarted immediately after surgery) before, during, and after coronary artery surgery. Group III is shown with a solid line, group IV with a broken line. There were no differences between the groups during the preoperative control periods. However, there were significant increments in RPP during intubation and the postoperative periods in group III patients compared to group IV patients.

From Oka Y et al: Clinical pharmacology of the new beta-adrenergic blocking drugs. Part 10. Beta-adrenoceptor blockade and coronary artery surgery, Am Heart J 99:255-269, 1980.

and the number of ischemic episodes in these patients actually decreased.[37] Beta-blockers are relatively contraindicated in patients with reactive airway disease or left-ventricular (LV) dysfunction. In these patients, if beta-blockade is indicated for other reasons, a trial of esmolol should be attempted.

Esmolol is a cardioselective beta-adrenoreceptor antagonist without intrinsic sympathomimetic activity.[72] Beta-receptor selectivity is a dose-dependent phenomenon that is relative rather than absolute; therefore, esmolol will have decreasing beta$_1$ selectivity with increasing dosage. Because of its short duration of action (elimination half-life of 9 minutes), any untoward events will quickly reverse with discontinuation. Studies evaluating the effectiveness of esmolol in patients with asthma support its cardioselective action. When esmolol was compared to placebo in a double-blind randomized crossover protocol, 10 patients (with mild asthma) had insignificant increases in airway reactivity while receiving the maximum infusion dose (300 μg/kg/min) of esmolol.[90] Because of the dose-dependent nature of beta-receptor selectivity, a lower dose achieving the

desired heart rate would be expected to elicit even less bronchoconstriction.

Information on the use of esmolol in patients with LV dysfunction is limited. In a study done on 10 patients—9 with a recent MI and all having angina—esmolol was found to be efficacious.[44] Left ventricular dysfunction was determined by MUGA scan, and baseline studies revealed that 5 patients had an EF of less than 25% and 5 patients had an EF of 25% to 36%. No patients were clinically in heart failure, and the mean PCWP was 11 mm Hg. Esmolol was infused at 2, 4, 8, 12, and 16 mg/min without reference to patient weight. A 2 mg/min infusion (equivalent to 30 μg/kg/min in a 70 kg person) showed a significant decrease in heart rate, from 91 ± 4 to 85 ± 4 beats per minute. Increasing the dosage caused a progressive decrease in heart rate, cardiac output, and ejection fraction. The drop in cardiac output was secondary to the decreased heart rate and occurred without any significant change in stroke volume. Blood pressure was maintained by an increase in systemic vascular resistance (SVR), and the angina present in all 10 patients was abolished at varying doses of esmolol. There does appear to be tremendous interpatient variability in the response to esmolol; therefore, careful titration of this drug is necessary in all patients, particularly those with LV dysfunction.

Another beta-blocker with specific indications in perioperative patients with ischemic heart disease is labetalol. The combined alpha and beta-adrenoreceptor blocking activity of this drug is ideal for hypertensive, tachycardiac patients with CAD. Labetalol is also beneficial in hypertension alone, because the reflex tachycardia that is common with other antihypertensives (for example, hydralazine, nitroprusside, and nifedipine) is blocked. The mechanism responsible for the hypotensive effect of labetalol is $alpha_1$ receptor antagonism, and additional arterial dilation mediated by $beta_2$ receptor agonist activity.[62] Labetalol also has antiarrhythmic effects, which have been demonstrated in ischemic and nonischemic models,[79] providing an excellent profile of activity in postoperative patients with CAD.

The hemodynamics that normally result from labetalol administration are a decrease in blood pressure, a decrease or no change in heart rate, and an increase or no change in cardiac output.[80] Overall coronary artery flow remains unchanged despite the lower blood pressure; therefore, coronary vascular resistance is decreased. Flow to left ventricular regions distal to severe coronary narrowing is decreased slightly, but in spite of this, patients experience less angina, exercise longer, and have less ST segment depression on ECG. Other studies have demonstrated a significant reduction in angina and silent myocardial ischemia with labetalol, and the effects seen are similar to a beta-blocker nifedipine combination.[81]

Labetalol can be administered as a bolus or by continuous infusion after a loading dose of 10 to 20 mg. When titrating a continuous infusion, rebolusing and increasing the infusion will obtain the desired effect more quickly. Labetalol has an elimination half-life of approximately 8 hours, so accumulation can occur.

Nitrates

Nitroglycerin prophylaxis for coronary ischemia has been practiced for many years. Patients with CAD are able to increase their angina threshold and improve their exercise tolerance by prophylactically taking nitroglycerin sublingually. This practice has been extrapolated to the operating room in an attempt to decrease ischemia in patients with CAD. Three studies have been published evaluating the effectiveness of 0.5 µg/kg/min and 1.0 µg/kg/min nitroglycerin administered before anesthetic induction and continued through surgery. Ischemia in these studies was assessed by continuous ECG or Holter monitoring. The studies by Thomson and Gallagher were done on CABG patients and were unable to demonstrate any overall difference in ischemia between IV nitroglycerin and placebo.[33,102] These authors did find less hypertension, more hypotension, and increased fluid requirements in the nitroglycerin group. The one improvement in ischemia noted in Gallagher's study was that with hypotension (MAP $\geq$ 20% below baseline), there was less ischemia in the nitroglycerin group than in the placebo group (15% versus 33%).

In contrast to these two studies, Coriat et al found significantly less ischemia when nitroglycerin was administered at 1.0 µg/kg/min than when it was given at 0.5 µg/kg/min.[18] The patients in this study also had less hypertension and increased fluid requirements in the high-dose group (1.0 µg/kg/min) than in the low-dose group. There are five major differences between this study and the previous two: (1) this study was done in noncardiac surgery patients (41 of 45 procedures were vascular surgery); (2) all patients in this study had stable, effort-related angina (in Gallagher's study 50% of the patients had unstable angina); (3) there was no invasive hemodynamic monitoring in 75% of Coriat's patients (correlation of blood pressure changes with ischemia is difficult); (4) the criteria for defining ischemia was more sensitive in Coriat's study, which may explain why 14 patients in Group 1 (0.5 µg/kg/min) with 18 episodes of ischemia had no perioperative infarctions; and (5) there was no control group for comparison. Instead, the authors (for ill-defined reasons) compare 0.5 versus 1.0 µg/kg/min nitroglycerin infusions. While it does have these drawbacks, this is the only study examining prophylactic nitroglycerin in noncardiac surgical patients. In this population (stable angina), prophylactic nitroglycerin may be beneficial. This study deserves to be repeated, this time with appropriate controls and hemodynamic monitoring. It should also be continued into the postoperative period, when these patients develop the greatest risk of ischemia and infarction (see Figure 17-6). Until then, the only conclusion that can definitely be made is that prophylactic nitroglycerin, given intraoperatively, decreases hypertension, increases hypotension, and increases intravenous fluid requirements.

Nitrates remain an important part of therapy for ischemic heart disease. Nitroglycerin enhances regional myocardial flow to ischemic areas, improves the ratio of endocardial to epicardial perfusion, increases oxygen tension in the subendocardium, and increases collateral flow.[68] The mechanism of the antianginal effect of nitrates is complex and probably involves a combination of coronary vasodilation, systemic venodilatation, and arterial vasodilation. Determining the specific site of action in a patient is difficult, and the site may vary depending upon the clinical situation. It is important that clinicians using nitrates establish an endpoint for their therapy; either resolution of pain, normalization of ECG changes, or preload reduction. Nitrates continued in the perioperative period for maintenance purposes should be dosed accordingly, and arbitrary higher dosing should be discouraged. Higher doses will lead to hemodynamic changes that can be detrimental and increase fluid requirements. In the intraoperative and immediate postoperative period only, intravenous ni-

troglycerin (NTG) should be used, because gastrointestinal absorption is unreliable and absorption of topical agents in hypothermic and rewarming patients is erratic. For conversion purposes, it is important to know the amount of nitroglycerin contained in common preparations. Transderm-Nitro and Nitro-Dur patches contain 0.5 mg of nitroglycerin/cm^2 and the Nitrodisc patch contains 0.625 mg/ cm^2,[101] 10 cm patches delivering 5 mg or 6.25 mg of nitroglycerin respectively over 24 hours. Nitropaste contains approximately 11.6 mg of nitroglycerin per inch of paste delivered over 6 hours when applied appropriately.[84]

The effect of varying doses of nitrates on the vasculature has been examined.[29] Doses of nitroglycerin as small as 75 to 150 μg delivered sublingually (duration of action 20 to 40 minutes) have been shown to significantly increase the diameter of epicardial coronary arteries, without any change in heart rate or mean aortic pressure. Increasing the dose to 450 μg in this study resulted in a small additional increase in coronary diameter, but at the same time caused an increased heart rate and decreased mean aortic pressure. Higher doses of nitroglycerin affect both venous and arterial vascular tone (Figure 17-

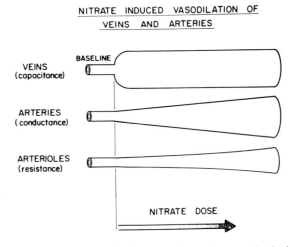

NITRATE INDUCED VASODILATION OF
VEINS AND ARTERIES

FIGURE 17-12. Hemodynamic effects of nitrates on the major vascular beds. At very low doses the venous or capacitance vessels are near maximally dilated. The systemic arteries begin to dilate at low doses; this is further accentuated with higher doses of nitrates. Systolic blood pressure begins to fall even in the absence of an effect on resistance vessels. Arteriolar vasodilation occurs only with very high nitrate concentrations, which are probably not achieved with usual clinical doses of these drugs.

From Abrams J: Hemodynamic effects of nitroglycerin and long-acting nitrates, Am Heart J 110:216-224, 1985.

12). At lower doses (30 to 40 μg/min), venodilation predominates, and a decrease in arterial resistance is often difficult to demonstrate because of reflex neurohormonal changes that occur.[97] Increasing the dose of nitroglycerin (greater than 250 μg/min) overrides the reflex changes and arterial vasodilation occurs. Hemodynamic responses to nitroglycerin may vary greatly from patient to patient depending upon the patient's volume status and underlying myocardial function. Any reflex tachycardia or hypotension that develops will attenuate the beneficial effects of nitroglycerin on myocardial ischemia. Efforts to block these changes have included the use of beta-blockers, volume infusion, and vasopressors. Borer demonstrated that nitroglycerin and phenylephrine together had a beneficial effect in patients with normal LV function suffering from acute myocardial infarction.[8]

Nitroglycerin has been used as an antihypertensive and was compared to nitroprusside in post-CABG patients. In a randomized crossover study, 14 of 17 patients obtained comparable decreases in MAP, with nitroglycerin infusions of less than 300 μg/min.[30] Three patients required over 1100 μg/min, and two had no satisfactory decrease in MAP. Higher cardiac outputs and lower intrapulmonary shunting were found in the nitroglycerin group than in the nitroprusside group. These effects, combined with the beneficial effects of nitroglycerin on coronary flow, make it preferable to nitroprusside for treating postoperative hypertension in *responsive patients* with CAD.

Tolerance to the action of nitrates has been recognized for several years, and experimental work has shown that this effect can be seen as early as 18 to 24 hours with continuous infusions.[1] The mechanisms responsible for this tolerance are currently being studied, and preliminary data suggests that depletion of sulfhydryl groups in vascular smooth muscle cells is partly responsible. This mechanism is supported by the fact that researchers have been able to partially reverse the tolerance that develops by administering *N*-acetylcysteine to patients.[65]

With tolerance developing so rapidly, the use of continuous intravenous nitroglycerin becomes complicated. If sulfhydryl depletion occurs sooner at higher doses (conjecture), then it is extremely important to use the lowest possible dose to obtain the desired effect. If continuous steady-state levels of nitroglycerin are responsible for the development of tolerance, then varying the dose administered or discontinuing the infusion for short periods may prove efficacious. The ideal approach will probably involve some interference with the mechanism at the cellular level.

Calcium Channel Blockers

With regard to continuation of calcium channel blockers during the perioperative period, there is conflicting evidence whether a withdrawal phenomenon occurs. In some patients, precipitation and worsening of myocardial ischemia, including infarction, has occurred with abrupt withdrawal of calcium channel blockers.[58] There are also anecdotal reports of sudden exaggerated hemodynamic responses postoperatively in patients acutely withdrawn from calcium antagonists. The mechanism for this response is reported by one group of authors to be an increased sensitivity of alpha$_2$ adrenoreceptors, leading to an increase in vascular tone, while others theorize that a direct vascular membrane process involving calcium channels is responsible for the observed increase in tone.[69] This "withdrawal phenomenon" does not occur in all patients, and its onset is variable, requiring up to one week in some patients. A study examining 81 patients withdrawn from either nifedipine or placebo was unable to demonstrate any hemodynamic differences perioperatively, and only those patients having angina at rest experienced an increase in symptoms.[39] These patients were considered by the authors to have a definite component of vasospasm to their CAD. Until this issue is resolved, I would recommend continuing these drugs preoperatively unless otherwise contraindicated.

The use of calcium channel blockers in intraoperative and immediate postoperative patients is limited to intravenous verapamil or sublingual nifedipine because of questionable gastrointestinal absorption. Verapamil has fewer vasodilating properties than nifedipine and more negative dromotropic and inotropic effects.[95] In patients on beta-blockers, intravenous verapamil can provoke serious conduction abnormalities and decreases in ventricular function.[95]

Nifedipine given sublingually (SL) has an onset of action within minutes. While the actual site of absorption remains arguable, the time of onset of activity is not. One study measured blood pressure every 5 minutes after giving 20 mg of nifedipine by this route to severely hypertensive patients.[55] There was a rapid and statistically significant drop in blood pressure every 5 minutes for 30 to 45 minutes, at which point the antihypertensive effect reached a plateau. The magnitude of the hypotensive effect from nifedipine is directly related to the pretreatment blood pressure. Normotensive volunteers were found to have a more attenuated drop in vascular resistance than hypertensive patients.[78] The vasodilation that occurs with nifedipine is limited to arterial vessels, with very little if any, effect on the venous system.[73] Several recent case reports have documented dramatic falls in blood pressure, precipitating angina and MI in patients given 10 mg of nifedipine sublingually.[75] Because it is administered sublingually, physicians tend to have a somewhat cavalier attitude toward nifedipine, but its onset of action is very similar to parenterally administered drugs, and close observation is required with its use.

The vasodilating action of nifedipine is countered in nonbeta-blocked patients by a reflex tachycardia. The increase in heart rate, combined with the afterload reduction, frequently leads to an increase in cardiac output. Because of its coronary vasodilating properties, nifedipine is useful in hypertensive postoperative patients with CAD, and particularly useful in patients who are bradycardic. Combined with beta-blockers, nifedipine does not increase the risk of conduction abnormalities and appears relatively safe in patients with decreased LV function.

Mechanical Devices

In certain situations where surgery is necessary because of malignancy, bowel obstruction or fractures, and the patient has either severe inoperable CAD or refuses CABG, intraaortic counterpulsation can be used. The intraaortic balloon pump, which provides excellent temporary support, can be placed in the OR immediately before surgery and can be removed within 72 hours. This type of support has been used effectively at some centers.[7]

SUMMARY

The successful management of surgical patients with CAD requires an understanding of the changes in myocardial oxygen supply and demand that occur perioperatively. I have described these hematologic, hemodynamic, and neurohumoral responses specific to the perioperative period. By manipulating these pathophysiologic processes with mechanical and pharmacologic agents, patients can be safely managed through this vulnerable period.

REFERENCES

1. Abrams J: Tolerance to organic nitrates, Circulation 74:1181–1185, 1986.
2. Arkins R, Smessaert AA, and Hicks RG: Mortality and morbidity in surgical patients with coronary artery disease, JAMA 190:485–488, 1964.
3. Arous EJ, Baum PL, and Cutler BS: The ischemic exercise test in patients with peripheral vascular disease, Arch Surg 119:780–783, 1984.
4. Baer S, Nakhjavan F, and Kajani M: Postoperative myocardial infarction, Surg Gynecol Obstet 120:315–322, 1965.
5. Becker RC and Underwood DA: Myocardial infarction in patients undergoing noncardiac surgery, Cleve Clin J Med 54:25–28, 1987.
6. Beven EG: Routine coronary angiography in patients undergoing surgery for abdominal aortic aneurysm and lower extremity occlusive disease, J Vasc Surg 3:682–684, 1986.
7. Bonchek LI and Olinger GN: Intra-aortic balloon counterpulsation for cardiac support during noncardiac operations, J Thorac Cardiovasc Surg 78:147–149, 1979.
8. Borer JS et al: Reduction in myocardial ischemia with nitroglycerin or nitroglycerin plus phenylephrine administered during acute myocardial infarction, N Engl J Med 293:1008–1012, 1975.
9. Boucher CA et al: Determination of cardiac risk by dipyridamole-thallium imaging before peripheral vascular surgery, N Engl J Med 312:389–394, 1985.
10. Bredbacka S et al: Pre- and postoperative changes in coagulation and fibrinolytic variables during abdominal hysterectomy under epidural or general anaesthesia, Acta Anaesth Scand 30:204–210, 1986.
11. Breslow MJ et al: Changes in T-wave morphology following anesthesia and surgery: a common recovery room phenomenon, Anesthesiology 64:398–302, 1986.
12. Calvin JE et al: Cardiac mortality and morbidity after vascular surgery, Can J Surg 29:93–97, 1986.
13. Cannon RO III et al: Angina caused by reduced vasodilator reserve of the small coronary arteries, J Am Coll Cardiol 6:1359–1373, 1983.
14. Carli F et al: An investigation of factors affecting postoperative rewarming of adult patients, Anaesthesia 41:363–369, 1986.
15. Carliner NH et al: Routine preoperative exercise testing in patients undergoing major noncardiac surgery, Am J Cardiol 56:51–58, 1985.
16. Cohn P: Detection and prognosis of the asymptomatic patient with silent myocardial ischemia, Am J Cardiol 61:4B–6B, 1988.

17. Coriat P et al: Clinical predictors of intraoperative myocardial ischemia in patients with coronary artery disease undergoing non-cardiac surgery, Acta Anaesth Scand 26:287–290, 1982.

18. Coriat P et al: Prevention of intraoperative myocardial ischemia during noncardiac surgery with intravenous nitroglycerin, Anesthesiology 61:193–196, 1984.

19. Crawford ES et al: Operative risk in patients with previous coronary artery bypass, Ann Thorac Surg 26:215–221, 1978.

20. Cucchiara RF et al: Evaluation of esmolol in controlling increases in heart rate and blood pressure during endotracheal intubation in patients undergoing carotid endarterectomy, Anesthesiology 65:528–531, 1986.

21. Cutler BS et al: Assessment of operative risk with electrocardiographic exercise testing in patients with peripheral vascular disease, Am J Surg 137:484–490, 1979.

22. Cutler BS and Leppo JA: Dipyridamole thallium 201 scintigraphy to detect coronary artery disease before abdominal aortic surgery, J Vasc Surg 5:91–100, 1987.

23. Deanfield JE et al: Myocardial ischemia during daily life in patients with stable angina: its relation to symptoms and heart rate changes, Lancet 2:753–758, 1983.

24. Detsky IS et al: Cardiac assessment for patients undergoing noncardiac surgery, Arch Intern Med 146:2131–2134, 1986.

25. Dripps RD, Lamont A, and Eckenhoff JE: The role of anesthesia in surgical mortality, JAMA 178:261–266, 1961.

26. Driscoll AC et al: Clinically unrecognized myocardial infarction following surgery, N Engl J Med 264:633–639, 1961.

27. Eagle KA et al: Dipyridamole-thallium scanning in patients undergoing vascular surgery, JAMA 257:2185–2189, 1987.

28. Epstein SE et al: Dynamic coronary obstruction as a cause of angina pectoris: implications regarding therapy, Am J Cardiol 55:61B–68B, 1985.

29. Feldman RI et al: Coronary arterial responses to graded doses of nitroglycerin, Am J Cardiol 43:91–97, 1979.

30. Flaherty JT et al: Comparison of intravenous nitroglycerin and sodium nitroprusside for treatment of acute hypertension developing after coronary artery bypass surgery, Circulation 65:1072–1077, 1982.

31. Frishman WH: Beta-adrenergic blocker withdrawal, Am J Cardiol 59:26F–32F, 1987.

32. Gage AA et al: Assessment of cardiac risk in surgical patients, Arch Surg 112:1488–1492, 1977.

33. Gallagher JD et al: Prophylactic nitroglycerin infusions during coronary artery bypass surgery, Anesthesiology 64:785–789, 1986.

34. Gerson MC et al: Cardiac prognosis in noncardiac geriatric surgery, Ann Intern Med 103:832–837, 1985.

35. Goldman L: Cardiac risks and complications of noncardiac surgery, Ann Intern Med 98:504–513, 1983.

36. Goldschlager N: Use of the treadmill test in the diagnosis of coronary artery disease in patients with chest pain, Ann Intern Med 97:383–388, 1982.

37. Gottlieb SO et al: Effect of the addition of propranolol to therapy with nifedipine for unstable angina pectoris: a randomized, double-blind, placebo-controlled trial, Circulation 73:331–337, 1986.

38. Gottlieb SO et al: Silent ischemia as a marker for early unfavorable outcomes in patients with unstable angina, N Engl J Med 314(19):1214–1219, 1986.

39. Gottlieb SO and Gerstenblith G: Safety of acute calcium antagonist withdrawal: studies in patients with unstable angina withdrawn from nifedipine, Am J Cardiol 55:27E–30E, 1985.

40. Halter JB, Pflug AE, and Porte D Jr: Mechanism of plasma catecholamine increases during surgical stress in man, J Clin Endocrinol Metab 45:936–944, 1977.

41. Hamsten A et al: Haemostatic function in myocardial infarction, Br Heart J 55:58–66, 1986.

42. Hertzer NR et al: Coronary artery disease in peripheral vascular patients, Ann Surg 199:223–233, 1984.

43. Homma S et al: Usefulness of oral dipyridamole suspension for stress thallium imaging without exercise in the detection of coronary artery disease, Am J Cardiol 57:503–508, 1986.

44. Iskandrian AS et al: Effects of esmolol on patients with left ventricular dysfunction, J Am Coll Cardiol 8:225–231, 1986.

45. Jeffrey CC et al: A prospective evaluation of cardiac risk index, Anesthesiology 58:462–464, 1983.

46. Kanto JH: Labetalol in the treatment of angina pectoris, Int J Clin Pharmacol Ther Toxicol 25:166–174, 1987.

47. Kaplan J: Cardiovascular physiology. In Miller R (editor): Anesthesia, ed 2, New York, 1986, Churchill Livingstone.

48. Kaplan JA and King SB III: The precordial electrocardiographic lead (V_5) in patients who have coronary artery disease, Anesthesiology 45:570–574, 1976.

49. Kaplan JA and Wells PH: Early diagnosis of myocardial ischemia using the pulmonary arterial catheter, Anesth Analg 60:789–793, 1981.

50. Klein HO et al: The early recognition of right ventricular infarction: diagnostic accuracy of the electrocardiographic V_4R lead, Circulation 67:558–565, 1983.

51. Kleinman B et al: Qualitative evaluation of coronary flow during anesthetic induction using thallium-201 perfusion scans, Anesthesiology 64:157–164, 1986.

52. Kotrly KJ et al: Intraoperative detection of myocardial ischemia with an ST segment trend monitoring system, Anesth Analg 63:343–345, 1984.

53. Kotter GS et al: Myocardial ischemia during cardiovascular surgery as detected by an ST segment trend monitoring system, J Cardiothorac Anesth 1:190–199, 1987.

54. Kruskal JB et al: Fibrin and fibrinogen-related antigens in patients with stable and unstable coronary artery disease, N Engl J Med 317:1361–1365, 1987.

55. Lacche A and Basaglia P: Hypertensive emergencies: effects of therapy by nifedipine administered sublingually, Curr Therap Res 34:879–887, 1983.

56. Leigh JM, Walter K, and Janaganathan P: Effect of preoperative anaesthetic visit on anxiety, Br Med J 2:987–989, 1977.

57. Leppo J et al: Serial thallium-201 myocardial imaging after dipyridamole infusion: diagnostic utility in detecting coronary stenoses and relationship to regional wall motion, Circulation 66:649–657, 1982.

58. Lette J et al: Rebound of vasospastic angina after cessation of long-term treatment with nifedipine, Can Med Assoc J 130(9):1169-1172, 1984.

59. Loeb HS et al: Effects of pharmacologically-induced hypertension on myocardial ischemia and coronary hemodynamics in patients with fixed coronary obstruction, Circulation 57:41–46, 1978.

60. Lowenstein E, Yusuf S, and Teplick RS: Perioperative myocardial reinfarction: a glimmer of hope—a note of caution, Anesthesiology 59:493–494, 1983.

61. Lunn JK et al: Arterial blood-pressure and pulse-rate responses to pulmonary and radial arterial catheterization prior to cardiac and major vascular operations, Anesthesiology 51:265–269, 1979.

62. MacCarthy EP and Bloomfield SS: Labetalol: a review of its pharmacology, pharmacokinetics, clinical uses and adverse effects, Pharmacotherapy 3:193–219, 1983.

63. Macintyre PE, Pavlin EG, and Dwersteg JF: Effect of meperidine on oxygen consumption, carbon dioxide production, and respiratory gas exchange in postanesthesia shivering, Anesth Analg 66:751–755, 1987.

64. Manelli M et al: A study on human adrenal secretion: measurement of epinephrine, norepinephrine, dopamine and cortisol in peripheral and adrenal venous blood under surgical stress, J Endocrinol Invest 5:91–95, 1982.

65. May DC et al: In vivo induction and reversal of nitroglycerin tolerance in human coronary arteries, N Engl J Med 317:805–809, 1987.

66. McCabe CJ et al: The value of electrocardiogram monitoring during treadmill testing for peripheral vascular disease, Surgery 89(2):183–186, 1981.

67. McCollum CH et al: Myocardial revascularization prior to subsequent major surgery in patients with coronary artery disease, Surgery 81:302–304, 1977.

68. McGregor M: The nitrates and myocardial ischemia, Circulation 66:689–692, 1982.

69. Mehta J and Lopez LM: Calcium-blocker withdrawal phenomenon: increase in affinity of alpha$_2$ adrenoreceptors for agonist as a potential mechanism, Am J Cardiol 58:242–246, 1986.

70. Modig J et al: Role of extradural and of general anaesthesia in fibrinolysis and coagulation after total hip replacement, Br J Anaesth 55:625–629, 1983.

71. Mohr R et al: Cardiac complications in vascular procedures: comparison of percutaneous angioplasty and surgery, Catheter and Cardiovascular Diagnosis 9:339–343, 1983.

72. Morganroth J: Esmolol: an ultrashort-acting beta-blocker for the ICU, Hospital Physician 23(5):23–32, 1987.

73. Mostbeck A, Partsch H, and Peschl L: Investigations on peripheral blood distribution. In Jatine and Lichtlen (editors): Proceedings of the 3rd International Adalat Symposium, Tokyo, 1976, University of Tokyo Press.

74. Oka Y et al: Beta-adrenoreceptor blockade and coronary artery surgery, Am Heart J 99:225–269, 1980.

75. O'Mailia JJ, Sander GE, and Giles TD: Nifedipine-associated myocardial ischemia or infarction in the treatment of hypertensive urgencies, Ann Intern Med 107:185–186, 1987.

76. Pasternack PF et al: The value of the radionuclide angiogram in the prediction of perioperative myocardial infarction in patients undergoing lower extremity revascularization procedures, Circulation 72 (suppl II):13-17, 1985.

77. Pasternack PF et al: The hemodynamics of beta-blockade in patients undergoing abdominal aortic aneurysm repair, Circulation 76(suppl III):1-7, 1987.

78. Pedersen OL, Christensen NJ, and Ramsch KD: Comparison of acute effects of nifedipine in normotensive and hypertensive man, J Cardiovasc Pharmacol 2:357–366, 1980.

79. Poqwizd SM, Sharma AD, and Corr PB: Influence of labetalol, a combined alpha and beta adrenergic blocking agent on the dysrhythmias induced by coronary occlusion and reperfusion, Cardiovasc Res 16:398–407, 1982.

80. Prida XE, Hill JA, and Feldman RL: Systemic and coronary hemodynamic effects of combined alpha- and beta-adrenergic blockade (labetalol) in normotensive patients with stable angina pectoris and positive exercise stress test responses, Am J Cardiol 59:1084–1088, 1987.

81. Quyyumi AA et al: Effects of combined alpha and beta adrenoreceptor blockade in patients with angina pectoris: a double blind study comparing labetalol with placebo, Br Heart J 53:47–52, 1985.

82. Raby KE et al: Detection of preoperative ischemia to assess cardiac risk in peripheral vascular surgery, Clin Res 36(3):349A, 1988.

83. Rao TLK, Jacobs KH, and El-Etr AA: Reinfarction following anesthesia in patients with myocardial infarction, Anesthesiology 59:499–505, 1983.

84. Reichek N et al: Sustained effects of nitroglycerin ointment in patients with angina pectoris, Circulation 50:348–352, 1974.

85. Roberts R and Sobel BE: Elevated plasma MB creatine phosphokinase activity, Arch Intern Med 136:421–424, 1976.

86. Rocco MB et al: Prognostic importance of myocardial ischemia detected by ambulatory monitoring in patients with stable coronary artery disease, Circulation 78:877–884, 1988.

87. Rodriguez JL et al: Physiologic requirements during rewarming: suppression of the shivering response, Crit Care Med 11:490–497, 1983.

88. Russell WJ et al: Changes in plasma catecholamine concentrations during endotracheal intubation, Br J Anaesth 53:837–839, 1981.

89. Selwyn A and Braunwald E: Ischemic heart disease. In Braunwald et al (editors): Harrison's principles of internal medicine, ed 11, 1987, McGraw-Hill Inc.

90. Sheppard D et al: Effects of esmolol on airway function in patients with asthma, J Clin Pharmacol 26:169–174, 1986.

91. Slogoff S and Keats AS: Does perioperative myocardial ischemia lead to postoperative myocardial infarction? Anesthesiology 62:107–114, 1985.

92. Slogoff S and Keats AS: Further observations on perioperative myocardial ischemia, Anesthesiology 65:539–542, 1986.

93. Smith JS et al: Intraoperative detection of myocardial ischemia in high-risk patients: electrocardiography versus two-dimensional transesophageal echocardiography, Circulation 5:1015–1021, 1985.

94. Sonntag H et al: Myocardial blood flow and oxygen consumption during high-dose fentanyl anesthesia in patients with coronary artery disease, Anesthesiology 56:417–422, 1982.

95. Soward AL, Vanhaleweyk GLJ, and Serruys PW: The haemodynamic effects of nifedipine, verapamil and diltiazem in patients with coronary artery disease: a review, Drugs 32:66–101, 1986.

96. Steen PA, Tinker JH, and Tarhan S: Myocardial reinfarction after anesthesia and surgery, JAMA 239:2566–2570, 1978.

97. Stewart DJ et al: Altered spectrum of nitroglycerin action in long-term treatment: nitroglycerin-specific

98. Szecsi E et al: Abrupt withdrawal of pindolol or metoprolol after chronic therapy, Br J Clin Pharmacol 13:3535–3575, 1982.

99. Szekeres L and Udvary E: Haemodynamic factors influencing myocardial ischaemia in a canine model of coronary artery stenosis: the effects of nitroglycerin, Br J Pharmacol 79:337–345, 1983.

100. Tarhan S et al: Myocardial infarction after general anesthesia, JAMA 220:1451–1454, 1972.

101. Thadani U et al: Transdermal nitroglycerin patches in angina pectoris, Ann Intern Med 105:485–492, 1986.

102. Thomson IR, Mutch WAC, and Culligan JD: Failure of intravenous nitroglycerin to prevent intraoperative myocardial ischemia during fentanyl-pancuronium anesthesia, Anesthesiology 61:385–393, 1984.

103. Tomatis LA, Fierens EE, and Verbrugge GP: Evaluation of surgical risk in peripheral vascular disease by coronary arteriography: a series of 100 cases, Surgery 71:429–435, 1972.

104. Topkins MJ and Artusio JF Jr: Myocardial infarction and surgery: a five year study, Anesth Analg 43:716–720, 1964.

105. Trager MA, Teinberg BI, and Kaplan JA: Right ventricular ischemia diagnosed by an esophageal electrocardiogram and right atrial pressure tracing, J Cardiothorac Anes 1:123–125, 1987.

106. von Knorring J: Postoperative myocardial infarction: a prospective study in a risk group of surgical patients, Surgery 90:55–60, 1981.

107. Waller JL et al: Hemodynamic responses to preoperative vascular cannulation in patients with coronary artery disease, Anesthesiology 56:219–221, 1982.

108. Walsh J et al: Premedication abolished the increase in plasma beta-endorphin observed in the immediate preoperative period, Anesthesiology 66:402–405, 1987.

109. Wells PH and Kaplan JA: Optimal management of patients with ischemic heart disease for noncardiac surgery by complementary anesthesiologist and cardiologist interaction, Am Heart J 102:1029–1037, 1981.

110. Wohlgelernter D et al: Regional myocardial dysfunction during coronary angioplasty, evaluation by two-dimensional echocardiography and 12-lead electrocardiography, J Am Coll Cardiol 7:1245, 1986.

111. Zeldin RA: Assessing cardiac risk in patients who undergo noncardiac surgical procedures, Can J Surg 27:402–404, 1984.

CHAPTER **18**

Arrhythmias Including SSS/Heart Block

NEAL T. SAKIMA

An arrhythmia may be defined as "any abnormality in the rate, regularity, or site of origin of the cardiac impulse, or disturbance in the conduction of that impulse such that the normal sequence of activation of atria and ventricles is altered."[39] Perioperative arrhythmias may reflect either appropriate physiologic responses to perioperative stress or inherent abnormalities of cardiac electrophysiologic function. Both anesthetic agents and surgical complications can contribute to the development of perioperative arrhythmias that may adversely affect cardiovascular function. This chapter will discuss the incidence of perioperative arrhythmias, the pathogenesis of these arrhythmias, and then specific arrhythmias and conduction disturbances in detail.

INCIDENCE OF PERIOPERATIVE ARRHYTHMIAS

In 1967, Kuner et al[66] published results from a series of 154 consecutive patients who had continuously recorded intraoperative electrocardiographic (ECG) monitoring. Excluding sinus tachycardia, 95 patients (61.7%) showed evidence of one or more arrhythmias (Table 18-1). Of the 195 arrhythmias seen, the majority were supraventricular in origin and involved accelerated pacemaker activity of usually nondominant cardiac tissues. This study did not comment on the hemodynamic impact of these rhythm disturbances. The high incidence of intraoperative arrhythmias suggests that these rhythm disturbances occur because of effects of anesthetics and

TABLE 18-1. Arrhythmias occurring during anesthesia and surgery

Type of arrhythmia	Percent of patients*
Wandering pacemaker	28%
Isorhythmic AV dissociation	22%
Nodal rhythm	19%
Premature ventricular contractions	18%
Sinus bradycardia	14%
Premature supraventricular contractions	12%
Paroxysmal supraventricular tachycardia	3%
Ventricular tachycardia	3%
Others (including atrial flutter and fibrillation, idioventricular rhythm, ventricular standstill and blocks)	6%

From Kuner et al: Cardiac arrhythmias during anesthesia, Dis Chest 52(5):580-587, 1967.
*Some patients had more than one arrhythmia.

surgical stress on the heart rather than reflecting underlying cardiac pathology.

Kuner found no difference in the incidence of arrhythmias between patients with and without preexisting cardiac disease (58.8% versus 62.0%, respectively). However, Vanik and Davis[126] reported a higher incidence of arrhythmias in patients with heart disease (34.9% versus 16.3%). Perhaps the discrepant findings can be explained by the findings of Bertrand et al[13] who found a similar incidence of supraventricular arrhythmias in patients with and without heart disease, but found an increased incidence of ventricular arrhythmias in patients with cardiac disease (60% versus 37%). Other investigators, however, report an increased incidence of both supraventricular and ventricular ectopic beats in patients with heart disease.[62] Thus the data support the conclusion that patients with preexisting cardiac disease have an increased incidence of ventricular arrhythmias and, possibly, supraventricular arrhythmias, suggesting that underlying cardiac disease can increase the susceptibility to anesthetic and stress-induced arrhythmias.

Further insight into mechanisms contributing to perioperative rhythm disturbances is provided by the finding of Kuner that intraoperative arrhythmias occur more commonly in intubated patients (72.2% versus 43.9%), presumably as a result of airway stimulation. This finding is supported by Bertrand et al,[13] who found that arrhythmias occurred most

commonly at the time of intubation and extubation. Airway manipulation is a potent stimulus for increased sympathetic tone, increased circulating catecholamines, and thus arrhythmogenesis. Katz and Bigger[60] reviewed 13 studies and found that the incidence of arrhythmias during intubation was quite variable (0% to 90%) and depended on the specific anesthetic agents used, the definition of an arrhythmia, and the method of recording and analyzing the arrhythmia. Reininkainen and Pontinen[97] compared the incidence of arrhythmias during intubation with different anesthetic techniques and found an incidence of 29% with halothane alone, 54% with halothane and succinylcholine, 17% with thiopental and succinylcholine, and 8% with thiopental, succinylcholine, and propranolol. This study suggests that succinylcholine increases the incidence of intubation related arrhythmias, at least when used with halothane, that halothane may be associated with a greater frequency of arrhythmias than thiopental, and that propranolol decreases the incidence of arrhythmias, presumably by attenuating the cardiac effects of sympathetic stimulation. Whether these differences are specifically caused by the agents involved, the susceptibility of the individual patient, or the differences in the depth of anesthesia is not known.

The above data suggest that both increased sympathetic tone and direct cardiac effects of general anesthetic agents contribute to the development of intraoperative arrhythmias. The use of regional anesthetic techniques, however, does not reduce the risk for developing intraoperative arrhythmias. Arrhythmias occurred with equal frequency in patients receiving general versus regional anesthesia in Kuner's series and in Vanik and Davis's series.[66,126] Similarly, Reininkainen and Pontinen[97] found a 14.5% incidence of arrhythmias during maintenance of general anesthesia (not including arrhythmias occurring during induction and intubation) versus a 17.6% incidence during epidural anesthesia. The incidence of arrhythmias during intubation, however, was 35.8%, and if these arrhythmias are included with those seen during maintenance of general anesthesia, then there was an increased incidence of arrhythmias during general anesthesia. Kimbrough et al[62] studied 18 men undergoing cystoscopies under local lidocaine anesthesia, half of whom subsequently had repeat cystoscopies under halothane general anesthesia and the other half of whom had epidural anesthesia for their repeat cystoscopies

TABLE 18-2. Comparison of cardiac rhythm in 92 cystoscopies in 18 men with respect to the type of anesthesia used

	18 men local anesthesia	9 men general anesthesia	9 men epidural anesthesia
Total cytoscopies	39	24	29
NUMBER OF CYSTOSCOPIES IN PATIENTS WITH:			
Ectopic beats of any type	24 (61.5%)	9 (37.5%)	11 (37.9%)
Ventricular ectopic beats	19 (48.7%)	2 (8.0%)	4 (13.8%)
Supraventricular ectopic beats	13 (33.3%)	9 (37.5%)	9 (31.0%)

From Kimbrough HM, Crampton RS, and Gillenwater JY: Cardiac rhythm in men during cystoscopy, J Urol 113:846-849, 1975.

(Table 18-2). The incidence of supraventricular and ventricular ectopic beats during the repeat cystoscopies was not significantly different between the two groups. However, the incidence of ventricular ectopic beats was greater during the first cystoscopy done with the local injection of lidocaine than with either general or epidural anesthesia. This suggests that there is no significant difference in the incidence of arrhythmias between general or regional anesthesia, but that stressors such as intubation and inadequate anesthesia increase the incidence of arrhythmias.

The incidence of arrhythmias may also depend on the type of inhalational anesthetic used. Ventricular arrhythmias, for example, are less common with enflurane and isoflurane than with halothane.* The studies of Forrest et al[37] suggest that isoflurane is associated with a very low incidence of intraoperative arrhythmias (Table 18-3). Perhaps of greater importance than the type of anesthetic agent are the findings of Forrest[37] and Dodd[30] that many arrhythmias observed intraoperatively are actually present on preoperative ECG recordings.

Arrhythmias can also occur in the postoperative period. Goldman[44] studied 916 consecutive patients over 40 years of age undergoing major noncardiac surgery and found a 4% incidence of new postoperative supraventricular tachyarrhythmias. The factors thought to be associated with the onset of new postoperative supraventricular tachyarrhythmias in these patients are listed in the box on p. 245. Although Goldman states that no deaths occurred as a direct result of the supraventricular tachyarrhythmias, there was a 49% mortality in patients who

*References 23, 26, 55-57, 96, 113, 122.

TABLE 18-3. Incidence of arrhythmias using isoflurane

	Induction*	Maintenance*
Atrial arrhythmias	3.6% (59%)	3.9% (53%)
Nodal arrhythmias	1.5% (22%)	2.1% (10%)
Ventricular arrhythmias	2.5% (33%)	2.3% (35%)

From Forrest JB et al: Clinical evaluation of isoflurane, Can Anaesth Soc J 29(suppl 1):S1-S59, 1982.
*The numbers in parentheses represent the percentages of patients who had the arrhythmia preoperatively.

developed supraventricular tachyarrhythmias postoperatively, presumably secondary to concurrent medical problems.

In contrast to the relatively low incidence of supraventricular tachyarrhythmias following general surgery, these rhythms, particularly atrial fibrillation, occur commonly following thoracic surgical procedures. A review of the literature by Krowka et al[64] revealed an incidence of postpneumonectomy arrhythmias ranging between 6% and 29%. In his own series of 236 consecutive patients, Krowka found that 95% of postpneumonectomy tachyarrhythmias occurred within 6 days after surgery, and only 4% occurred intraoperatively. Risk factors associated with postpneumonectomy arrhythmias include intrapericardial dissection and interstitial or perihilar edema. Patients with postpneumonectomy arrhythmias had a significantly increased 30 day mortality compared to those patients who did not have arrhythmias (25% versus 7%).

In summary, perioperative arrhythmias are common. The majority of these arrhythmias are supra-

Factors contributing to the onset of new postoperative supraventricular tachyarrhythmias
Acute cardiac events Severe congestive heart failure or pulmonary edema Myocardial infarction Myocardial ischemia without infarction Cardiac arrest Pericardial tamponade
Major infection Pneumonia Peritonitis Positive blood cultures
Hypotensive event preceding supraventricular tachycardia Therapy with adrenergic agents Acute hemorrhage and hypovolemia
Anemia (hematocrit less than 30%)
Metabolic derangements Hypokalemia Acidosis (pH $\leq$ 7.25)
Medications New intravenous therapy (droperidol, sodium nitroprusside, dopamine, and epinephrine) High dose therapy with parenteral bronchodilator drugs
Hypoxemia (PaO$_2$ $\leq$ 60 mm Hg) **Abnormal temperature without major infection** Hypothermia Fever
From Goldman L: Supraventricular tachyarrhythmias in hospitalized adults after surgery, Chest 73(4):450-454, 1978.

ventricular. Patients with preexisting heart disease are more likely to have ventricular dysrhythmias than patients without heart disease. Surgical stress and airway manipulation both appear to be causally related to the development of intraoperative arrhythmias, and certain anesthetic agents may increase the likelihood of their occurrence. None of the large series published in the literature address the hemodynamic consequences of these arrhythmias and thus the clinical importance of these common complications is not known.

PATHOGENESIS OF PERIOPERATIVE ARRHYTHMIAS

While most arrhythmias in nonsurgical settings are the result of intrinsic cardiac disease, arrhythmias that develop in the perioperative period are usually caused by either stress-induced changes in autonomic tone or the effects of anesthetic agents on the heart. This section will discuss both these topics in detail.

The Autonomic Nervous System and the Heart

Increased sympathetic tone may be caused by anxiety, pain, hypoxia, hypercarbia, hypovolemia, or hypotension. While every effort may be made to avoid or treat these reversible causes of increased sympathetic tone, the stress response associated with anesthesia and surgery will increase sympathetic tone even under optimal conditions. Treating this increased sympathetic tone prophylactically with beta-adrenergic blockers has been shown to decrease the incidence of arrhythmias.[49,129] However, beta blockade will also blunt appropriate compensatory increases in sympathetic tone. The section on sinus tachycardia discusses the use of prophylactic beta-blockade in detail.

Altered parasympathetic tone may contribute to arrhythmias during the perioperative period. Surgical manipulation or pressure on the carotid sinus can cause an increase in vagal tone with a resultant bradycardia. Gastrointestinal manipulation, vomiting, traction on the extraocular muscles, or eyeball compression can also induce a vagal reflex.[127] Drugs such as the anticholinesterases, which are used to reverse neuromuscular blockade, cause an increase in parasympathetic tone and must be used with an anticholinergic agent such as atropine or glycopyrrolate to prevent bradycardia.

Atropine has been used prophylactically in patients scheduled for ophthalmic surgery because of the high incidence of bradyarrhythmias from the oculocardiac reflex (OCR). In a study by Bosomworth et al,[16] premedication with intramuscular atropine 30 to 120 minutes preoperatively was ineffective in blocking the OCR, but intravenous atropine given just before the operation was effective. However, atropine may produce an undesirable tachycardia or ventricular dysrhythmia.[4,125] Prophylactic atropine is, therefore, not routinely recommended, and the bradyarrhythmias are treated only if and when they occur. Glycopyrrolate is probably as effective as atropine in blocking the OCR, produces less tachycardia, but has a slower onset time.[82] Retrobulbar block has been used with variable success in preventing the OCR.[11,16,75,116] However, the retrobulbar block itself may elicit the OCR and has the added risk of traumatic injury during placement of the block.

Anesthetic Agents and the Heart

Inhalational agents. Halothane, enflurane, and isoflurane decrease automaticity in isolated sinus node preparations* resulting in a decreased heart rate. In vivo, halothane, enflurane, and isoflurane also decrease heart rate by decreasing sympathetic tone[50,100] and by blunting baroreflex mediated increases in heart rate.[31,63,110,115] Enflurane and isoflurane depress baroreceptor function less than halothane.[32,35,85] The increased heart rate that is sometimes seen during isoflurane anesthesia may be caused by both decreased suppression of the baroreceptor reflex[63,110,115] and decreased suppression of sympathetic nervous system activity.[35]

Halothane and enflurane prolong atrioventricular (AV) conduction in isolated rabbit hearts[91] and in intact dogs.[3] This effect is blocked with atropine and propranolol, suggesting that AV slowing by inhalation agents may be an indirect effect mediated through the autonomic nervous system.[3] High concentrations of halothane and enflurane prolong intraventricular and intraatrial conduction times, and this effect is exacerbated by acidosis.[91] Halothane, enflurane, and isoflurane also increase His-Purkinje system (HPS) conduction time.[3] Although these effects theoretically could produce heart block in patients with underlying conduction system disease, clinical studies have shown that this is not the case.[10,41,102,133]

Premature ventricular complexes (PVCs) occur more commonly with halothane than with other inhalational anesthetics.† Although the mechanism is not completely elucidated, the threshold for catecholamine induced PVCs is lower with halothane than with other anesthetic agents. Drug interactions can also increase the incidence of arrhythmias. For example, halothane increases ventricular irritability in aminophylline pretreated dogs,[122] and this effect is more common with acute rather than chronic aminophylline loading.[95] Concomitant use of halothane

*References 15, 72, 91, 94, 99.
†References 21, 26, 55-57, 96, 113, 122.

with drugs that block reuptake of norepinephrine, such as tricyclic antidepressants, may sensitize the heart to epinephrine-induced ventricular ectopy. The combination of halothane and pancuronium can cause severe ventricular dysrhythmias in dogs on chronic tricyclic therapy.[34] Although not proven to be equally dangerous in humans, this combination of agents should probably be avoided, if possible. The widespread availability of equally effective alternatives to halothane make it possible to avoid many of these arrhythmogenic drug interactions by using another agent.

A lower dose of epinephrine is required to induce ventricular ectopy when halothane is combined with tricyclic antidepressants compared to enflurane.[130] There are case reports of patients receiving tricyclic antidepressants who have prolonged episodes of severe arrhythmias during anesthesia and surgery.[93] However, a case-control study of patients with cardiac disease showed a similar incidence of perioperative arrhythmias in patients taking or not taking tricyclic antidepressants.[83] This finding may be explained by a study that showed that while the incidence of epinephrine-induced arrhythmias in halothane anesthetized dogs increases with imipramine pretreatment for a short period of time, the arrhythmogenic dose of epinephrine is not significantly different from untreated dogs when the imipramine is given for 6 weeks before being studied.[119]

Although nitrous oxide is not considered to be an arrhythmogenic agent, Roizen[101] suggests an association between this agent and episodes of intraoperative accelerated AV junctional rhythm. This association may be the result of sympathomimetic effects of nitrous oxide. However, this association remains unproven, and given the usual insignificant hemodynamic impact of this arrhythmia, no changes in practice patterns are recommended.

Neuromuscular blocking agents and the heart. Succinylcholine produces muscle relaxation by depolarizing nicotinic acetylcholine neuromuscular receptors. It also stimulates cholinergic receptors in both sympathetic and parasympathetic ganglia.[40] In low doses, succinylcholine may have a negative chronotropic effect that is blocked by either atropine or nicotinic ganglionic blocking drugs. Repeat doses of succinylcholine are also associated with bradycardia.[1,71,109] This may be caused by succinylmonocholine, a metabolite of succinylcholine that may enhance vagal sensitivity or have direct muscarinic effects on the sinus node.[1,109,132]

In larger doses, a positive chronotropic response can occur that appears to be mediated by adrenergic receptors.[67,132] Succinylcholine also appears to lower the threshold for catecholamine-induced ventricular dysrhythmias under anesthesia in both monkeys and dogs.[78] It is not known whether a lower threshold for ventricular ectopy or increased sympathetic tone accounts for the observation of Reininkainen and Pontinen[97] that halothane anesthetized patients intubated with succinylcholine have an increased incidence of arrhythmias compared to patients intubated without succinylcholine.

Nondepolarizing muscle relaxants bind to smooth muscle nicotinic receptors and act as competitive antagonists. Pancuronium may cause tachycardia by blocking cardiac muscarinic receptors[108] and by stimulating sympathetic ganglia.[70] Pancuronium may also have direct effects on the heart to increase automaticity.[54] Vecuronium and atracurium do not cause significant changes in heart rate at the doses used clinically.* This may make patients more vulnerable to bradycardic episodes with vagal stimulation.[20,59,106,121] Glycopyrrolate given just before the induction of anesthesia has been shown to be effective in preventing the majority of bradycardic episodes in general surgical patients who receive vecuronium during isoflurane/nitrous oxide anesthesia.[25] The risk of bradycardia must be weighed against the risk of inducing excessive tachycardia when deciding to use such a prophylactic regimen.

Reflex tachycardia may occur because of hypotension induced by the ganglionic blockade and histamine release caused by tubocurarine, and to a lesser extent, by metocurine.[17] Although vagal blockade by tubocurarine has been demonstrated in the cat at doses comparable to those causing neuromuscular blockade,[107] the change in heart rate seen in man is small and is associated with a decrease in blood pressure consistent with the reflex tachycardia mentioned previously.[24,123]

All the anticholinesterases that are used to reverse nondepolarizing neuromuscular blockade have parasympathomimetic properties and can cause bradycardia. This complication can be avoided by combining anticholinesterases and anticholinergic agents according to the pharmacodynamic characteristics of each. Edrophonium, for example, has a more rapid onset of action than neostigmine, and atropine has a more rapid onset of action than glycopyrrolate.[27] Clinical studies show that the combinations of edrophonium/atropine and neostigmine/glycopyrrolate produce greater heart rate stability than edrophonium/glycopyrrolate and neostigmine/atropine, respectively.* Pyridostigmine has a slower onset of action than neostigmine[27] and the combination of pyridostigmine/glycopyrrolate produces less of a change in heart rate than pyridostigmine/atropine.[46]

MANAGEMENT ISSUES RELATING TO PERIOPERATIVE ARRHYTHMIAS

The remainder of this chapter is devoted to specific arrhythmias that either occur frequently in the perioperative period or, alternatively, present important management questions. The following topics will be addressed: (1) intraoperative nodal arrhythmias; (2) management of patients with malignant ventricular ectopy; (3) postoperative atrial fibrillation; (4) sinus tachycardia; (5) indications for prophylactic pacing before sugery; (6) management of patients with permanent pacemakers; and (7) arrhythmias associated with pulmonary artery catheter placement. Myocardial ischemia is discussed in another chapter, and for the purposes of this section, it is assumed that ischemia has been ruled out as an etiology of the problem under discussion.

Nodal Rhythm

Accelerated nodal rhythm occurs commonly during anesthesia and surgery. It appears to be the result of an interaction between increased sympathetic tone and electrophysiologic effects of anesthetic agents. Accelerated nodal rhythms are less commonly encountered in nonsurgical settings and, thus this rhythm disturbance is distinctly an "anesthetic" phenomenon.

Lindgren[68] found a 63% incidence of AV junctional rhythms in children undergoing adenotonsillectomy under halothane/thiopental anesthesia, with lower incidence noted in those patients receiving enflurane/thiopental or in those patients having only adenoidectomy (see Table 18-4). Kuner's series[66] included a broad range of ages, anesthetics, and surgical procedures, and had only a 19% incidence of intraoperative nodal rhythm. However, many instances of isorhythmic dissociation and wandering pacemaker were noted that may have actually been accelerated nodal rhythms.

*References 7, 46, 51, 103, 118.

*References 5, 80, 81, 90, 104.

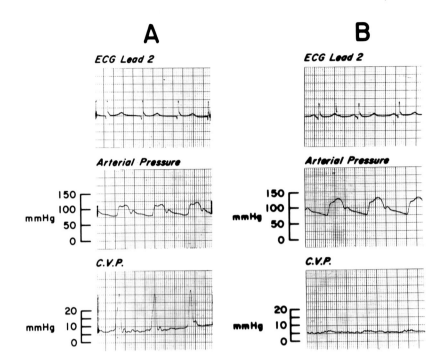

FIGURE 18-1. Electrocardiogram and arterial blood pressure and central venous pressure tracings recorded intraoperatively. *A*, During accelerated junctional rhythm. *B*, Following conversion to sinus rhythm after administration of propranolol. Note absence of P waves on ECG and presence of canon A waves on central venous pressure tracing during junctional rhythm. Paper speed 25 mm/s.

From Breslow MJ, Evers AS, and Lebowitz P: Successful treatment of accelerated junctional rhythm with propranolol: possible role of sympathetic stimulation in the genesis of this rhythm disturbance, Anesthesiology 62:180-182, 1985.

TABLE 18-4.   Incidence of nodal rhythms

	Tonsillectomy and adenoidectomy	Adenoidectomy
Halothane and pentothal	63%	10%
Enflurane and pentothal	26%	24%

From Lindgren L: ECG changes during halothane and enflurane anaesthesia for ENT surgery in children, Br J Anaesth 53:653-661, 1981.

Accelerated nodal rhythms appear to be caused by selective sensitization of perinodal pacemaker cells by anesthetic agents to sympathetic nervous system stimulation such that increases in sympathetic tone (or decreases in parasympathetic tone) result in a nodal rate in excess of the sinus rate. Consistent with this mechanism, acute increases in surgical stimulation or administration of pancuronium or atropine can induce the arrhythmia while administration of beta adrenergic blockers, cholinergic agonists (including succinylcholine), or agents that increase reflex parasympathetic tone by increasing blood pressure, such as phenylephrine, can restore sinus rhythm.

Since accelerated nodal rhythms are always faster than the immediately preceding sinus rate, the hemodynamic impact of this rhythm disturbance is caused by the loss of the atrial kick, which accounts for approximately 15% of the cardiac output. However, in patients with noncompliant ventricles, it may account for up to 50% of the cardiac output.[14,48] In healthy patients, intraoperative accelerated nodal rhythms rarely require therapy. Frequently, the only clue to the presence of this arrhythmia is the presence of cannon A waves on the central venous pressure tracing (Figure 18-1). However, in patients with significant underlying heart disease, this rhythm disorder can result in significant hypotension and require therapy.

Propranolol (0.25 to 0.5 milligrams) usually restores sinus rhythm.[18] Changing anesthetic agents or adjusting the depth of anesthesia can also terminate the accelerated nodal rhythm. However, when hypotension is severe, phenylephrine or a similar alpha-adrenergic agonist will not only increase blood pressure via peripheral vasoconstriction, but it can also restore sinus rhythm by increasing the reflex vagal tone.

Far less commonly, bradycardic junctional escape rhythms (typically at 40 to 50 beats per minute) are encountered during anesthesia. A vagolytic agent such as atropine may be used in this setting to increase either the sinus rate or the nodal rate. Similarly, a sympathomimetic agent such as ephedrine may be used.

Premature Ventricular Complexes

Ventricular ectopy, a common intraoperative rhythm disturbance, may represent ongoing chronic ectopy rather than a consequence of anesthesia and surgery.[30,37] Surgical trauma, however, increases sympathetic tone, and can either exacerbate or induce premature ventricular complexes (PVCs). In addition, the potent inhalational anesthetics sensitize the heart to catecholamines and lower the threshold for ventricular irritability.

Despite a tendency toward increased ventricular ectopy in the perioperative period, ventricular tachycardia and ventricular fibrillation appear to be uncommon, even in patients with prior malignant ventricular ectopy on chronic suppressive therapy. However, specific data on this class of patients are not available.

Whether antiarrhythmic therapy should be continued through the perioperative period is unclear. Many antiarrhythmic drugs prolong conduction in the AV node or HPS. While potent inhalational anesthetic agents also prolong these conduction times, potential augmentation of this effect by antiarrhythmic therapy does not appear to be clinically important and therapy should probably be continued throughout the perioperative period. One exception to this recommendation is the patient on a Class I-A antiarrhythmic agent with a prolonged QT interval and a history of torsade de pointes. These patients should have their therapy decreased or discontinued to normalize their QT interval preoperatively to min-

imize the risk of inducing torsade de pointes intraoperatively.[128]

When a patient is unable to take oral medications during the perioperative period, a parenteral form of the drug should be used. If no parenteral formulation is available, an alternative drug in the same class should be considered. In the latter situation, a cardiology consultation should be obtained to aid in choosing an appropriate regimen. Table 18-5 lists the major classes of antiarrhythmic drugs, the elimination half-life for each, the usual oral dosing intervals, and whether or not a parenteral formulation is available.

Ventricular ectopy, which develops in the perioperative period, is a common problem for which definitive management is difficult to recommend. Whether observation in an intensive care unit or treatment with antiarrhythmic drugs is indicated is not clear from the available literature. Because increased sympathetic nervous system activity is common in this setting, many clinicians administer beta-adrenergic receptor antagonists. Rigorous examination of this practice has not been performed. Reversible causes of increased sympathetic nervous tone should be treated before instituting therapy with beta-adrenergic blockers or lidocaine.

Postoperative Atrial Fibrillation

Postoperative supraventricular tachycardias, such as atrial fibrillation, are not common in the postoperative period, but, when present, are associated with a high mortality.[44] These arrhythmias probably reflect either severe underlying disease or significant surgical complications. A possible exception to this may be patients who undergo resection of pulmonary tissue in whom the incidence of atrial fibrillation ranges from 3% to 16%.* Some studies report an increased incidence of postoperative arrhythmias in patients after pneumonectomy when compared to patients undergoing lobectomy,[23,86] but other studies report a similar incidence with both procedures.[19,42,58,112] There is no correlation between preoperative pulmonary function tests and postoperative arrhythmias,[61,64] but there is an increased incidence of postoperative arrhythmias in patients with preoperative angina pectoris or congestive heart failure[86] and in patients with chest radiographs showing interstitial or perihilar edema.[64] Local trauma and irritation may also be a factor since intrapericardial

*References 23, 42, 58, 64, 86.

TABLE 18-5. Antiarrhythmic drugs

Class	Elimination half-life	Usual oral dosing interval	Parenteral form availability
I-A			
Disopyramide	6-8 hours	6-8 hours	no
Procainamide	2-4 hours	4-6 hours	yes
Quinidine	3-19 hours	6 hours	yes
I-B			
Lidocaine	1.5-2 hours	—	yes
Mexilitene	6-17 hours	6-8 hours	no
Tocainide	13-15 hours	6-12 hours	no
I-C			
Encainide	1-3 hours	6-8 hours	no
Flecainide	12-27 hours	12 hours	no
II			
Esmolol	9 minutes	—	yes
Metoprolol	3-4 hours	6-24 hours	yes
Propranolol	3-4 hours	6-8 hours (SR form-24 hours)	yes
III			
Amiodarone	40-55 days	24 hours	yes
Bretylium	4-17 hours	—	yes
IV			
Verapamil	3-12 hours	8-12 hours (SR form-24 hours)	yes
OTHER			
Digoxin	34-44 hours	24 hours	yes

From McEvoy GK (editor): American Hospital Formulary Drug Information 88, Bethesda, Md, 1988, American Society of Hospital Pharmacists, Inc; Frishman WH; Med Clin North Am 72(1):37-81, 1988; Michelson EL and Dreifus LS: Med Clin North Am; 72(2):275-319, 1988; and Woosley RL and Funck-Brentano C: Am J Cardiol 61:61A-69A, 1988.

dissection has been correlated with postpneumonectomy arrhythmias.[64] Krowka et al[64] found no correlation between increasing age and the incidence of arrhythmias after pneumonectomy, and noted a significantly increased 30 day mortality in those patients who did have arrhythmias (25% versus 7%). It is unclear whether this increased mortality depends upon the presumed etiology of the arrhythmia (cardiac disease, pulmonary disease, or local irritation).

Although prophylactic digitalization has been recommended in patients undergoing pulmonary resection, there are no prospective, randomized studies to support this recommendation. There are also studies showing an increased incidence of intraoperative[126] and postoperative[58] arrhythmias in patients who have received prophylactic digitalization. Based on these studies, digitalization for arrhythmia prophylaxis cannot be recommended, although digoxin may be used to optimize preoperative cardiovascular status before thoracotomy.

Treatment of postoperative atrial fibrillation is directed toward controlling the ventricular response, restoring sinus rhythm, and avoiding embolic complications. Digoxin remains the principal drug used to control the ventricular response in patients in atrial fibrillation, but it may not affect the likelihood of conversion to normal sinus rhythm.[36] Vigorous digitalization can increase ectopic ventricular activity after electrical cardioversion, although animal data suggest that the incidence of postcardioversion ventricular ectopy is not increased in the absence of ECG evidence of digoxin toxicity. Verapamil can also be used to control the ventricular response. Pretreatment with calcium chloride can decrease the hypotensive effect of verapamil without compromising its antiarrhythmic effect.[47] Beta-adrenergic blocking agents may also be used to control the ventricular response.

After the ventricular response is controlled, chemical cardioversion may be required with a Class I-A antiarrhythmic agent such as procainamide or quinidine. In the presence of hypotension, congestive heart failure or angina, electrical cardioversion should be performed.

The risk of embolism in patients with atrial fibrillation of short duration has not been well defined. In nonsurgical patients, it is probably safe to cardiovert without anticoagulation within 3 to 7 days after the onset of the atrial fibrillation.[29,33] However, postoperative patients are in a hypercoagulable state[87] and it has not been determined whether this recommendation can be applied to the surgical patient. If a patient requires emergency cardioversion, anticoagulation for 1 to 4 weeks after cardioversion has been recommended in patients who have had the atrial fibrillation for greater than several days because of a risk of late embolic complications.[33,52] However, the risk of late embolic complications after atrial fibrillation has not been defined in the postoperative patient, and it must be weighed against the risk of surgical bleeding.

Sinus Tachycardia

Sinus tachycardia is common during anesthesia and surgery and is almost universal in the postoperative period. Although not generally defined as an arrhythmia, it can precipitate myocardial ischemia in patients with coronary artery disease and may require treatment. Since increased sinus rate is almost always caused by increased sympathetic tone, beta-adrenergic receptor antagonists offer a specific means of slowing the heart rate. The choice of which agent to use depends on the clinical setting. During surgery, rapid changes in surgical stimulation relative to anesthetic depth can result in transient increases in heart rate. Use of a long acting beta-blocker may be ill-advised because subsequent decreases in sympathetic tone or unexpected blood loss can quickly result in decreased blood pressure and cardiac output, and persistent beta-blockade can attenuate normal compensatory increases in heart rate and contractility.

In the past, propranolol was the only parenteral beta-adrenergic blocker available. There are now several parenteral agents available with beta-1 selectivity and a shorter duration of action. While the beta-1 selective blockers have less of an effect on pulmonary function than nonselective agents, they still can impair pulmonary function in a dose-dependent fashion and may cause bronchospasm at low doses in patients with reactive airways.[38,73]

Esmolol, an ultra-short acting beta-1 selective adrenergic blocker, effectively attenuates the tachycardia associated with intubation without adversely affecting cardiac index in patients undergoing coronary revascularization.[43,76,88] Esmolol also safely attenuates tachycardia in ASA I to IV patients undergoing noncardiac surgery.[98] However, it has no effect on heart rate in patients who are on beta-adrenergic blockers preoperatively.[28] In the postoperative patient, esmolol can be used as a titratable beta-adrenergic blocker to control heart rate in patients whose clinical status may change rapidly.

Labetolol, a nonselective beta and selective alpha-1 adrenergic blocker, also blocks the tachycardic response to intubation.[53] It is longer acting than esmolol and is therefore potentially more hazardous to use for this purpose than esmolol. Clinically, labetolol is used primarily as a parenteral antihypertensive agent and is especially useful in patients with an associated tachycardia. Of note, labetolol has less bronchoconstricting effect than propranolol in patients with asthma.[114]

Metoprolol, a beta-1 selective adrenergic blocker, has a relatively long half-life (3 to 4 hours) and has not been used widely for acute therapy of sinus tachycardia in the perioperative period. As a prophylactic agent in dental patients without significant cardiac disease, it decreases heart rate and decreases the incidence of PVCs.[49,129] Pasternak et al[92] showed that prophylactic metoprolol in patients undergoing abdominal aortic aneurysm repair decreased intraoperative and postoperative heart rates, decreased the incidence of PVCs, and decreased the incidence of perioperative myocardial infarction (3.1% in the metoprolol group versus 17.6% in the control group). The cardiac index was decreased in the metoprolol treated group immediately after unclamping of the aorta and immediately postoperatively by 15% and 19%, respectively. However, there was no significant difference in cardiac index before or during aortic cross-clamping, or from 6 to 48 hours postoperatively. These results must be interpreted with some caution since historical controls were used and the study was not prospective, blinded, or randomized. Further studies will be needed to establish the efficacy of prophylactic beta-adrenergic blockade in patients with coronary artery disease undergoing major noncardiac surgery.

Prophylactic Intraoperative Pacing

Indications for prophylactic cardiac pacing during anesthesia and surgery are incompletely defined. Symptomatic patients who meet the requirements for permanent pacemaker insertion occasionally come to the hospital for surgery and should have a temporary (and permanent) pacemaker placed. Patients with complete heart block who normally have adequate escape rhythms should probably have prophylactic pacing. Similarly, patients with sick sinus syndrome may progress to sinus bradycardia and sinus arrest, and require pacing since these bradyarrhythmias are typically resistant to drug therapy.[6] In contrast, patients with preexisting bundle-branch block, including bifascicular block with or without coexisting first degree AV block, do not appear to be at high risk to develop complete heart block, and pacing is generally not recommended.[10,41,102,133]

The recent introduction of several new methodologies have increased the options for intraoperative pacing. The available choices are shown in the box above, right. Placement of a transvenous pacing wire is the most direct method of temporarily pacing either the atrium or ventricle. Atrial pacing maintains the atrial kick and adds significantly to the cardiac index.[7] However, it cannot be used in the presence of an AV block unless a ventricular pacing wire is also used. An atrial pacing wire is more difficult to place than a ventricular wire, although neither necessarily requires fluoroscopy for placement.[69]

For the patient who requires a pulmonary artery catheter, a specialized pacing pulmonary artery catheter is a convenient method to obtain both atrial and ventricular pacing capabilities. However, Zaidan and Freniere[134] found that in cardiac surgical patients, successful atrial capture was achieved in only 89.2% of patients, ventricular pacing in 93.8% of patients, and A-V sequential pacing in 87.7% of patients. Also, pacing thresholds were approximately 4 mA for both atrial and ventricular capture which is much higher than the thresholds of less than 1 mA that are usually obtained with a properly placed pacing wire in direct contact with the endocardium.[65] In addition, the position of the pacing electrodes is fixed relative

---

Methods of temporary pacing
Transvenous pacing wire Pacing pulmonary artery catheter "Paceport" pulmonary artery catheter Esophageal pacing External pacing

to the tip of the pulmonary artery catheter, and it may not be possible to position the catheter such that it wedges properly and captures at the same time. The "Paceport" pulmonary artery catheter attempts to overcome these disadvantages by having a pacing wire pass through a port in the catheter. Thus, the wire can be positioned independently of the tip of the pulmonary artery catheter to obtain capture.

Esophageal pacing has been used primarily for atrial pacing. Ventricular pacing via the esophagus is not reliably successful even with high output stimuli.[9] Esophageal pacing does not require invasion of the vascular system, but experience with its use in the perioperative period is limited at this time and it requires equipment that is not routinely available in most operating rooms.

Transcutaneous temporary pacing has been shown to be a safe and effective technique in the operating room.[12] It can be used in conscious patients, but Zoll et al[136] found that 11% of their patients had "intolerable" discomfort with its use. Transcutaneous pacing is noninvasive, but it does require special equipment that is not routinely available in operating rooms.

Management of Patients with Permanent Pacemakers

The most common permanent pacemakers in current use are VVI, DVI, and DDD pacemakers.[22] A VVI pacemaker paces the ventricle (V), senses beats in the ventricle (V), and is inhibited (I) when the natural heart rate is greater than the heart rate at which the pacemaker is set. A DVI pacemaker paces both the atrium and the ventricle (D), senses beats in the ventricle (V), and is inhibited (I) when the natural heart rate is greater than the rate at which the pacemaker is set. DDD pacemakers may pace both the atrium and the ventricle (D), senses beats in both the atrium and the ventricle (D), and is both inhibited when the natural heart rate is greater than

TABLE 18-6.   Five position pacemaker code

Position	Category	Letters
I	Chamber(s) paced	V = Ventricle
		A = Atrium
		D = Double
II	Chamber(s) sensed	V = Ventricle
		A = Atrium
		D = Double
		O = None
III	Mode of re-sponse(s)	T = Triggered
		I = Inhibited
		D = Double
		O = None
IV	Programmable functions	P = Programmable (rate and/or output)
		M = Multi-programmable
		O = None
V	Special tachy-arrhythmia functions	B = Bursts
		N = Normal rate competition
		S = Scanning
		E = External

the pacemaker rate, and can trigger a ventricular paced beat after a preceding atrial beat (D). Table 18-6 more fully describes the nomenclature of permanent pacemakers.

Proper perioperative pacemaker management must account for interference with pacemaker sensing and for failure to capture the paced beats. Since unipolar pacemakers measure the potential difference between an intracardiac electrode and an indifferent electrode on the pulse generator, they are vulnerable to inhibition by electrical potentials generated by skeletal muscle.[22,89,135] In the ambulatory setting myopotentials from the pectoral muscles usually do not exceed 4 mV, while the intraventricular cardiac potential measured is usually at least 10 mV in amplitude.[22] Therefore, it should be possible to eliminate interference from myopotentials by keeping the sensitivity above 4 mV but below the amplitude of a normal cardiac depolarization potential. Myopotential inhibition can occur with bipolar electrical systems, but it is unusual and suggests possible pacemaker malfunction resulting from defective insulation of the catheter electrodes or penetration of the electrode through the heart allowing myopotentials from the diaphragm to be sensed.[22]

Electrocautery devices may suppress pacemaker activity and should be avoided when possible. If electrocautery must be used, the ground plate should be located such that the current path will be kept away from the pulse generator and intracardiac electrode(s).[135] The active tip of the electrocautery should remain at least 15 centimeters away from the pulse generator because ventricular fibrillation can be induced if the electrocautery current is conducted down the lead to the heart.[135]

If it is anticipated that electrical interference will render the demand mode of a pacemaker ineffective, the pacemaker should be placed on an asynchronous mode (VOO = ventricular pacing, no sensing, and no inhibition). Some pacemakers incorporate an interference mode during which they automatically go into an asynchronous mode.[22] The risk of inducing ventricular fibrillation by competing rhythms is small as long as there is low energy output from the generator, hypoxia is avoided, and electrolyte and acid-base balance is maintained.[89]

Factors that increase the pacing threshold and cause failure to capture include changes in pH, PO_2, PCO_2, and potassium, and the use of antiarrhythmic agents, including propranolol and procainamide.[135] Electrode displacement and subcutaneous emphysema isolating the indifferent electrode on the pulse generator are other causes of pacemaker failure.[117] In contrast, decreased cardiac conduction threshold from myocardial ischemia, increased sympathomimetic amines, and hypoxia may induce ventricular fibrillation.[89]

Arrhythmias Associated With Pulmonary Artery Catheter Placement

Placement of pulmonary artery catheters is a common cause of perioperative arrhythmias. Shah et al[111] reported a 72% incidence of arrhythmias (PVCs in 70.7% and PACs in 1.3%) in a series of 6,245 patients. Persistent PVCs occurred in only 3.1% of patients and these were treated successfully with 50 to 100 milligrams of lidocaine. Sprung[120] found that advanced ventricular arrhythmias (defined as 3 or more consecutive ventricular beats) occurred more commonly in the presence of myocardial infarction or ischemia, hypoxemia (PO_2 less than 60 mm Hg), and acidosis (pH less than or equal to 7.20). Shock, hypocalcemia, and hypokalemia may also predispose to ventricular arrhythmias. Prophylactic lidocaine does not decrease the incidence of ventricular ectopy during preoperative PA catheter placement.[105] These data suggest that most arrhythmias seen during preoperative PA catheter placement are transient and do not require therapy. Severe ventricular ectopy can usually be easily treated with lidocaine.

Pulmonary artery catheter placement may cause right bundle-branch block (RBBB). Shah et al[111] observed that three patients who developed a new RBBB (0.05%) and one of 113 patients who had a preexisting left bundle branch block (LBBB) developed complete heart block. The incidence of RBBB during right heart catheterization in patients with preexisting LBBB has been reported by other investigators to be significantly higher (as high as 23% [2]) than that observed by Shah. However, that study involved patients undergoing electrophysiologic testing that uses stiffer catheters than those used for pulmonary artery catheterization. In a study of critically ill medical patients by Sprung et al[120], 5% of patients developed new RBBB, but new RBBB did not occur in any of the eight patients with preexisting LBBB. The incidence of RBBB observed in this study is similar to that found by Thompson et al[124] in preoperative cardiac surgical patients (5%). Morris et al[84] studied 47 MICU and CCU patients with LBBB undergoing 82 pulmonary artery catheterizations. There were five episodes of complete heart block, but none of them were associated with placement of the pulmonary artery catheter. Since the incidence of complete heart block in patients with LBBB is quite low, most clinicians do not use prophylactic pacemaker placement before pulmonary artery catheter placement. One should, however, be aware of the risk of complete heart block and be prepared to treat it should it occur. In the absence of a preexisting LBBB, the development of a RBBB during pulmonary artery catheter insertion does not require specific therapy.

Correctly positioning a pulmonary artery catheter following pacemaker wire insertion is often difficult and may require fluoroscopy. Some practitioners circumvent this problem by employing pulmonary artery catheters with pacing potential. However, these catheters do not function until the pulmonary artery catheter is properly positioned in the pulmonary artery and they, therefore, would not be useful for heart block encountered during the insertion procedure.

REFERENCES

1. Abdul-Rasool IH, Sears DH, and Katz RL: The effect of a second dose of succinylcholine on cardiac rate and rhythm following induction of anesthesia with etomidate or midazolam, Anesthesiology 67:795-797, 1987.
2. Akhtar M et al: Induction of iatrogenic electrocardiographic patterns during electrophysiologic studies, Circulation 56:60-65, 1977.
3. Atlee JL et al: Conscious-state comparisons of the effects of inhalation anesthetics of specialized atrioventricular conduction times in dogs, Anesthesiology 64:703-710, 1986.
4. Averill KH and Lamb LE: Less commonly recognized actions of atropine on cardiac rhythm, Am J Med Sci 237:304-318, 1959.
5. Azar I et al: The heart rate following edrophonium-atropine and edrophonium-glycopyrrolate mixtures, Anesthesiology, 59:139-141, 1983.
6. Barnes PK et al: Comparison of the effects of atracurium and tubocurarine on heart rate and arterial pressure in anaesthetized man, Br J Anaesth 55:91S-94S, 1983.
7. Befeler B et al: Cardiovascular dynamics during coronary sinus, right atrial, and right ventricular pacing, Am Heart J 81(3):372-380, 1971.
8. Belic N and Talano JV: Current concepts in sick sinus syndromes. II. ECG manifestations and diagnostic and therapeutic approaches, Arch Intern Med 145:722-726, 1985.
9. Benson DW: Transesophageal electrocardiography and cardiac pacing: state of the art, Circulation, 75(suppl III):86-90, 1987.
10. Berg GR and Kotler MN: The significance of bilateral bundle-branch block in the preoperative patient, Chest 59(1):62-67, 1971.
11. Berler DK: The oculocardiac reflex, Am J Ophthalmol 56:954-959, 1963.
12. Berliner D et al: Transcutaneous temporary pacing in the operating room, JAMA 254:84-86, 1985.
13. Bertrand CA et al: Disturbances of cardiac rhythm during anesthesia and surgery, JAMA 216(10):1615-1617, 1971.
14. Boba A: Significant effects on the blood pressure of an apparently trivial atrial dysrhythmia, Anesthesiology 48:282-283, 1978.
15. Bosnjak ZJ and Kampine JP: Effects of halothane, enflurane, and isoflurane on the SA node, Anesthesiology, 58:314-321, 1983.
16. Bosomworth PP, Ziegler CH, and Jacoby J: The oculo-cardiac reflex in eye muscle surgery, Anesthesiology 19(1):7-10, 1958.
17. Bowman WC: Non-relaxant properties of neuromuscular blocking drugs, Br J Anaesth 54:147-160, 1982.

18. Breslow MJ, Evers AS, and Lebowitz P: Successful treatment of accelerated junctional rhythm with propranolol: possible role of sympathetic stimulation in the genesis of this rhythm disturbance, Anesthesiology 62:180-182, 1985.

19. Burman SO: The prophylactic use of digitalis before thoracotomy, Ann Thorac Surg 14(4):359-368, 1972.

20. Carter ML: Bradycardia after the use of atracurium, Br Med J 287:247-248, 1983.

21. Casson WR and Jones RM: Cardiac rate and rhythm during anaesthesia for dental extraction. A comparison of halothane, enflurane, and isoflurane, Br J Anaesth 57:476-481, 1985.

22. Castellanos A et al: Pacemaker-induced arrhythmias. In Mandel WJ (editor): cardiac arrhythmias: their mechanisms, diagnosis, and treatment, Philadelphia, 1987, JB Lippincott Co.

23. Cohen MG and Pastor BH: Delayed cardiac arrhythmias following noncardiac thoracic surgery, Dis Chest 32:435-440, 1957.

24. Coleman AJ et al: The immediate cardiovascular effects of pancuronium, alcuronium, and tubocurarine in man, Anaesthesia 27(4):415-422, 1972.

25. Cozanitis DA, Pouttu J, and Rosenberg PH: Bradycardia associated with the use of vecuronium. A comparative study with pancuronium with and without glycopyrronium, Anaesthesia 42:192-194, 1987.

26. Cripps TP and Edmondson RS: Isoflurane for anaesthesia in the dental chair. A comparison of the incidence of cardiac dysrhythmias during anaesthesia with halothane and isoflurane, Anaesthesia 42:189-191, 1987.

27. Cronnelly R and Morris RB: Antagonism of neuromuscular blockade, Br J Anaesth 54:183-194, 1982.

28. de Bruijn N:, Croughwell N, and Reeves JG: Hemodynamic effects of esmolol in chronically beta-blocked patients undergoing aortocoronary bypass surgery, Anesth Analg 66:137-144, 1987.

29. DeSilva RA et al: Cardioversion and defibrillation, Am Heart J 100(6):881-895, 1980.

30. Dodd RB, Sims WA, and Bone DJ: Cardiac arrhythmias observed during anesthesia and surgery, Surgery 51:440-447, 1962.

31 Duke PC, Fownes D, and Wade JG: Halothane depresses baroreflex control of heart rate in man, Anesthesiology 46:184-187, 1977.

32. Duke PC, Hill K, and Trosky S: The effect of isoflurane and isoflurane with nitrous oxide anesthesia on baroreceptor reflex control of heart rate in man, Anesthesiology 57(suppl 3A):A41, 1982.

33. Dunn M et al: Antithrombotic therapy in atrial fibrillation, Chest 89(suppl):68S-74S, 1986.

34. Edwards R et al: Cardiac responses to imipramine and pancuronium during anesthesia with halothane or enflurane anesthesia, Anesthesiology 50:421-425, 1979.

35. Eger EI, II: The pharmacology of isoflurane, Br J Anaesth 56:71S-99S, 1984.

36. Falk RH et al: Digoxin for converting recent-onset atrial fibrillation to sinus rhythm. A randomized, double-blinded trial, Ann Intern Med 106(4):503-506, 1987.

37. Forrest JB et al: Clinical evaluation of isoflurane, Can Anaesth Soc J 29(suppl 1):S1-S59, 1982.

38. Frishman WH: Beta-adrenergic blockers, Med Clin North Am 72(1):37-81, 1988.

39. Gadsby DC and Wit AL: Normal and abnormal electrical activity in cardiac cells. In Mandel, WJ (editor): Cardiac arrhythmias: their mechanisms, diagnosis, and management, Philadelphia, 1987, JB Lippincott Co.

40. Galindo AH and Davis TB: Succinylcholine and cardiac excitability, Anesthesiology 23:32-40, 1962.

41. Gertler MM et al: Cardiovascular evaluation in surgery. I. Operative risk in cancer patients with bundle branch block, Surg Gynecol Obstet 99:441-450, 1954.

42. Ghosh P and Pakrashi BC: Cardiac dysrhythmias after thoracotomy, Br Heart J 34:374-376, 1972.

43. Girard D et al: The safety and efficacy of esmolol during myocardial revascularization, Anesthesiology 65:157-164, 1986.

44. Goldman L: Supraventricular tachyarrhythmias in hospitalized adults after surgery, Chest 73(4):450-454, 1978.

45. Gregoretti SM, Sohn YJ, and Sia RL: Heart rate and blood pressure changes after ORG NC45 (vecuronium) and pancuronium during halothane and enflurane anesthesia, Anesthesiology 56:392-395, 1982.

46. Gyermek L: Clinical studies on the reversal of the neuromuscular blockade produced by pancuronium bromide. I. The effects of glycopyrrolate and pyridostigmine, Curr Ther Res 18(3):377-386, 1975.

47. Haft JI and Habbab MA: Treatment of atrial arrhythmias: effectiveness of verapamil when preceded by calcium infusion, Arch Intern Med 146:1085-1089, 1986.

48. Haldeman G and Schaer H: Haemodynamic effects of transient atrioventricular dissociation in general anaesthesia, Br J Anaesth 44:159-162, 1972.

49. Hanna MH, Heap DG, and Kimberley APS: Cardiac dysrhythmia associated with general anaesthesia for oral surgery, Anaesthesia 38:1192-1194, 1983.

50. Hickey RF and Eger EI, II: Circulatory pharmacology of inhaled anesthetics. In Miller RD (editor): Anesthesia, New York, 1986, Churchill Livingstone.

51. Hilgenberg JC and Stoelting RK: Haemodynamic effects of atracurium in the presence of potent inhalation agents, Br J Anaesth 58:70S-74S, 1986.

52. Huerta BJ and Lemberg L: Anticoagulation in atrial fibrillation, Heart Lung 14(5):521-523, 1985.

53. Inada E et al: Effect of labetolol on the hemodynamic response to intubation: a controlled randomized double-blind study, Anesthesiology 67(3A):A31, 1987.

54. Jacobs HK et al: Cardiac electrophysiologic effects of pancuronium, Anesth Analg 64:693-699, 1985.

55. Joas TA and Stevens WC: Comparison of the arrhythmic doses of epinephrine during forane, halothane, and fluroxene anesthesia in dogs, Anesthesiology 35:48-53, 1971.

56. Johnston RR, Eger EI, II, and Wilson C: A comparative interaction of epinephrine with enflurane, isoflurane, and halothane in man, Anesth Analg 55:709-712, 1976.

57. Jones RM: Clinical comparison of inhalation anaesthetic agents, Br J Anaesth 56:57S-69S, 1984.

58. Juler GL, Stemmer EA, and Connolly JE: Complications of prophylactic digitalization in thoracic surgical patients, J Thorac Cardiovasc Surg 58(3):352-360, 1969.

59. Karhunen U, Nilsson E, and Brander P: Comparison of four non-depolarizing neuromuscular blocking drugs in the suppression of the oculocardiac reflex during strabismus surgery in children, Br J Anaesth 57:1209-1212, 1985.

60. Katz RL and Bigger JT: Cardiac arrhythmias during anesthesia, Anesthesiology 33(2):193-213, 1970.

61. Keagy BA et al: Correlation of pre-operative pulmonary function testing with clinical course in patients after pneumonectomy, Ann Thorac Surg 36(3):253-257, 1983.

62. Kimbrough HM, Crampton RS, and Gillenwater JY: Cardiac rhythm in men during cystoscopy, J Urol 113:846-849, 1975.

63. Kotorly KJ et al: Baroreceptor reflex control of heart rate during isoflurane anesthesia in humans, Anesthesiology 60:173-179, 1984.

64. Krowka MJ et al: Cardiac dysrhythmia following pneumonectomy, Chest 91(4):490-495, 1987.

65. Krueger SK et al: Temporary pacemaking by general internists, Arch Intern Med 143:1531-1533, 1983.

66. Kuner J et al: Cardiac arrhythmias during anesthesia, Dis Chest 52(5):580-587, 1967.

67. Leiman BC, Katz J, and Butler BD; Mechanisms of succinylcholine-induced arrhythmias in hypoxic or hypoxic:hypercarbic dogs, Anesth Analg 66:1292-1297, 1987.

68. Lindgren L: ECG changes during halothane and enflurane anaesthesia for ENT surgery in children, Br J Anaesth 53:653-662, 1981.

69. Littleford PO and Pepine CJ; A new temporary atrial pacing catheter inserted percutaneously into the subclavian vein without fluoroscopy: a preliminary report, PACE 4:458-464, 1981.

70. Loh L: The cardiovascular effects of pancuronium bromide, Anaesthesia 25(3):356-363, 1970.

71. Lupprian KG and Churchill-Davidson HC: Effect of suxamethonium on cardiac rhythm, Br Med J 1:1774-1777, 1960.

72. Lynch C, III, Vogel S, and Sperelakis N: Halothane depression of myocardial slow action potentials, Anesthesiology 55:360-368, 1981.

73. McDevitt DG: Pharmacologic aspects of cardioselectivity in a beta-blocking drug, Am J Cardiol 59:10F-12F, 1987.

74. McEvoy GK (editor): American Hospital Formulary Service Drug Information 88, Bethesda, Md, 1988, American Society of Hospital Pharmacists, Inc.

75. Mendelblatt FI, Kirsch RE, and Lemberg L: A study comparing methods of preventing the oculocardiac reflex, Am J Ophthalmol 53:506-512, 1962.

76. Menkhaus PG et al: Cardiovascular effects of esmolol in anesthetized humans, Anesth Analg 64:327-334, 1985.

77. Michelson EL and Dreifus LS: Newer antiarrhythmic drugs, Med Clin North Am 72(2):275-319, 1988.

78. Miller RD and Savarese JJ: Pharmacology of muscle relaxants and their antagonists. In Miller RD (editor): Anesthesia, New York, 1986, Churchill Livingstone.

79. Miller RD et al: Clinical pharmacology of vecuronium and atracurium, Anesthesiology 61:444-453, 1984.

80. Mirakhur RK: Antagonism of the muscarinic effects of edrophonium with atropine or glycopyrrolate, Br J Anaesth 57:1213-1216, 1985.

81. Mirakhur RK, Dundee JW, and Clarke RSJ: Glycopyrrolate-neostigmine mixture for antagonism of neuromuscular block: comparison with atropine-neostigmine mixture, Br J Anaesth 49:825-829, 1977.

82. Mirakhur RK et al: IM or IV atropine or glycopyrrolate for the prevention of the oculocardiac reflex in children undergoing squint surgery, Br J Anaesth 54:1059-1063, 1982.

83. Moir DC et al: Cardiotoxicity of amitriptyline, Lancet 2:561-564, 1972.

84. Morris D, Mulvihill D, and Lew YW: Risk of developing complete heart block during bedside pulmonary artery catheterization in patients with left bundle-branch block, Arch Intern Med 147:2005-2010, 1987.

85. Morton M, Duke PC, and Ong B: Baroreflex control of heart rate in man: awake and during enflurane and enflurane-nitrous oxide anesthesia, Anesthesiology 52:221-223, 1980.

86. Mowry FM and Reynolds EW, Jr: Cardiac rhythm disturbances complicating resectional surgery of the lung, Ann Intern Med 61:688-695, 1964.

87. Muller R and Musikic P: Hemorheology in surgery- A review, Angiology 38:581-592, 1987.

88. Newsome LR et al: Esmolol attenuates hemodynamic responses during fentanyl-pancuronium anesthesia for aortocoronary bypass surgery, Anesth Analg 65:451-456, 1986.

89. O'Neill MJ and Davis D: Pacemakers in noncardiac surgery, Surg Clin North Am 63(5):1103-1112, 1983.

90. Ostheimer G: A comparison of glycopyrrolate and atropine during reversal of nondepolarizing neuromuscular block with neostigmine, Anesth Analg 56(2):182-186, 1977.

91. Ozaki S et al: Electrophysiologic effects of enflurane and halothane on isolated rabbit hearts in the presence and absence of metabolic acidosis, Anesth Analg 64:1060-1064, 1985.

92. Pasternak PF et al: The hemodynamics of beta-blockade in patients undergoing abdominal aortic aneurysm repair, Circulation 76(suppl III):III-1-III-7, 1987.

93. Plowman PE and Thomas WJW: Tricyclic antidepressants and cardiac dysrhythmias during dental extraction, Anaesthesia 29:576-578, 1974.

94. Porius AJ and van Zwieten PA: Quantitative evaluation of the cardiodepressive action of halothane and some related drugs in isolated heart muscle: comparison with in vivo circumstances, Arch Int Pharmacodyn 205:134-143, 1973.

95. Prokocimer PG et al: Epinephrine arrhythmogenicity is enhanced by acute, but not chronic aminophylline administration during halothane anesthesia in dogs, Anesthesiology 65(1):13-18, 1986.

96. Raj PP, Tod MJ, and Jenkins MT: Clinical comparison of isoflurane and halothane anesthetics, South Med J 69:1128-1132, 1976.

97. Reininkainen M and Pontinen P: On cardiac arrhythmias during anesthesia, Acta Med Scand 180(suppl 457):1-35, 1966.

98. Reves JG and Flezzani P: Perioperative use of esmolol, Am J Cardiol 56:57F-62F, 1985.

99. Reynolds AK, Chiz JF, and Pasquet AF: Halothane and methoxyflurane: a comparison of their effects on cardiac pacemaker fibers, Anesthesiology 33:602-610, 1970.

100. Roizen MF, Horrigan RW, and Frazer BM: Anesthetic dose blocking adrenergic (stress) and cardiovascular responses to incision—MAC-BAR, Anesthesiology 54:390-398, 1981.

101. Roizen MF, Plummer GO, and Lichtor JL: Nitrous oxide and dysrhythmias, Anesthesiology 66:427-431, 1987.

102. Rooney SM, Goldiner PL, and Muss E: Relationship of right bundle-branch block and marked left axis deviation to complete heart block during general anesthesia, Anesthesiology 44(1):64-66, 1976.

103. Rupp SM, Fahey MR, and Miller RD: Neuromuscular and cardiovascular effects of atracurium during nitrous oxide-fentanyl and nitrous oxide-isoflurane anaesthesia, Br J Anaesth 55:67S-70S, 1983.

104. Salem MG and Ahearn RS: Atropine of glycopyrrolate with neostigmine 5 mg: a comparative dose-response study, J R Soc Med 79(1):19-21, 1986.

105. Salmenpera M, Peltola K, and Rosenberg P: Does prophylactic lidocaine control cardiac arrhythmias associated with pulmonary artery catheterization? Anesthesiology 56:210-212, 1982.

106. Salmenpera M et al: Cardiovascular effects of pancuronium and vecuronium during high-dose fentanyl anesthesia, Anesth Analg 62:1059-1064, 1983.

107. Savarese JJ: The autonomic margins of safety of metocurine and d-Tubocurarine in the cat, Anesthesiology 50:40-46, 1979.

108. Saxena PR and Bonta IL: Specific blockade of cardiac muscarinic receptors by pancuronium bromide, Arch Intern Pharmacodyn 189:410-412, 1972.

109. Schoenstadt DA and Whitcher CE: Observations on the mechanism of succinylcholine-induced cardiac arrhythmias, Anesthesiology 24:358-362, 1963.

110. Seagard JL et al: Effects of isoflurane on the baroreceptor reflex, Anesthesiology 59:511-520, 1983.

111. Shah KB et al: A review of pulmonary artery catheterization in 6,245 patients, Anesthesiology 61:271-275, 1984.

112. Shields TW and Ujiki GT: Digitalization for prevention of arrhythmias following pulmonary surgery, Surg Gynecol Obstet 126:743-746, 1968.

113. Sigurdsson GH et al: Cardiac arrhythmias in non-intubated children during adenoidectomy. A comparison between enflurane and halothane anesthesia, Acta Anaesth Scand 27:75-80, 1983.

114. Skinner C, Gaddie J, and Palmer KNV: Comparison of intravenous AH5158 (ibidomide) and propranolol in asthma, Br Med J 2:59-61, 1975.

115. Skovsted P and Sapthavichaikul S: The effects of isoflurane on arterial pressure, pulse rate, autonomic nervous activity, and barostatic reflexes, Can Anaesth Soc J 24:304-314, 1977.

116. Smith RB, Douglas H, and Petruscak J: The oculocardiac reflex and sino-atrial arrest, Can Anaesth Soc J 19(2):138-142, 1972.

117. Smith SA, Weissberg PL, and Tan L: Permanent pacemaker failure due to surgical emphysema, Br Heart J 54:220-221, 1985.

118. Sokoll MD et al: Safety and efficacy of atracurium (BW33A) in surgical patients receiving balanced or isoflurane anesthesia, Anesthesiology 58:450-455, 1983.

119. Spiss CK, Smith CM, and Maze M: Halothane-epinephrine arrhythmias and adrenergic responsiveness after chronic imipramine administration in dogs, Anesth Analg 63:825-828, 1984.

120. Sprung CL et al: Advanced ventricular arrhythmias during bedside pulmonary artery catheterization, Am J Med 72:203-208, 1982.

121. Starr NJ, Sethna DH, and Estafanous FG: Bradycardia and asystole following the rapid administration of sufentanil with vecuronium, Anesthesiology 64(4):521-523, 1986.

122. Stirt JA, Berger JM, and Sullivan SF: Lack of arrhythmogenicity of isoflurane following administration of aminophylline in dogs, Anesth Analg 62:568-571, 1983.

123. Stoelting RK: The hemodynamic effects of pancuronium and d-Tubocurarine in anesthetized patients, Anesthesiology 36(6):612-615, 1972.

124. Thompson IR et al: Right bundle-branch block and complete heart block caused by the Swan-Ganz catheter, Anesthesiology 51:359-362, 1979.

125. Thurlow AC: Cardiac dysrhythmias in outpatient dental anaesthesia in children. The effect of prophylactic intravenous atropine, Anaesthesia 27(4):429-435, 1972.

126. Vanik PE and Davis HS: Cardiac arrhythmias during halothane anesthesia, Anesth Analg 47:299-307, 1968.

127. Waxman MB, Wald RW, and Cameron D: Interactions between the autonomic nervous system and tachycardias in man, Clin Cardiol 1(2):143-185, 1983.

128. Weiskopf M and Stead SW: Polymorphous ventricular tachycardia during coronary artery bypass surgery, Anesthesiology 64:392-394, 1986.

129. Whitehead MH, Whitmarsh VB, and Horton JN: Metoprolol in anaesthesia for oral surgery, Anaesthesia 35:779-782, 1980.

130. Wong KC et al: Influence of imipramine and pargyline on the arrhythmogenicity of epinephrine during halothane, enflurane, or methoxyflurane anesthesia in dogs, Life Sci 27:2675-2678, 1980.

131. Woosley RL and Funck-Brentano C: Overview of the clinical pharmacology of antiarrhythmic drugs, Am J Cardiol 61:61A-69A, 1988.

132. Yasuda I et al: Chronotropic effects of succinylcholine and succinylmonocholine on the sinoatrial node, Anesthesiology 57:289-292, 1982.

133. Zagatti G et al: Cardiac pacing as prophylaxis in surgical operations, G Ital Cardiol 1(suppl 8):50-54, 1978.

134. Zaidan JR and Freniere S: Use of a pacing pulmonary artery catheter during cardiac surgery, Ann Thorac Surg 35(6):633-636, 1983.

135. Zamost B and Benumof JL: Anesthesia in the geriatric patient. In Katz J, Benumof J, and Kadis LB (editors): Anesthesia and uncommon diseases: pathophysiologic and clinical correlations, Philadelphia, 1981, WB Saunders Co.

136. Zoll PM et al: External non-invasive temporary cardiac pacing: clinical trials, Circulation 71:937-944, 1985.

CHAPTER 19

Asthma and Chronic Obstructive Lung Disease

SANDRALEE A. BLOSSER
PETER ROCK

Patients with asthma or chronic obstructive pulmonary disease are at risk for exacerbation of these conditions when undergoing anesthesia and surgical procedures and have a high incidence of postoperative atelectasis and pneumonia. This chapter presents an approach to accurate preoperative assessment, anesthetic options, and a guide to perioperative management that will minimize the risk to the patient with asthma and chronic obstructive pulmonary disease. Before the presentation of specific management strategies, the pathophysiology of these diseases is reviewed. A theme of this chapter will

259

be the paucity of outcome studies in the area of lung disease and anesthesia. Clinical studies have identified the types of patients prone to respiratory complications as well as surgical procedures that are more likely to cause postoperative pulmonary complications. We are readily able to identify patients, types of surgery, and categories of morbidity that may occur. However, studies demonstrate that this morbidity is only modestly altered with perioperative interventions.

ASTHMA
Mechanisms

Asthma occurs or has occurred in up to 5% of the population.[31] It is defined by the American Thoracic Society as a clinical syndrome, characterized by hyperresponsiveness of the trachea and bronchi to various stimuli, and variable obstruction of the airways that changes in severity spontaneously or as a result of therapy.[2] Bronchoconstriction results from bronchial smooth muscle contraction and muscular hyperplasia and hypertrophy and is accompanied by submucosal edema, denuded epithelium, eosinophilic infiltrates, and hypersecretion of mucus.[38] The clinical manifestations of asthma are dyspnea, cough, and wheezing. Respiratory distress is often rapidly reversible with bronchodilators but can progress to severe prolonged episodes of airway obstruction. Between exacerbations, the patient may be symptom free.

Asthma is a heterogenous disease that is usually classified according to the stimuli that precipitate an exacerbation. Idiosyncratic or intrinsic asthma often occurs in older individuals who lack features that suggest an immunologic basis for their disease (no history of allergy, negative results to skin tests, and normal IgE levels). Allergic or extrinsic asthma is associated with childhood onset, a positive family history, skin allergy, rhinitis, and elevated serum IgE levels. Environmental factors that may precipitate bronchospasm because of hyperreactivity of the tracheobronchial tree include viral upper respiratory tract infection, occupational exposures, pollutants found in urban areas, physical stimulation, exercise, emotional stress, aspirin, and cold air.

One mechanism of hyperirritability is triggering of tissue mast cells. Direct antigen–mast cell interaction in the mucosa, or receptor-mediated mast cell activation, results in release of chemical mediators such as histamine (acting on H_1 receptors to constrict

bronchi), proteolytic enzymes, chemotactic factors, and prostaglandin metabolites.[34] In select instances, H_2 receptors may be responsible for inhibitory control feedback of mediator release.

The autonomic nervous system has also been implicated in the pathogenesis of reactive airways.[34] Increased parasympathetic tone primarily affects the larger airways and seems to mediate the rapid reflex increases in bronchial tone with airway instrumentation during anesthesia and surgery discussed later in detail.[5] Alpha-adrenergic stimulation results in bronchial smooth muscle constriction, while $beta_2$-receptor stimulation causes bronchodilation. Adrenergic tone, however, does not appear normally to affect airway tone significantly, since major sympathetic blockade (spinal or epidural anesthesia) does not produce clinically recognizable bronchospasm from an unopposed parasympathetic system.

Sympathetic nervous system effects on the lung are primarily regulated by circulating epinephrine. Alpha-receptor-induced bronchoconstriction is mild.[34] Bronchodilation resulting from $beta_2$-receptor stimulation may be mediated by receptor activation of adenylate cyclase, which increases intracellular concentration of cyclic AMP.[34] Decreases in intracellular cyclic AMP cause increased mediator release. Cyclic AMP is degraded by phosphodiesterases and inhibition of this leads to increased cyclic AMP. This mechanism may explain theophylline-related bronchodilation. It has also been suggested that methylxanthines cause bronchodilation by blocking adenosine receptors.[8] A study by Fraser et al suggests that autoantibodies to beta-adrenergic receptors may play a role in the pathophysiology of asthma.[24] Walden et al also found that alpha-adrenergic blockade may be helpful in preventing bronchospasm in patients with exercise and cold air–induced asthma.[85]

Pathophysiology

Bronchospasm and mucus production cause increased airway resistance, airflow obstruction, and decreased flow rate and volume of exhaled gas (FEV_1, the volume of gas exhaled in the first second of a forced expiration). Air trapping and hyperinflation of the lungs occur. Increases in residual volume, functional residual capacity (FRC), and total lung capacity are observed. Lung compliance decreases at these high volumes. Work of breathing increases as a result of decreased compliance, increased airway resistance, and mechanical disadvantage of the respiratory muscles related to increased lung volumes. Hypoxemia may occur as airway obstruction leads to redistribution of ventilation and development of ventilation-perfusion inequality. Oxygen delivery may be decreased at a time when the increased work of breathing causes an increase in oxygen consumption. An increased ratio of dead space to tidal volume can lead to wasted ventilation so that increased minute ventilation is required to maintain adequate alveolar ventilation. When adequate ventilation cannot be maintained, either because of respiratory muscle fatigue or obtundation, hypercarbia develops, which may further affect respiratory muscles and blunt the ability to maintain the required minute ventilation.

CHRONIC OBSTRUCTIVE PULMONARY DISEASE (COPD)
Mechanisms

Chronic obstructive pulmonary disease is a common disorder that is estimated to occur in approximately 1% to 3% of the U.S. population.[31] It includes chronic bronchitis and emphysema, which, although different entities, often occur together because of a common cause (smoking). COPD differs from asthma in that there may be components of reversible and irreversible obstruction to airflow. The major site of airflow obstruction is the small airways. Cigarette smoking and, to a lesser extent, occupational or environmental exposures are responsible for nearly all cases of COPD. Mechanisms by which these factors cause COPD are incompletely understood but may include an imbalance between proteases and antiproteases, which results in destruction of the lung matrix.[88]

COPD may be suspected and diagnosed on clinical grounds and can be readily confirmed by spirometric demonstration of airflow obstruction, that is, the ratio of FEV_1 to FVC (forced vital capacity) is less than 0.80. The type of COPD is determined by clinical criteria. Chronic bronchitis is defined by the American Thoracic Society as "a clinical disorder characterized by cough and excessive production of mucus present on most days for at least 3 months in the year for not less than 2 successive years."[2] Patients with chronic bronchitis have airway narrowing from hyperplasia and hypertrophy of the mucus-producing glands in the submucosa of the large airways and the goblet cells of the smaller airways. They exhibit inflammation, edema, peribronchial fibrosis,

mucous plugs, and increased smooth muscle in the airways.

In contrast to chronic bronchitis, emphysema can only be diagnosed with certainty by histologic examination. On microscopic examination the lung shows distention of airspaces distal to the terminal bronchiole and destruction of alveolar septa. The airway narrows because of the loss of radial traction. Emphysema is classified according to whether there is centriacinar or panacinar involvement. Both are usually present in varying degrees in the same lung. As a result of destruction and distention of airspaces there is usually a mismatch of ventilation ($\dot{V}$) and perfusion ($\dot{Q}$). Areas with large airspaces and destroyed parenchyma have few capillaries and thus high $\dot{V}/\dot{Q}$ ratios (dead-space type pathophysiology). Areas in the periphery often have small, crowded alveoli and preserved capillary beds. These latter gas exchange units have low $\dot{V}/\dot{Q}$ ratios and contribute to hypoxemia (shuntlike effects).

Pathophysiology

Clinical evidence of obstruction may be absent when chronic bronchitis and emphysema are mild, but obstruction is always present when the patient is symptomatic.[39] Loss of lung tissue and elastic recoil may result in dynamic collapse of the airway in expiration. Symptoms and signs may include dyspnea, cough, sputum production, and wheezing. The consequences of increased airway resistance are decreased gas flow and increased residual volume. These changes increase the work of breathing and lead to diaphragmatic fatigue and respiratory failure. Unlike asthma, emphysema and chronic bronchitis are largely irreversible processes. With smoking cessation, many chronic bronchitic patients will stop cough and sputum production, but destroyed lung parenchyma is not restored to normal.

Patients with COPD frequently have abnormal arterial blood gases. Arterial hypoxemia may be secondary to carbon dioxide retention as well as $\dot{V}/\dot{Q}$ inequality. The $PaCO_2$, which reflects alveolar ventilation, may be normal or high, depending on the ratio of minute ventilation to "wasted ventilation." Some patients respond to the increased work of breathing by appropriately increasing minute ventilation, keeping their $PaCO_2$ normal, while some hypoventilate with a resultant high $PaCO_2$ and lower PaO_2. Differences in peripheral or central chemoreceptor sensitivity as well as in muscle strength may explain the variation in $PaCO_2$ observed in patients. It should not be assumed, however, that all patients with COPD have a decreased ventilatory drive. Recent studies using the airway occlusion technique to assess ventilatory drive in mechanically ventilated patients with COPD actually demonstrate an increased ventilatory drive.[68] Presumably, the failure to be weaned from mechanical ventilation under these conditions reflects mechanical or pathophysiologic factors (for example, noncompliant lungs, large ratio of dead space to tidal volume) that impede weaning rather than diminished respiratory drive.

Pulmonary hypertension and right ventricular failure are late complications of COPD. Elevations in pulmonary artery pressure are caused by alveolar hypoxia and subsequent pulmonary arterial constriction as well as decreased vessel cross-sectional area secondary to parenchymal destruction.

PREOPERATIVE EVALUATION

Preoperative evaluation identifies the presence and severity of lung disease and provides a basis for designing therapeutic interventions to ensure that the patient is in optimal condition before the proposed anesthesia and surgery. If the proposed operation is elective, interventions can be planned and the operation scheduled in an attempt to reduce operative risk. For emergent surgical procedures information gained from the preoperative evaluation will determine what therapeutic interventions are required immediately before and during surgery. There is little evidence, however, that outcome is improved by "optimizing" the condition of patients with underlying lung disease for either elective or emergency surgery.

History

Certain historical features are of value in determining the severity of a patient's respiratory disease and in planning appropriate perioperative therapy. Frequency and intensity of bronchospasm, short-term and/or long-term asthmatic therapy, hospitalizations for treatment, including intubation and mechanical ventilation, should be sought. Prior history of hospitalization for bronchospasm or respiratory failure, steroid use, and history of mechanical ventilation suggest severe disease. The amount of cigarettes smoked and the number of years the patient has used tobacco products is important. Information

concerning the nutritional status can be elicited from the patient. Cardiac disorders may be associated with chronic lung disease, and symptoms suggestive of either congestive heart failure or coronary artery disease may require further evaluation. Any current therapy, including medications and oxygen administration, must be documented. Changes in the character of cough and sputum may suggest a recent respiratory infection, either bacterial or viral.

Physical Examination

Use of accessory muscles, prolonged expiratory phase, and the barrel chest configuration are seen in only a minority of patients with emphysema, while patients with chronic bronchitis are often overweight and cyanotic. Obesity increases the risk of postoperative pulmonary complications.[33] An asthmatic patient, between episodes, may have no clinical findings on physical examination, or wheezing and rhonchi may be present even if there are no other symptoms such as shortness of breath or cough. Evidence of right-sided heart failure should be sought, such as peripheral edema, RV heave, loud or widely split P2, and neck vein distention.

Chest X-ray Examination

Airflow obstruction is highly correlated with the level of the right dome of the diaphragm when it is at or below the seventh rib anteriorly on PA x-ray examination. A cardiac silhouette with a transverse diameter of less than 11.5 centimeters is also highly specific, as is a retrosternal airspace (on the lateral view) of greater than 4.4 centimeters.[9] These parameters have low sensitivity, and airflow obstruction often exists with a "normal" chest x-ray examination. Hyperlucency and bronchial markings do not appear to be valuable indicators.[9] If RV failure is present, the pulmonary arteries are often prominent and the cardiac silhouette may be enlarged. The chest x-ray examination in asthma is not diagnostic, although hyperinflation may be seen if the patient is symptomatic. The value of the *routine* chest x-ray examination in asymptomatic patients (not just patients with lung disease) has been questioned. However, it is frequently of value in patients with underlying lung disease to exclude pneumonia, pneumothorax, or pleural effusion as a cause of dyspnea, and it serves as a basis of comparison should perioperative complications occur.

Laboratory Studies

There may be an increase in sputum and blood eosinophilia during an acute asthmatic attack, but these are not specific for asthma. In COPD, an elevated serum bicarbonate may be an indication of chronic respiratory acidosis. Polycythemia may be a clue to chronic hypoxemia and in rare cases, may require phlebotomy (see Chapter 24). Arterial blood gas analysis will usually reveal whether the patient is chronically hypercapnic or hypoxic. A PaO_2 of less than 60 mm Hg correlates with pulmonary hypertension.[41] Hypercapnia ($PaCO_2$ of greater than 45 mm Hg) is correlated with an increased risk of perioperative complications.[81]

Pulmonary Function Tests

Preoperative pulmonary function tests (PFTs) are done to identify the type and severity of pulmonary disease. While there are many different types of tests that can be obtained, simple spirometry before and after bronchodilators is usually all that is necessary (Figure 19-1). Dyspnea is assumed to occur at an FEV_1 less than 2 L,[17] exertional dyspnea develops when the FEV_1 falls below 50% of predicted, and dyspnea at rest occurs when the FEV_1 is less than 25% of predicted.[7] In asthma, emphysema, and chronic bronchitis the FVC decreases less than the FEV_1 resulting in a FEV_1/FVC ratio less than 0.80. Certainly, the preoperative finding of dyspnea in a patient (especially if it is new) should prompt further evaluation and perhaps even deferral of elective surgery in some cases.

The degree of spirometric abnormality correlates with the incidence of postoperative complications such as atelectasis and pneumonia.[81] Predictors of risk include the FEV_1 and the maximal breathing

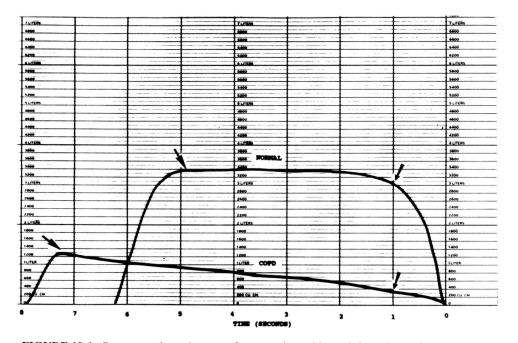

FIGURE 19-1. Representative spirograms from a patient without airflow obstruction *(upper trace)* and from a patient with COPD *(lower trace)*. Time in seconds is on the abscissa and exhaled volume on the ordinate. The FEV_1 is shown by the small arrows; FVC by the large arrows. Note that the tracing from the normal individual has a plateau. No such plateau is evident in the tracing from the patient with COPD. Finally, note the reduction in the FEV_1/FVC ratio in the patient with COPD; this ratio is over 0.80 in the normal patient.

capacity (MBC). An FEV_1 of less than 1 L and an MBC of less than 50% predicted are associated with a high risk of perioperative respiratory complications.[81] The combination of an FEV_1/FVC ratio of less than 65% predicted and an FVC of less than 70% predicted has also been found to highly correlate with postoperative complications.[26] While these are valuable indices, there is no one value of a preoperative pulmonary function test that absolutely contraindicates surgery. Spirometry in an asthmatic may be normal between exacerbations or may reveal unsuspected airflow obstruction. If there is a significant (greater than 15%) improvement with bronchodilators during testing, such therapy should be instituted or intensified.[42] Patients with COPD who are given bronchodilators may have minimal improvement on spirometry but show clinical improvement.

Not every preoperative patient with known or suspected COPD requires spirometry. Certainly, PFTs frequently confirm what is already suspected on the basis of the history and physical exam. Also, while postoperative pulmonary complications are correlated with abnormal PFTs, these tests have not been shown to be superior, as predictors, to clinical findings.[46a] Nonetheless, we believe that spirometry is useful in many patients. In most instances spirometry is a bedside test. It is simple and noninvasive. It allows one to quantitate the degree of a patient's disability. Most importantly, spirometry is valuable as a guide to therapy. Patients who have an improvement in the FEV_1 or FVC with bronchodilators should be started on or continue to receive these agents. This improvement would be difficult if not impossible to quantitate clinically. Also, the recovery and pulmonary function from surgery may be determined by spirometry, which may result in changes in therapy.

Electrocardiogram and Arrhythmias

Right-sided heart chamber enlargement or cor pulmonale may be suggested by electrocardiographic findings (right axis deviation, right ventricular hypertrophy, or right atrial enlargement) (see box above, right).[53] The electrocardiographic findings of right-sided heart enlargement are insensitive but specific. The electrocardiogram may also reveal arrhythmias. A correlation has been noted between the types of arrhythmias observed and the clinical status of patients with COPD. During acute exacerbations or respiratory failure and in the postoperative period,

---

Electrocardiographic signs of right ventricular hypertrophy

1. Right axis deviation
   ($> +110°$)
2. Early R-wave progression
   ($R/S >1$ and V1 and time to intrinsicoid deflection > 0.03 sec, $R/S <1$ in V5, V6)
3. Altered repolarization in right precordial leads
   (ST segment depression and inverted T-wave V1-V2)
4. Normal QRS interval

---

supraventricular tachycardia is common, whereas ventricular arrhythmias are more common when the pulmonary disease is stable.[6] Multifocal atrial tachycardia (MAT), an otherwise unusual rhythm disturbance, is frequently encountered in patients with COPD, and is exacerbated by aminophylline. It is characterized by changing P-wave morphology and variable PP and RR intervals. Recent data suggest that this rhythm can be controlled effectively (slowing of rate, not conversion to sinus rhythm) by verapamil.[47,67] Many etiologic factors of this arrhythmia may be involved, including hypoxemia, drugs (digitalis, sympathomimetics, aminophylline), coronary artery disease, and procedures such as bronchoscopy, pulmonary artery catheter insertion, and tracheal suctioning. Arrhythmias in COPD patients are associated with a poor overall prognosis.[80]

PREOPERATIVE INTERVENTIONS
Pulmonary Toilet

Preoperative respiratory toilet can educate patients about postoperative measures and increase cooperation with treatment. These measures include chest percussion and vibration, postural drainage, deep breathing, coughing, and incentive spirometry. The combination of these measures appears to be beneficial for acutely ill patients with large volumes of secretions and/or lobar atelectasis although the delivery of this chest physical therapy may be associated with bronchospasm and hypoxemia. Postural drainage alone and directed coughing alone may be effective, while there are no data showing a beneficial effect of percussion or vibration alone[43] (see Chapter 15).

Hydration and Nutrition

The effect of hydration status on clearance of secretions is unclear. A dehydrated patient is more likely to be hemodynamically unstable during surgery. Malnutrition predisposes to perioperative respiratory failure, pneumonia, and sepsis, and is associated with increased mortality. Poor caloric and protein intake is associated with impaired pulmonary defense mechanisms, destruction of pulmonary parenchyma, decreased diaphragmatic muscle mass and strength, decreased inspiratory muscle strength, and inability to sustain adequate ventilation.[62] The influence of malnutrition and nutritional repletion on perioperative morbidity and mortality is discussed in detail in Chapter 29.

Medications

Current medications and level of compliance with the medical regimen should be determined and appropriate drug levels obtained (Table 19-1). Many patients with reversible airway disease are on both inhaled and oral bronchodilators. Administration of beta$_2$ agonists via aerosol (as opposed to parenteral administration) increases bronchial selectivity, results in fewer side effects than non-beta$_2$ selective drugs or other routes of administration, and is considered to be the route of choice.

Methylxanthines are generally less potent than beta-agonists. Plasma concentrations of 10 to 20 μg/ml are therapeutic. It is important to measure the blood level of theophylline, however, because it may vary widely in reponse to a given dose. In the acutely ill patient a change in level may be observed from day to day without any obvious change in clinical status, in association with other conditions, and with administration of other drugs (Table 19-2). There is little additional benefit from higher blood levels of theophylline, and the incidence of side effects rises markedly.[54] A recent review of theophylline suggests that it may not be efficacious when used as the sole agent in treating an asthmatic attack.[50]

Theophylline has other properties in addition to direct airway effects. It acts to improve mucous clearance by accelerating mucociliary transport,[87] stimulates the central nervous system respiratory center located in the medulla, improves diaphragmatic muscle function,[55] mildly increases cardiac contractility, is a diuretic, and is a pulmonary vasodilator. Some advocate starting all patients with asthma on intravenous aminophylline the night be-

fore surgery.[35] We do not do this routinely because the therapeutic-to-toxic ratio is small, and because better bronchodilation with fewer side effects may be achieved with inhaled beta$_2$ agonists. Also, methylxanthines in combination with surgically induced increases in levels of catecholamines and volatile anesthetic agents can lead to ventricular ectopy. Thus, we strongly recommend inhalational therapy preoperatively for those patients with asthma or COPD who are not already receiving these agents.

Anticholinergic drugs produce bronchodilation by blocking the parasympathetic nervous system and are effective against irritant bronchoconstriction. They have little effect on mediator-induced constriction and are more effective with COPD than with asthma.[59] Although newer anticholinergic aerosols (ipratropium bromide) have a slower onset of action than inhaled sympathomimetics, they have a longer duration of action. Use of glucocorticoids as therapeutic agents in asthma and COPD is controversial. These agents can reduce inflammation and edema in the airway but are not bronchodilators. Indications and dosage are not well established. Accepted usage includes acute illness (bronchospasm or exacerbation of COPD) that is worsening or not resolving despite appropriate therapy. The effects of glucocorticoids on the airway may not be seen for 6 or more hours following the first dose, so they are not immediately helpful in acute bronchospasm. If the patient is receiving steroids they should be continued during the perioperative period and increased if necessary to mimic the normal stress response. Inhaled steroids are effective in treating bronchospasm but not in the acute setting. They may avoid some of the systemic side effects seen with parenteral administration such as adrenal suppression. However, adrenal suppression can occur when inhaled steroids are used at high doses (over 1500 μg/day).[72] Such doses are not commonly used and parenteral glucocorticoids are not routinely given (for example, stress dose coverage) to a patient on the usual doses of inhaled steroids who is not receiving oral steroid therapy.

In selected asthmatic patients preoperative administration of steroids (for example, 100 mg hydrocortisone the night before and the day of surgery) may be of benefit in preventing perioperative bronchospasm as steroids may reduce bronchial hyperreactivity. Even single doses of steroids used in the emergency room setting have been found to be of

TABLE 19-1. Pharmacologic agents for bronchospasm

Drug	Route	Acuity	Comments
Methylxanthines	PO	Chronic asthma and COPD	Serum levels 10-20 μg/ml Levels may vary widely
	IV	Acute bronchospasm	Adjunct to Beta$_2$ agonists May cause MAT Interact with halothane to cause ventricular ectopy
Beta$_2$ agonists	Inhaled	Acute or chronic bronchospasm	Sole treatment in some cases Education necessary for proper inhalation technique Frequent doses to reach distal airways Potential for tachycardia
Anticholinergics	Inhaled	Acute or chronic bronchospasm	Better for COPD than asthma Slower onset than beta$_2$ agonists Preventative Effective against reflex or irritant bronchospasm
Cromolyn	Inhaled	Chronic asthma	Asthma therapy More effective in young than elderly Takes weeks to be effective Not for acute episodes
Corticosteroids	PO, IV, Inhaled	Chronic or acute COPD or asthma	Antiinflammatory Not a bronchodilator, reduces hyperreactivity Multiple systemic side effects Takes hours to work
Lidocaine	IV, Inhaled	Acute broncospasm	May be given through endotracheal tube For reflex bronchoconstriction Serum levels of 1.5-5 μg/ml

TABLE 19-2. Clearance of methylxanthines

Decreased	Increased
Cirrhosis	Youth (children)
Pulmonary edema	Cigarette smoking
Prematurity	Phenytoin
Cimetidine	Ingestion of charbroiled meat
Erythromycin	
Allopurinol	

benefit.[51] However, the lack of a well-controlled study on the perioperative use of steroids and outcome in bronchospastic patients makes this speculative.

If the patient is receiving cromolyn sodium it should be continued preoperatively. It would not be beneficial to initiate such therapy in the preoperative period because several weeks of therapy may be needed before an effect is seen. This compound may act by inhibiting degranulation of mast cells and by inhibiting nonspecific bronchial hyperreactivity and is most helpful in atopic asthma to prevent exacerbations. Antihistamines are not clinically useful, perhaps because histamine is not the sole mediator in bronchospasm.

Patients with COPD are frequently placed on antibiotics either to treat an infection (purulent bronchitis or pneumonia) or prophylactically in an effort to suppress the bacterial colonization that occurs in these patients. If time permits, it may be of value to prescribe antibiotics several days before surgery in an effort to decrease the quantity and thickness of the sputum. Expectorants and mucolytic agents have not been shown to add to therapy and may actually cause bronchospasm.[52]

TABLE 19-3.   Premedication

Drug class	Use	Respiratory effect
Benzodiazepines	Reduce anxiety	Mild depression of respiratory drive—worse with IV route
	Sedation	No effect on airway resistance or flow rates
Barbiturates	Sedation	Minimal respiratory depression in premed doses
H_1 antagonists	Sedation	Decreased manifestations of histamine release
	Dry secretions	
H_2 antagonists	Increase gastric pH	Possible augmentation of histamine-induced bronchospasm (does not appear to be a clinically significant issue)
Narcotics	Analgesia	Depressed respiratory drive
	Sedation	Histamine release (morphine, meperidine)
		Chest wall rigidity (fentanyl)
Anticholinergics	Dry secretions	Decreased tracheal mucous velocity
	Decreased gastric volume	Increase dead space

Premedication

Premedication is a general term that includes sedatives, drying agents, and other drugs administered to the patient before the induction of anesthesia (Table 19-3). Premedication reduces anxiety, provides analgesia, decreases excessive secretions, and decreases the risk of pneumonia should aspiration of gastric contents occur. In addition to these positive attributes of premedication, there is a risk of respiratory depression in patients with lung disease if sedation is not carefully managed. The benzodiazepines reduce anxiety, produce sedation, and cause mild depression of ventilatory drive. When given intravenously they increase respiratory depression.[14] Airway resistances and flows are not affected and cardiovascular effects are minimal.[14] Barbiturates and droperidol in premedicant doses cause minimal respiratory depression and are effective orally.[75] Antagonists of the histamine$_1$ receptor have sedative and drying properties, and may reduce systemic manifestations of histamine release.[28]

The opiates are all respiratory depressants. Even in the awake patient there is a depressed response to carbon dioxide resulting in decreased alveolar ventilation.[73] Morphine can cause a release of histamine and potentially precipitate bronchospasm, but this does not appear to be a clinically significant phenomenon.[65] By virtue of its histamine-releasing properties, morphine can also reduce blood pressure and cause venodilation. Fentanyl, which is sometimes given intravenously during intravascular catheter insertion for additional sedation before the induction of anesthesia, does not cause release of histamine and therefore does not affect bronchomotor tone. It can, however, be associated with chest-wall rigidity and decreased respiratory system compliance (especially when given rapidly and in association with nitrous oxide). The decreased compliance may be profound enough to require control of the airway.[74]

Anticholinergic medications will decrease respiratory tract secretions that may be associated with coughing, laryngospasm, and bronchospasm during induction and maintenance of anesthesia. Doses used for premedication are not large enough to prevent reflex bronchoconstriction directly. These agents may, however, decrease tracheal mucous velocity and contribute to the retention of secretions.[1] Atropine does not alter the response to carbon dioxide but does dilate large airway passages, so that dead-space is increased and an increased minute ventilation is required to maintain PCO_2.[73] Atropine can also cause sinus tachycardia, possibly resulting in multifocal atrial tachycardia. Glycopyrolate causes less tachycardia and less sedation. It also decreases the volume and acidity of gastric secretions, which are increased by theophylline.[23]

Preoperative antagonism of histamine$_2$ receptors can increase gastric pH, thus decreasing the severity of aspiration pneumonitis should it occur. Theoretically, administration of an H_2 receptor blocker can result in bronchoconstriction from loss of inhibitory feedback by H_2 receptors on mediator release (and unopposed H_1 receptor activity). In one animal study H_2 blockers in clinically relevant concentrations augmented histamine-induced bronchoconstriction, ranitidine having less of an effect than cimetidine.[45] In man it has been shown that while orally administered cimetidine does not itself cause bronchospasm, it can increase sensitivity to bronchospasm induced by histamine.[79] Once again, no human studies are available on bronchoconstriction related to H_2 blockade preoperatively and it is worth repeating that H_1 blockers are not routinely used to treat bronchospasm. Metoclopramide speeds gastric emptying by stimulating motility of the gastrointestinal tract and relaxing the pyloric sphincter, and may be used preoperatively to decrease gastric volume. It has no respiratory side effects. We do not routinely use H_2 blockers preoperatively. However, they are used whenever the risk of aspiration of gastric contents is increased (full stomach, hiatal hernia, or bowel obstruction).

Oxygen Therapy

It is clear from many studies that continuous oxygen therapy is beneficial for the patient with hypoxemia characterized by a resting PaO_2 of less than 55 to 60 mm Hg.[22,56] Patients with severe COPD may be on chronic oxygen therapy and this must be continued during the preoperative period. The patient with COPD who has chronic hypoxemia and is not on oxygen may even benefit from short-term therapy.[22] If the procedure is elective, the surgery should be deferred to allow the patient to receive several weeks of continuous home oxygen therapy to improve intellectual functioning, relieve polycythemia, reduce pulmonary artery pressures, and treat congestive heart failure. The theoretic basis of this recommendation is sound; nevertheless, there are *no* studies in hypoxemic patients who are not on chronic oxygen therapy that demonstrate that preoperative oxygen administration reduces perioperative morbidity or mortality.

Specific Management Issues

Cigarette smoking. Significant pulmonary disease is associated with more than 20 pack-years of smoking, and postoperative respiratory morbidity is greater in patients who smoke more than 10 cigarettes a day.[57] Short-term abstinence (48 hours) decreases carboxyhemoglobin levels (3% to 15% in smokers) to those of nonsmokers (less than 2.5%), abolishes the effects of nicotine on the cardiovascular system, and improves respiratory ciliary beating.[57] Abstinence of 1 to 2 weeks is required to decrease sputum volume, and 4 to 6 weeks for improvement in symptoms and function.[57] The combination of preoperative and postoperative treatment, including cessation of smoking for several days, antibiotics for evidence of infection, chest physical therapy, humidity, and bronchodilator drugs, has been shown to decrease pulmonary complications postoperatively.[76] Note that this study does not demonstrate that preoperative preparation alone or cessation of cigarette smoking alone can alter perioperative morbidity. Rather, such preoperative treatment *in combination* with postoperative measures may alter outcome. The effects, if any, of preoperative measures are unknown.

Acute pulmonary infection. If there is evidence of acute pulmonary infection, surgery should be delayed if possible until it has subsided. General anesthetic agents can impair mucociliary clearance[48] (see Chapter 15) and predispose to pulmonary aspiration of gastric contents, both of which may exacerbate underlying lung disease. In addition, impaired cough and atelectasis, which occur in almost all patients postoperatively, will delay resolution of a pneumonia. The benefits of deferral of elective surgery have not been clearly demonstrated; nevertheless, deferral seems a logical course. Airway hyperreactivity produced by viral illness is present for at least 3 weeks following symptomatic recovery and therefore, bronchospasm may occur in the operating room setting even after a patient has clinically recovered from a viral upper respiratory infection.[21]

Persistent wheezing. A common issue is that of the wheezing patient who is scheduled for surgery the next day. Conservative management would dictate that any patient in less than optimal condition should not have surgery. This is not to say that the patient must be "cured" but rather that the patient be in the "best" attainable condition. However, we are not aware of any studies indicating a reduction in risk if preoperative wheezing or an asthmatic exacerbation is controlled before surgery. In the current climate of cost-containment it is neither practical nor reasonable to automatically defer elective surgery in all such cases.

We recommend that the patient with bronchospasm be intensively treated with inhaled bronchodilators (every 3 to 4 hours). It is customary to use beta$_2$ adrenergic agents because of their more rapid onset and possible increased efficacy, but it would be acceptable to use an inhaled anticholinergic as well. Parenteral steroids can be used but with the recognition that there may be adverse effects on wound healing. A theophylline infusion may be started, but it is imperative to monitor serum levels; a value close to 10 μg/ml is ideal. Although dose-dependent bronchodilation occurs with theophylline, there is little clinical benefit and marked disadvantage to higher serum levels. Tobacco use must be discontinued immediately. Any evidence of an associated infection such as purulent bronchitis should be treated with appropriate antimicrobial drugs and should cause elective surgery to be delayed.

Many patients will improve under this regimen. Clearly, patients who show no improvement by clinical measurements (dyspnea, wheezing, inspiratory/expiratory (I/E) ratio, or respiratory rate) or laboratory tests (spirometry, blood gases, chest x-ray examination) should have nonemergency surgery deferred. Patients who show marked improvement are still at risk for perioperative bronchospasm because the airways remain hyperreactive for several weeks after an asthmatic exacerbation. The decision to proceed with surgery must balance the risk of perioperative bronchospasm with the urgency of the surgery.

Congestive heart failure and coronary artery disease. Heart failure is an independent risk factor for anesthesia.[30] Patients with COPD are at risk for the development of cor pulmonale, and should be carefully evaluated for this condition. Peripheral edema, ascites, paroxysmal nocturnal dyspnea, and orthopnea suggest the presence of cor pulmonale. In addition, cigarette smoking is associated with an increased risk of coronary artery disease, which should be suspected in patients with COPD. Patients with coronary artery disease may be on digoxin, diuretics, and antianginal medications, which will need to be continued in the perioperative period.

Suitability for pulmonary resection. Patients scheduled for thoracotomy and lung resection are at increased risk for postoperative problems and should be specifically evaluated to establish the likelihood of adequate postoperative respiratory function. This evaluation attempts to measure the amount of pulmonary function that will remain after a variable amount of lung tissue is removed or, in the worst case, if a pneumonectomy is performed. A preoperative FVC of less than 1.7 L or FEV_1 of less than 1.2 L, predicted postoperative FEV_1 of less than 800 ml, maximum breathing capacity of less than 50% predicted, or inability to complete a 60 watt exercise protocol indicate a poor postoperative prognosis.[26,61] Split function testing using a double-lumen endotracheal tube is rarely done nowadays, having been replaced by isotope scanning. Similarly, while temporary balloon occlusion of the pulmonary artery provides important information, it, too, is rarely performed as it requires a specially constructed device and expertise not readily available.

The perfusion scan permits measurement of the amount of perfusion each segment of lung receives and this measurement can then be used to estimate postoperative FEV_1. These data have been used to estimate resectability (by the above criteria). Two simpler methods are also available to estimate post-resection lung function. Egeblad recently described a system of evaluation based on preoperative spirometry, bronchoscopic and radiographic findings.[20] Also, the lateral position test can be used to predict postpneumonectomy lung function.[86] The indices listed above represent guidelines as to resectability; there are no absolute values below which a patient is destined to be a pulmonary cripple. Over the last 20 years the limits of acceptable pulmonary function that are deemed to prohibit surgery have been progressively lowered. Also, other factors may assume equal or greater weight in the determination of resectability. These factors include associated systemic diseases such as chronic liver or kidney disease, morbid obesity, malnutrition, coronary artery disease, psychologic status, and level of family support.

The Effect of Interventions On Perioperative Morbidity

It is commonly accepted that patients with COPD are at increased risk for postoperative pulmonary complications (PPC). Latimer et al in 1971 summarized several series and determined that pneumonia and atelectasis occurred frequently. Higher rates were observed after operations on the abdomen and thorax and lower rates of complications were observed after surgery on other regions. Overall, rates of PPC were as high as 70%.[46] Stein et al found a PPC rate of 3.3% in patients with normal spirometry compared to a PPC rate of 70% in patients with abnormal spirometry.[76] Gold et al[29] studied 148 patients with COPD who underwent general anesthesia with either halothane or isoflurane. In this study

TABLE 19-4. Predicators of postoperative pulmonary complications*

Parameter	Value
Maximal breathing capacity (MBC)	<50% predicted
FEV$_1$	<1 liter
FVC	<70% predicted
FEV$_1$/FVC	<65% predicted
PaO$_2$	>45 mm Hg
PaCO$_2$	<60 mm Hg

*Complications defined as atelectasis or pneumonia.

approximately 15% of patients had atelectasis and almost 10% of patients had either a pleural effusion or pneumonia.

It seems clear from these and other such studies[32,89] that patients with underlying lung disease are at increased risk for postoperative pulmonary complications (Table 19-4). However, there are methodologic problems with these studies. The determination of COPD is usually based on clinical and not spirometric or other quantifiable criteria. Control groups may not be included. The type of postoperative care is not specified. A prospective study has yet to be performed in which a large number of normal individuals and patients with a predetermined degree of spirometrically defined dysfunction undergo similar surgery, anesthesia, and postoperative care, and in whom PPCs are compared.

The few studies that examine the effects of perioperative interventions on outcome indicate that these may decrease postoperative complications. Stein et al looked at the effects of a variety of perioperative measures in patients with COPD.[76] They found that pulmonary complications were reduced, but this study was not randomized. Furthermore, this study did not specifically examine preoperative interventions. Tarhan et al reviewed the hospital charts of over 60,000 patients who had received a general anesthetic over a 3-year period.[78] They identified 464 patients with "lung disease," and of these "some type" of preoperative preparation was employed in 227. Those who had this preparation had a lesser incidence of pulmonary complications. However, this study was retrospective and there is no control group. Further, the type of preoperative preparation was not standardized. Finally, the manner in which patients were identified as having lung disease is not specified and it seems likely that patients were iden-

tified as having COPD on the basis of clinical findings rather than spirometry. It is likely that not all patients having surgery who had COPD were identified by this process and therefore this study probably reports a select group of patients.

Celli et al looked at the role of lung expansion *postoperatively* in the prevention of postoperative pulmonary complications.[10] In this study incentive spirometry and similar manuevers did reduce the number of patients with postoperative complications (cough, sputum production, fever, or tachycardia). Again, this study looked at postoperative measures not preoperative ones. Stock et al compared the effects of CPAP, incentive spirometry, and a regimen of cough and deep breathing on postoperative atelectasis and pneumonia.[77] They concluded that all three regimens were effective in decreasing pneumonia and attributed this to frequency and intensity of respiratory care rather than the use of a specific modality.

Thus there is very little information on the issue of preoperative interventions by themselves in patients with COPD. Although it is intuitively pleasing to assume that preoperative measures will reduce postoperative complications, it remains to be proven. Current outpatient regimens for COPD frequently employ bronchodilators, antibiotics, and corticosteroids. In such patients, inpatient preoperative "tuning up" may be unnecessary. The value of such a regimen in preventing postoperative pulmonary complications in an untreated patient remains to be demonstrated although it seems a logical course.

INTRAOPERATIVE MANAGEMENT
Monitoring

Pulse oximetry and capnography are noninvasive and continuous monitors of arterial hemoglobin oxygen saturation and alveolar carbon dioxide concentration respectively (see Chapter 7). An arterial catheter provides much useful information at very low risk to the patient.[25,71] Indications for arterial catheterization include surgery or operative positions that require frequent arterial blood gases, preexisting blood gas abnormalities, and anticipated need to carefully follow postoperative ventilation and oxygenation.

Central venous catheterization may be helpful during surgery requiring large bore access or when large fluid fluxes are anticipated. In those patients in whom pulmonary artery hypertension exists, right atrial

TABLE 19-5. Effect of intraoperative position

Lateral	$\dot{V}/\dot{Q}$ inequality, worsened by open chest
	potential for spillage from "up" lung to dependent lung
Prone	No impairment if abdominal wall free to move
Trendelenburg	Reduced FRC
	Increased pulmonary blood volume
	Elevated pulmonary artery pressures
	Possible increase in left atrial pressures

pressures may not reflect left atrial pressures, and in such patients a pulmonary artery catheter may be of value.

Effect of Intraoperative Position

Operative site will influence the anesthetic plan because of its effect on pulmonary function (Table 19-5) (see Chapter 15). In thoracic surgery the major problems include surgically induced pneumothorax, open chest ventilation in the lateral position (in which most nonvascular chest surgery is performed), and aspiration of secretions or blood from one lung to the other. Double-lumen endotracheal tubes can protect against aspiration from one lung to the other and allow selective ventilation of either lung. In the lateral decubitus position there is greater blood flow to the dependent lung than the nondependent lung.[3] In the anesthetized patient receiving mechanical ventilator therapy, there is poorer ventilation to the dependent lung.[40,70] This effect is observed independent of the state of muscle relaxation or underlying lung disease. The superior lung is relatively less perfused but better ventilated than the dependent lung. This results in $\dot{V}/\dot{Q}$ inequality, which can be partially corrected by positive end-expiratory pressure (PEEP).[70] When the chest is opened, $\dot{V}/\dot{Q}$ mismatch may further worsen as there is increased ventilation of the upper lung. Double-lumen endobronchial tubes allow selective addition of PEEP to the dependent lung, continuous positive airway pressure (CPAP) to the nondependent and nonventilated lung (that is, the lung undergoing surgery), and combinations of these modalities. When the nondependent lung is not ventilated, for purposes of surgical exposure, hypoxic pulmonary vasoconstriction

(HPV) diverts blood flow to the ventilated lung, resulting in a variable degree of shunting that is on on the order of 20%.[3] In general, in this position, the elimination of carbon dioxide is not a problem.

Other positions used during surgery may also affect ventilation and oxygenation. In a properly positioned prone patient where the abdominal wall is free to move there is no impairment of respiratory function. The normal reduction in FRC observed in anesthetized patients is made worse by the Trendelenburg position. In this position, the abdominal contents push the diaphragm into the chest, causing an even greater decrease in FRC than that which normally occurs in an anesthetized patient in the supine position. An increase in pulmonary blood volume may also occur as a result of the head down position, as much of the lung is below the level of the left atrium, and this will tend to increase the amount of the lung that is in zone 3 (that is, pulmonary artery pressure > left atrial pressure > alveolar pressure). Patients with elevated pulmonary artery pressures do not tolerate this position well, because pulmonary artery pressure is further increased. In addition, patients with elevated left atrial pressures may develop pulmonary edema when placed in this position.

Regional Versus General Anesthesia

It is commonly believed that a regional anesthetic is indicated and general anesthesia less desirable in patients with lung disease (Table 19-6). Unfortunately, there are no data to support this belief. Clinical studies are needed, in a randomized fashion and in a well-defined group of patients with either COPD or asthma, to examine the effect on outcome of anesthetic technique. Nonetheless, one can still identify the advantages and disadvantages of each with respect to patients with underlying lung disease, even if precise clinical end-point data are unavailable.

Regional anesthetics include subarachnoid (spinal), extradural (epidural), and major nerve blocks (brachial plexus). These techniques do not usually require airway manipulation and are less likely to produce bronchospasm or bronchorrhea. Muscle relaxants are not required and thus will not contribute to postoperative respiratory depression. Judicious use of sedatives usually results in minimal alterations in blood gases. Inhalational anesthetics are not required and ventilatory control is not affected. However, these techniques are not suitable for all surgical

TABLE 19-6.   Regional versus general anesthesia

	Advantages	Disadvantages
Regional	Muscle relaxant not required Airway not instrumented Ventilatory control unaffected Minimal alterations in ABGs	Requires cooperative patient Airway not controlled May need sedatives Unable to suction secretions Potential for respiratory embarassment with "high block"
General	Renders patient "cooperative" Airway controlled Ability to suction secretions (if intubated) Applicable to all patients and procedures	May require muscle relaxants Respiratory depression Airway instrumentation

procedures or positions, and they require cooperative patients. Also, airway control is assumed but not ensured. Brachial plexus block for surgery on an upper extremity may produce unintentional pneumothorax. Unintentional blockade of high thoracic or cervical motor segments by spinal or epidural anesthesia may result in intercostal muscle weakness with impaired cough and atelectasis, or even diaphragmatic weakness, with consequent respiratory failure. Expertise in these anesthetic techniques is required to avoid problems. Finally, even in the best of hands, regional anesthetics are occasionally unsuccessful, requiring adoption of a general anesthetic technique.

General anesthesia requires neither special instruments nor procedures. It ensures patient cooperation and control of the airway and permits suctioning of airway secretions. Disadvantages include the occasional need for muscle relaxants, respiratory depression from general anesthetic agents, and possible induction of severe bronchospasm as a result of airway manipulation. No one technique is always best. Clearly, the anesthetic plan must be tailored to the individual patient, type of surgery, and intraoperative position. Those seeking a "magic wand" will be disappointed.

Choice of Anesthetic Agent

The induction of anesthesia can be accomplished by intravenous and/or inhalational medications but, regardless of agent, there will be changes in the respiratory system that include blunted responses to hypoxemia and hypercarbia, reduced alveolar ventilation, increased work of breathing secondary to decreased respiratory system compliance, and an increased volume of secretions (Table 19-7).

Both the hypocapnic bronchoconstrictor reflex, which has been clearly demonstrated in animals but is less clearly established in man, and which acts to decrease ventilation to poorly perfused areas, and hypoxic pulmonary vasoconstriction (HPV), which shunts blood away from poorly ventilated areas, serve to match ventilation and perfusion. Inhalational anesthetics depress both these compensatory mechanisms.[83] A recent study by Benumof et al concerning the effect on HPV of the volatile inhalational anesthetics found that although these agents inhibited HPV slightly it was not a clinically significant effect.[4] Therefore, inhalational anesthetics are not contraindicated during one-lung anesthesia. Similarly, intravenous anesthetics do not seem to affect HPV and are frequently used during one lung anesthesia. Cardiac output is also usually decreased by inhalational anesthetics, which results in decreased pulmonary blood flow.

Oxygen in high concentration is delivered to the patient during induction and before endotracheal intubation to "denitrogenate" the lungs so that a possible period of apnea will not result in desaturation (the FRC will serve as a reservoir of oxygen). The time required to denitrogenate the lungs is variable and depends on regional time constants of emptying (inhomogeneity of ventilation within the lung). For healthy patients this may be accomplished by several large (vital capacity) breaths, whereas patients with COPD may require up to 10 minutes of normal breathing. The hypercarbic patient who depends on the hypoxemic drive for ventilation may experience respiratory depression during this maneuver and the anesthesiologist may need to assist ventilation.

TABLE 19-7.   Effects of anesthetic agents on the respiratory system

Agent	Respiratory effects
Volatile anesthetics	Reduced alveolar ventilation (decreased TV, increased rate)
	Increased secretions
	Depressed hypoxic pulmonary vasoconstriction
	Depressed hypocapneic bronchoconstriction
	Blunted response to hypoxemia and hypercarbia
	Bronchodilation
Nitrous oxide	No effect on bronchomotor tone
	Depresses response to hypoxia but no effect on response to hypercarbia
	Diffuses into closed or poorly ventilated spaces
Barbiturates	Minimal respiratory depression when used in sedative doses but apnea when used to induce anesthesia
	Depressed response to hypercarbia
Narcotics	Respiratory depression (decreased rate and decreased minute volume)
	Blunted response to hypoxemia and hypercarbia
Ketamine	Chest wall rigidity (fentanyl)
	Sympathomimetic-bronchodilator
	No effect on response to hypercarbia and hypoxemia, respiration maintained
	Increases airway secretions
Etomidate	Apnea when used to induce anesthesia
	No effect on bronchomotor tone

The volatile inhalational anesthetics (halothane, enflurane, and isoflurane) all depress ventilation, and this effect is enhanced in patients with COPD.[60] Even at low concentrations (less than 1%) these agents also depress the hyperpneic responses to carbon dioxide and to hypoxemia.[44] The depressed ventilatory response to hypoxia can be critical in patients with COPD who may be stimulated to breathe by hypoxia. In general, inhalational anesthetics reduce tidal volume and increase respiratory rate with an overall effect of decreased alveolar ventilation and increased $PaCO_2$.[28]

As noted previously, the inhalational anesthetics are bronchodilators acting through depression of reflexes and direct smooth-muscle relaxation.[37] Enflurane and isoflurane, because they are more irritating than halothane, may cause more coughing and secretions when a patient is incompletely anesthetized. An inhalational induction is an effective way to avoid bronchospasm, provided the airway is not instrumented until the anesthesia is deep, and provided that the patient is not at risk for aspiration of gastrointestinal contents. All volatile anesthetic agents are effective in preventing and reversing bronchospasm.[37] These agents are all myocardial depressants. Halothane sensitizes the myocardium to

catecholamines, is associated with arrhythmias, and may predispose to ventricular arrhythmias in the presence of a high theophylline level.[63]

Nitrous oxide has no effect on bronchomotor tone. Usually used in inhaled concentrations of greater than 50% of the inspired gas it limits the maximum FiO_2 deliverable and thus is not suitable for use in patients who require a high FiO_2 to prevent hypoxemia. When this agent is discontinued it rapidly leaves the body (a result of its low blood solubility) and can transiently lower alveolar PO_2. This phenomenon, termed diffusion hypoxia, is not limited to patients with lung disease. To avoid its occurrence, all patients should be placed on a FiO_2 of 1.0 at the time the nitrous oxide is discontinued. Nitrous oxide does not depress the response to carbon dioxide but does depress the response to hypoxia.[40] This agent can diffuse into closed or poorly communicating gas spaces (pneumothorax, bleb, bulla) and cause them to expand, leading to dangerous hemodynamic consequences. Therefore, it should be used with caution, or not at all, in patients with bullous disease.

Ultra-short-acting barbiturates are commonly used for induction and have marked effects on the respiratory system. Apnea occurs after a moderate dose

(2 to 4 mg/kg IV, thiopental). The response to CO_2 is depressed and hypoxia becomes a stimulus for breathing.[40] Preoxygenation may therefore (infrequently) increase the respiratory depression associated with barbiturates. Although thiopental anesthesia has been associated with bronchoconstriction in animals, more recent studies have suggested that it is the instrumentation of the airway that precipitates laryngospasm and bronchospasm and not the barbiturate itself.[42] Secretions are not increased with this drug.

Narcotics are used to induce and maintain anesthesia. They usually result in hypoventilation and can blunt or abolish the response to hypercapnia and to hypoxemia.[28] Etomidate, a steroidal induction agent, does not usually cause cardiovascular depression and is thus useful in patients with heart disease. Like the barbiturates, it causes apnea when used for the induction of anesthesia. It has not been associated with bronchoconstriction although it will not prevent airway manipulation-induced bronchoconstriction.[28] It has been reported to produce temporary adrenal suppression.[84]

Ketamine can be used to induce and maintain anesthesia. When it is used as an induction agent, anesthesia develops somewhat more slowly than with barbiturates or etomidate, but this agent is useful in asthmatic patients. Ketamine has a sympathomimetic effect and prevents increases in airway resistance and bronchospasm in animals with allergic asthma.[36] Hypoxic and hypercarbic stimulation to ventilation is maintained. This drug increases heart rate, cardiac output, blood pressure, and myocardial oxygen consumption. It is not recommended for use in patients with cor pulmonale or ischemic heart disease. Ketamine also increases airway secretions, which can be controlled with an anticholinergic.

Endotracheal Intubation

Instrumentation of the airway, which may precipitate bronchospasm, can often be avoided through the use of mask anesthesia or use of regional anesthetic techniques. If, however, there is risk of aspiration of gastric contents or blood from the operative field (as in head and neck procedures or gastrointestinal surgery), or if the location of surgery and/or positioning of the patient contraindicates mask anesthesia, an endotracheal tube must be used. Neuromuscular blockade is commonly used to facilitate placement of the endotracheal tube and provide muscle relaxation during surgery. Muscle relaxants have little direct effect on the pulmonary system, with the exception of d-tubocurarine and atracurium, which may release histamine and cause bronchospasm. d-Tubocurarine has been found to increase airway resistance in man.[12] Succinylcholine will not relieve bronchospasm, as it does not block smooth muscle contraction. Muscle relaxants may contribute to atelectasis, $\dot{V}/\dot{Q}$ inequality, and hypoxemia.[82] Just before intubation, lidocaine may be used to help reduce or prevent bronchospasm; the IV route (1 to 3 mg/kg) may have advantages over the aerosol or topical route as the latter may induce bronchospasm.[18] Lidocaine acts by depressing airway reflexes that lead to bronchospasm.

It is well appreciated that COPD patients who suffer an exacerbation and require intubation may be difficult to wean from mechanical ventilation. This difficulty often relates to the underlying pathophysiology that may be impaired ventilatory mechanics, fatigued muscles of respiration, or nutritional deficiencies. It is traditional practice to view tracheal intubation as a "last step" in the management of a patient with COPD and respiratory failure. In the acute surgical setting, however, it is inappropriate to view intubation as a maneuver that will necessarily lead to inability to extubate at the end of a procedure and hence lead to long-term ventilatory dependence. Only if the underlying pathophysiology is worsened will tracheal intubation necessitate long-term ventilatory assistance. Thus, if $\dot{V}/\dot{Q}$ inequality from atelectasis or fluid overload can be avoided, if muscle mechanics are not depressed by residual muscle relaxants or diaphragmatic dysfunction that accompanies upper abdominal surgery, and if ventilatory drive is not excessively affected by residual anesthetic agents, postoperative extubation should be easily accomplished. Even if these conditions are not achieved there is no reason that the patient cannot be returned to close to the baseline conditions that prevailed before surgery, as these changes resolve. Furthermore, most of the above problems are not the result of intubation per se; they may necessitate postoperative ventilatory support even if intraoperative intubation was not employed.

Management of Ventilation and Oxygenation

Ventilation during surgery should be adjusted to maintain the blood gases close to the baseline range of the patient. Providing adequate time for exhalation is important in patients with obstructive airways disease to allow the lungs to empty and thus avoid "breath-stacking."[58] Air should be warmed and humidified, since cold dry air may be a stimulus for bronchospasm.[16] Use of devices to create positive pressure on exhalation can reduce the amount of airway collapse and atelectasis. Excessive airway pressures, however, should be avoided because of the possibility of rupturing a bleb, resulting in pneumothorax. General anesthesia decreases the ventilatory response to CO_2, and, in patients with preexisting lung disease, may lead to unacceptable hypercarbia if the patient is allowed to breathe spontaneously without assistance.

Hypercapnic patients have elevated levels of cerebrospinal fluid bicarbonate so that the pH of this fluid is relatively normal even with the chronically elevated $PaCO_2$. If at the end of surgery the arterial PCO_2 is not allowed to return to baseline levels, a CSF alkalosis will result and hypoventilation may be a consequence. While there is little reason to allow hypercapnia during anesthesia and surgery, the $PaCO_2$ must be near baseline values when extubation is contemplated. Similarly, it is common to maintain the PaO_2 at levels greater than baseline during surgery in an attempt to ensure adequate oxygen transport to the tissues. Careful reduction in the inspired concentration of oxygen at the end of surgery or when extubation is possible will allow the PaO_2 to return to a level that is both safe and does not result in hypoventilation.

Treatment of Intraoperative Bronchospasm

Bronchospasm developing during surgery is not necessarily related to preexisting reactive airways disease. Other causes of wheezing should be considered, such as pulmonary edema, endobronchial intubation, pneumothorax, aspiration, and drug reactions. Once these have been eliminated as a cause, there are several therapeutic options. Deepening the inhalational anesthetic may relieve the bronchoconstriction. Inhaled bronchodilators can be given directly into the inspiratory limb of the breathing circuit. These agents include both sympathomimetics (metaproterenol, albuterol) and anticholinergics (atropine, ipratropium). The former have few systemic side effects and are rapidly effective (5 to 10 minutes). The latter are particularly effective in blocking the parasympathetic stimulation associated with airway instrumentation but have an onset time

of about 30 minutes and would be better given during the preoperative period to blunt or prevent bronchospasm related to laryngoscopy or intubation. Both of these therapies are dependent upon adequate ventilation to deliver the drug to smaller airways. Successive inhalations of bronchodilator, 10 to 15 minutes apart, may reach obstructed airways better. Severe bronchospasm may necessitate an increase in the concentration of inspired oxygen. Pulse oximetry is helpful in detecting a decrease in hemoglobin saturation quickly and noninvasively. Bronchospasm in an intubated patient is also effectively treated with a volatile anesthetic, which then serves two purposes: providing anesthesia and controlling bronchospasm directly.

If these measures fail to control the bronchospasm, a theophylline infusion or parenteral sympathomimetic, or both, should be used; however, failure to control bronchospasm frequently reflects inadequate inhaled bronchodilator therapy. Terbutaline (beta$_2$ agonist) may be given subcutaneously with an onset of action of 30 to 60 minutes, but may cause tachycardia. Epinephrine subcutaneously and isoproterenol as an intravenous infusion are quite efficacious in acute exacerbations of asthma but may cause tachycardia and hypertension.[66] These drugs should be used cautiously, if at all, in any patient, especially one with hypertension or coronary artery disease or who is elderly. These agents, which can produce ventricular ectopy alone, are even more arrhythmogenic when used in combination with theophylline and volatile inhalational anesthetics. They are rarely used in a perioperative setting in adults. The treatment of bronchospasm occasionally may take hours, and attempting to speed its resolution by using toxic agents may have more morbidity than benefit. In severe bronchospasm the goal is to maintain adequate oxygenation; hypercarbia that is unaccompanied by hypoxemia or acidosis is unlikely to cause harm.[15] Most often, rather than resorting to epinephrine, the patient's lungs should be ventilated as permitted by the bronchospasm and supplemental oxygen should be administered to ensure adequate oxygenation.

Steroids do not help in the acute situation in the operating room, but if bronchospasm appears to be prolonged and refractory, they may be helpful for postoperative management. Lidocaine may be given as an aerosol or as an intravenous bolus or drip to depress reflex bronchoconstriction related to airway manipulation.[19] It should be used at the same blood concentration as for cardiac arrhythmias. Because of lidocaine-induced suppression of cough reflex and mucus transport, secretions may accumulate in the lungs. These will need to be suctioned to prevent atelectasis and pneumonia.

Intraoperative Hypoxemia

Intraoperative hypoxemia can be divided into several diagnostic categories. First, hypoxemia may result from a reduction in inspired oxygen concentration especially if nitrous oxide is used. Modern anesthesia practice dictates use of an oxygen analyzer in the inspiratory limb of the breathing circuit and use of "fail-safe" systems designed to prevent delivery of a hypoxic gas mixture. Second, hypoventilation (including disconnection of the breathing circuit or esophageal intubation), by raising arterial and thus alveolar CO_2, may contribute to hypoxemia. Third, rebreathing is a common cause of elevated PCO_2, as anesthetic breathing systems usually involve partial rebreathing and include a carbon dioxide absorber in the circuit. If this absorber fails, carbon dioxide levels in the inspired gas will increase. Fourth, actual shunting of blood may accompany an endobronchial intubation resulting in areas of lung that are perfused but not ventilated. Finally, ventilation-perfusion inequality is probably responsible for most other cases of hypoxemia under anesthesia. Examples of these conditions include secretions, bronchospasm, pleural effusions, pneumothorax, and atelectasis secondary to surgical retractors or position.

Timing of Extubation

At the end of surgery the decision must be made to either extubate the patient or transfer him or her to the intensive care unit for mechanical ventilation. This decision is based on the preoperative pulmonary function tests, arterial blood gases, type of surgery, and the operative course. Factors associated with a higher risk of pulmonary complications are anesthetic time (greater than 2 to 3 hours), upper abdominal and chest incisions, repeated general anesthesia within a 12-month period and, importantly, an elevated preoperative $PaCO_2$.[78] If extubation is performed the muscle relaxant must be reversed. Neostigmine can precipitate bronchospasm and increase secretions, but these effects are avoided by concomitant use of atropine. Patients with hyper-

reactive airways often have endotracheal extubation performed under deep anesthesia (except when there is a contraindication), to prevent the development of bronchospasm. Rarely is the decision to admit the patient to the intensive care unit postoperatively made at the end of surgery, and this decision is not necessarily predicated on the need for postoperative ventilation but rather on the need for further therapy and observation.

POSTOPERATIVE CONSIDERATIONS

Immediate postoperative management starts with the recognition of patients and types of procedures that have the greatest risk of complications. Abnormalities of pulmonary function and gas exchange after abdominal and thoracic surgery should be expected even in healthy patients. Ideally, patients with significant lung disease should be managed in an intensive care unit after surgery. The endotracheal tube may be left in place to facilitate removal of secretions and ensure that the patient is awake and strong enough to breathe without assistance, particularly if the type of surgery predisposes to worsened respiratory function and there was impaired preoperative function. Benefits of leaving the endotracheal tube in place, which include a secure airway, a route to suction airway secretions, and ensuring adequate ventilation and oxygenation, must be balanced against the risks, which include precipitation of bronchospasm, increased work of breathing, infection, and agitation requiring sedation.

Effect of Operative Site

Pulmonary complications following thoracic surgery may be more frequent than after abdominal surgery.[33] Patients undergoing upper abdominal surgery are at greater risk of pulmonary complications than those having lower abdominal surgery. The vital capacity decreases approximately 60% after an upper abdominal procedure and about 40% after lower abdominal procedures.[13] Over a 3-week period, vital capacity returns to baseline. Postoperatively, FRC decreases, reaching a nadir at 18 to 24 hours. In upper abdominal surgery it decreases 30% and in lower abdominal surgery about 10%, returning to baseline within 2 weeks. This decrease in FVC and FRC puts patients with pulmonary disease at a higher than usual risk of respiratory failure. Those undergoing nonthoracic and nonabdominal surgery are at much less risk of pulmonary complications.

During the early postoperative period, residual anesthesia, postoperative pain medications, and hypoventilation can interact to produce arterial hypoxemia and hypercarbia, necessitating close observation by trained personnel. Furthermore, the observed postoperative reduction in FRC below closing capacity, which results in small airway closure, can lead to atelectasis and hypoxemia. Finally, with abdominal operations, there is postoperative diaphragmatic dysfunction and cough is impaired, which can lead to retention of secretions. Total prevention of these changes is not possible, so the goal of therapy is to minimize the abnormalities.[13] A discussion of different therapeutic options can be found in Chapter 15.

Pain Relief

Although surgically induced changes in lung function are not entirely the result of pain and splinting, data indicate that this mechanism is important,[13] and postoperative pain management is an important part of the care of patients with severe lung disease. Parenteral narcotics have been used for many years and are quite efficacious, particularly when given in a setting that provides close observation by trained personnel and that permits adequate dosing. Pain relief may be achieved by methods other than parental narcotics. Intercostal nerve blocks give 4 to 6 hours of relief for thoracotomy or upper abdominal surgery with less depression of peak air flow than with parenteral narcotics. A promising area of postoperative pain control is the use of epidural or intrathecal narcotics. There may be a greater decrease in FEV_1 and FVC following surgery in patients receiving parenteral narcotics than in those receiving epidural narcotics, but this is not a consistent finding. Likewise, epidural narcotics may decrease peak expiratory flow less than intercostal block or parenteral narcotic.[11] Respiratory depression can occur following epidural or intrathecal narcotic administration, with maximum effects at 6 to 10 hours persisting for as long as 24 hours, and necessitating close observation of the patient during that period. A promising area of investigation is the use of intrapleural local anesthetics.[64]

Postoperative Hypoxia

Postoperative hypoxia may be particularly difficult to manage in patients with COPD or asthma. Respiratory depression secondary to residual anesthetic, muscle relaxant, and the effect of narcotics may contribute to hypoxemia, as does atelectasis and lung edema. Because these patients may ventilate on the basis of hypoxic drive, management requires careful attention to the level of inspired oxygen and PaO_2.

Medications

Medications, including bronchodilators, steroids, and antibiotics, should be continued postoperatively. Care must be taken to avoid and/or monitor the interactions of other drugs with theophylline. Beta-blockers should be used with care as they may precipitate bronchospasm. Labetalol and esmolol may prove sufficiently beta$_2$ selective to permit their use in patients with reactive airways.[27,49,69] Other important measures in the postoperative period may include chest physical therapy, incentive spirometry, postural drainage, and adequate hydration.

SUMMARY

Safe anesthetic management of patients with underlying lung disease necessitates an understanding of the underlying pathophysiology, the respiratory system changes that result from the surgical procedure and anesthesia, and the therapeutic interventions available. On the basis of this knowledge a rational anesthetic plan is determined for each patient. As clinical studies are performed in some of the areas discussed we may be able to further refine our care of these patients.

REFERENCES

1. Annis P, Landa J, and Lichtiger M: Effects of atropine on velocity of tracheal mucous in anesthetized patients, Anesthesiology 44:74-77, 1976.
2. American Thoracic Society Definitions, Am Rev Respir Dis 136:225-244, 1987.
3. Benumof J: One lung ventilation and hypoxic pulmonary vasoconstriction, Anesth Analg 64:821-833, 1985.
4. Benumof J, Augustine S, and Gibbons J: Halothane and isoflurane only slightly impair arterial oxygenation during one lung ventilation in patients undergoing thoracotomy, Anesthesiology 67:910-915, 1987.
5. Boushey HA et al: Bronchial hyperreactivity, Am Rev Respir Dis 121:389-413, 1980.
6. Brashear RE: Arrhythmias in patients with chronic obstructive pulmonary disease, Med Clin North Am 68:969-981, 1984.
7. Braunwald E et al (editors): Harrison's principles of internal medicine, ed 11, New York, 1987, McGraw-Hill Book Co.

8. Bukowsky M, Nakatsu K, and Munt P: Theophylline reassessed, Ann Intern Med 101:63-73, 1984.

9. Burki NK and Krumpelman JL: Correlation of pulmonary function with the chest roentgenogram in chronic airway obstruction, Am Rev Respir Dis 121:217-223, 1980.

10. Celli B, Rodriguez K, and Snider G: A controlled trial of intermittent positive pressure breathing, incentive spirometry, and deep breathing exercises in preventing pulmonary complications after abdominal surgery, Am Rev Respir Dis 130:12-15, 1984.

11. Coleman DL: Control of postoperative pain: nonnarcotic and narcotic alternatives and their effect on pulmonary function, Chest 92:520-528, 1987.

12. Crago R et al: Respiratory flow resistance after curare and pancuronium, measured by forced oscillations, Can Anaesth Soc J 19:607-614, 1972.

13. Craig DB: Postoperative recovery of pulmonary function, Anesth Analg 60:46-52, 1981.

14. Dalen J et al: The hemodynamic and respiratory effects of diazepam (Valium), Anesthesiology 30:259-263, 1969.

15. Darioli R and Perret C: Mechanical controlled hypoventilation in status asthmaticus, Am Rev Respir Dis 129:385-387, 1984.

16. Deal EC et al: Airway responsiveness to cold air and hyperpnea in normal subjects and in those with hay fever and asthma, Am Rev Respir Dis, 121:621-628, 1980.

17. Diener C and Burrows B: Further observations on the course and prognosis of chronic obstructive lung disease, Am Rev Respir Dis 111:719-724, 1975.

18. Downes H and Hirshman CA: Lidocaine aerosols do not prevent allergic bronchoconstriction, Anesth Analg 60:28-32, 1981.

19. Downes H, Gerber N, and Hirshman CA: IV lignocaine in reflex and allergic bronchoconstriction, Br J Anaesth 52:873-878, 1980.

20. Egeblad K et al: A simple method for predicting pulmonary function after lung resection, Scand J Thorac Cardiovasc Surg 20:103-107, 1986.

21. Empey DW et al: Bronchial hyperreactivity after upper respiratory tract infection, Am Rev Respir Dis 113:131-139, 1976.

22. Fletcher EC and Levin DC: Cardiopulmonary hemodynamics during sleep in subjects with chronic obstructive pulmonary disease, Chest 85:6-14, 1984.

23. Foster LJ, Trudeau WL, and Goldman AL: Bronchodilator effects on gastric acid secretion, JAMA 241:2613-2615, 1979.

24. Fraser CM, Venter JC, and Kaliner M: Autonomic abnormalities and autoantibodies to beta-adrenergic receptors, N Engl J Med 305:1165-1170, 1981.

25. Gardner R et al: Percutaneous indwelling radial artery catheters for monitoring cardiovascular function, N Engl J Med 290:1227-1231, 1974.

26. Gass GD and Olsen GN: Preoperative pulmonary function testing to predict postoperative morbidity and mortality, Chest 89:127-135, 1986.

27. George RB et al: Comparison of the effects of labetalol and hydrochlorthiazide on the ventilatory function of hypertensive patients with asthma and propranolol sensitivity, Chest 88:815-818, 1985.

28. Gilman A et al (editors): The pharmacological basis of therapeutics, ed 7, New York, 1985, MacMillan Publishing Co.

29. Gold M, Schwam S, and Goldberg M: Chronic obstructive pulmonary disease and respiratory complications, Anesth Analg 62:975-981, 1983.

30. Goldman L: Cardiac risks and complications of noncardiac surgery, Ann Intern Med 98:504-513, 1983.

31. Guenter CA and Welch MH (editors): Pulmonary medicine, ed 2, Philadelphia, 1982, JB Lippincott Co.

32. Hanson G, Drablos PA, and Steinert R: Pulmonary complications, ventilation and blood gases after upper abdominal surgery, Acta Anaesth Scand 21:211-215, 1977.

33. Harmon E and Lillington G: Pulmonary risk factors in surgery, Med Clin North Am 63:1289-1298, 1979.

34. Hirshman CA: Airway reactivity in humans, Anesthesiology 58:170-177, 1983.

35. Hirshman CA: ASA 1984 Annual Refresher Course Lectures 138:1-7.

36. Hirshman CA et al: Ketamine block of bronchospasm in experimental canine asthma, Br J Anaesth, 51:713-717, 1979.

37. Hirshman CA et al: Mechanism of action of inhalation anesthesia on airways, Anesthesiology 56:107-111, 1982.

38. Hogg JC: The pathology of asthma, Chest 87:152S-153S, 1985.

39. Hugh-Jones P and Whimster W: The etiology and management of disabling emphysema, Amer Rev Respir Dis 117:343-378, 1978.

40. Kaplan JA: Thoracic Anesthesia, New York, 1983, Churchill Livingstone.

41. Keller CA et al: Pulmonary hypertension in chronic obstructive pulmonary disease, Chest 90:185-192, 1986.

42. Kingston HG and Hirshman CA: Perioperative management of the patient with asthma, Anesth Analg 63:844-855, 1984.

43. Kirilloff LH et al: Does chest physical therapy work? Chest 88:436-444, 1985.

44. Knill RL and Gelb AW: Ventilatory responses to hypoxia and hypercapnia during halothane sedation and anesthesia in man, Anesthesiology 49:244-251, 1978.

45. Koga Y, Iwatsuki N, and Hashimoto Y: Direct effects of H_2-receptor antagonists on airway smooth muscle and on responses mediated by H_1- and H_2-receptors, Anesthesiology 66:181-185, 1987.

46. Latimer RG et al: Ventilatory patterns and pulmonary complications after upper abdominal surgery determined by preoperative and postoperative computerized spirometry and blood gas analysis, Am J Surg 122:622-632, 1971.

46a. Lawrence VA, page CP, and Harris GD: Preoperative spirometry before abdominal operations. A critical appraisal of its predictive value, Arch Intern Med 149:280-285, 1989.

47. Levine JH, Michael JR and Guarnieri T: Treatment of multifocal atrial tachycardia with verapamil, N Engl J Med 312:21-25, 1985.

48. Lichtiger M, Landa J, and Hirsch J: Velocity of tracheal mucus in anesthetized women undergoing gynecologic surgery, Anesthesiology 42:753-756, 1975.

49. Light R, Chetty K, and Stansbury D: Comparison of the effects of labetalol and hydrochlorothiazide on the ventilatory function of hypertensive patients with mild chronic obstructive pulmonary disease, Am J Med 68:109-114, 1983.

50. Littenberg B: Aminophylline treatment in severe, acute asthma. A meta-analysis, JAMA 259:1678-1684, 1988.

51. Littenberg B and Gluck E: A controlled trial of methylprednisolone in the emergency treatment of acute asthma, N Engl J Med 314:150-152, 1986.

52. Lourenco RV and Cotromanes E: Clinical aerosols. I. Characterization of aerosols and their diagnostic uses, Arch Intern Med 142:2163-2172, 1982.

53. Mariott HJL: Practical electrocardiography, ed 7, Baltimore, 1983, Williams & Wilkins.

54. McFadden ER: Introduction: methylxanthine therapy and reversible airway obstruction, Am J Med 79(suppl 6A):1-4, 1985.

55. Murciano D et al: Effects of theophylline on diaphragmatic strength and fatigue in patients with chronic obstructive pulmonary disease, N Engl J Med 311:349-353, 1984.

56. Nocturnal Oxygen Therapy Trial Group: Continuous or Nocturnal Oxygen Therapy In Hypoxemic Chronic Obstructive Lung Disease, Ann Intern Med 93:391-398, 1980.

57. Pearce AC and Jones RM: Smoking and anesthesia: preoperative abstinence and perioperative morbidity, Anesthesiology 61:576-584, 1984.

58. Pepe P and Marini J: Occult positive end-expiratory pressure in mechanically ventillated patients with airflow obstruction, Am Rev Respir Dis 126:166-170, 1982.

59. Petrie GR and Palmer K: Comparison of aerosol ipratropium bromide and salbutamol in chronic bronchitis and asthma, Br Med J 1:430-432, 1975.

60. Pietak S et al: Anesthetic effects on ventilation in patients with chronic obstructive pulmonary disease, Anesthesiology 42:160-166, 1975.

61. Reichel J: Assessment of operative risk of pneumonectomy, Chest 62:570-576, 1972.

62. Rochester DF and Esau SA: Malnutrition and the respiratory system, Chest 85:411-415, 1984.

63. Roizen MF and Stevens WC: Multiform ventricular tachycardia due to the interaction of aminophylline and halothane, Anesth Analg 57:738-741, 1978.

64. Rosenberg P et al: Continuous intrapleural infusion of bupivacaine for analgesia after thoracotomy, Anesthesiology 67:811-813, 1987.

65. Rosow C et al: Histamine release during morphine and fentanyl anesthesia, Anesthesiology 56:93-96, 1982.

66. Rossing TH et al: Emergency therapy of asthma: comparison of the acute effects of parenteral and inhaled sympathomimetics and infused aminophylline, Am Rev Respir Dis 122:365-371, 1980.

67. Salerno DM et al: Intravenous verapamil for treatment of multifocal atrial tachycardia with and without calcium pretreatment, Ann Intern Med 107:623-628, 1987.

68. Sasson C et al: Airway occlusion pressure: an important indicator for successful weaning in patients with chronic obstructive pulmonary disease, Am Rev Respir Dis 135:107-113, 1987.

69. Sheppard D et al: Effects of esmolol on airway function in patients with asthma, J Clin Pharmacol 26:169-174, 1986.

70. Shim C et al: Positional effects on distribution of ventilation in chronic obstructive pulmonary disease, Ann Intern Med 105:346-350, 1986.

71. Slogoff S, Keats A, and Arlund C: On the safety of radial artery cannulation, Anesthesiology 59:42-47, 1983.

72. Smith MJ and Hodson ME: Effects of long term inhaled high dose beclomethasone dipropionate on adrenal function, Thorax 38:676-681, 1983.

73. Smith T et al: Effects of premedicant drugs on respiration and gas exchange in man, Anesthesiology 28:883-890, 1967.

74. Sokoll M, Hoyt J, and Gergis S: Studies in muscle rigidity, nitrous oxide, and narcotic analgesic agents, Anesth Analg 51:16-20, 1972.

75. Soroker D et al: Respiratory function following premedication with droperidol or diazepam, Anesth Analg, 57:695-699, 1978.

76. Stein M and Cassara EL: Preoperative pulmonary evaluation and therapy for surgery patients, JAMA 211:787-790, 1970.

77. Stock MC et al: Prevention of postoperative pulmonary complications with CPAP, incentive spirometry, and conservative therapy, Chest 87:151-157, 1985.

78. Tarhan S et al: Risk of anesthesia and surgery in patients with chronic bronchitis and chronic obstructive pulmonary disease, Surgery 74:720-726, 1973.

79. Tashkin D et al: Effect of orally administered cimetidine on histamine- and antigen-induced bronchospasm in subjects with asthma, Am Rev Respir Dis, 125:691-695, 1982.

80. Thomas A and Valabhji P: Arrhythmia and tachycardia in pulmonary heart disease, Br Heart J 31:491-495, 1969.

81. Tisi GM: Preoperative identification and evaluation of the patient with lung disease, Med Clinic North Am 71:399-412, 1987.

82. Tokics L et al: Lung collapse and gas exchange during general anesthesia: effects of spontaneous breathing, muscle paralysis, and positive end-expiratory pressure, Anesthesiology 66:157-167, 1987.

83. Voelkel NF: Mechanisms of hypoxic pulmonary vasoconstriction, Am Rev Respir Dir 133:1186-1195, 1986.

84. Wagner RL et al: Inhibition of adrenal steroidogenesis by the anesthetic etomidate, N Engl J Med 310:1415-1421, 1984.

85. Walden S et al: Effect of alpha-adrenergic blockade on exercise induced asthma and conditioned cold air, Am Rev Respir Dis 130:357-362, 1984.

86. Walkup R et al: Prediction of postoperative pulmonary function with the lateral position test, Chest 77:24-27, 1980.

87. Wanner A: Effects of methylxanthines on airway mucociliary function, Am J Med 79(suppl 6A):16-21, 1985.

88. Wewers MD and Gadek JE: The protease theory of emphysema, editorial, Ann Intern Med 107:761-763, 1987.

89. Wightman J: A prospective survey of the incidence of postoperative pulmonary complications, Br J Surg 55:85-91, 1968.

CHAPTER 20

Hypertension

MICHAEL J. BRESLOW
MICHAEL LISH

It is estimated that 60 million Americans (28% of the population) have hypertension, which is adequately controlled in only a small fraction of these people.[40,75,78] Risks associated with chronic hypertension include stroke, myocardial infarction, congestive heart failure, and renal failure.[42,56] This chapter discusses hypertension as a risk factor for perioperative morbidity and mortality, addresses preoperative assessment and management of the hypertensive patient, reviews the pathogenesis of intraoperative and postoperative hypertension, and reviews drugs available for treating perioperative hypertension.

HYPERTENSION AND PERIOPERATIVE RISK

Hypertension is a chronic disease with the following end-organ effects that may adversely affect perioperative outcome: (1) altered cerebral blood flow autoregulation, (2) myocardial hypertrophy, (3) atherosclerotic vascular disease, and (4) vascular intimal proliferation. First, cerebral blood flow regulation is altered by chronic hypertension[68] (Figure 20-1). Cerebral vessels constrict or dilate in response to changes in arterial blood pressure to keep cerebral blood flow constant (autoregulation). This compensatory mechanism sustains normal cerebral blood flow in nonhypertensive patients until blood pressure falls below approximately 50 mm Hg.[34,61] Chronic hypertension is associated with a rightward shift of the cerebral autoregulatory curve, so that decreases in cerebral blood flow occur at higher blood pressures. This change is of clinical relevance since perioperative reductions of arterial blood pressure that are tolerated by other patients may decrease cerebral blood flow in hypertensive patients.[47,68] Animal studies indicate that effective long-term antihypertensive therapy restores cerebral autoregulation to normal.[72]

A second effect of chronic hypertension, myocardial hypertrophy, occurs as a result of the increased work the heart must perform. Myocardial hypertrophy increases myocardial oxygen consumption, decreases coronary vasodilator reserve,[6] and alters the coronary autoregulatory response curve.[36]

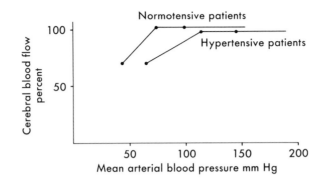

FIGURE 20-1. Mean curves of autoregulation of cerebral blood flow (CBF) in normotensive and severely hypertensive human subjects. Each curve is defined by the mean values of resting blood pressure, the lower limit of CBF autoregulation, and the lowest tolerated blood pressure. The curve from the hypertensive patients is shifted to the right on the blood pressure axis.

Reprinted with permission from Standgaard S: Circulation 53:720–727, 1976.

These changes predispose to myocardial ischemia in susceptible patients. In addition, when hypertension is severe and/or prolonged, the increased work load imposed on the heart can result in congestive heart failure. Third, hypertension is an independent risk factor for the developoment of coronary artery disease. Coronary intimal injury from longstanding hypertension predisposes to cholesterol deposition, atheroma formation, and vascular occlusion. The decrease in the death rate from myocardial infarction observed over the past decade is probably, in part, caused by improved treatment of chronic hypertension.[23] Finally, intimal proliferation occurs in the penetrating arteries of kidney and brain in patients with longstanding hypertension (Figure 20-2). The vascular lumen is narrowed, and a high incidence of renal failure and lacunar stroke are observed in hypertensive patients. Successful antihypertensive therapy can decrease the incidence of most hypertension-related vascular complications.[9,73]

Because of these serious end-organ changes, hypertensive patients might be expected to have an increased incidence of myocardial infarction, congestive heart failure, stroke, and renal failure in the perioperative time. However, it has not been clearly shown that these complications occur with greater frequency in hypertensive surgical patients. Whether this lack of evidence reflects the paucity of adequately controlled studies or a true lack of association of hypertension with these perioperative

problems is not known. Studies detailing the perioperative course of hypertensive patients are reviewed in the following paragraph.

Reports from the first half of this century suggested that perioperative mortality was markedly greater in hypertensive patients than in patients without hypertension.[57,66] None of these studies, however, corrected for the effects of underlying medical problems which may have independently increased perioperative risk. Of equal importance, anesthetic and surgical practice have improved over the years, reducing perioperative risk for all patients.

Using multivariate analysis techniques, Goldman et al[32] identified prior myocardial infarction and preoperative congestive heart failure (but not hypertension) as independent predictors of perioperative cardiac death, myocardial infarction, heart failure, and arrhythmias. These findings must be interpreted with caution. Although hypertension may not be an independent predictor, the well-documented causal relationship between hypertension and both coronary artery disease and congestive heart failure suggests that hypertensive patients will have a greater risk of perioperative cardiac complications than healthy controls. Their findings do suggest, however, that hypertension does not increase perioperative risk in patients with underlying coronary artery disease or congestive heart failure. Goldman did not distinguish between patients with treated hypertension and those in whom the condition was untreated; and no conclusion concerning effects of untreated hypertension

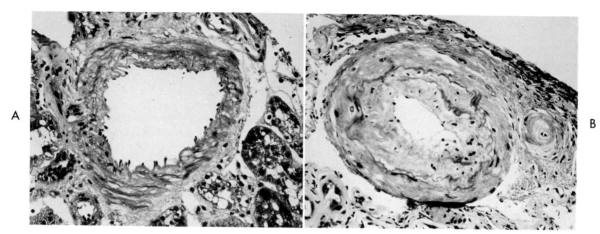

FIGURE 20-2. Medium size interlobular renal arteries from normal (**A**) and hypertensive (**B**) patients. Note intimal proliferation and narrowing of lumen in vessels from the hypertensive patient.

on perioperative outcome can be made. Assidao et al[5] and Towne and Bernhard[70] reported a greater incidence of neurologic deficits in patients who became hypertensive after carotid endarterectomy, but neither study determined whether postoperative hypertension causes neurologic deficits or is simply a marker for neurologic injury. Although postoperative hypertension is more common in previously hypertensive patients,[29,63] a causal relationship between preoperative hypertension and postoperative neurologic deficits has not been established. The role of hypertension in development of perioperative acute renal failure has not been evaluated. In one study, patients who discontinued antihypertensive therapy preoperatively had lower postoperative urine outputs than hypertensive patients who continued their medications through surgery, but no association with acute renal failure was reported.[64]

To summarize, chronic untreated hypertension increases the risk for development of atheromatous coronary, cerebral, and renal vascular diseases. Patients with these end-organ diseases are at risk for further ischemic injury during the perioperative period. Although hypertension has not been clearly shown to increase perioperative ischemic risk in patients with vascular disease, hypertensive patients are more hemodynamically labile than normotensive patients in the perioperative period,[64] leading many practitioners to postpone elective surgery in poorly controlled hypertensive patients.

PREOPERATIVE ASSESSMENT AND MANAGEMENT

Any hypertensive patient should be carefully assessed preoperatively to determine the presence and severity of coronary, cerebral, and renal diseases. Findings of left ventricular hypertrophy, congestive heart failure, retinopathy, or renal insufficiency usually require special perioperative management strategies that are discussed in detail elsewhere in this book. Blood pressure must be taken in both arms to avoid inappropriate management based on blood pressure readings taken from an arm supplied by an atheromatous subclavian artery.[44] An elevated preoperative blood pressure may reflect either the stress of upcoming surgery, inadequate antihypertensive therapy, or poor compliance with the medical regimen. Blood pressure recordings during current and previous hospitalizations, retinal and cardiac exam and electrocardiographic signs of left ventricular hypertrophy provide some information regarding the long-term adequacy of antihypertensive therapy. There is no general agreement concerning perioperative management of poorly treated or untreated hypertensive patients. Prys-Roberts et al[58] reported that patients with poorly controlled hypertension had an increased incidence of perioperative ischemia, and these data are used by some to justify postponement of elective surgery. In contrast, Goldman et al[31] found no increased incidence of cardiovascular complications in untreated hypertensive patients, providing ammunition for those who believe that it is safe to proceed with elective procedures in such patients. Both studies have been widely criticized. Neither study randomized hypertensive patients to treated and untreated groups, and it is unlikely that such data will be forthcoming to permit definitive recommendations. Most practitioners anesthetize mildly hypertensive patients but delay elective surgery in severely hypertensive patients. In any case, rapid preoperative restoration of blood pressure to normal using potent, quick-acting drugs is not an appropriate substitute for initiation of a stable and effective antihypertensive regimen in elective surgical patients. The changes in cerebrovascular autoregulation that occur in chronically hypertensive patients may predispose to cerebral ischemic injury during rapid return of blood pressure to normal.[47,68]

Most surgical patients with chronic hypertension are receiving antihypertensive therapy. Antihypertensive agents are listed in the box above, right. Although continuation of antihypertensive drugs throughout the perioperative period is felt to promote hemodynamic stability,[59] and is the current standard of care, many of these agents have other effects that may influence perioperative management.

Diuretics

Diuretics have been first line antihypertensive agents for many years. Chronic diuretic therapy can cause hypokalemia and hypovolemia, and some agents such as the thiazides, may prolong the duration of action of muscle relaxants.[53] Total body potassium stores are markedly depleted during chronic use of some diuretic agents. However, hypokalemia does not appear to increase the risks for perioperative arrhythmias,[37] and rapid infusions of potassium solutions the night before surgery are not indicated. Diuretics may complicate fluid management, and some patients appear to require continued diuretic therapy to maintain urine output throughout the perioperative period (diuretic dependency). These complications are probably not prevented by omitting diuretics the morning before surgery since many of these agents have a long duration of action.

Beta-Adrenergic Antagonists

Cardiovascular mortality is less in hypertensive patients who are treated with beta-blockers,[38,69] and use of these agents has increased in recent years. Beta-blockers should be continued throughout the

---

Antihypertensive agents

Diuretics
Beta-adrenergic receptor antagonists
Vasodilators
   Direct—hydralazine
   Alpha-adrenergic antagonists—prazosin
   Calcium blockers—nifedipine
   Angiotensin converting enzyme inhibitors—
     captopril, enalopril
   Norepinephrine depletors
     guanethidine—peripheral only
     reserpine—peripheral and central
$Alpha_2$-agonists
   Clonidine
   Alpha-methyldopa

---

perioperative period—a recommendation strongly supported by published data.[3,18,35,54] Chronic administration of beta-blockers increases cellular expression of beta receptors, and this effect may enhance sensitivity to beta-agonist stimulation upon withdrawal.[1,30] The heart rate responses to isoproterenol in normal volunteers before, during, and after propranolol administration are shown in Figure 20-3.[12] Propranolol (40 mg taken orally every 6 hours) almost completely blocked the heart rate response to infused isoproterenol, but 24 and 48 hours after propranolol withdrawal, isoproterenol increased heart rate to twice the levels observed before beginning beta-blockade. Although this report only shows supersensitivity to beta-agonist stimulation 24 to 36 hours after beta-blocker withdrawal, Prys-Roberts et al observed significant increases in heart rate following laryngoscopy in patients on chronic beta-blocker therapy unless beta-blockers were administered the morning of surgery.[60] The potential value of perioperative beta-blockade is highlighted by the recent report that hypertensive patients who were given a single dose of a beta-blocker preoperatively had a reduced incidence of intraoperative ischemic events.[67] Complications of beta-blockade, such as myocardial depression and bradycardia, are rarely observed in patients receiving perioperative beta-blockade. Bolling et al[11] reported that postoperative nitroprusside requirements correlated directly with plasma propranolol levels in coronary artery bypass patients. The authors suggested that loss of $beta_2$-receptor-mediated vasodilation in these patients ex-

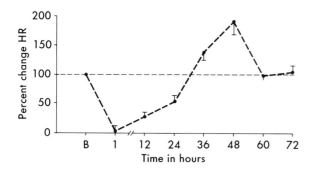

FIGURE 20-3. Percent change in heart rate (HR) caused by isoproterenol administration before (B) and up to 72 hours after 160 mg daily of oral propranolol in six normal volunteers. * = Significantly less than the prepropranolol baseline (P < 0.05); ** = significantly greater than the prepropranolol baseline (P < 0.05).

Reprinted with permission from Boudoulas H et al: Ann Intern Med 87:433–36, 1977.

acerbated the hypertensive response to increased perioperative sympathetic nervous system activity. But this conclusion is doubtful; no attempt was made to exclude the possibility that propranolol therapy simply served as a marker for preoperative hypertension.

Vasodilators

Data to assess the benefits and hazards of vasodilator agents (for example, calcium blockers) in the perioperative period are not available. While continuation of vasodilator therapy probably improves perioperative blood pressure control, these agents could, theoretically, attenuate compensatory vasoconstriction during hemorrhage. Despite widespread use of calcium channel blockers as antianginal agents, perioperative administration of these drugs does not appear to decrease the incidence of intraoperative ischemic episodes.[19] Calcium channel blockers potentiate neuromuscular blockade[45.79] and have been reported to reduce anesthetic requirements.[52] Little data exist on perioperative use of angiotensin converting enzyme (ACE) inhibitors. Colson et al reported normal blood pressure regulation in nine patients undergoing coronary artery bypass grafting.[20] ACE inhibitors can produce azotemia in nonsurgical patients with renal artery stenosis by reducing efferent arteriolar tone and decreasing glomerular capillary pressure,[39] but whether ACE inhibitors alter the incidence of perioperative renal

insufficiency is unknown. Intraoperative splanchnic hypoperfusion is correlated with development of perioperative complications[25] and since angiotensin II appears to be the principal mediator of splanchnic vasoconstriction,[7] perioperative use of ACE inhibitors may possibly be beneficial in high risk patients. Reserpine and guanethidine deplete norepinephrine from sympathetic nerve terminals and cause vasodilation. Both agents attenuate the vasoconstriction response to indirect-acting vasopressors and augment the response to direct-acting sympathomimetic agents.[16] Reserpine depletes central as well as peripheral catecholamines and decreases anesthetic requirements.[53]

Drugs that decrease central sympathetic outflow. Clonidine, a centrally acting alpha$_2$-agonist, decreases sympathetic outflow and lowers blood pressure. Although severe rebound hypertension after clonidine withdrawal has been reported in nonsurgical settings,[17,62] postoperative cessation of clonidine in clonidine-treated patients does not appear to increase risk for hypertensive complications. Transdermal clonidine permits administration of the drug throughout the perioperative period, but transdermal pharmacokinetics require 48 hours to achieve peak blood levels, and the patch must be applied several days before surgery.[77] Clonidine significantly reduces anesthetic requirements,[26] and high-dose alpha$_2$-agonists have been reported to have anesthetic effects.[65] Like clonidine, alpha-methyldopa also decreases blood pressure and reduces anesthetic requirements by decreasing central sympathetic outflow.

INTRAOPERATIVE HYPERTENSION

Intraoperative hypertension is often a manifestation of inadequate anesthetic depth in relation to the level of noxious stimulation. Imbalances between anesthetic depth and stimulation are often a result of abrupt and unanticipated changes in surgical stimulation, inability to rapidly alter anesthetic depth because of long half-lives of many anesthetic agents, deliberate avoidance of excessive anesthetic depth, or inadequate analgesic therapy on emergence from anesthesia. Other causes of intraoperative hypertension include hypervolemia, baroreceptor denervation during carotid endarterectomy[13,48] or radical neck dissection,[55] aortic crossclamping, unrecognized pheochromocytoma, and hypothermia. The

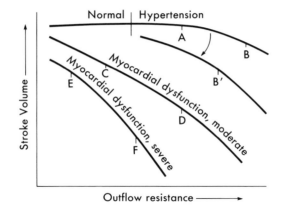

FIGURE 20-4. Relation of left ventricular stroke volume to systemic outflow resistance in normal and diseased hearts. A family of curves may be described, depending on the severity of the myocardial disease. If cardiac function is normal, a rise in resistance results in hypertension, since cardiac output remains fairly constant. Heart failure in a hypertensive patient could be shown either by a move to point *B*, a high resistance with normal function, or point *B'*, which represents a shift to a slightly depressed ventricular-function curve. When myocardial dysfunction is more severe, as shown by the lower two curves, blood pressure is no longer directly determined by resistance since stroke volume and resistance are inversely related. Consequently, arterial pressure may be similar at points *E* and *F* despite marked differences in cardiac output and resistance.

Reprinted with permission from N Engl J Med 297:27–31, 1977.

cause of intraoperative hypertension should ideally be identified before antihypertensive drug therapy is begun.

Overzealous treatment of hypertension may be as deleterious as hypertension itself. Commonly cited reasons for intraoperative antihypertensive therapy include: prevention of myocardial ischemia, reduction of afterload to augment cardiac output, prevention of excessive surgical bleeding, and avoidance of acute neurologic injuries. While these may be appropriate justification for instituting antihypertensive therapy in certain settings, they do not support widespread use of antihypertensive agents intraoperatively. Elevated arterial blood pressures increase myocardial oxygen consumption; however, Buffington et al found that, for any given heart rate, myocardial ischemic episodes were more common at lower rather than at higher blood pressures.[15] Fremes et al[28] noted increased myocardial lactate extraction as mean arterial blood pressure (MAP) decreased from 119 to 97 mm Hg, but when MAP was further decreased to 80 mm Hg lactate production occurred. Reduction of afterload with vasodi-

lators to improve myocardial performance is likely to increase cardiac output significantly only in patients with impaired ventricular function. Normal patients have only minimal reduction in myocardial performance as afterload increases (Figure 20-4). Potent vasodilators can also reduce ventricular preload and adversely affect cardiac output.

Treatment of intraoperative hypertension to limit surgical bleeding has not been thoroughly evaluated. Deliberate hypotension clearly assists in maintaining a blood-free surgical field during microscopic surgery on the middle ear,[43] and reduces blood loss during certain orthopedic and urologic operations.[2,22] Case reports suggest that hypertension increases bleeding in patients having either coronary artery bypass grafting[74] or facial surgery.[51] However, data do not exist on which to base recommendations of specific levels of blood pressure at which bleeding is best controlled. Probably such therapy is unnecessary for most general surgery patients.

Prevention of acute neurologic catastrophes is perhaps the most common rationale for antihypertensive therapy in the operating room. However, intraoper-

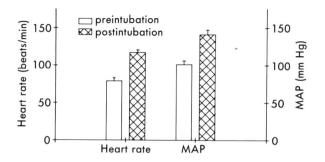

FIGURE 20-5. Heart rate and mean arterial blood pressure (MAP) before and after laryngoscopy and intubation.

Adapted from Laurito CE et al: Anesth Analg 67:389–392, 1988.

TABLE 20-1. Interventions to modulate hemodynamic changes during laryngoscopy and intubation

Agent	Effect on HR response	Effect on BP response	Ref
Lidocaine			
IV or aerosol	No	No	44
Esmolol	Yes	Partial	20
Labetalol (low dose)			
10 to 20 mg	Yes	No	39
Labetalol (high dose)			
70 mg	Yes	Partial	9,47

ative cerebral vascular accidents are rarely reported except during carotid endarterectomy or cardiopulmonary bypass. Narrowing of cerebral vessels and altered cerebral autoregulation in patients with chronic hypertension may increase the risk for ischemic events during acute antihypertensive therapy. Accordingly, patients must be carefully selected and treatment must be goal-directed to achieve specific beneficial effects and avoid the hazards of overzealous blood pressure reduction.

Skillful anesthesiologists reduce the likelihood of intraoperative hypertension by anticipating upcoming noxious events and constantly titrating anesthetic depth to the level of stimulation. During laryngoscopy, however, hypertension is extremely difficult to control (Figure 20-5). Laryngoscopy and intubation are brief, but profoundly stimulating experiences, which are invariably followed by little or no stimulation during the time the patient is "prepped and draped." After "standard" thiopental induction, laryngoscopy and intubation increase both heart rate (15 to 40 beat/min) and mean arterial blood pressure (40 to 50 mm Hg),[21,41,46,49] and greater increases are observed in patients requiring emergent surgery.[10] Many studies have evaluated strategies to attenuate this hemodynamic response (Table 20-1). The results of these studies can be summarized as follows: (1) blood pressure is more difficult to control than heart rate, (2) high doses of beta-blockers are required to attenuate the rise in blood pressure, (3) labetalol, a combined alpha-adrenergic and beta-adrenergic receptor antagonist, is no more effective than esmolol,

a short-acting beta$_1$-selective antagonist, and (4) lidocaine has no effect on the hemodynamic response. Because of its efficacy and short half-life, esmolol appears to be the drug of choice to blunt the hemodynamic responses to laryngoscopy. Labetalol can be used, but the large dose requirement and long half-life produce undesirable adrenergic blockade throughout the operative period. High-dose narcotic anesthetics also quite effectively prevent hemodynamic changes during laryngoscopy, but this technique frequently requires prolonged postoperative ventilation. Small doses of supplemental narcotics may blunt the hemodynamic response to laryngoscopy. Recent evidence suggests that intranasal nitroglycerine (2 mg) also effectively prevents the hypertensive response.[50]

Hypertension also occurs commonly at the end of surgery when anesthetic depth must be decreased to allow the patient to awaken. Anesthetics are usually terminated before the end of surgery to prevent prolonged postoperative somnolence, and a relative imbalance between anesthetic depth and surgical stimulation can result in hypertension. This effect is particularly important when intraoperative narcotic administration is inadequate to provide analgesia as brain levels of volatile anesthetics decrease and awakening occurs.

POSTOPERATIVE HYPERTENSION

Postoperative hypertension occurs in 5% to 10% of recovery room admissions after routine elective surgical procedures[24,29] and hypertension is more common in patients who are hypertensive preoperatively.[29,63] However, the incidence of hypertension approaches 50% after operations on the abdominal aorta,[31] extracranial cerebral vessels,[5,48] and coronary vessels.[27,76] Perioperative alterations in blood pressure correlate directly with serum catecholamine levels,[33] and these findings implicate adrenergic hyperactivity in the pathogenesis of this common problem. A recent study in our institution found that epidural morphine decreased pain, attenuated the sympathetic nervous system response to surgery, and reduced the incidence of postoperative hypertension in patients having aortic surgery.[14] Neither increased activity of the renin-angiotensin system nor pituitary secretion of vasopressin appear to mediate postoperative hypertension.[8,75] Carotid baroreceptor denervation probably contributes to the high incidence of hypertension after either carotid endarterectomy or radical neck dissection,[12,48,55] and a cardiac afferent reflex may mediate a hypertensive response in cardiac surgical patients postoperatively.[27]

Anxiety and pain can contribute to increased sympathetic nervous system activity postoperatively, and measures to minimize these effects may decrease the incidence of hypertension. Anderson[4] recently reported that extensive preoperative consultation with the patient to review common perioperative events decreases the incidence of hypertension following cardiac surgery. Many studies have documented the inadequacy of common analgesic regimens in surgical patients (see Chapter 13), and improved analgesic strategies can also decrease the incidence of postoperative hypertension. Vanstrum et al[11] found

that intrathecal morphine, for example, provides superior analgesia and reduces need for nitroprusside therapy after coronary artery bypass surgery. These data are consistent with our finding that epidural morphine decreases the incidence of hypertension following aortic surgery.[14] Measures aimed at reducing anxiety and pain should be routinely employed in all patients, and special measures should be considered for patients who are likely to be adversely affected by postoperative hypertension. Specific antihypertensive agents should be used only if problematic hypertension persists despite adequate anxiety and pain relief.

ANTIHYPERTENSIVE AGENTS USED IN THE PERIOPERATIVE PERIOD

Antihypertensive agents commonly used in the perioperative period are listed in Table 20-2. Although sublingual and transdermal routes of administration are possible, abnormalities of gastrointestinal function and need for rapid titration require that most of these agents be given parenterally. Short-acting agents are preferred for intraoperative use since hemodynamic conditions may change rapidly and unpredictably. Many anesthetic agents depress heart rate and cardiac contractility, and antihypertensive agents with these actions should be used with caution intraoperatively. Longer-acting agents are preferred for effective and consistent blood pressure control postoperatively when sympathetic tone, heart rate, and cardiac output are increased. Antihypertensive agents which depress heart rate and cardiac

TABLE 20-2.   Antihypertensive agents used in the perioperative period

Name	Route of administration	Type of agent	Comments
Nitroprusside	IV	Vasodilator	Potent arterial dilator, short half-life, dose not to exceed 10 μg/kg/min
Nitroglycerine	IV	Vasodilator	Predominantly venodilator
Labetalol	IV	Alpha and beta-adrenergic antagonist	Excellent drug for postoperative hypertension
Esmolol	IV	Beta-adrenergic antagonist	Short half-life, B₁ selective
Nifedipine	Sublingual	Ca⁺⁺ blocker	Can cause reflex tachycardia
Hydralazine	IV, IM	Vasodilator	Frequently causes increased heart rate
Alpha-methyldopa	IV	Decreases central sympathetic outflow	Can cause drowsiness, slow onset of action
Clonidine	Transdermal	Decreases central sympathetic outflow	48° to achieve steady-state plasma levels

output are frequently desirable postoperatively (see Chapter 17).

Nitroprusside, an arterial dilator with an extremely short half-life, is used for rapid adjustment of blood pressure during changing intraoperative hemodynamic conditions. Use of nitroprusside is limited by the need for a pump infusion system, a dedicated central venous catheter, continuous monitoring of blood pressure, frequent alterations in dose, and a high incidence of transient episodes of hypertension and hypotension. Excessive doses can result in cyanide toxicity. Nitroglycerine, predominantly a venodilator, is not a particularly effective antihypertensive agent. Hydralazine, a direct-acting vasodilator, is limited by a long half-life and high incidence of both hypotension and tachycardia. Direct chronotropic stimulation and baroreflex-mediated increases in heart rate make hydralazine a poor antihypertensive choice in patients with coronary artery disease, unless concomitant beta-blockade is used. Labetalol, a combined alpha and beta-blocker, decreases blood pressure with little change in heart rate. An initial dose of 2.5 to 5 mg for intraoperative use (smaller than that listed in the package insert) is recommended to avoid hypotension and to minimize long-term effects. Slow administration of 10 to 20 mg over 15 to 20 minutes generally results in gradual and predictable reductions of blood pressure postoperatively. Larger doses can be used if needed, and may have a more prolonged duration of action. Esmolol, a pure beta-blocker with a very short half-life, can be used alone or in combination with vasodilators to treat perioperative hypertension. Other drugs such as sublingual nifedipine, alpha-methyldopa, and transdermal clonidine can also be used for perioperative hypertensive therapy. Large doses of nifedipine should be avoided since treatment of overdose is difficult. The dose, duration of action, and antihypertensive effects of parenteral alpha-methyldopa are similar to those of the orally administered drug. While not well-suited for treatment of acute postoperative hypertension, alpha-methyldopa may be of value in the chronically hypertensive patient who requires prolonged parenteral therapy postoperatively.

SUMMARY

Although hypertension is common among surgical patients, many questions remain concerning the perioperative implications of this disease. Furthermore, despite the prevalence of intraoperative and postoperative hypertension, confusion exists concerning indications for treatment and optimal management regimens. These unresolved questions are highly important, however, since perioperative treatment of hypertension is very expensive and probably results in significant morbidity. The challenge is to conduct rigorous studies to answer many of the unresolved issues in this area.

REFERENCES

1. Aarons RD et al: Elevation of B-adrenergic receptor density in human lymphocytes after propranolol administration, J Clin Invest 65:949–957, 1980.
2. Ahlerling TE, Henderson JB, and Skinner DG: Controlled hypotensive anesthesia to reduce blood loss in radical cystectomy for bladder cancer, J Urol 129:953–954, 1983.
3. Alderman EL et al: Coronary artery syndromes after sudden propranolol withdrawal, Ann Intern Med 81:625–627, 1974.
4. Anderson EA: Preoperative preparation for cardiac surgery facilitates recovery, reduces psychological distress, and reduces the incidence of acute postoperative hypertension, J Consult Clin Psychol 55(4):513–520, 1987.
5. Asiddao CB, Donegan JH, and Whitesell RC: Factors associated with perioperative complications during carotid endarterectomy, Anesth Analg 8:631–638, 1982.
6. Bache RJ et al: Effect of maximal coronary vasodilation on transmural myocardial perfusion during tachycardia in dogs with left ventricular hypertrophy, Circ Res 49:742–750, 1981.
7. Bailey RW et al: Protection of the small intestine from nonocclusive mesenteric ischemic injury due to cardiogenic shock, Amer J of Surg 153:108–116, 1987.
8. Balley DR et al: The renin-angiotensin-aldosterone system during cardiac surgery with morphine-nitrous oxide anesthesia, Anesthesiology 42:538–544, 1975.
9. Berglund G et al: Coronary heart disease after treatment of hypertension, Lancet 1:1–5, 1978.
10. Bernstein JS et al: Beat-by-beat cardiovascular responses to rapid sequence induction in human: effects of labetalol, Anesthesiology 67:A32, 1987.
11. Bolling SF et al: Propranolol induced postoperative hypertension following coronary artery bypass grafting, J Thorac Cardiovasc Surg 87(1):112–119, 1984.
12. Boudoulas H et al: Hypersensitivity to adrenergic stimulation after propranolol withdrawal in subjects, Ann Intern Med 87:433–436, 1977.
13. Bove EL et al: Hypotension and hypertension as consequences of baroreceptor dysfunction following carotid endarterectomy, Surgery 85:633–637, 1979.

14. Breslow MJ et al: Epidural morphine decreases post-operative hypertension by attenuating sympathetic nervous system hyperactivity, JAMA 261:3577-3581, 1989.
15. Buffington CW: Impaired systolic thickening associated with halothane in the presence of a coronary stenosis is mediated by changes in hemodynamics, Anesthesiology 64:632-640, 1986.
16. Burn JH and Rand MJ: Actions of sympathomimetic amines on animals treated with reserpine, J Physiol (Lond) 144:314-336, 1958.
17. Campbell BC and Reid JL: Regimen for the control of blood pressure and symptoms during clonidine withdrawal, Int J Clin Pharmacol Res 5:215-222, 1985.
18. Caralps JM et al: Results of coronary artery surgery in patients receiving propranolol, J Thorac Cardiovasc Surg 67:526-530, 1974.
19. Chung FC et al: Calcium channel blockade does not offer adequate protection from perioperative myocardial ischemia, Anesthesiology 69:343-347, 1988.
20. Colson P et al: Effect of preoperative renin-angiotensin system blockade on hypertension following coronary surgery, Chest 93(6):1156-1158, 1988.
21. Ebert J et al: Effect of esmolol on the heart and blood pressure response during endotracheal intubation, Anesthesiology 67:A30, 1985.
22. Eerola R et al: Controlled hypotension and moderate haemodilution in major hip surgery, Ann Chir Gynaecol 69:109-113, 1979.
23. The effect of treatment on mortality in mild hypertension. Hypertension Detection and Follow-up Program Cooperative Group, N Engl J Med 307:976-980, 1983.
24. Eltringham RJ: Complications in the recovery room, J Royal Soc Med 72:278-280, 1979.
25. Fiddian-Green RG and Baker S: Predictive value of the stomach wall pH for complications after cardiac operations: comparison with other monitoring, Critical Care Medicine 15(2):153-156, 1987.
26. Flacke JW et al: Reduced narcotic requirement by clonidine with improved hemodynamic and adrenergic stability in patients undergoing coronary bypass surgery, Anesthesiology 67:11-19, 1987.
27. Fouad FM et al: Possible role of cardioaortic reflexes in post coronary bypass hypertension, Am J Cardiol 44:866-872, 1979.
28. Fremes SE et al: Effects of postoperative hypertension and its treatment, J Thorac Cardiovasc Surg 86:47-56, 1983.
29. Gal TJ and Cooperman LH: Hypertension in the immediate postoperative period, Br J Anaesth 47:70-74, 1975.
30. Glaubiger G and Lefkowitz RJ: Elevated B-adrenergic receptor numbers after chronic propranolol treatment, Biochem Biophys Res Commun 78:720-725, 1977.
31. Goldman C and Caldera DL: Risks of general anesthesia and elective operation in the hypertensive patient, Anesthesiology 50:285-292, 1979.
32. Goldman L et al: Cardiac risk factors and complications in non-cardiac surgery, Medicine 57:357-370, 1978.
33. Halter JB, Pflug AE, and Porte D, Jr: Mechanism of plasma catecholamine increases during surgical stress in man, J Clin Endocrinol Metab 45:936-944, 1977.
34. Harper Am et al: The influence of sympathetic nervous activity on cerebral blood flow, Arch Neurol 27:1-6, 1972.
35. Harrison DC and Alderman EL: Discontinuation of propranolol therapy. Cause of rebound angina pectoris and acute coronary events, Chest 69:1-2, 1976.
36. Harrison DG et al: The effect of hypertension and left ventricular hypertrophy on the lower range of coronary autoregulation, Circulation 77(5):1108-1115, 1988.
37. Hirsch I et al: The overstated risk of preoperative hypokalemia, Anesth Analg 67(2):131-136, 1988.
38. Hjalmarson A et al: Effect on mortality of metoprolol in acute myocardial infarction, Lancet 2:823-827, 1981.
39. Hricik DE et al: Captopril-induced functional renal insufficiency in patients with bilateral renal-artery stenoses or renal artery stenosis in a solitary kidney, N Engl J Med 308:373-376, 1983.
40. Hypertension prevalence and the status of awareness, treatment, and control in the United States: Final report of the subcommittee on definition and prevalence of the 1984 joint national committee, Hypertension F:457-468, 1985.
41. Inada E et al: Effect of labetalol on the hemodynamic response to intubation: a controlled randomized double-blind study, Anesthesiology 67:A31, 1987.
42. Kannel WB: Role of blood pressure in cardiovascular morbidity and mortality, Prog Cardiovasc Dis 17:5-25, 1974.
43. Kerr AR: Anaesthesia with profound hypotension for middle ear surgery, Br J Anaesth 49:447-452, 1977.
44. Kirkendall WM, Feinleib M, and Mark AC: American Heart Association recommendations for human blood pressure determination by sphygmomanometer, Circulation 62:1146-1155, 1980.
45. Kraynack BJ, Lawson NW, and Gintautas J: Verapamil reduces indirect muscle twitch amplitude and potentiates pancuronium in vitro, Anesthesiology 57:A265, 1982.
46. Laurito CE et al: Effects of aerosolized and/or intravenous lidocaine on hemodynamic responses to laryngoscopy and intubation in outpatients, Anesth Analg 67:389-392, 1988.
47. Ledingham JGG and Rajagopalan B: Cerebral complications in the treatment of accelerated hypertension, Quart J Med 48:25-41, 1979.

48. Lehv MS, Salzman EW, and Silen W: Hypertension complicating carotid endarterectomy, Stroke 1:307-313, 1970.

49. Leslie JB et al: Ablation of the hemodynamic responses to tracheal intubation with preinduction intravenous labetalol, Anesthesiology 57:A30, 1987.

50. Mahajan RP et al: Intranasal nitroglycerin and intraocular pressure during general anesthesia, Anesth Analg 67:631–636, 1988.

51. Mara JE and Baker JL, Jr: Hypertension and haematomas: prophylaxis with apresoline, Br J Plastic Surg 30(2):169–170, 1977.

52. Maze M and Mason DM: Verapamil decreases the MAC for halothane in dogs, Anesth Analg 62:274, 1983.

53. Miller RD, Way WL, and Eger EI, II: The effects of alpha-methyldopa, reserpine, and guanethidine on minimum alveolar anesthetic requirement (MAC), Anesthesiology 29:1153–1158, 1968.

54. Miller RR et al: Propranolol withdrawal rebound phenomenon-exacerbation of coronary events after abrupt cessation of antianginal therapy, N Engl J Med 293:416–418, 1975.

55. McGuirt WF and May JS: Postoperative hypertension associated with radical neck dissection, Arch Otolaryng Head Neck Surg 113:1098–1100, 1987.

56. McKee PA et al: The natural history of congestive heart failure: the Framingham study, N Engl J Med 284:1441–1447, 1971.

57. O'Hare JP and Hoyt L: Surgery in nephritic and hypertensive patients, N Engl J Med 200:1292–1295, 1929.

58. Prys-Roberts C, Meloache R, and Foex P: Studies of anesthesia in relation to hypertension. 1. Cardiovascular responses of treated and untreated patients, Br J Anaesth 43:122–137, 1971.

59. Prys-Roberts C et al: Hypertension and anesthesia. Fifty years on, Anesthesiology 50:281–284, 1979.

60. Prys-Roberts C et al: Studies of anesthesia in relation to hypertension. V. Adrenergic beta-receptor blockade, Br J Anaesth 45:671–681, 1973.

61. Purves MJ (editor): Physiology of cerebral circulation, Cambridge, Mass, 1972, Cambridge University Press.

62. Reid JL et al: Clonidine withdrawal in hypertension—changes in blood pressure and plasma and urinary noradrenaline, Lancet 1:1171–1174, 1977.

63. Roberts AJ et al: Systemic hypertension associated with coronary artery bypass surgery, J Thorac Cardiovasc Surg 74:846–859, 1977.

64. Ryhanen P et al: Changes during and after anesthesia in treated and untreated hypertensive patients, Ann Chir Gyn 67(5):180–184, 1978.

65. Segal IS et al: Dexmedetomidine diminishes halothane anesthetic requirements in rats through a postsynaptic alpha$_2$ adrenergic receptor, Anesthesiology 69:818–823, 1988.

66. Sprague HB: The heart in surgery. An analysis of the results of surgery on cardiac patients during the past ten years at The Massachusetts General Hospital, Surg Gynecol Obstet 49:54–58, 1929.

67. Stone JG et al: Myocardial ischemia in untreated hypertensive patients: effect of a single small oral dose of a beta-adrenergic blocking agent, Anesthesiology 68:495–500, 1988.

68. Strandgaard S: Autoregulation of cerebral blood flow in hypertensive patients. The modifying influence of prolonged antihypertensive treatment on the tolerance to acute, drug-induced hypertension, Circulation 53:720–727, 1976.

69. Timolol-induced reduction in mortality and reinfarction in patients surviving acute myocardial infarction. The Norwegian Multicenter Study Group, N Engl J Med 304:801–807, 1981.

70. Towne JB and Bernhard VM: The relationship of postoperative hypertension to complications following carotid endarterectomy, Surgery 88(4):575–580, 1980.

71. Vanstrum GS, Bjornson KM, and Ilko R: Postoperative effects of intrathecal morphine in coronary artery bypass surgery, Anesth Analg 67(3):261–267, 1988.

72. Varstrup S et al: Chronic antihypertensive treatment restores normal autoregulation to the cerebral circulation in the rat, Acta Neurol Scand 65(Suppl 90):164–165, 1982.

73. Veterans Administration Cooperative Study Group on Antihypertensive Agents: Effects of treatment on morbidity in hypertension. II. Results in patients with diastolic blood pressure averaging 90 through 114 mm Hg, JAMA 213:1143–1152, 1970.

74. Viljoen JF, Estafanous FG, and Tarazi RC: Acute hypertension immediately after coronary artery surgery, J Thorac Carciovasc Surg 71(4):548–550, 1976.

75. Vital and Health Statistics: Heart disease in adults: United States—1960-62, Series II, No 6, Washington DC, 1964, US Dept of Health, Education and Welfare.

76. Wallach R et al: Pathogenesis of paroxyamal hypertension developing during and after coronary bypass surgery: a study of hemodynamic and humoral facators, Am J Cardiol 46:559–565, 1980.

77. Weber M: Transdermal antihypertensive therapy. Clinical and metabolic considerations, Am Heart J 112:906–912, 1986.

78. Wilber JA and Barrow JG: Reducing elevated blood pressure: experience found in a community, Minn Med 52:1303–1305, 1969.

79. Williams JP et al: Verapamil potentiates the neuromuscular blocking effects of enflurane in vitro, Anesthesiology 59:A276, 1983.

CHAPTER **21**

Diabetes and Other Endocrine Disorders

LUCILLE W. KING
DOUGLAS S. SNYDER

Diabetes mellitus
    Perioperative risk
    Effect of anesthesia and surgery on glucose
        homeostasis
    Perioperative management
Hyperthyroidism
Hypothyroidism
Pheochromocytoma
Adrenal insufficiency

This chapter will discuss perioperative management of patients with endocrine diseases, including diabetes mellitus, hyperthyroidism and hypothyroidism, pheochromocytoma, and adrenal insufficiency. Unlike many diseases, endocrine disorders do not affect one specific organ system but rather have diffuse effects on all organ systems. With the exception of diabetes mellitus, untreated endocrine disorders are infrequently encountered in the operating room; therefore, assessment of perioperative risk for these patients is difficult. End-organ effects of each of several different endocrine disorders are reviewed, with special attention to issues relevant to the perioperative period. Existing literature concerning perioperative risk assessment and management strategies is reviewed, and recommendations for management will be outlined.

DIABETES MELLITUS

Diabetes mellitus is a common, chronic disease. The prevalence of type II diabetes (adult onset) is approximately 1% to 5% in the United States, and type I diabetes (juvenile onset) affects an additional 0.5%. An estimated 200,000 new cases of diabetes are diagnosed each year.[106] Diabetes can lead to significant complications—ones involving the cardiovascular, renal, and nervous systems—which may contribute to surgical morbidity and mortality. In addition, diabetes may adversely affect wound healing and increase susceptibility to infection. This section reviews factors that increase perioperative risk, examines the effects of perioperative stress on glucose homeostasis, and presents guidelines for management of diabetic patients in the perioperative period.

292

Perioperative Risk

Cardiac. In diabetic patients, coronary artery disease (CAD) occurs earlier in life and more frequently, and it may account for more than half of all deaths.[106] A recent study from Finland found that newly diagnosed type II diabetic men were 1.7 times more likely to have had a myocardial infarction than age-matched nondiabetic controls, and diabetic women were 4.4 times more likely. Chest pain and ischemic EKG changes were approximately twice as common among the diabetic patients as among the control patients.[148] Anginal symptoms are often absent and thus are an unreliable index of myocardial ischemia in diabetic patients.[91] Accordingly, all diabetics having surgery should be treated as if they have CAD (see Chapter 12). Diabetic patients can also develop cardiomyopathy and have congestive heart failure in the absence of significant coronary artery disease. Pathologic studies show PAS-positive glycoprotein, fibrosis, and microaneurysms in the myocardium.[46] The cause of this cardiomyopathy is unknown. Preoperative evaluation should specifically seek symptoms suggestive of early congestive heart failure, because this may necessitate an altered management approach.

Renal. Diabetic nephropathy is clinically evident in 50% of diabetics after 20 years of disease,[106] and hypertension is seen in approximately 70% of diabetics.[32] Hyperkalemia in the setting of mild/moderate azotemia may be caused by hyporeninemic hypoaldosteronism[32] or type 4 renal tubular acidosis. There are few data on the perioperative implications of these abnormalities of potassium excretion. Preoperative high or high normal serum potassium levels, however, probably indicate a need for intraoperative and postoperative monitoring of potassium levels, since perioperative increases in catabolism can lead to significant hyperkalemia. Asymptomatic bacteriuria is common in diabetic patients[32] and should be treated before elective surgery. Diabetic patients are at increased risk of developing acute renal failure following the administration of iodinated contrast agents, particularly when the onset of the disease occurs before the age of 40, the creatinine value is greater than 2.0 mg/dl, or there is evidence of other vascular disease.[87] The general recommendation is to keep these patients well hydrated during such procedures, but this is not clearly protective.[87]

Autonomic Nervous System. Diabetic patients frequently develop peripheral and autonomic neuropathy. Autonomic neuropathy involving the gastrointestinal tract may delay gastric emptying, impair esophageal and intestinal motility,[32] and increase the risk for aspiration during intubation. Autonomic neuropathy has also been associated with increased intraoperative swings in blood pressure and heart rate and an increased need for vasopressor therapy.[17] Intraoperative cardiorespiratory arrest has been reported in diabetic patients with autonomic neuropathy during anesthesia for minor procedures.[98] Although the mechanism responsible for cardiorespiratory arrest is not known, these reports suggest that patients with severe autonomic neuropathy may constitute a previously unrecognized high-risk group. Screening for autonomic neuropathy includes checking for postural changes in blood pressure and for vagal nerve abnormalities. The most sensitive index for vagal nerve dysfunction is the loss of beat-to-beat variation in heart rate during deep breathing (Figure 21-1). Vagal neuropathy is often indicative of more widespread abnormalities of the autonomic nervous system.[106]

Infections. Infection in diabetics is an important cause of morbidity and mortality. Infections such as malignant external otitis, rhinocerebral mucormycosis, emphysematous pyleonephritis, papillary necrosis, and emphysematous cholecystitis are almost exclusively seen in diabetics.[157] Diabetics may also be predisposed to gram-negative and staphylococcal pneumonia, gram-negative sepsis and group B streptococcal bacteremia.[157] In one report gram-negative sepsis occurred in 7% of postoperative diabetic patients, compared to an incidence of less than 1% in nondiabetic patients. The most common organism was *Escherichia coli,* and the most common source was the urinary tract.[1] Diabetes is an independent risk factor that increases mortality from Gram-negative bacteremia.[67]

Diabetics seem to have defective mobilization of inflammatory cells and defective phagocytosis and bactericidal activity by polymorphonuclear leukocytes.[94] One retrospective clinical study found a direct correlation between prevalence of infection and the mean plasma glucose level in diabetic patients.[109] These same authors reported less intracellular bactericidal activity by activated leukocytes against *E. coli* and *Staphylococcus aureus,* and lower serum opsonic activity in poorly controlled diabetic patients than in either nondiabetic control subjects or well-controlled diabetic patients. Control of blood glucose

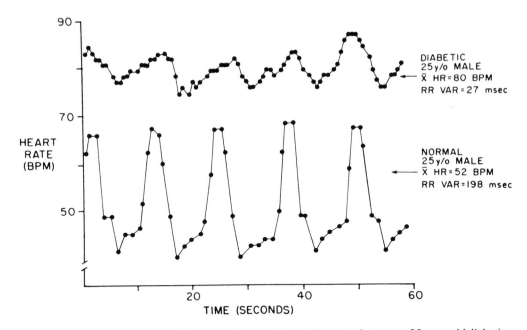

FIGURE 21-1. Comparison of the beat-to-beat variation in heart rate between a 25-year-old diabetic male and an age matched control. The faster rate and reduced variation indicate loss of vagal function in the diabetic male.

From Porter D and Halter JB: Textbook of endocrinology, Philadelphia, 1981, WB Saunders Co.

may, therefore, be important in prevention of infections and for maintenance of host resistance.[109] In support of this recommendation, Nolan et al[94] found that the bactericidal function of granulocytes from diabetics improved with better glycemic control.[94]

The perioperative implication of these abnormalities of white blood count (WBC) function is that diabetics have a greater frequency of surgical wound infections. The large study of Cruse and Foord[23] reported surgical wound infections in 10.7% of diabetics, compared to 1.8% of nondiabetic patients.[23] Although Polk et al[104] suggest that this greater incidence may reflect the presence of additional independent risk factors for infection, such as age and obesity, a recent Italian study, of approximately 1000 subjects who underwent total hip replacement (which excluded aged and obese patients) found the surgical wound infection rate to be 11% in diabetics and 2% in nondiabetic patients.[149]

Wound Healing. Defects in wound healing, including (1) poor collagen formation, (2) poor tensile strength, (3) depressed leukocyte function, (4) diminished capillary ingrowth, and (5) diminished fibroblast proliferation, are described in experimental models of diabetes.[83,156] Administration of insulin, even without restoration of euglycemia, improved all these parameters.[83,156] Whether these abnormalities are associated with clinically important problems in wound healing in diabetic patients is not known.

Miscellaneous. Insulin-dependent diabetics may be at increased risk for postoperative venous thromboembolism. Bergquist et al[8] prospectively studied 83 patients undergoing renal transplantation with plethysmography and thermography on postoperative days 7 and 21. Forty percent of the diabetics developed thrombosis compared with 14% of nondiabetic patients.[8]

Diabetic patients with a history of NPH insulin usage are probably at increased risk for major reactions to protamine, which is used for reversal of systemic heparinization. Hypotension, requiring intravenous catecholamine treatment, occurred in 7 of 651 patients who received protamine after cardiac catheterization. Four of these reactions occurred in the 15 NPH insulin-dependent diabetics. No adverse reactions occurred in diabetic patients who had never taken NPH insulin.[133] Nell and Thomas[90] found protamine antibodies in 122 (38%) of 319 NPH insulin-treated diabetics, whereas only 8% of diabetics treated with protamine-free lente insulin and 2.5% of controls had such antibodies.[90] These patients are theoretically at increased risk for anaphylactoid reactions to protamine. However, a recent prospective study[72] found only a 2% incidence (1 of 50 patients) of clinical reactions to protamine in NPH insulin–dependent diabetic patients.[72]

Effect of Anesthesia and Surgery on Glucose Homeostasis

Stress-induced hyperglycemia occurs in nondiabetic patients during burns, sepsis, trauma, and myocardial infarction.[106] Surgery inflicts a similar stress and also frequently results in hyperglycemia. In one study of 12 nondiabetic patients undergoing gastrectomy, blood glucose rose from an average of 80 mg/dl to 145 mg/dl[145]; in another study of patients having elective abdominal surgery, the blood glucose levels of nondiabetic patients rose from approximately 135 mg/dl preoperatively to about 270 mg/dl. In this latter study, the blood glucose levels of the diabetic patients rose from approximately 200 mg/dl to 350 mg/dl during laparotomy.[38] The mechanisms responsible for elevations in blood glucose during stress have been extensively studied and are reviewed next.

The major hormone that acts to reduce blood glucose levels is insulin. Counterregulatory hormones, including glucagon, epinephrine, norepinephrine, cortisol, and growth hormone, raise blood glucose levels by decreasing peripheral glucose utilization and by increasing proteolysis, lipolysis, gluconeogenesis, and glycogenolysis.[106] During surgical stress, these counterregulatory hormones rise. Goldberg et al[38] demonstrated that glucagon rises from approximately 150 pg/ml to approximately 300 pg/ml by 5 hours following elective abdominal surgery; growth hormone peaks at >30 ng/ml by 45 minutes intraoperatively from a baseline of 3 ng/ml; and cortisol rises to about 30 μg/dl from a baseline of 10 μg/dl.[38] The hormonal responses of both diabetic

and control patients were similar.[38] Norepinephrine and epinephrine levels increase fourfold to sixfold intraoperatively.[91] Epinephrine levels returned to normal within 6 to 12 hours after surgery, but norepinephrine levels remain elevated for several days.[22,116]

Eigler et al,[28] in a series of studies in conscious dogs, elucidated how these counterregulatory hormones interract to produce hyperglycemia. Glucose metabolism was studied during separate and combined infusions of glucagon, epinephrine, and cortisol at rates sufficient to achieve plasma levels comparable to those observed in severe physiologic stress. Glucagon increased glucose production by 65% but also increased glucose clearance and resulted in only minimal increases in blood glucose. Epinephrine increased glucose production only slightly but decreased glucose clearance, and blood glucose increased 33%. Infusion of glucagon and epinephrine together produced an exaggerated glycemic response because of increased glucose production and decreased glucose clearance. Cortisol alone had no effect on glucose production. However, simultaneous infusion of all three hormones produced a glycemic response four times greater than the sum of the responses to the individual hormones. Thus the effect of glucagon and epinephrine on glucose production was sustained and amplified by cortisol, whereas epinephrine decreased glucose clearance by inhibiting insulin secretion.[28,31]

Shamoon et al[123] performed similar studies in healthy human subjects. When all three hormones were infused simultaneously, the magnitude of the increase in plasma glucose was three times the sum of the increases observed with the individual hormones. Epinephrine inhibited glucose clearance despite a onefold to twofold increase in insulin levels (see Figure 21-2).[123] It is important to note that stress hyperglycemia does not require a preexisting abnormality in insulin secretion.[31] When insulin deficiency is present, stressful stimuli may result in hyperketonemia, as well as in hyperglycemia.[13]

Stress hyperglycemia during surgery is not seen when regional anesthesia is used. Presumably this is because neural afferents from the site of tissue injury are blocked, and increases in plasma, norepinephrine, epinephrine, growth hormone, and cortisol do not occur.[29,44,101] Postoperatively, however, when regional analgesia wears off, pain-induced in-

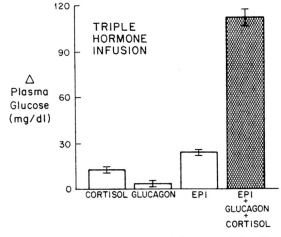

FIGURE 21-2. Demonstration of the synergistic effect on blood glucose levels in human subjects when cortisol, epinephrine, and glucagon are infused *simultaneously,* as compared to the effect of *single hormone infusions* when these hormones are infused separately.

From Shamoon H et al: Synergistic interactions among antiinsulin hormones in the pathogenesis of stress hyperglycemia in humans. J Clin Endocrinol Metab 52:1235-1241, 1981.

creases in stress hormones and glucose levels may occur. Whether late rises in blood glucose might be prevented or attentuated by aggressive regimens for postoperative analgesia, such as peridural opiate administration, is not known.

Perioperative Management

While intraoperative hypoglycemia and its potential for serious neurologic consequences must be avoided, there is evidence that hyperglycemia can also have an adverse impact in the perioperative period and that aggressive control of blood sugar is indicated. Hyperglycemia can impair in vivo leukocyte function, impair wound healing, and contribute to the increased incidence of wound infections in diabetics. Uncontrolled diabetes can also lead to electrolyte disturbances, osmotic diuresis, and ketoacidosis. Experimental studies suggest that hyperglycemia sensitizes cerebral tissues to ischemic injury.[125]

Although many regimens have been proposed to achieve glycemic control in the perioperative period in insulin-dependent diabetic patients, few studies compare the effectiveness of different protocols. The most commonly used regimen administers one half to two thirds of the daily insulin dose as NPH insulin preoperatively and gives dextrose solutions intraoperatively.[105] While simple to employ, this protocol does not prevent intraoperative hyperglycemia.

In a study by Walt et al,[154] 5% of patients receiving preoperative insulin therapy developed significant hyperglycemia ($>$400 mg/dl) and this incidence was not different from that observed in patients receiving no preoperative insulin and no intraoperative dextrose. Of note, 3 of 58 patients receiving preoperative insulin in this study developed hypoglycemia despite intraoperative glucose infusion.[154] Failure of preoperative insulin to prevent hyperglycemia was also reported by Goldberg et al.[38] Patients having abdominal surgery had mean serum glucose levels of 390 $\pm$ 80 mg/dl 3 hours after skin incision. Similarly, mean blood glucose levels exceeded 300 mg/dl in a study by Taitelman et al,[141] and 2 of 13 patients required additional insulin because of markedly increased blood glucose levels.[38] Hypoglycemia was not observed in either of these latter two studies.[38,154]

It should not be surprising that a simple, fixed regimen of preoperative insulin is not uniformly effective. The magnitude and duration of the stress response varies with the type of surgical procedure and the nature of the anesthetic. Regional anesthetic techniques can significantly attenuate intraoperative rises in stress hormones,[29,44,101] and high-dose narcotic techniques can also blunt the stress response.[35] Thus the degree and duration of perioperative hyperglycemia will vary considerably from patient to patient. This variability is likely also to be influenced by the adequacy of preoperative glycemic control.

In an effort to achieve adequate glycemic control during the perioperative period, investigators have studied the effectiveness of intraoperative insulin administration by continuous infusion or by intermittent intravenous boluses. Walts et al[154] measured hourly glucose levels in patients who received neither insulin nor glucose preoperatively, but who received glucose infusion at a rate of 6.25 g/hr intraoperatively. Patients were given intravenous bolus injections of regular insulin (10 units) every 2 hours during surgery if blood glucose values exceeded 200 mg/dl. No patient had a rise in plasma glucose, but hypoglycemia occurred in 2 of the 33 patients studied.[154]

Myers et al[85] reported another example of insulin

titration. Regular insulin was given intravenously before induction of anesthesia and then at hourly intervals during surgery according to a protocol based on blood glucose determinations. At the end of surgery blood glucose in these patients (194.9 ± 42 mg/dl) was significantly lower than in patients given standard preoperative insulin and supplemental subcutaneous insulin every 2 hours by sliding scale (360 ± 104) mg/dl. Hypoglycemia did not occur with this regimen.[85]

There are relatively few reports on the use of continuous insulin infusions intraoperatively. Taitelman et al[141] reported that 2 of 6 patients receiving a continuous insulin infusion at 2 units per hour required alterations of insulin and dextrose infusion rates to avoid hypoglycemia.[141] In another study, Goldberg et al[38] found that continuous intraoperative insulin infusion (1 unit per hour) resulted in lower plasma glucose levels compared to conventional preoperative insulin therapy, but the differences were not statistically significant.[38] There was no hypoglycemia. These two studies suggest that continuous insulin regimens offer potentially superior glycemic control but they require monitoring blood glucose levels and altering the infusion rate as needed.

Finally, a technique using simultaneous infusion of insulin (3.2 units/hr), glucose (10% dextrose, 10 g/hr), and potassium (10 mEq/500 ml 10% dextrose) has been proposed. Combined use of glucose and insulin has been advocated to reduce the risk of hypoglycemia or hyperglycemia during alterations in infusion rate. Although these authors report good glycemic control,[143] a study from another institution failed to confirm this.[12] Furthermore, this regimen appears to be quite cumbersome, since the entire infusate must be changed to alter the insulin-to-glucose ratio.

In summary, intraoperative insulin administration appears to result in superior glycemic control. This approach, however, requires rapid and accurate determinations of blood glucose levels and the ability to accurately titrate insulin, since alterations in infusion rate will likely be necessary. Whether the additional expense and time commitment of this approach is truly justified remains to be determined. Although there are few data to indicate that perioperative hyperglycemia adversely affects outcome, hyperglycemia can complicate fluid and electrolyte management, lead to ketoacidosis or hyperosmolar coma, and may adversely affect wound healing. The use of regional anesthetic techniques may be an attractive alternative, since stress-induced hyperglycemia is significantly reduced with conduction blockade. Despite the widespread use of preoperative intermediate insulin regimens, these techniques do not result in optimal glycemic control and are not without risk for producing hypoglycemia.

Routine use of intraoperative insulin and glucose is probably unnecessary in the diet-controlled diabetic patient. Oral hypoglycemic medications should be withheld on the day of surgery, except for chlorpropamide, which should be discontinued on the day before surgery because of its long half-life. Blood glucose levels should be checked frequently in the postoperative period and treated with regular insulin for values greater than 250 mg/dl according to a sliding scale. Human or purified pork insulin preparations are recommended to minimize antibody production and the potential development of insulin resistance or allergy, should insulin be required in the future.[87]

Perioperative management of the diabetic patient requires careful evaluation of end-organ dysfunction and recognition of risks associated with these abnormalities. Neuroendocrine responses to surgical trauma require management strategies to minimize hyperglycemia and to avoid hypoglycemia.

HYPERTHYROIDISM

Perioperative recognition of hyperthyroidism is the key to successful management of this complex physiologic and biochemical abnormality. The condition is characterized by increased production of triiodothyronine and/or tetraiodothyronine, and patients typically are initially seen between the ages of 20 and 40 years. Hyperthyroidism occurs more frequently in females and the most common cause is Graves' disease (diffuse toxic goiter).[34,131] Although palpable abnormalities of the thyroid gland may suggest the possibility of hyperthyroidism,[40,152] diagnosis is based on signs and symptoms with confirmation by laboratory testing.

Signs and symptoms reflect the systemic effects of excessive thyroid hormone, which increases the rate of biochemical reactions, total body oxygen consumption, and heat production. These changes result in clinical manifestations including sweating, vasodilation, and tachycardia. Nevertheless, subtle manifestations such as weight loss, listlessness, apathy, or psychiatric abnormalities mandate a high index of suspicion, especially in the elderly. Serum T4 should be interpreted with a T3 resin uptake to correct for changes in binding proteins; a serum T3 level may be the best confirmatory laboratory test.[40]

Hyperthyroidism increases cardiac output and heart rate and may cause arrhythmias. Cardiac output is increased in excess of metabolic requirements, and this effect may be partially mediated by vasodilation of skin and muscle.[131] Similar hyperdynamic circulatory changes are common with sympathetic nervous system hyperactivity, but thyroid hormones alone appear to mediate these effects in hyperthyroidism. Although the number of beta-adrenergic receptors is increased by persistently elevated levels of thyroid hormone, serum catecholamines are not increased and the cardiovascular responsiveness to catecholamines is not altered in hyperthyroidism.[60,82]

Animal studies suggest that hyperthyroidism predisposes to perioperative hepatotoxicity. When rats were pretreated with T3 and anesthetized with either 1.8% enflurane or 1% halothane in 21% oxygen, 24% of the animals in the enflurane group and 92% of the animals in the halothane group developed centrilobular hepatic necrosis. The authors speculated that decreased splanchnic blood flow during anesthesia resulted in relative ischemia to the hypermetabolic hepatocytes.[9,160] Although hyperthyroid patients have been found to have a higher incidence of elevation in LDH levels, they do not appear to have an increased incidence of postoperative hepatic dysfunction.[121] Of interest, the antithyroid drug propylthiouricil may be hepatotoxic, and methimazole may cause cholestatic jaundice. Glycogen synthesis is reduced in hyperthyroidism, and decreased glycogen content may predispose to hepatic pathologic factors. Although further prospective studies are needed to clarify this issue, hyperthyroid patients do not appear to have an increased risk of postoperative hepatic dysfunction.

Preoperative examination should include careful evaluation of the airway for tracheal compression or deviation by a large goiter, which may make intubation difficult. Preoperative x-ray examination may help reveal abnormal neck anatomy and retrosternal extension of the thyroid gland. Mirror laryngoscopy is useful to assess vocal cord movement.[84] Hyperthyroidism has no known direct pulmonary effects, but respiratory insufficiency may develop in compromised individuals, since increased metabolism increases carbon dioxide production. Table 21-1 summarizes end-organ effects of hyperthyroidism.

Theoretic considerations suggest that preoperative and intraoperative drugs that accentuate the signs of hyperthyroidism should be avoided. Atropine, for example, may prevent sweating, and both cyclopropane and ether increase serum catecholamines and should be avoided.[96] Drugs that undergo extensive biotransformation into toxic substances such as methoxyflurane should also be avoided.[131] Increased intraoperative blood loss has been reported in hyperthyroid surgical patients. Special attention to eye care intraoperatively is important to prevent corneal ulceration, since 5% of hyperthyroid patients have proptosis.

Many recommendations for preoperative preparation of hyperthyroid patients have been made. Propylthiouracil (PTU), iodine, hydrocortisone, and beta-adrenergic blockers decrease thyroid hormone levels or block peripheral effects. One hundred to 300 mg of PTU orally every 8 hours blocks oxidation, organification, and coupling of thyroid hormone and also blocks peripheral conversion of T4 to T3. PTU will generally produce clinical improvement in 1 to 2 weeks and a euthyroid state in 6 to 7 weeks.[129] After PTU is started, potassium iodide (5 drops orally three times daily) can be added to block thyroid hormone release and inhibit organification. Sodium iodide (1 g intravenously every 8 to 12 hours) can be substituted for saturated solution of potassium iodide (SSKI). Hydrocortisone (100 mg intravenously every 8 hours) decreases T4 and extrathyroidal T3 production and protects against potential decreased adrenal reserve. Propranolol administered orally or intravenously can be titrated using the heart rate as the end point.[40,131] Beta-adrenergic blockade is hazardous in congestive heart failure,

TABLE 21-1. End-organ effects of hyperthyroidism

Metabolic rate	Increased
Cardiovascular function	Hyperdynamic, increased cardiac output, dysrhythmias, cardiac insufficiency
Respiratory function	Increased CO_2 production reflecting hypercatabolism
Renal function	Presumably unimpaired
CNS function	Apathy, emotional lability

but cardiac function may improve in the profoundly tachycardic patient if heart rate is slowed.[50] Occasionally, therapy needs to be guided by determinations of cardiac output. Esmolol, a newer beta-adrenergic blocker, may be ideal in this situation because it has a very short half-life and can be titrated by continuous intravenous infusion. Reserpine or guanethidine may be substituted if beta blockade is not tolerated.

The most dangerous complication of hyperthyroidism in surgical patients is thyroid storm, which usually develops within 6 to 18 hours postoperatively and lasts for several days.[131,153] Before antithyroid and adrenergic-blocking drugs were used to prepare these patients for thyroidectomy, storm occurred in 10% to 32% of hyperthyroid patients and had a high mortality.[40,80,153] Treatment of thyroid storm with iodine alone had a mortality rate of 60% to 70%, but when steroids and beta-adrenergic blocking agents were added, mortality was reduced to 25% of patients.[54,131,153] Propranolol alone does not reliably prevent thyroid storm.[30] If thyroid storm is triggered in the perioperative time, rapid recognition and treatment is required. Manifestations include hyperpyrexia, tachycardia, and severe hypotension, but these features do not distinguish storm from malignant hyperthermia (MH). CPK levels are typically decreased in thyrotoxicosis and increased in MH.[92] It is critical to make a correct diagnosis, because specific life-saving therapy differs for each disease. In addition to decreasing thyroid hormone levels and blocking their systemic effects, supportive strategies in storm include fluid therapy, oxygen, and mechanical cooling devices. Aspirin should be avoided because it displaces T4 from binding proteins and may increase metabolic rate.[40]

HYPOTHYROIDISM

Documented hypothyroidism occurs in 0.5% to 0.8% of the adult population, but undiagnosed or untreated disease probably occurs more frequently. Untoward events associated with anesthesia and surgery in these patients include hypotension, cardiac arrest, and increased sensitivity to drugs, with prolonged unconsciousness and coma.* This section reviews the perioperative problems associated with hy-

pothyroidism and presents management strategies that may reduce morbidity and mortality.

Hypothyroidism is an insidious disease, and diagnosis requires a high index of suspicion. Forty percent to 50% of cases are caused by previous thyroid resection or radioactive iodine treatment, and many patients with hypothyroidism are inadequately treated.[88] Symptoms include lethargy, intolerance to cold, hoarseness, constipation, dry skin, impairment of memory, and apathy. Examination may reveal hoarseness, periorbital edema, lateral thinning of the eyebrows, brittle hair, dry skin, goiter, hypothermia, bradycardia, and prolongation of the relaxation phase of deep tendon reflexes.[88,135] The physical findings that are statistically predictive of hypothyroidism are deep tendon reflex changes, husky voice, and dry skin.[55] Cardiomegaly, pleural effusion, ascites, and peripheral edema may mimic congestive heart failure. The constellation of decreased consciousness, spontaneous hypothermia, hypoventilation, and congestive heart failure suggests the presence of myxedema coma.

Diagnosis of signs and symptoms must be confirmed by appropriate laboratory testing. Primary hypothyroidism may be divided into subclinical, mild, or overt categories. In subclinical hypothyroidism the patient is asymptomatic with normal T4 levels and a mildly elevated thyroid-stimulating hormone (TSH) level. In mild hypothyroidism, the patient may have nonspecific symptoms such as hair loss and constipation, with a low T4 level and an elevated TSH level. Overt hypothyroidism is characterized by obvious clinical manifestations, with profoundly reduced T4 levels, and a metabolic rate only 55% to 60% of normal.[88]

Myocardial depression may be associated with the hypothyroid state. Although low circulating concentrations of thyroid hormone have been associated with reversible conversion of beta-adrenergic to alpha-adrenergic receptors, there is no direct evidence for reduced cardiac responsiveness to exogenous catecholamines.[25] Myxedematous infiltration of the myocardium, alterations in sarcoplasmic reticulum function, and reduced myosin ATPase activity contribute to decreased contractility.[137] Cardiac output is reduced because of decreased heart rate and stroke volume.[52] Systolic time intervals correlate directly with the clinical severity of hypothyroidism. In overt hypothyroidism, for example, left ventricular ejection time is shortened and the preejection

*References 1, 21, 49, 66, 95, 122.

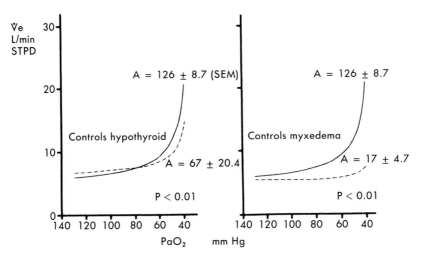

FIGURE 21-3. Hypoxic ventilatory drive was moderately depressed in the hypothyroid group but markedly depressed in the myxedema group.

From Zwillich CW et al: Ventilatory control and myxedema and hyperthyroidism, NEJM 292:662-665, 1975.

period is increased.[11] Despite these abnormalities, hypothyroidism is rarely responsible for overt heart failure, and the presence of congestive failure suggests underlying heart disease.[52,88] However, negative inotropic agents such as potent inhalation anesthetics may seriously impair myocardial function in hypothyroid patients.

In addition to direct effects on myocardial function, 60% of patients with overt hypothyroidism develop protein- and mucin-rich pericardial effusions. However, tamponade is rare because of the gradual rate of fluid accumulation. EKG changes in hypothyroidism include sinus bradycardia, flattening or inversion of T waves in lead II, and low amplitude P, QRS, and T waves. Careful preoperative assessment of cardiovascular function and reserve is required in hypothyroid patients.[88]

Pulmonary complications are common in hypothyroidism, but controversy exists regarding the mechanisms involved. Maximum breathing capacity and diffusing capacity are reduced in overt hypothyroidism, and both parameters improve with return to a euthyroid state.[158] Hypoxic and hypercapneic ventilatory drives are markedly reduced (Figures 21-3 and 21-4), but this response does not appear to result from mechanical ventilatory dysfunction, since spirometric measurements are only minimally

reduced in myxedematous patients and are usually normal in mildly hypothyroid patients.[160] Respiratory failure associated with myxedema is usually associated with obesity, unrelated intrinsic lung disease, or coma.[70,160]

A variety of other abnormalities in hypothyroidism have important perioperative consequences. Hypothyroid patients are exquisitely sensitive to drugs that depend on metabolic transformation for their elimination, such as narcotics. Free water clearance is impaired and patients may develop hyponatremia. Adynamic ileus, megacolon, and delayed gastric emptying are associated with severe hypothyroidism. Hypothyroid patients are also prone to develop hypoglycemia, anemia, and hypothermia.[2,88] In addition, concomitant adrenal insufficiency occurs in some hypothyroid patients, which could potentially result in perioperative cardiovascular instability. See Table 21-2 for a listing of systemic effects of hypothyroidism.

Replacement of thyroid hormone is usually accomplished slowly. Although plasma levels of T3, T4, and TSH can be corrected fairly quickly, reversal of organ-specific abnormalities may be surprisingly slow. Normal T3 levels do not ensure reversal of thyroid myopathy. Abnormal muscle biopsies have been noted for 7 to 15 months following initiation

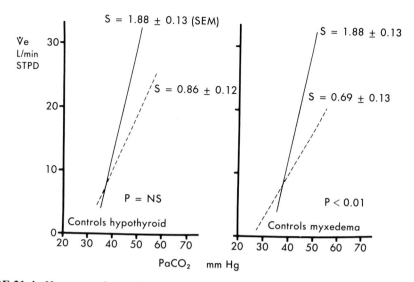

FIGURE 21-4. Hypercapneic ventilatory drive was depressed in both hypothyroid and myxedema groups, but the latter to a significant degree.

From Zwillich CW et al: Ventilatory control and myxedema and hyperthyroidism NEJM 292:662-665, 1975.

TABLE 21-2. End-organ effects of hypothyroidism

Metabolic rate	Reduced; 55% to 60% of normal in overt hypothyroidism
Cardiovascular function	Reduced; ↓ LVET, ↑ preejection period, ↓ cardiac output (↓ HR, ↓ SV, ↑ PVR), probable baroreceptor dysfunction
Respiratory function	Impaired hypoxic ventilatory drive
	Impaired hypercapneic ventilatory drive
	Impaired diffusing capacity for CO
Renal function	Impaired free water clearance ↓ GFR, CrCl, tubular transport
CNS function	Depressed (myxedema coma, end-stage)

of replacement therapy. Recovery of hypoxic ventilatory drive is variable and depends on the severity of the initial disease process. In one study[159], mildly hypothyroid patients demonstrated normal responsiveness to hypoxia in 3 weeks, whereas myxedematous patients required 3 to 6 months for recovery (Figure 21-5). Hypercapneic ventilatory response

did not improve with hormonal replacement.[70,160]

When administered intravenously, a single bolus of T4 produces peak increases in basal metabolic rate in 10 to 12 days. In contrast, an intravenous bolus of T3 increases basal metabolic rate much more quickly (36 to 72 hours), and some investigators have reported a maximal effect as early as 6 hours.[88,135] Bolus doses of T3 can exceed tissue storage capacities and transiently elevate plasma levels sufficiently to cause cardiovascular complications including angina, arrhythmias, and sudden death.[2] If thyroid hormone must be given intravenously, as for myxedema, it is recommended that it be given as T4.

Establishing a euthyroid state in patients before elective anesthesia and surgery is generally recommended to avoid postoperative central nervous system depression, to promote wound healing, and to facilitate recovery. A notable exception to this recommendation is the hypothyroid patient with symptomatic coronary artery disease. Hay et al[47] reported no perioperative morbidity or mortality in untreated hypothyroid patients undergoing coronary bypass surgery, whereas four of nine patients who received thyroid replacement before surgery suffered preoperative myocardial infarctions. A later study of seven patients with incapacitating angina and severe hy-

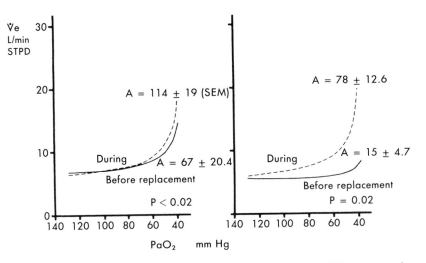

FIGURE 21-5. Hypoxia ventilatory drive increased significantly with thyroid hormone replacement in both hypothyroid *(left)* and myxedema *(right)* groups.

From Zwillich CW et al: Ventilatory control and myxedema and hyperthyroidism NEJM 292:662-665, 1975.

pothyroidism noted uneventful perioperative courses when limited thyroid replacement was administered before coronary revascularization and full replacement followed surgery.[99] In a review of 50 patients with coexisting hypothyroidism and coronary artery disease, Levine et al[69] concluded that judicious use of propranolol and thyroid hormone frequently failed to control either ischemic symptoms or hypothyroidism and suggested that coronary bypass grafting should assume a dominant role in management.

Careful intraoperative management of the hypothyroid patient should result in a safe and uneventful course. The dosages of sedative and narcotic drugs may be titrated to desired clinical effects when the patient is awake to minimize prolonged postoperative somnolence. Supplemental corticosteroids should be considered, if adequate adrenal reserve has not been demonstrated preoperatively. Preoperative neutralization of gastric acid with H_2 antagonists or use of agents that increase gastric emptying may reduce the risks associated with pulmonary aspiration of acidic gastric contents. Slow induction of anesthesia with cricoid pressure may be safer than a rapid-sequence induction, because the former technique simultaneously minimizes the possibility of abrupt hypotension and provides airway protection.

An awake intubation may be indicated in severe overt hypothyroidism. Care must be taken to avoid inadvertent hypocarbia during controlled ventilation, since CO_2 production is reduced at low metabolic rates.

Following induction, a variety of agents can be employed to maintain anesthesia. Despite the general clinical impression that anesthetic requirements are reduced, hypothyroidism does not appear to reduce the dose of volatile drugs necessary to prevent skeletal muscle responses to noxious stimuli. However, volatile agents in usual doses may cause excessive hypotension as a result of associated underlying myocardial depression, attenuated baroreceptor function, and hypovolemia. Careful observation of hemodynamic parameters and early recognition of congestive heart failure are essential throughout the operative course.

Hypothermia is a common problem in normal patients during anesthesia and surgery, and defective thermogenic mechanisms increase the susceptibility to hypothermia in hypothyroidism.[66] Since increased mortality has been associated with hypothermia in hypothyroid patients,[33] body temperature must be continually monitored and every effort made to prevent loss of body heat intraoperatively.

Several studies have evaluated the perioperative outcome of hypothyroid patients. In a retrospective report[71], hypothyroid patients had a higher prevalence of preoperative risk factors such as hypertension and anemia, but did not differ from control patients with regard to intraoperative temperature, blood pressure, need for vasopressors, time to extubation, fluid requirements, electrolyte imbalances, or incidence of arrhythmias. Postoperatively, the incidence of pulmonary complications, myocardial infarction, sepsis, need for prolonged ventilatory assistance, and the length of time to hospital discharge were also similar to that of control patients. Despite reports of decreased platelet adhesiveness and low levels of clotting factors, bleeding problems were not encountered. The authors concluded that it is safe to proceed with surgery in mild-to-moderate hypothyroidism, but they could not address the advisability of operation in severe disease because of the limited number of such patients in their study.[155] In contrast, a prospective analysis of perioperative outcome reported an increased incidence of intraoperative hypotension and heart failure in hypothyroid patients. Postoperatively, hypothyroid patients had a higher incidence of gastrointestinal and neuropsychiatric problems and had a lower incidence of fever, despite comparable rates of infection. Hypothyroid patients were similar to control subjects when analyzed for perioperative blood loss, duration of hospitalization, anesthetic recovery time, wound healing, pulmonary complications, and death.[69]

In summary, hypothyroid patients are probably more sensitive than are normal individuals to the adverse effects of anesthetic agents. Careful management of patients with mild-to-moderate hypothyroidism should result in a good outcome, should preoperative replacement therapy not be possible or advisable. Inadequate data exist concerning outcome in severely hypothyroid patients. These patients should be considered to be at high risk, and only truly emergent procedures should be performed before correction of thyroid hormone status.

PHEOCHROMOCYTOMA

Pheochromocytomas are catecholamine-secreting tumors that arise in the adrenal medulla or along the paravertebral sympathetic chain from the pelvis to the base of the skull.[37] These tumors occur in 0.1% of all hypertensives,[126] and mainly release norepinephrine.[23a] Pheochromocytomas are usually diagnosed in patients between the ages of 30 and 50 years, 10% are bilateral, and 10% to 30% are malignant, some with catecholamine-secreting metastases.[53,135]

Preoperative diagnosis and management of pheochromocytomas are important to avoid increased perioperative mortality. Reports from the 1960s cited perioperative mortality rates of 50% in undiagnosed patients and 26% mortality when the diagnosis was established preoperatively.[39,132] Recent studies, however, report much lower mortality figures (4% in patients who were not treated preoperatively with alpha-adrenergic blocking agents) and attribute the improved outcome to better anesthetic management.[26,120] Careful preoperative preparation is strongly recommended to minimize intraoperative hemodynamic disturbances and their sequelae. In addition, patients with chronically elevated levels of circulating catecholamines develop systemic abnormalities, such as cardiomyopathy and hypertension, that also require special perioperative management.

A high index of suspicion is necessary to make a diagnosis of pheochromocytoma. These tumors occur independently, in association with other functional endocrine tumors (multiple endocrine neoplasia syndromes types II and III), and in patients with neurocutaneous syndromes such as Von Recklinghausen's disease and Von Hippel–Lindau disease.[126] Clinical presentation is quite variable; symptoms are influenced by the type of catecholamine secreted. Approximately 50% of patients develop persistent hypertension with intermittent exacerbations. Other symptoms include headache, palpitations, diaphoresis, nausea, vomiting, weight loss, tremulousness, visual disturbances, and personality changes such as anxiety and psychosis. Orthostatic hypotension is also common and probably reflects reduced intravascular volume. If beta-adrenergic effects predominate, tachyarrhythmias occur at normal or reduced arterial blood pressure. Symptoms may last for minutes to hours, are episodic or sustained, and are often provoked by activity.[53] End-organ effects of pheochromocytoma are presented in Table 21-3.

Diagnosis is made by biochemical confirmation of excess catecholamine production. The most commonly used tests, which are relatively easy to perform and readily available, involve measurement of urinary catecholamines or their metabolites, vanillyc mandelic acid and total metanephrines. Urinary metanephrines probably are more reliable than either

TABLE 21-3. End-organ effects of pheochromocytoma

Metabolic rate	Reflects catecholamine effects
Cardiovascular function	Reflects catecholamine effects; tachy-dysrythmias; orthostatic hypotension reflecting intravascular volume depletion, cardiac insufficiency
Respiratory system	Unimpaired
Renal function	Possibly impaired secondary to hypertension
CNS function	Emotional lability, somnolence postoperatively

urinary vanillyc mandelic acid or free catecholamines.[16] Determination of plasma catecholamines may be more reliable in detecting the presence of pheochromocytoma, but the exact role in diagnosis is subject to debate. Plasma catecholamine levels of 1000 pg/ml or less during periods of hypertension exclude the diagnosis. Levels of 1000 or 2000 pg/ml are equivocal, and levels greater than 2000 pg/ml are diagnostic.[14] Provocative and suppression tests are available to evaluate catecholamine levels in the equivocal range, but these tests may be of questionable value because of concerns for reliability and patient safety.[15,43,53]

Perioperative Management

Definitive end points for optimal preoperative preparation of patients with pheochromocytoma remain elusive. Roizen et al[115] proposed the following criteria to define adequate therapy: (1) arterial blood pressure not greater than 164/90 on more than two measurements over a 48-hour period, (2) orthostatic hypotension present, but blood pressure greater than 80/45, (3) ECG free from ST-segment and T-wave changes for a minimum of 2 weeks, and (4) no more than one premature ventricular contraction every 5 minutes. To achieve these or other similar goals, a variety of alpha- and beta-adrenergic blocking agents have been used.

Alpha-adrenergic blocking agents treat arterial hypertension, as well as counteract venoconstrictive effects of high circulating catecholamines. The nonselective alpha blocker, phenoxybenzamine, is most commonly used because of its long half-life (>24 hours). The usual initial dose of 20 to 40 mg per day by mouth is subsequently increased by 10 to 20 mg per day until both symptoms and blood pressure are controlled. These effects require 10 to 14 days at an average dose of 60 to 250 mg per day.[27] Prazosin, a selective alpha I blocker, may offer a potential advantage over phenoxybenzamine because it does not interfere with presynaptic adrenergic receptor-mediated inhibition of norepinephrine release[53] but has the disadvantage of a shorter half-life.[151] Beta blockers are commonly added to the regimen to control tachycardia and dysrhythmias.[59] Beta blockade without preestablished alpha blockade can precipitate severe pressor effects as a result of prevention of beta-mediated vasodilation. The need for beta blockers is somewhat dependent on the type of catecholamine secreted, and epinephrine-secreting tumors are more likely to require such therapy. The usual required dose of propranolol is 80 to 120 mg/day, but some patients with epinephrine-secreting tumors may require up to 480 mg/day. An alternative approach used in some centers is to pretreat patients with alpha-methyltyrosine to inhibit tyrosine hydroxylase conversion of tyrosine to dihydroxyphenylalanine (DOPA) and thus limit the rate of catecholamine production. Use of this agent is preferable in patients who either prove refractory to standard therapies or in whom beta blockade is contraindicated.

A number of studies have attempted to evaluate the utility of preoperative pharmacologic preparation of patients with pheochromocytoma. Comparison of 51 pretreated patients (phenoxybenzamine at an average dose of 160 mg/day; eight patients also received beta blockers) with 11 untreated historic controls showed a reduced incidence of "excessive blood-pressure variations." However, alpha blockade was frequently incomplete, since 69% of patients had systolic pressures greater than 175 mm Hg during surgery. Beta blockade did not reduce the incidence of arrhythmias.[132] A series of 4 patients pretreated with prazosin (one patient also received labetalol) found that three of four patients required additional vasodilators during tumor manipulation. No patient had excessive tachycardia or arrhythmias, perhaps because of blockade of postsynaptic myocardial alpha I adrenergic receptors.[27] Consistent with this, prazosin has been shown to be more effective than L-metoprolol, a selective beta I blocking agent, in decreasing the arrhythmogenic dose of epinephrine in halothane-anesthetized dogs.[77] One theoretical and often cited disadvantage of adrenergic blockade is that it may make tumor localization more difficult by masking hemodynamic changes associated with manipulation at surgery. However, blood pressure variations with tumor palpation appear to be similar in pretreated and untreated patients,[26] most likely because these transient large increases in agonist concentration successfully compete for receptor occupancy and activation.

Alpha and beta blockers should be continued up to and including the day of surgery. Regional anesthesia has been used successfully for both pheochromocytoma resection and other surgical procedures in patients with pheochromocytoma.[58] Although it has been hypothesized that sympathetic blockade from spinal or epidural techniques may enhance adrenergic receptor sensitivity to circulating catecholamines or predispose to hypotension on withdrawal of catecholamines following resection, there are few data to support these contentions.[53] General anesthesia is the most commonly used technique and has been successfully administered with a variety of anesthetic agents. Halothane, enflurane, and isoflurane all cause a dose-dependent decrease in circulating catecholamine concentrations, but halothane lowers the threshold of the heart to the arrhythmogenic effects of circulating epinephrine[57]. The dose of epinephrine (submucosal) required to produce PVCs in 50% of normal patients anesthetized with either halothane, enflurane, or isoflurane was 2.1, 10.9, and 6.7 μg/kg, respectively; these findings suggest that arrhythmias may be more common in patients with pheochromocytoma who are anesthetized with halothane, and this agent should probably not be used. Droperidol has been proposed as a worthwhile addition to the anesthetic regimen in patients with pheochromocytoma. However, it can have both beneficial and adverse effects. Droperidol antagonizes the pressor effects of catecholamines and decreases the incidence of arrhythmias.[138] It interferes with reuptake of norepinephrine by postganglionic sympathetic nerve endings and can also directly stimulate release of catecholamines. There are reports of significant hypertensive episodes after droperidol administration in patients with pheochromocytoma.[10,138] Muscle relaxants are usually required for pheochromocytoma resection. Vecuronium, because it has no ganglionic blocking effects, may be the agent of choice. In clinically effective doses (0.08 mg/kg), pancuronium is a weak ganglionic blocker and can be safely used. However,

there are reports of severe hypertension after large doses of pancuronium (0.15 mg/kg),[58] which may be secondary to catecholamine release from preadrenergic nerve endings, as shown in a dog model. Because of its marked anticholinergic effects, gallamine should be avoided; succinylcholine should probably not be used because it may stimulate sympathetic ganglia or contribute to catecholamine release with muscle fasciculation.[27] Several other commonly used intraoperative drugs, such as morphine, curare, and atracurium, may indirectly increase circulating catecholamines by releasing histamine, and their use should probably be avoided when possible.

Intraoperative tumor manipulation and tumor removal can result in rapid fluctuations in arterial blood pressure, produce arrhythmias, and cause large variations in blood glucose concentration. Timing and anticipation of these events are important and require communication between surgeon and anesthesiologist. Rapid detection and appropriate treatment of hemodynamic changes are probably improved by frequent intravascular measurement of arterial and pulmonary capillary wedge pressures and cardiac output. Hypertension can be treated with either sodium nitroprusside or phentolamine, but tachyphylaxis and longer duration of action can limit the usefulness of the latter agent. Tumor vein ligation is often associated with significant reductions in arterial blood pressure as a result of both decreased systemic vascular resistance and venodilation. Short-term administration of alpha agonists and fluid administration may be required. Intraoperative use of autotransfusion devices can inadvertently cause hypertension if catecholamine levels in autotransfused blood are high; additional wash cycles may prevent this problem.[111,127]

Ventricular arrhythmias are usually treated with lidocaine, although amiodarone has been used to treat both supraventricular and ventricular arrhythmias.[128] Beta blockade may be useful for treatment of tachycardia and arrhythmias. Esmolol, a selective beta I blocker with a short half-life, may be particularly well suited for such therapy. Hyperglycemia is common before excision of pheochromocytoma, whereas hypoglycemia can develop after tumor resection. These usual trends may be affected by adrenergic drug therapy, and blood sugar should be closely monitored during and after an operation.

Prolonged somnolence and greatly reduced analgesic requirements after pheochromocytoma resection have been reported, but explanations for these phenomena are unknown. While plasma catecholamines may not return completely to normal levels for several days after resection, postoperative hypertension is usually caused by pain or intravascular fluid overload. In rare cases, residual pheochromocytoma or inadvertent renal artery ligation may explain persistent postoperative hypertension.[27,53,86]

In summary, perioperative management of patients with pheochromocytoma is challenging. Proper preoperative preparation is important but will often not completely prevent significant intraoperative hemodynamic lability. Accordingly, close monitoring and timely and appropriate use of potent vasoactive agents are necessary.

ADRENAL INSUFFICIENCY

Addison's disease is an uncommon disease, and rarely do untreated patients present for surgery. It should, however, be considered in the differential diagnosis of unexplained perioperative hypotension. In contrast, patients with iatrogenic suppression of the hypothalamic-pituitary-adrenal (HPA) axis commonly require surgery. It is standard dogma that patients receiving long-term steroid therapy are at risk for developing acute perioperative adrenal insufficiency unless supraphysiologic replacement therapy is administered. This section will address the following issues: (1) duration of steroid therapy that produces HPA axis suppression, (2) time course for recovery of HPA axis following withdrawal of steroid therapy, (3) evaluation of the integrity of the HPA axis, and (4) guidelines for perioperative glucocorticoid coverage.

Axelrod[5] reviewed numerous studies regarding the responsiveness of the HPA axis to provocative tests in patients receiving long-term steroid therapy. Abnormal responses to ACTH or to metyrapone can be observed after only 3 days of glucocorticoid exposure. Streck and Lockwood[136] found that the cortisol response to either insulin-induced hypoglycemia or to ACTH administration was significantly reduced in normal men after exposure to prednisone (25 mg, twice daily) for 2 days. Although it is impossible to define precisely the shortest duration or the smallest dose of steroids that will produce HPA suppression, suppression clearly can develop early after exogenous administration. Axelrod[5] concluded that any patient who received the equivalent of 20 to 30 mg of prednisone daily for more than a week may have developed HPA suppression.

It may take up to 12 months for complete recovery of the HPA axis after prolonged high-dose glucocorticoid therapy. To define the natural history of recovery of the HPA axis following long-term suppression with corticosteroids, Graber et al[42] made serial measurements of HPA function over 12 months in eight patients with Cushing's syndrome after resection of adrenal tumors and in a separate group of six patients after withdrawal of long-term, high-dose steroids. Both ACTH and corticosteroid levels were initially low in these patients (Figure 21-6). During the second through the fifth months, ACTH levels rose to supranormal levels, but plasma 17-OH corticosteroids and the adrenal response to ACTH remained below normal. Corticosteroid levels rose to normal in the sixth to ninth months, but persistent supranormal levels of ACTH suggested ongoing reduced responsiveness of the adrenal gland. After more than 9 months, most patients had normal levels of corticosteroids and ACTH and normal adrenal responses to ACTH. Thus hypothalamic-pituitary function is the first component of the HPA axis to return to normal after chronic suppression; this is followed by return of adrenocortical function. Of greatest relevance to the present discussion, HPA suppression may persist for a year after a course of supraphysiologic glucocorticoid therapy.[5]

The intravenous ACTH stimulation test is a safe, simple, and reliable means of evaluating the HPA axis before surgery in patients who have received glucocorticoid therapy. Kehlet and Binder[64] demonstrated that the preoperative cortisol response to 250 μg of ACTH in patients previously on glucocorticoid therapy was an excellent predictor of the maximal cortisol response observed during general anesthesia and surgery (Figure 21-7). Thus markedly impaired cortisol secretion during surgery is unlikely to occur if a normal adrenal response to ACTH is demonstrated preoperatively.[64]

If such preoperative testing cannot be done, it must be assumed that the patient who received high-dose glucocorticoid treatment for 2 to 3 weeks within the preceding year is at risk to develop adrenocortical insufficiency during surgical stress. The current recommended schedule for corticosteroid supplementation is outlined in the box on p. 310.[73,87] The recommendation of 300 mg of hydrocortisone daily is based on approximations of the maximal daily glucocorticoid output of the adrenal glands,[73] rather than

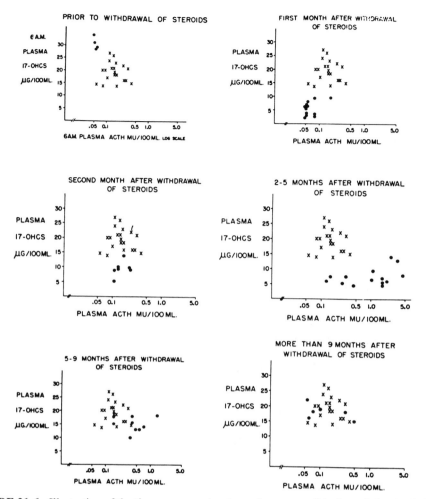

FIGURE 21-6. Illustration of the time course and pattern of recovery of the hypothalamic pituitary adrenal axis.

From Graber et al: Natural history of pituitary-adrenal recovery following long-term suppression with corticosteroids. J Clin Endocrinol Metab 25:11-16, 1965.

on studies that critically assess actual requirements during stress.

Some authors have suggested lower dosages for stress coverage. Kehlet[65] estimated normal cortisol secretion to be approximately 75 to 100 mg during the first 24 hours after surgery and proposed a schedule of 25 mg of soluble cortisol intravenously on induction of anesthesia, followed by 100 mg cortisol intravenously every 24 hours until oral intake is possible after major surgery. Symreng et al[140] used this regimen of steroid replacement in six patients who had impaired cortisol responses to ACTH before sur-

gery. None of these patients developed cardiovascular instability in the perioperative period. Cortisol levels during surgery were actually slightly higher in the treated group than in the control group of patients who had normal preoperative cortisol response to ACTH.

Recently, Udelsman et al[146] studied the clinical effects of different replacement dosages of glucocorticoids in adrenalectomized monkeys undergoing cholecystectomy. Monkeys were given hydrocortisone at either 0.1, 1.0, or 10 times the physiologic replacement dose. The mortality rate was increased

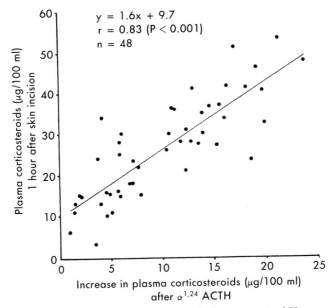

FIGURE 21-7. Comparison between the adrenocortical response to 250 mcg of ACTH and the hypothalamic-pituitary-adrenocortical response to major surgery, measured one hour after skin incision.

From Kehlet H and Binder C: Value of an ACTH test in assessing hypothalamic-pituitary-adrenocortical function in glucocorticoid-treated patients. Br Med J 2:147-149, 1973.

Glucocorticoid coverage for surgery

1. Hydrocortisone phosphate or hemosuccinate, 100 mg IM, on call to the operating room
2. Hydrocortisone phosphate or hemisuccinate 50 mg IM or IV in recovery room and every 6 hours for the next 3 doses
3. Decrease to 25 mg every 6 hours for 24 hours if postoperative recovery is satisfactory
4. Taper to maintenance dosage over next 3 to 5 days
5. Increase cortisol dosage to 200 to 400 mg over 24 hours if fever, hypotension, or other complications occur

From Baxter JD and Tyrell JB: The adrenal cortex. In Endocrinology and metabolism, Felig P et al, editors: New York, 1981, McGraw-Hill Book Co, p 462.

---

in the subphysiologically treated group but not in animals receiving normal physiologic doses. The perioperative outcome of the physiologically treated animals was similar in all respects to either the supraphysiologic group or sham-operated controls. The authors concluded that physiologic glucocorticoid re-

placement is adequate perioperative treatment and that hypercortisolemia following surgical stress may not be necessary. Kehlet and Binder[63] attempted to evaluate the need for supraphysiologic steroid replacement by withholding steroids in 104 glucocorticoid-treated patients who underwent elective surgical procedures. Perioperative plasma corticosteroid levels in approximately 50% of these patients were reduced when compared to levels obtained from 42 normal control subjects who had similar operations. Although eight patients developed hypotension during surgery that was unexplained by the operative course, only one had an associated low plasma corticosteroid level. These data suggest that the risk of acute adrenal insufficiency in glucocorticoid-treated patients undergoing surgery is low. Thus present recommendations for perioperative steroid replacement are probably excessive. While some glucocorticoid coverage seems prudent, actual dose requirements are unknown. One hundred milligrams of cortisol daily in divided doses would seem to be adequate, but definitive recommendations cannot be made without detailed confirmatory studies.

In summary, patients may have suppression of the HPA axis if they have received supraphysiologic dosages of glucocorticoids for 2 to 3 weeks within the past 12 months. The ACTH stimulation test accurately and reliably assesses the integrity of the HPA axis, since responsiveness of the adrenal gland is the last to recover. Patients who are shown to be or who are suspected to be adrenally insufficient should receive glucocorticoid coverage during the perioperative period.

REFERENCES

1. Abbott TR: Anesthesia in untreated myxoedema: report of 2 cases, Br J Anesth 39:510-514, 1967.
2. Anderson A and Hausmann W: Triiodothyronine in myxoedema coma (letter), Lancet 2:999, 1956.
3. Arai T et al: Use of nicardipine in the anesthetic management of pheochromocytoma, Anesth Analg 65:706-708, 1986.
4. Ariyan S and Halasz NA: The incidence of postoperative gram-negative shock in diabetics, Am J Med Sci 254:808-815, 1967.
5. Axelrod L: Glucocorticoid therapy, Medicine 5:39-65,
6. Babad AA and Eger EI: The effects of hyperthyroidism and hypothyroidism on halothane and oxygen requirements in dogs, Anesthesiology 29:1087-1093, 1968.
7. Bell GM et al: End-organ responses to thyroxin therapy in subclinical hypothyroidism, J Clin Endocrinol 22:83-89, 1985.
8. Bergqvist D et al: Juvenile diabetes mellitus—a risk factor for postoperative venous thromboembolism: Acta Med Scand 217:307-308, 1985.
9. Berman ML et al: Isoflurane and enflurane-induced hepatic necrosis in triiodothyronine-pretreated rats, Anesthesiology 58:1-5, 1983.
10. Bittar DA: Innovar-induced hypertensive crisis in patients with pheochromocytoma, Anesthesiology 50:366-369, 1979.
11. Bough EW et al: Myocardial function and hypothyroidism. Relation to disease severity and response to treatment, Arch Intern Med 138:1476-1480, 1978.
12. Bowen DJ et al: Perioperative management of insulin-dependent diabetic patients. Use of continuous intravenous infusion of insulin-glucose-potassium solution, Anesthesiology 37:852-855, 1982.
13. Bratusch-Marrain PR: Insulin-counteracting hormones: their impact on glucose metabolism, Diabetologia 24:74-79, 1983.
14. Bravo EL et al: Circulating and urinary catecholamines in pheochromocytoma: diagnostic and pathophysiologic implications, N Engl J Med 301:682-686, 1979.
15. Bravo EL et al: Clonidine-suppression test: a useful aid in the diagnosis of pheochromocytoma, N Engl J Med 305:623-626, 1981.
16. Bravo EL and Gifford RW Jr: Pheochromocytoma: diagnosis, localization and management, New Engl J Med 311:1298-1303, 1984.
17. Burgos LG et al: Increased intraoperative cardiovascular morbidity in diabetics with autonomic neuropathy, Anesthesiology 67(3A):A66, 1987.
18. Burr WA et al: Serum triiodothyronine in reverse triiodothyronine concentrations after surgical operation, Lancet 2:1271-1279, 1975.
19. Burrow GN: Hyperthyroidism during pregnancy, N Engl J Med 298:150-153, 1978.
20. Canary JJ et al: The effects of oral and intramuscular administration of reserpine in thyrotoxocosis, N Engl J Med 257:435-442, 1957.
21. Catz B and Russell S: Myxedema, shock, and coma, Arch Intern Med 108:407-417, 1961.
22. Chernow et al: Hormonal responses to graded surgical stress, Arch Intern Med 147:1273-1278, 1987.
23. Cruse PJE et al: A five-year prospective study of 23,649 surgical wounds, Arch Surg 107:206-209, 1973.
23a. Cryer PE: Physiology and pathophysiology of the human sympathoadrenal neuroendocrine system, N Engl J Med 303:436-444, 1980.
24. Davis PJ and Davis FB: Hyperthyroidism in patients over the age of 60 years. Clinical features in 85 patients, Medicine 53:161-181, 1974.
25. Donaghue K et al: Cardiac function in acute hypothyroidism, Eur J Nucl Med 11:147-149, 1985.
26. Desmonts JM et al: Anaesthetic management of patients with phaechromocytoma. A review of 102 cases, Br J Anaesth 49:991-998, 1977.
27. Desmonts JM and Marty J: Anaesthetic management of patients with phaeochromocytoma, Br J Anaesth 56:781-789, 1984.
28. Eigler N et al: Synergistic interactions of physiologic increments of glucagon, epinephrine, and cortisol in the dog. A model for stress-induced hyperglycemia, J Clin Invest 63:114, 1979.
29. Engquist A et al: The blocking effect of epidural analgesia on the adrenocortical and hyperglycemic responses to surgery. Acta Anaesth Scand 21:303-335, 1977.
30. Eriksson et al: Propranolol does not prevent thyroid storm, N Engl J Med 296:263-264, 1977.
31. Felig P et al: Hormonal interactions in the regulation of blood glucose, Rec Prog Horm Res 35:501-529, 1979.
32. Felig P et al: The endocrine pancreas: diabetes mellitus. In Felig Petal, editors: Endocrinology and metabolism, New York, 1981, McGraw-Hill.
33. Forestoer CF: Coma in myxedema, Arch Intern Med 111:734-743, 1963.

34. Furszyfer JL et al: Grave's disease in Olmsted County Minnestoa, 1935-1967, Mayo Clin Proc 45:636-644, 1970.

35. George J: Clin Endocrinol Metab, 1974.

36. Giesecke AH et al: Urinary epinephrine and nor-epinephrine during innovar-nitrous oxide anesthesia in man, Anesthesiology 28:701-704, 1967.

37. Gilsanz FJ et al: Cardiomyopathy and pheochromocytoma, Anaesthesia 38:888-891, 1983.

38. Goldberg NJ et al: Insulin therapy in the diabetic surgical patient: metablic and hormone response to low dose insulin infusion, Diabetes Care 4:279-284, 1981.

39. Goldfien A: Pheochromocytoma: diagnosis and anesthetic and surgical management, Anesthesiology 24:462-471, 1963.

40. Goldmann DR: Surgery in patients with endocrine dysfunction, preoperative consultation, Med Clin North Am 71:499-509, 1987.

41. Goldstein S and Killip T III: Catecholamine depletion and thyrotoxicosis. Effect of guanethidine on cardiovascular dynamics, Circulation 31:219-227, 1965.

42. Graber AL et al: Natural history of pituitary-adrenal recovery following long-term suppression with corticosteroids, J Clin Endocrinol 25:11-16, 1965.

43. Halter JB et al: Clonidine-suppression test for the diagnosis of pheochromocytoma (letter), N Engl J Med 306:49-50, 1982.

44. Halter JB, Pflug AE, and Porte D: Mechanism of plasma catecholamine increases during surgical stress in man, J Clin Endocrinol Metab 45:936, 1977.

45. Hamaji M et al: Anaesthetic management with morphine in phaeochromocytoma, Can Anaesth Soc J 31:681-686, 1984.

46. Hamby RI et al: Diabetic cardiomyopathy, JAMA 229:1749-1754, 1974.

47. Hay ID et al: Thyroxin therapy in hypothyroid patients undergoing coronary revascularization: a retrospective analysis, Ann Int Med 95:456-457, 1981.

48. Hjortrup A et al: Influence of diabetes mellitus on operative risk, Br J Surg 72:783-785, 1985.

49. Holvey DN et al: Treatment of myxedema coma with intravenous thyroxin, Arch Intern Med 113:89-96, 1964.

50. Howitt G and Rowlands DJ: Beta-sympathetic blockade in hyperthyroidism, Lancet 1:628-631, 1966.

51. Howitt G et al: Myocardial contractility, and the effects of beta-adrenergic blockade in hypothyroidism and hyperthyroidism, Clin Sci 34:485-495, 1968.

52. Ibbertson HK: Hypothyroidism, Pharmacol Ther 2:177-196, 1977.

53. Hull CJ: Phaeochromocytoma. Diagnosis, preoperative preparation and anaesthetic management, Br J Anaesth 58:1453-1468, 1986.

54. Ingbar SH: Thyrotoxic storm, N Engl J Med 274:1242-1254, 1966.

55. James ML: Endocrine disease in anesthesia. A review of anesthetic management in pituitary, adrenal and thyroid diseases, Anaesthesia 25:232-252, 1970.

56. James MFM: The use of magnesium sulfates in the anesthetic management of pheochromocytoma, Anesthesiology 62:188-190, 1985.

57. Johnston RR, Eger EI, and Wilson C: A comparative interaction of epinephrine with enflurane, isoflurane, and halothane in man, Anesth Analg 55:709-712, 1976.

58. Jones RM and Hill AB: Severe hypertension associated with pancuronium in a patient with a phaeochromocytoma, Can Anaesth Soc J 28:394-396, 1981.

59. Juan D: Pharmacologic agents in the management of pheochromocytoma, South Med J 75:211-216, 1982.

60. Katz J, Bensmof I, and Kadis LB: Anesthesia and uncommon diseases. Pathophysiologic and clinical correlations, Philadelphia, 1981, WB Saunders Co.

61. Kaufman BH et al: Pheochromocytoma in the pediatric age group: current status, J Pediatr Surg 18:879-884, 1983.

62. Kay et al: Elevated plasma vasopressin (AVP) levels during resection of pheochromocytomas, Surgery 100:1150-1153, 1986.

63. Kehlet H and Binder C: Adrenocortical function and clinical course during and after surgery in unsupplemented glucocorticoid-treated patients, Br J Anaesth 45:1043-1048, 1973.

64. Kehlet H and Binder C: Value of an ACTH test in assessing hypothalamic-pituitary-adrenocortical function in glucocorticoid-treated patients, Br Med J 2:147-149, 1973.

65. Kehlet H: A rational approach to dosage and preparation of parenteral glucocorticoid substitution therapy during surgical procedures, Acta Anaesth Scand 19:260-264, 1975.

66. Kim JM and Hackman L: Anesthesia for untreated hypothyroidism: report of three cases, Anesth Analg 56:299-302, 1977.

67. Kreger BE et al: Gram-negative bacteremia. IV. Reevaluation of clinical features and treatment in 612 patients, Am J Med 68:344-355, 1980.

68. Ladenson PW, Goldenheim PD, and Ridgway EC: Rapid pituitary and peripheral tissue responses to intravenous triiodothyronine in hypothyroidism, J Clin Endocrinol 56:1252-1259, 1983.

69. Ladenson PW et al: Complications of surgery in hypothyroid patients, Am J Med 77:261-266, 1984.

70. Levelle JP, Jopling MW, and Sklar GS: Perioperative hypothyroidism: an unusual postanesthetic diagnosis, Anesthesiology 63:195-197, 1985.

71. Levine HD: Compromise therapy in the patient with angina pectoris and hypothyroidism. A clinical assessment, Am J Med 69:411-418, 1980.

72. Levy JH et al: Prospective evaluation of risk of protamine reactions in patients with NPH insulin-dependent diabetes, Anesth Analg 6:739-742, 1986.

73. Liddle G: The adrenal cortex. In Williams RH, editor: Textbook of endocrinology, Philadelphia, 1981, WB Saunders Co.

74. Lidgren L: Postoperative orthopaedic infections in patients with diabetes mellitus, Acta Orthop Scand 44:149-151, 1973.

75. Mackin JF, Canary JJ, and Pittman CS: Thyroid storm and its management, New Engl J Med 291:1396-1398, 1974.

76. Marshall K: Anesthetic management of the patient undergoing resection of a pheochromocytoma. Thirty-eighth Annual Refresher Course Lectures and Clinical Update Program, 1987, 154:1-6.

77. Maze M and Smith CM: Identification of receptor mechanism mediating epinephrine-induced arrythmias during halothane anesthesia in the dog, Anesthesiology 59:322-326, 1983.

78. Mihm FG: Pulmonary artery pressure monitoring in patients with pheochromocytoma, Anesthesiology 57:A42, 1982 (abstract).

79. Mihm FG: Pulmonary artery pressure monitoring in patients with pheochromocytoma, Anesth Analg 62:1129-1133, 1983.

80. McArthur JW et al: Thyrotoxic crisis: an analysis of the 36 cases seen at the Massachusetts General Hospital during the past twenty-five years, JAMA 134:868-874, 1974.

81. McBrien DJ and Hindle W: Myxoedema and heart-failure, Lancet 1:1066-1068, 1963.

82. McDevitt DG et al: The role of the thyroid in the control of heart rate, Lancet 1:998-1000, 1968.

83. McMurry JF Jr: Wound healing with diabetes mellitus, Surg Clin North Am 64:769-778, 1984.

84. Mercer DM and Eltringham RJ: Anesthesia for thyroid surgery, ENT 64:35-42, 1985.

85. Meyers EF et al: Perioperative control of blood glucose in diabetic patients: a two-step protocol, Diabetes Care 9:40-46, 1986.

86. Miller D and Robblee JA: Perioperative management of a patient with malignant pheochromocytoma, Can Anaesth Soc J 32: 278-282, 1985.

87. Molitch ME: Endocrinology. In Molitch ME, editor: Management of medical problems in surgical patients, Philadelphia, 1982, FA Davis Co.

88. Murkin JM: Anesthesia and hypothyroidism: a review of thyroxine physiology, pharmacology, and anesthetic implications, Anesth Analg 61:371-383, 1982.

89. Murray JF: Hyperpyrexia of uncertain origin, Br J Anaesth 50:387-388, 1978.

90. Nell LJ et al: Frequency and specificity of protamine antibodies in diabetic and control subjects, Diabetes 37:172-176, 1988.

91. Nesto RW et al: Angina and exertional myocardial ischemia in diabetic and non-diabetic patients: assessment by exercise thallium scintigraphy, Ann Intern Med 108:170-175, 1988.

92. Nevins MA et al: Pitfalls in interpreting serum creatine phosphokinase activity, JAMA 224:1382-1387, 1973.

93. Newmark SR, Himathongkam T, and Shane JM: Hyperthyroid crisis, JAMA 230:592-593, 1974.

94. Nolan CM et al: Further characterization of the impaired bactericidal function of granulocytes in patients with poorly controlled diabetes, Diabetes 27:889-894, 1978.

95. Nordquist et al: Myxedema coma and CO_2 retention, Acta Med Scand 166:189-194, 1960.

96. Oyama T: Endocrine responses to anesthetic agents, Br J Anaesth 45:276-281, 1973.

97. Page MM and Watkins PJ: The heart in diabetes: autonomic neuropathy and cardiomyopathy, Clin Endocrinol Metab 6:377-388, 1977.

98. Page MM and Watkins PJ: Cardiorespiratory arrest and diabetic autonomic neuropathy, Lancet 14-16, 1978.

99. Paine TD et al: Coronary arterial surgery in patients with incapacitating angina pectoris and myxoedema, Am J Cardiol 40:226-231, 1977.

100. Partamian JO and Bradley RF: Acute myocardial infarction in 258 cases of diabetes, N Engl J Med 273:455-461, 1965.

101. Pflug AE and Halter JB: Effect of spinal anesthesia on adrenergic tone and the neuroendocrine responses to surgical stress in humans, Anesthesiology 55:120-126, 1981.

102. Pietros RJ et al: Cardiovascular responses in hyperthyroidism: the influence of adrenergic receptor blockades, Arch Intern Med 129:426-429, 1972.

103. Plumpton FS et al: Corticosteroid treatment and surgery, Anaesthesia 24:12-18, 1969.

104. Polk HC et al: Operating room-acquired infection: its epidemiology and prevention, Surg Ann 9:83-101, 1977.

105. Podolsky S: Management of diabetes in the surgical patient, Med Clin North Am 66:1361-1372, 1982.

106. Porte D and Halter JB: The endocrine pancreas and diabetes mellitus. In Williams RH, editor: Textbook of endocrinology, Philadelphia, 1981, WB Saunders.

107. Ram CVS, Meese R, and Hill SC: Failure of alpha-methyltyrosine to prevent hypertensive crisis in

pheochromocytoma, Arch Intern Med 145:2114-2115, 1985.

108. Ramsay ID: Muscle dysfunction in hyperthyroidism, Lancet 2:931-934, 1966.

109. Rayfield EJ et al: Infection and diabetes: the case for glucose control, Am J Med 72:439-450, 1982.

110. Remine WH et al: Current management of pheochromocytoma, Ann Surg 179:740-748, 1974.

111. Rice MJ, Violante EV, and Kreluli JF: Effect of autotransfusion on catecholamine levels during pheochromocytoma resection, Anesthesiology 67:1017, 1987.

112. Robson NJ: Emergency surgery complicated by thyrotoxicosis and thyrotoxic periodic paralysis, Anesthesiology 40:27-31, 1985.

113. Roizen MF: A prospective randomized trial of four anesthetic techniques for resection of pheochromocytoma (abstract), Anesthesiology 57:A43, 1982.

114. Roizen MF et al: The effect of alpha-adrenergic blockade on cardiac performance and tissue oxygen delivery during excision of pheochromocytoma, Surgery 94:941-945, 1983.

115. Roizen MF: Endocrine abnormalities and anesthesia: implications for the anesthesiologist. Refresher Course in Anesthesiology, 13:161-177, 1984.

116. Rutberg HE et al: Effects of the extradural administration of morphine, or bupivacaine, on the endocrine response to upper abdominal surgery, Br J Anaesth 56:233-238, 1984.

117. Schimmel M and Utiger RD: Thyroidal and peripheral production of thyroid hormones: review of recent findings and their clinical implications, Ann Int Med 87:760-768, 1977.

118. Schlesinger MG, Garci SL, and Saxe IH: Studies in nodular goiter. Incidence of thyroid nodules in routine necropsies in a nongoitrous region, JAMA 110:1638-1641, 1938.

119. Schnelle N et al: Anesthesia for surgical treatment of pheochromocytoma, Surg Clin North Am 45:991-1001, 1965.

120. Scott HW Jr et al: Pheochromocytoma: present diagnosis and management, Ann Surg 183:587-593, 1976.

121. Seino H et al: Postoperative hepatic dysfunction after halothane or enflurane anesthesia in patient with hyperthyroidism, Anesthesiology 64:122-125, 1986.

122. Senior RM et al: The recognition and management of myxoedema coma, JAMA 217:61-65, 1971.

123. Shamoon H et al: Synergistic interactions among antiinsulin hormones in the pathogenesis of stress hyperglycemia in humans, J Clin Endocrinol Metab 52:1235-1241, 1981.

124. Shanks RG et al: Controlled trial of propranolol in thyrotoxicosis, Lancet 1:993-994, 1969.

125. Sieber FE et al: Glucose: a reevaluation of its intra-operative use, Anesthesiology 67:72-81, 1987.

126. Sjoerdsma A et al: Pheochromocytoma: current concepts of diagnosis and treatment, Ann Int Med 65:1302-1326, 1966.

127. Smith DF, Mihm FG, and Mefford I: Hypertension after intraoperative autotransfusion in bilateral adrenalectomy for pheochromocytoma, Anesthesiology 58:182-184, 1983.

128. Solares G et al: Amiodarone, phaeochromocytoma and cardiomyopathy, Anaesthesia 41:186-190, 1986.

129. Solomon DH: Hyperthyroidism: antithyroid drug treatment. In Werner SC and Ingbar SH, editors: The thyroid, ed 3, New York, 1971, Harper and Row.

130. Stamm WE et al: Epidemiology of nosocomial infections due to gram-negative bacilli: aspects relevant to development and use of vaccines, J Infect Dis 136:S151-S160, 1977.

131. Stehling LC: Anesthetic management of the patient with hyperthyroidism, Anesthesiology 41:585-595, 1974.

132. Stenstrom G, Haljamae H, and Tisell LE: Influence of preoperative treatment with phenoxybenzamine on the incidence of adverse cardiovascular reactions during anaesthesia and surgery for phaeochromocytoma, Acta Anaesthesiol Scand 29:797-803, 1985.

133. Stewart WJ et al: Increased risk of severe protamine reactions in NPH insulin-dependent diabetics undergoing cardiac catheterization, Circulation 70:788-792, 1984.

134. Stirt JA et al: Atracurium in a patient with pheochromocytoma, Anesth Analg 64:547-550, 1985.

135. Stoelting RB and Dierdorf JF, editors: Anesthesia and co-existing disease, New York, 1983, Churchill Livingstone.

136. Streck WF and Lockwood DH: Pituitary adrenal recovery following short-term suppression with corticosteroids, Am J Med 66:910-914, 1979.

137. Suko J: The calcium pump of cardiac sarcoplasmic reticulum. Functional alterations at different levels of thyroid states in rabbits, J Physiol (Lond) 228:563-582, 1973.

138. Sumikawa K and Amakata Y: The pressor effect of droperidol on a patient with pheochromocytoma, Anesthesiology 46:359-361, 1977.

139. Suzukawa M et al: Use of isoflurane during resection of pheochromocytoma, Anesth Analg 62:100-103, 1983.

140. Symreng T et al: Physiological cortisol substitution of long-term steroid-treated patients undergoing major surgery, Br J Anaesth 53:949-953, 1981.

141. Taitelman U et al: Insulin in the management of the diabetic surgical patient, JAMA 237:658-660, 1977.

142. Theilen EO, Wilson WR, and Tutunji FJ: The acute

hemodynamic effects of alpha-methyldopa thyrotoxic patients and normal subjects, Metabolism 12:625-630, 1963.

143. Thomas DJB et al: Insulin-dependent diabetes during the perioperative period, Anaesthesia 39:629-637, 1984.

144. Toft AD et al: Thyroid function after surgical treatment of thyrotoxocosis. A report of 100 cases tested with trapanolon before operation, N Engl J Med 298:643-647, 1978.

145. Tsuji H et al: Inhibition of metabolic responses to surgery with beta-adrenergic blockade, Br J Surg 67:503-505, 1980.

146. Udelsman R et al: Adaptation during surgical stress: a reevaluation of the role of glucocorticoids, J Clin Invest 77:1377-1381, 1986.

147. Utiger RD: Decreased extrathyroidal triiodothyronine production in nonthyroidal illness: benefit or harm? Am J Med 69:807-810, 1980.

148. Uusitupa M et al: Prevalence of coronary heart disease, left ventricular failure and hypertension in middle-aged, newly diagnosed type 2 (non-insulin-dependent) diabetic subjects, Diabetologia 28:22-27, 1985.

149. Vannini P et al: Diabetes as pro-infective risk factor in total hip replacement, Acta Diabetol Lat 21:275-280, 1984.

150. Vater M, Achola K, and Smith G: Catecholamine responses during anaesthesia for phaeochromocytoma, Br J Anaesth 55:357-360, 1983.

151. Vellar ID et al: Pheochromocytoma: a review of the St. Vincent's Hospital, Melbourne Experience (1969-1984) and of recent advances in management, Aust New Zealand J Surg 55:463-470, 1985.

152. Vinik AI, Pimstone BL, and Hoffenberg R: Sympathetic nervous system blocking in hyperthyroidism, J Clin Endocrinol Metab 28:725-727, 1968.

153. Waldstein SS et al: A clinical study of thyroid storm, Ann Int Med 52:626-642, 1960.

154. Walts LF et al: Perioperative management of diabetes mellitus, Anesthesiology 55:104-109, 1981.

155. Weinberg AD et al: Outcome of anesthesia in surgery and hypothyroid patients, Arch Intern Med 143:893-897, 1983.

156. Weringer EJ et al: Effects of insulin on wound healing in diabetic mice, Acta Endocrinol 99:101-108, 1982.

157. Wheat LJ: Infection and diabetes mellitus, Diabetes Care 3:187-197, 1980.

158. Wilson WR and Bedell GN: The pulmonary abnormalities in myxedema, J Clin Invest 39:42-55, 1960.

159. Wood M et al: Halothane-induced hepatic necrosis in triiodothyronine-pretreated rats, Anesthesiology 52:470-476, 1980.

160. Zwillich CW et al: Ventilatory control and myxedema and hypothyroidism, N Engl J Med 292:662-665, 1975.

CHAPTER 22

Pregnancy

ANDREW P. HARRIS
MICHAEL J. SENDAK

Pregnant patients require anesthesia and surgery for three reasons: (1) correction of surgical problems unrelated to pregnancy, (2) surgical therapy for pregnancy-related problems, and (3) delivery of the child. Surgical diseases unrelated to pregnancy that occur with greater frequency in pregnant patients include trauma, breast masses, appendicitis, and ovarian torsion. The most common pregnancy-related disease requiring surgery is cervical incompetence. Surgical delivery of the child by cesarean section occurs in ever-increasing numbers. Compared to nongravid patients, perioperative morbidity and mortality are only slightly increased in pregnant patients, but there is substantial risk to the fetus.

The primary perioperative concern is safe care of both the mother and child. To safeguard the fetus, familiarity with normal maternal and fetal physiology and knowledge of potential adverse effects of anesthesia and anesthetic agents on each is necessary. The fetus is at risk because of possible teratogenic effects of anesthetic agents, inadvertent induction of premature labor, and compromised placental function. Finally, for the mothers, maternal hemodynamic diseases unique to pregnancy such as toxemia and peripartum cardiomyopathy can increase perioperative risk and require special management.

MATERNAL PHYSIOLOGIC CHANGES OF PREGNANCY
Cardiovascular

The major maternal cardiovascular changes occurring during pregnancy are listed in Table 22-1.* Cardiac output progressively increases throughout

*References 4, 24, 32, 34, 42, 44.

314

TABLE 22-1. Cardiovascular changes associated with term pregnancy

Blood volume	Increases 44% to 48%
Plasma volume	Increases 50%
Red blood cell mass	Increases 25%
Cardiac output	Increases 40% to 50%
Stroke volume	Increases 30%
Heart rate	Increases 15%
Total peripheral resistance	Decreases 20% to 25%
Mean arterial blood pressure	No change or slight decrease
Central venous pressure	No change
Femoral venous pressure (supine)	Increases to 24 cm H_2O

gestation to values that are 40% to 50% above non-pregnant values. Increased cardiac output is caused by increased blood volume, increased heart rate (by 12 to 15 beats per minute), increased stroke volume, and decreased systemic vascular resistance. These changes are well tolerated in normal patients, but patients with underlying cardiac disease may require inotropic or diuretic support in the middle and last trimester to prevent heart failure.

Cardiac output increases still further during labor, 15% during the latent phase, 30% during the active phase, and 45% during the expulsive phase.[43] Each contraction raises cardiac output an additional 10% to 25% as 300 to 500 ml of blood are squeezed from the uterus into the central circulation. After delivery, cardiac output may be 80% higher than prelabor values, and returns to normal over several days. Therefore, patients with underlying heart disease may initially exhibit cardiac dysfunction during labor and delivery and remain at increased risk for decompensation in the immediate postpartum week.

Although arterial blood pressure remains normal during pregnancy in most women, increases in the compliance of the central circulation occasionally results in lower than normal blood pressures, which do not indicate cardiac dysfunction, hypovolemia, or hemorrhage. Hypertension should be regarded as a sign of impending toxemia of pregnancy (discussed later). Central venous, mean arterial, and mean pulmonary artery occlusion pressures remain within the nonpregnant (normal) range during gestation.

Blood volume increases progressively throughout gestation, and is 44% to 48% higher than normal volumes at term. Increased red blood cell mass and plasma volume do not contribute equally to blood volume expansion. Plasma volume increases 50% by term, but red blood cell volume increases only 25%, resulting in the "physiologic" anemia of pregnancy. Hemoglobin concentrations as low as 10 to 11 g/dl are considered normal in pregnancy. As with other hemodynamic changes, blood volume returns to normal within the first few postpartum weeks. After delivery, assuming that blood loss is not excessive, hematocrit often increases spontaneously as blood volume contracts to normal.

Mechanical effects of the enlarging uterus alter the appearance of the electrocardiogram (ECG). Increasing uterus size causes cephalad displacement of the diaphragm and shifts the heart upward, leftward and anteriorly. The ECG may show left axis deviation, and reversible ST, T, and Q wave changes appear (especially in the inferior leads). Perioperative ECGs should be interpreted in light of these changes.

Uterine enlargement also compresses the abdominal aorta and inferior vena cava. Although aortic compression can compromise distal blood flow as a result of reduced perfusion pressure, these changes are rarely significant. However, in contrast, uterine compression of the inferior vena cava (IVC) frequently increases femoral venous pressure, dilates venous channels, and decreases venous return to the heart. While complete IVC occlusion occurs in 83% of near-term parturients in the supine position,[23] increased return of blood to the right side of the heart via collateral flow (azygos, perivertebral, and ovarian veins) and baroreceptor-mediated increases in heart rate and vascular tone prevent hypotension in most patients. The "supine hypotensive syndrome" (pallor, sweating, nausea, hypotension, and altered mentation) develops in 5% to 10% of near-term parturients because of inadequate compensation. These patients tend to develop profound hypotension with low-volume hemorrhage or sympathectomy, the latter most commonly seen following epidural anesthesia. When blood pressure is maintained as a result of sympathetically mediated vasoconstriction in these patients, the accompanying reductions in uterine blood flow (secondary to uterine artery constriction) may compromise fetal well-being. IVC compression also produces pooling and stasis of venous blood in the lower extremities and predisposes to phlebitis and venous varicosities during pregnancy.

Because of the potential adverse effects of aortocaval compression, the parturient should not be allowed to lie supine for any length of time after the twentieth week of gestation. Leftward tilt of the maternal pelvis should be maintained throughout the perioperative period to shift the uterus off the vertebral column and prevent compression of the inferior vena cava. Uterine displacement can be accomplished by: (1) inserting a wedge under the right hip and buttock, (2) tilting an operating table 15 to 20 degrees to the left, or (3) repositioning the uterus manually. Without proper patient positioning, the administration of anticholinergics, vasopressors, and intravenous fluids is often ineffective in normalizing uterine blood flow even if maternal blood pressure is corrected. If significant compression persists, the patient should be placed in a full left or right lateral position.

Hematologic

As mentioned earlier, red blood cell mass increases less than plasma volume during pregnancy, and hematocrit and hemoglobin concentration decrease. The white blood cell count is slightly elevated.[33] There is usually a steady increase in platelet count to greater than 300,000/mm^3 at term; however, some patients have a fall in platelet count toward term.[33] Fibrinogen concentration increases to almost twice normal by term.[17] The concentrations of most other clotting factors also progressively increase (with the exception of factor XIII) and antithrombin-III levels decrease.[17] These changes result in a hypercoagulable state during pregnancy. While this may act to prevent excessive blood loss from the uterus following delivery, it has also been cited as a cause for thromboembolic events associated with pregnancy.

Amniotic fluid has thromboplastin-like activity, and consumptive coagulopathy and disseminated intravascular coagulation (DIC) may follow release of amniotic fluid into the circulation. The uterus can be a source of plasminogen activator, and injury to the uterus may also result in coagulopathy.

Respiratory

Many mechanical, hormonal, and metabolic changes of pregnancy affect respiratory function. At term, the anteroposterior and transverse thoracic diameters increase. Despite cephalad displacement of the diaphragm, total lung capacity, vital capacity, inspiratory capacity, and inspiratory reserve volume change only slightly from nonpregnant values (Table 22-2).[4] However, functional residual capacity (FRC), expiratory reserve volume, and residual volume decrease 20%. If FRC decreases below closing volume, airway collapse, ventilation/perfusion mismatching, and hypoxemia can occur. Since general anesthesia also decreases FRC and impairs oxygenation, pregnant patients are at an increased risk for hypoxemia in the perioperative period following general anesthesia. These abnormalities are further accentuated in the supine position.

Progesterone increases metabolic rate, tidal volume, and respiratory rate; as a result, minute ventilation increases by 50% in pregnancy. Alveolar ventilation increases in excess of the increased CO_2 production, and $PaCO_2$ values of 28 to 32 mm Hg are common at term. Because $PaCO_2$ decreases, alveolar (and therefore arterial) PO_2 may exceed 100 mm Hg. Renal compensation for respiratory alkalosis decreases the serum bicarbonate concentration, thus serum pH remains normal. Circulatory or respiratory decompensation in pregnancy quickly results in both profound hypoxemia (for the reasons cited above) as well as metabolic acidosis (results from a diminished buffer base in the blood).

TABLE 22-2. Respiratory changes associated with term pregnancy

Minute ventilation	Increases 50%
Alveolar ventilation	Increases 70%
Tidal volume	Increases 40%
Respiratory rate	Increases 15%
Airway resistance	Decreases 36%
Oxygen consumption	Increases 20%
Total lung capacity	Decreases 5%
Inspiratory capacity	Increases 5%
Inspiratory reserve volume	No change
Vital capacity	No change
Residual volume	Decreases 20%
Functional residual capacity	Decreases 20%
$PaCO_2$	Decreases to 28 to 32 mm Hg
PaO_2	Increases slightly
pH	No change
Serum bicarbonate	Decreases to 18 to 24 meq/l

Renal

Renal blood flow increases as much as 50% in pregnancy. Glomerular filtration rate (GFR), effective renal plasma flow (ERPF), filtration fraction (GFR/ERPF), and creatinine clearance also increase markedly.[10] The upper limits of normal for serum creatinine and urea nitrogen values are lower (0.8 mg/dl and 13 mg/dl respectively) in pregnancy, and usual normal values may indicate renal dysfunction in the parturient. Since renal excretion of drugs is enhanced, maintenance drug dosage may need to be increased in pregnant patients, especially for drugs that depend predominantly on renal clearance.

Increased filtration rate of solute appears to overwhelm renal tubular absorptive capacity, resulting in glucosuria and aminoaciduria. In patients with normal glucose tolerance during pregnancy, 24-hour urine glucose excretion increases fivefold to tenfold over normal nonpregnant values,[25] and this effect is accentuated in patients with carbohydrate intolerance. Perioperative infusion of dextrose-containing fluids often results in severe hyperglycemia and osmotic diuresis. Blood glucose monitoring is preferred perioperatively, since qualitative testing of urine may be misleading. Urinary protein excretion increases from less than 100 mg in nonpregnant patients to 300 to 500 mg per 24 hours during pregnancy.[26] In a parturient with preexisting kidney disease, increased proteinuria may not indicate progression of the underlying renal dysfunction. Proteinuria and glucosuria may enhance susceptibility to urinary tract infections.

Gastrointestinal

The stomach is pushed into the left dome of the diaphragm by the gravid uterus and rotated by as much as 45 degrees. The combination of increased intragastric pressure and gastroesophageal incompetence predispose to gastric reflux. Cephalad and posterior displacement of the pylorus by the expanding uterus retards gastric emptying. All of these changes are exacerbated by twin gestation, polyhydramnios, obesity, head-down position, fundal pressure, and succinylcholine-induced fasiculations. Increased progesterone and decreased motility further diminish lower esophageal sphincter tone as well as delay gastric emptying.

Gastric volume and acidity increase in pregnancy, and the anatomic changes described above permit gastric contents to exit the stomach more easily through the esophagus than through the pylorus. During periods of unconsciousness or heavy sedation, all parturients are considered at risk for pulmonary aspiration of gastric contents by either passive regurgitation or active vomiting. Aspiration of gastric contents is the leading cause of peripartum maternal anesthetic death,[11] and maternal mortality from this complication has not declined over the last two decades.[41] Even in patients undergoing elective cesarean section (fasted overnight), 43% had gastric volumes of greater than 25 ml and gastric pH of less than 2.5,[7] thereby placing them at increased risk of acid aspiration pneumonitis. Perioperative precautions should be taken to prevent acid aspiration. These include (1) rapid sequence induction or awake intubation when general anesthesia is planned, (2) avoidance of excessive sedation, and (3) aspiration chemoprophylaxis with antacids, H_2 antagonists, or metaclopromide.

Clinically insignificant elevations of serum glutamic-oxaloacetic transaminase (SGOT), serum glutamic-pyruvic transaminase (SGPT), lactic acid dehydrogenase (LDH), alkaline phosphatase, and cholesterol are common during gestation and labor. The prothrombin time, serum bilirubin, and hepatic blood flow remain normal. When liver enzyme tests are markedly out of range, they should be further evaluated, since toxemia and fatty liver of pregnancy are serious, potentially life-threatening diseases. Hepatic production of pseudocholinesterase is probably normal during pregnancy, but increased blood volume decreases serum concentration and results in a 24% decrease in pseudocholinesterase activity at term.[38] This decrease in serum pseudocholinesterase activity slightly prolongs neuromuscular blockade after succinylcholine, but this effect is usually clinically insignificant.

Neurologic

Compared to nongravid controls, the concentration of volatile anesthetic required to produce anesthesia decreases 25% to 40% in pregnant ewes near term.[30] The etiologic cause of this lowered anesthetic requirement remains unclear, but may relate to elevated progesterone and/or endorphins present in the central nervous system during gestation. The volatile anesthetic agents may therefore produce stupor or unconsciousness in the parturient at lower inspiratory concentrations than one might expect, and result in unexpectedly prolonged emergence from general anesthesia.

Local anesthetic requirements for regional analgesia and anesthesia are also reduced. To achieve the same level of sensory blockade with epidural anesthesia administration in pregnancy, a 20% to 30% smaller dose of local anesthetic than that required in the nonpregnant patient is used. Acid-base changes in the CSF, increases in nerve tissue sensitivity to local anesthetics, and decrease in volume of the epidural space resulting from epidural venous engorgement may account for these observations. With subarachnoid block, decreased volume of CSF, elevated CSF pressure, changes in CSF proteins, increased neurosensitivity and/or enhanced cephalad spread of the anesthetic may account for the 30% to 50% reduction in local anesthetic requirement. The effective dose for subarachnoid and epidural narcotics is also lower in pregnant patients. Bromage et al[5] report that 7.5 mg of epidural morphine is the lowest effective dose for postoperative pain relief after lower abdominal surgery in nonobstetric patients, but 5 mg epidural morphine has been found effective for pain relief following cesarean section.[35]

FETAL CONSIDERATIONS

Safeguarding fetal well-being is a major goal of perioperative management of the pregnant patient. Many potential physiologic and pharmacologic perturbations occur that can interfere with fetal well-being. These include, but are not limited to: (1) fetal hypoxia and asphyxia, (2) preterm labor, (3) central nervous system alterations resulting from drugs administered to the mother that cross the placenta, and (4) the potential for teratogenicity from maternally administered medications.

Fetal Hypoxia and Asphyxia

Fetal hypoxia is defined as functional organ injury resulting from decreased oxygen availability to tissues on the cellular level. The end result of hypoxia is failure of intracellular oxidative metabolic functions as reflected by production of a metabolic acidosis (for example, lactic acid derived from anaerobic metabolism). In contrast, fetal asphyxia is defined as the combination of decreased oxygen delivery and inadequate CO_2 removal, usually on a systemic basis. Asphyxia results in a combination of respiratory and metabolic acidosis, and is frequently accompanied by a shocklike circulatory pattern.

In animal studies, fetal hypoxia at near term rarely results in permanent cerebral malfunction as an isolated finding. Oxygen transport to the fetal brain is "autoregulated," with arterial oxygen content being a major determinant of cerebral blood flow. As arterial oxygen content falls, the fetal brain increases both oxygen extraction and cerebral blood flow to preserve cerebral integrity. The difference between arterial and venous oxygen content decreases, but cerebral vascular resistance decreases.[21] By the time these compensatory mechanisms are overwhelmed, hypoxia has already resulted in cellular damage to other vital organ systems such as the heart or kidneys, which have either a much higher intrinsic O_2 demand, or a less well-protected blood flow during hypoxemia.

In contrast, asphyxial events may result in brain damage. Total asphyxial events usually result in death. Central nervous system damage following prolonged partial asphyxia depends upon the length of insult and the gestational age. In term infants, generalized cerebral edema and flattening of gyri occur, resulting in generalized cerebral atrophy and diffuse neurologic dysfunction.[29] If the partial asphyxia is prolonged, death usually results. An asphyxiated preterm fetus develops a more localized pattern of cellular damage, typically subependymal germinal matrix/intraventricular hemorrhage or periventricular leukomalacia. Spastic diplegia, the most frequently observed cerebral palsy in preterm infants, is a result of this regional pathologic change.[29]

The multiple potential origins of both fetal hypoxia and asphyxia need to be appreciated so that they can be prevented or ameliorated. Fetal hypoxia can occur as the result of either (1) hypoxemia with decreased, normal, or even slightly increased organ blood flow, or (2) normoxemia with decreased organ blood flow. Since oxygen transfer across the placenta is a gradient-driven process, any factor that decreases maternal uterine arterial oxygen content will decrease oxygen transport across the placenta to the fetus and result in fetal hypoxemia. Maternal arterial oxygen desaturation may occur from any respiratory problem associated with an increased alveolar-arterial oxygen gradient, and special care must be taken to ensure adequate oxygenation. Ideally, maternal arterial oxygen saturation should be monitored continuously throughout the perioperative period.

Shift of the maternal oxyhemoglobin dissociation curve to the left (lower P_{50}) may also diminish O_2

transfer across the placenta. Normally, fetal P_{50} is 6 to 8 mm Hg lower than maternal P_{50}, and this gradient promotes oxygen transfer from maternal to fetal blood, which binds oxygen with greater affinity. The maternal oxyhemoglobin dissociation curve can be left-shifted by hyperventilation, adversely affecting fetal O_2 transfer. Maternal P_{50} is also decreased in toxemia, but mechanisms responsible for this shift are unclear, although an increase in carbonmonoxyhemoglobin has been noted.[22]

Asphyxial events occur when both O_2 delivery to the fetus and CO_2 removal from the fetus are compromised. The two origins of these conditions are (1) inadequate placental perfusion (maternal or fetal) or (2) diminished intrinsic placental function. On the maternal side, assuming laminar flow characteristics, intervillous placental blood flow (the largest component of uterine blood flow at term) can be approximated by the equation:

$$Q = \frac{\pi}{8} \cdot \frac{\Delta P \cdot r^4}{\eta \cdot l}$$

where:

> Q is blood flow
> ΔP is the perfusion pressure gradient
> r is the vessel radius
> η is the blood viscosity
> l is the vessel length

Thus intervillous blood flow can be decreased acutely by factors that: (1) decrease perfusion pressure, (2) decrease perfusing artery radius, (3) increase blood viscosity, or (4) increase perfusing artery length. In clinical situations the predominant factors affecting intervillous blood flow are perfusion pressure and arterial vessel radius, since blood viscosity and vessel length are rarely acutely altered.

Perfusion pressure can be decreased by several mechanisms. First, uterine artery pressure can be decreased by aortic compression from uterine enlargement. "Downstream" increases in venous vascular pressure can likewise result in diminished uterine perfusion pressure. Femoral venous pressure can rise to 24 cm of water dring IVC occlusion,[4] and elevated venous pressure may be transmitted back to the uterine circulation to compromise perfusion. Uterine hypoperfusion can also result from maternal hypotension induced by general and/or regional anesthetics (iatrogenic hypotension). Finally, increased intrauterine pressure itself (that is, during uterine contraction) can become the functional downstream pressure and limit uterine flow.

The uterine arterial vessel radius is a function of both intrinsic tone and the presence or absence of extrinsic compression. Intrinsic uterine vessel tone is primarily modulated through alpha-adrenergic receptors. Any physiologic stimulus that results in alpha-adrenergic stimulation will tend to decrease uterine artery vessel radius thereby decreasing blood flow to the placenta. Alpha-adrenergic stimulation often occurs as a result of either baroreceptor-mediated responses to hypotension or catecholamine responses to "stress" (see Chapter 14). Decreases in uterine perfusion during hypotension are often greater than can be accounted for by the drop in perfusion pressure and likely reflect additional baroreceptor-mediated vasoconstriction. Several studies have also indicated that physical and psychologic stress in the parturient can elicit a vasoconstrictive response in the uterine vasculature and decrease uterine perfusion.[16,28,39] Good preoperative medication, adequate anesthesia, and careful attention to postoperative pain relief are necessary to minimize this stress response when surgery is required in pregnant patients. Finally, uterine vessel size can also be decreased by extrinsic compression of the vessels as they pass through the wall of the contracting uterus. If this results in fetal distress, tocolytic agents can be administered to relax the uterus and thereby improve placental perfusion.

On the fetal side of the placenta, the most common cause of hypoperfusion is mechanical compression of the umbilical arteries. Because flow in the fetal umbilical circulation (even during stress) appears directly related to perfusion pressure,[15] and vasoconstriction only occurs in the presence of extremely high (probably supraphysiologic) levels of circulating catecholamines or vasoconstrictors, decreases in umbilical blood flow resulting from causes other than mechanical cord compression or generalized fetal circulatory collapse are rare. Chronic, intermittent, or continuous mechanical obstruction of the umbilical vessels results in fetal asphyxia. Fetuses are placed at risk for umbilical artery obstruction when uterine contractions occur and when the amniotic fluid volume is decreased.

Intrinsic malfunction of the placenta leading to impaired gas exchange occurs in several disease states including placental abruption, toxemia of pregnancy, and postterm pregnancy. Whenever surgery is undertaken in these patients, careful fetal monitoring should be performed perioperatively, since the fetus is at increased risk of asphyxia secondary to the underlying placental abnormalities.

Iatrogenic placental inadequacy can also develop if bicarbonate is administered to the mother. Bicarbonate administration increases $PaCO_2$ in both mother and infant, but since bicarbonate does not readily cross the placenta, it cannot buffer fetal acidosis. The acute increase in maternal $PaCO_2$ following bicarbonate administration temporarily halts diffusion-driven transplacental CO_2 transport, and fetal respiratory acidosis ensues. Since bicarbonate is usually only given during maternal hemodynamic instability when the risk of fetal metabolic acidosis is increased, the ensuing increases in fetal $PaCO_2$ often exacerbate preexisting fetal metabolic acidosis. Therefore, bicarbonate should not be administered to an acidotic mother without careful consideration of fetal risks.

Whenever fetal hypoxia or asphyxia is suspected, fetal monitoring should be undertaken. This is true in the preoperative, intraoperative, and postoperative periods. The diagnosis of impaired fetal oxygenation is usually made by observing the secondary effects of hypoxemia on the fetal heart rate. Fetal heart rate is controlled by the brain stem via sympathetic and parasympathetic autonomic pathways, as well as by intrinsic automaticity of the myocardial conducting system. Under conditions of hypoxemia, there are both brainstem-mediated chemoreceptor responses as well as changes in tonic autonomic activity from the brainstem. As acidosis progresses, intrinsic myocardial automaticity may also decrease.

Therefore, several characteristics of the fetal heart rate pattern can be indicative of fetal distress. These include fetal tachycardia, fetal bradycardia, fetal periodic decelerations, and decreased fetal heart rate variability. Fetal tachycardia usually occurs secondary to infection or maternal fever, but can, rarely indicate fetal distress. More often, persistent fetal bradycardia (defined as a heart rate below 100) is associated with fetal distress and indicates the need to consider intervention if a viable fetus is present. Periodic fetal heart rate decelerations, especially those which directly follow uterine contractions (for example, "late" decelerations) also are indicative of fetal distress. Fetal heart rate variability is the result of moment-to-moment changes in parasympathetic and sympathetic outflow from the brain stem. The result of this modulation is the appearance of an irregular baseline heart rate (Figure 22-1), quite different from that seen in the normal adult. As the fetal brain stem becomes hypoxic, the "fine tuning" of fetal heart rate disappears, and the fetal heart rate trace loses its variability (Figure 22-2). The fetal heart rate may also lose its variability in the presence of either a fetal sleep state or drugs that cause sedation or sleep in the fetus (for example, narcotics,

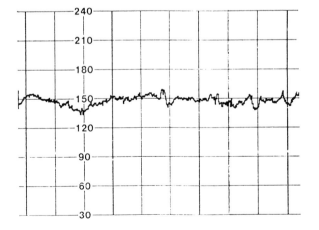

FIGURE 22-1. A sample fetal heart rate tracing is depicted. Both the baseline fetal heart rate and the variability are normal. The tracing encompasses a 3-minute time interval.

biturates). Although none of the fetal heart rate changes by themselves are very specific, when combinations occur they can signal impending asphyxia.

Preterm Labor

Anesthesia and surgery during gestation are associated with an increased risk of preterm labor. The most common cause of preterm labor in such patients is physical manipulation of the uterus during intraabdominal procedures. There is considerable controversy as to which type of anesthesia (general or regional) is best at limiting the risk of preterm labor during or after surgery in the pregnant patient. Most volatile anesthetic agents (halothane, isoflurane, and enflurane) relax uterine muscle and may thus protect the uterus against preterm contraction during intraabdominal surgical procedures. Despite this theoretical benefit, there is no evidence that either general anesthesia (using a potent inhalational agent) or regional anesthesia improve outcome or reduce the incidence of preterm delivery following surgery during pregnancy.

Parturients having intraabdominal surgical procedures should be advised that preterm delivery is a potential outcome. Monitoring of uterine activity by direct visualization of the uterus during surgery, or by tocodynamometry perioperatively, should be performed to detect preterm labor. Steps should be taken to monitor for this occurrence so that pharmacologic therapy can be initiated if necessary. Ritodrine or terbutaline (beta₂ sympathomimetic agents) may be useful acutely to prevent or stop preterm labor perioperatively. Intravenous magnesium sulfate may also be efficacious in this setting.

Pharmacologic Effect of Drugs on the Fetus

When they are given to the parturient just before delivery of the infant, pharmacologic agents that alter CNS function may also produce neurologic effects in the newborn. Because of functional similarities between the blood-brain barrier and the placental "barrier," one should follow the general rule that if a drug is active in the maternal central nervous system it will both cross the placenta and be active in the fetus. The fetal central nervous system is not as well developed as the adult and is more sensitive to depressant drugs such as sedatives and narcotic agonists. Meperidine, for example, is frequently used as a narcotic analgesic during labor. Meperidine readily crosses the placenta to the fetus. One product of meperidine metabolism, normeperidine, is very slowly excreted by the fetus and may cause sedation, seizures, or alter ventilatory response to CO_2 postnatally. Infants born several hours after administration of meperidine to the mother may be more depressed than one would normally expect.

Several classes of drugs have effects on the newborn infant after maternal administration. All narcotic agonists may be associated with newborn respiratory depression, and treatment with specific narcotic antagonists such as naloxone is indicated whenever this depression is clinically significant. Di-

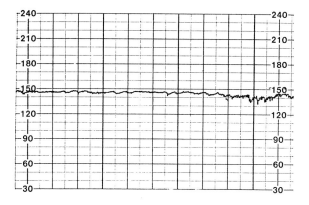

FIGURE 22-2. Although the baseline fetal heart rate is normal in this tracing, the variabilty is decreased. Although this could indicate fetal stress, this change could also be caused by an anesthetic-induced fetal sleep state (see text).

azepam may disrupt central thermal regulation in the newborn. Hypnotic agents such as the barbiturates can lead to depressed infants at birth. Ketamine, when used in doses exceeding 1 mg/kg, causes muscle rigidity in the newborn[20] and may complicate basic supportive measures such as endotracheal intubation and artificial respiration. Finally, prophylactic antibiotics administered before clamping of the umbilical cord may result in neonatal antibiotic concentrations that may interfere with bacteriologic diagnoses in the newborn period.

Teratogenic Effect of Drugs on the Fetus

In the human fetus, major organ development is complete by the thirteenth week of gestation with the exception of ongoing gamete formation and central nervous system differentiation and myelinization. Theoretically, teratogenesis involving organ systems other than the central nervous system or the reproductive tract should be temporally limited to the first trimester, and drugs administered after this trimester are unlikely to cause problems with organogenesis.

Animal models are frequently used to study the first trimester teratogenic effect of drugs. When analyzing animal studies to determine the teratogenic potential of drugs, it must be kept in mind that there are marked interspecies differences in the teratogenic effects of drugs. As an example, thalidomide, clearly a human teratogenic agent, was benign when tested in rats. Only repeat testing in other animal models and, of course, the results following clinical use in humans revealed its marked teratogenicity. Another difficulty in interpreting animal studies arises from the need to extrapolate from the large doses used in most animal studies down to the much smaller doses employed in clinical practice. For these reasons, statements regarding drug-induced teratogenicity in humans, based on nonprimate animal research, may or may not be valid.

Among anesthetic agents studied in humans, the only class of drug implicated to have teratogenic potential is the benzodiazepines. Cleft lip and/or palate malformation may occur in children after maternal administration of benzodiazapines in the first trimester.[37] All other commonly used anesthetic agents have either not been studied in large enough series, or have no remarkable teratogenic potential following *acute* administration to humans.

Chronic administration of anesthetic gases, even at subanesthetic concentrations, has been studied.

> **Signs and symptoms associated with severe preeclampsia**
>
> 1. Systolic blood pressure over 160, diastolic blood pressure over 110
> 2. Headache, mental confusion, scotomata
> 3. Abdominal pain
> 4. Pulmonary edema
> 5. Oliguria (<400 ml/24 hr)
> 6. Proteinuria (>5 gm/24 hr)
> 7. Thrombocytopenia (<100,000/mm³)

Although the results are inconclusive, chronic administration of nitrous oxide and potent inhalation agents may have teratogenic effects. For instance, studies measuring the miscarriage rate among operating room personnel indicate that female personnel who are chronically exposed to trace concentrations of anesthetic gases have miscarriage rates higher than their nonoperating room counterparts.[36] The miscarriage rate among wives of male anesthesiologists is also increased,[1] an observation suggesting that anesthetic agents have adverse effects on gametes as well.

MEDICAL PROBLEMS UNIQUE TO PREGNANCY
Toxemia of Pregnancy

Toxemia of pregnancy occurs in 5% of pregnancies and is defined as hypertension with edema and/or proteinuria. Preeclampsia describes toxemia of pregnancy without convulsions; patients with convulsions are termed eclamptic. Toxemia always occurs after the midpoint of gestation and is classified as either mild, moderate, or severe. This classification depends on the severity of hypertension and proteinuria and the presence of absence of associated signs. The characteristics associated with severe preeclampsia are listed in the box above, right.

Untreated toxemia may result in congestive heart failure, hypertensive crises, intracerebral hemorrhage, seizures, pulmonary aspiration, and acute renal insufficiency. A worrisome complication of severe preeclampsia is development of the HELLP syndrome, which consists of *h*emolysis, *e*levated *l*iver enzymes and hepatic damage, and thrombocytopenia (*low p*latelets). Hemorrhagic coagulopathy develops in up to 20% of patients with HELLP syndrome, and a marked increase in maternal and perinatal mortality have been noted. Accurate diagnosis and initiation of appropriate therapy is required to decrease the incidence of these serious complications.

Physiologically, toxemia is characterized by generalized vasoconstriction, decreased intravascular blood volume, and increased hematocrit (a hemoconcentration effect). Intervillous blood flow in the placenta is decreased, and intrauterine growth retardation can result. Nonobstetric surgery is rare in moderate to severe toxemia, because the definitive treatment of the underlying toxemia is delivery of the infant and removal of the placenta. However, in all patients having surgery after the twentieth week of pregnancy, the presence of toxemia should be ruled in or out, since the diagnosis has a profound potential impact on perioperative management.

Preoperative evaluation of a toxemia patient requires definition of the functional state of each organ system involved. Accurate blood pressure measurement and monitoring is key, since hypertension is an integral part of the disease and acute hypertensive crises can occur. Serum creatinine concentration will frequently be elevated above normal pregnancy values, and creatinine clearance is decreased. Serum liver enzyme concentration should be measured to

determine whether the HELLP syndrome is present or developing. A coagulation profile should be obtained, with special consideration given to the platelet count. If the platelet count is less than $100,000/mm^3$, coagulopathy can be considered to be present, since the bleeding time will almost always be prolonged. When the platelet count is $100,000/mm^3$ to $150,000/mm^3$, a bleeding time should be obtained in patients who exhibit signs of severe toxemia, since qualitative platelet dysfunction may also be present. Central nervous system hyperexcitability can be estimated by serially quantitating patellar and biceps deep tendon reflexes. Therapeutic levels of anticonvulsive medication should be achieved before surgery in all but extremely emergent circumstances. In emergency circumstances, an induction dose of barbiturate should provide an adequate and immediate (albeit short-lived) anticonvulsant effect.

Despite total body salt and water retention, intravascular volume is depleted in most patients with toxemia of pregnancy.[18] Foley catheterization of the bladder and measurement of urine output can assist in assessing intravascular volume status. Occasionally, central venous or pulmonary artery catheter-

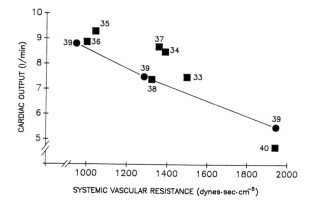

FIGURE 22-3. The hemodynamic findings of eight published studies of toxemic patients are shown on this graph. The range of systemic vascular resistance noted is wide, but a clear tendency to improved cardiac output (CO) at lower systemic vascular resistance (SVR) is present. Shnider SM et al show the change in SVR and CO observed following volume expansion (middle point) and volume expansion plus vasodilator therapy (left-hand point) in 10 otherwise untreated, nonlaboring preeclamptic patients. All the other studies included patients who had already received fluid therapy, magnesium, or other vasodilators, and were either in labor or were postpartum.

Benedetti TJ, Kates R and William V: Am J Obstet Gynecol 152:330-334, 1985; Benedetti TJ et al: Am J Obstet Gynecol 136:465-470, 1980; Cotton DB et al: Am J Obstet Gynecol 158:523-529, 1988; Clark SL et al: Am J Obstet Gynecol 154:490-494, 1986; Groenendijk R, Trimbos JBMJ, and Wallenburg HCS: Am J Obstet Gynecol 150:232-236, 1984; Hankins GDV et al: Am J Obset Gynecol 150:506-512, 1984; Phelan JP and Yurth DA: Am J Obstet Gynecol 144:17-22, 1982; and Strauss RG et al: Obstet Gynecol 55:170-174, 1980.

ization may be required to guide fluid therapy. When pulmonary artery catheterization is performed, most patients with toxemia of pregnancy demonstrate hyperdynamic left ventricular performance.[8] However, a subset of patients (usually severe preeclamptics) demonstrate depression of left and/or right ventricular function despite normal to high filling pressures.[6]

Data collected from eight individual studies* are plotted in Figure 22-3 to show the relationship between systemic vascular resistance and cardiac output in severe preeclamptics. There is a wide range of calculated systemic vascular resistances among the studies, and one might conclude that this simply represents physiologic variability. However, one major difference between the studies was the presence or absence of volume expansion and/or vasodilator therapy during the hemodynamic measurement. In those studies demonstrating moderate or markedly elevated systemic vascular resistance, patients tended to be on magnesium sulfate anticonvulsant therapy alone, or on no therapy at all. In contrast, those patients demonstrating only slightly elevated systemic vascular resistance (and higher cardiac output), tended to be receiving magnesium sulfate therapy, vasodilators, and fluid therapy. Groenendijk et al[13], in fact, demonstrated increasing cardiac output and lowered systemic vascular resistance sequentially in a group of 10 nonlaboring parturients as they were first given volume expansion and then vasodilator therapy (see Figure 22-3). In all, these studies suggest the importance of measuring cardiac output, calculating systemic vascular resistance, and basing therapeutic interventions on these hemodynamic variables to optimize systemic perfusion.

As far as anesthetic management is concerned, epidural anesthesia is the method of choice in preeclamptics. Although it has been suggested that spinal anesthesia is inappropriate in toxemics, there is no scientific evidence to support this contention as long as intravascular volume has been normalized. If general anesthesia is necessary, careful attention must be given to aspects of anesthetic management during which blood pressure elevation is a risk since cerebrovascular bleeds are the leading cause of death in toxemic patients. On induction and emergence, blood pressure control using parenteral agents is frequently necessary if severe hypertension is to be

*References 2,3,6,8,13,14,31,40.

avoided. Postoperative pain relief is likewise important, and intraspinal narcotics should be considered. If nondepolarizing muscle relaxants are used as part of perioperative care, the potential effect of concomitant magnesium sulfate use should be taken into account in dosing and reversing the muscle relaxant.

The ongoing risks of seizures, coagulopathy, and cardiorespiratory compromise mandate careful perioperative evaluation and monitoring. Complications of toxemia can occur in the postpartum period, since it can take weeks for normal organ function to return. The patient is especially at increased risk of seizures for the first 48 hours postpartum, and should have continued anticonvulsant prophylaxis for at least part of the postpartum period.

Cardiomyopathy of Pregnancy

In the absence of preexisting heart disease, peripartum cardiomyopathy is defined as cardiomyopathy that presents between the last month of pregnancy and the sixth postpartum month. Infectious, metabolic, and toxic cardiomyopathies must be excluded. Patients with peripartum cardiomyopathy usually have signs and symptoms consistent with congestive heart failure including fatigue, dyspnea on exertion, and peripheral edema. They may have chest pain, hemoptysis, and cough. Blood pressure may be elevated, normal, or decreased. Hemodynamic studies demonstrate elevated right and left heart filling pressures with diminished cardiac output.[19] Echocardiography reveals global left ventricular systolic dysfunction.[19] The long-term prognosis of this disease is poor, with reported mortality rates exceeding 50%.[9] Although perioperative risks in these patients have never been studied, the high mortality of the disease mandates appropriate identification and treatment.

Treatment modalities for peripartum cardiomyopathy include bed rest, digoxin, diuretics, and sodium restriction. Vasodilator therapy has been advocated, and intravenous inotropic support may be useful. Melvin et al[27] and Ghosh et al[12] found beneficial responses to immunosuppression therapy in 5 patients, 2 of whom had endomyocardial biopsy evidence of inflammatory reaction. These findings suggest that endomyocardial biopsy may be useful when planning medical therapy for this condition. If cardiac decompensation persists despite treatment, heart transplantation may provide the only means of survival. Anticoagulation to prevent systemic embolization may be required, but full anticoagulation during pregnancy is controversial, and subcutaneous heparin (which does not cross the placental barrier) may be preferable.

When patients present for surgery in the third trimester with the diagnosis of peripartum cardiomyopathy, appropriate anesthetic management is controversial. If the patient presents for delivery, induction of labor with an abbreviated second stage has been advocated. Such patients should receive adequate analgesia to minimize the pain of labor and reduce the stress response. Cesarean section should be used when deemed necessary. In patients with congestive heart failure and pulmonary edema of unclear etiologic origin, right-sided heart catheterization is advisable before the initiation of any anesthetic. If general anesthesia is planned, use of agents that do not cause myocardial depression is important. If a patient with peripartum cardiomyopathy presents for surgery other than delivery, either during or following pregnancy, these same precautions regarding anesthetic technique and monitoring apply.

SUMMARY

The unique aspects of maternal and fetal physiology need to be considered whenever caring for pregnant patients. Careful attention to providing optimal fetal conditions without compromising maternal well-being is necessary. This will frequently require more monitoring of the mother in the perioperative period than would normally be performed in young relatively healthy patients, as well as familiarity with the specificities of fetal monitoring. Cooperation and communication among all the subspecialists involved—the surgeon, obstetrician, anesthesiologist, intensivist, and neonatologist—is essential to provide the best possible perioperative care for both patients.

REFERENCES

1. Askrog V and Harvald B: Teratogen effect of inhalation anesthetics, Nord Med 83:498-500, 1970.
2. Benedetti TJ, Kates R, and Williams V: Hemodynamic observations in severe preeclampsia complicated by pulmonary edema, Am J Obstet Gynecol 152:330-334, 1985.
3. Benedetti TJ et al: Hemodynamic observations in severe pre-eclampsia with a flow-directed pulmonary artery catheter, Am J Obstet Gynecol 136:465-470, 1980.
4. Bonica JJ: Obstetric analgesia and anesthesia, Amsterdam, 1980, The World Federation of Societies of Anaesthesiologists.
5. Bromage PR, Camporesi E, and Chestnut D: Epidural narcotics for postoperative analgesia, Anesth Analg 59:473-480, 1980.
6. Clark SL et al: Severe preeclampsia with persistent oliguria: management of hemodynamic subsets, Am J Obstet Gynecol 154:490-494, 1986.
7. Cohen SE et al: Does metoclopramide decrease the volume of gastric contents in patients undergoing cesarean section? Anesthesiology 61:604-607, 1984.
8. Cotton DB et al: Hemodynamic profile of severe pregnancy-induced hypertension, Am J Obstet Gynecol 158:523-529, 1988.
9. Cunningham FG et al: Peripartum heart failure: idiopathic cardiomyopathy or compounding cardiovascular events? Obstet Gynecol 67:157-168, 1987.
10. Davison JM and Noble MCB. Serial changes in 24 hour creatinine clearance during normal menstrual cycles and the 1st trimester of pregnancy, Br J Obstet Gynaecol 88:10, 1980.
11. Finn WF: Maternal welfare - Nassau County, New York, 1957-1981. (review), Obstet Gynecol Surv 39:127-133, 1984.
12. Ghosh JC, Neelakantan C, and Chhetri MK. Peripartal cardiomyopathy: a clinical and haemodynamic study, Indian Heart J 26:213-218, 1974.
13. Groenendijk R, Trimbos JBMJ, and Wallenburg HCS. Hemodynamic measurements in preeclampsia: preliminary observations, Am J Obstet Gynecol 150:232-236, 1984.
14. Hankins GDV et al: Longitudinal evaluation of hemodynamic changes in eclampsia, Am J Obstet Gynecol 150:506-512, 1984.
15. Harris AP et al: Cerebral and peripheral circulatory responses to intracranial hypertension in fetal sheep, Circ Res (in press), 1989.
16. Hasaart TH and de Haan J: Effect of continuous infusion of norepinephrine on maternal pelvic and fetal umbilical blood flow in pregnant sheep, J Perinat Med 14:211-218, 1986.
17. Hathaway WE and Bonnar J: Coagulation in pregnancy. In Hathaway WE and Bonnar J (editors): Perinatal coagulation, New York, 1978, Grune & Stratton, Inc.
18. Hays PM, Cruikshank DP, and Dunn LJ: Plasma volume determination in normal and preeclamptic pregnancies, Am J Obstet Gynecol 151:958-966, 1985.
19. Homans DC: Peripartum cardiomyopathy, N Engl J Med 312:1432-1437, 1985.
20. Janeczko GF, El-Etr AA, and Younes S: Low-dose ketamine anesthesia for obstetrical delivery, Anesth Analg 53:828-831, 1974.

21. Jones MD et al: Fetal cerebral oxygen consumption at different levels of oxygenation, J Appl Physiol 43(6):1080-1084, 1977.

22. Kambam JR et al: Effect of pre-eclampsia on carboxyhemoglobin levels: a mechanism for a decrease in P_{50}, Anesthesiology 68:433-434, 1988.

23. Kerr MG, Scott DB, and Samule E: Studies of the inferior vena cava in late pregnancy, Br Med J 1:532-533, 1964.

24. Lees MM, Taylor SH, and Scott DB: A study of cardiac output at rest throughout pregnancy, J Obstet Gynaecol Br Commonw 74:319-328, 1967.

25. Lind T and Hytten FE: The excretion of glucose during normal pregnancy, J Obstet Gynaecol Br Common 79:961, 1972.

26. Lindheimer MD and Katz AI: The kidney in pregnancy. In Brenner BM and Rector FC (editors): The kidney, ed 3, Philadelphia, 1986, WB Saunders Co.

27. Melvin KR et al: Peripartum cardiomyopathy due to myocarditis, N Engl J Med 307:731-734, 1982.

28. Myers RE: Maternal psychological stress and fetal asphyxia: a study in the monkey, Am J Obstet Gynecol 122:47-59, 1975.

29. Niswander KR: Asphyxia in the fetus and cerebral palsy. In Pitkin RM and Zlatnik FJ (editors): 1983 Year book of obstetrics and gynecology, Chicago, 1983, Year Book Medical Publishers, Inc.

30. Palahniuk RJ, Shnider SM, and Eger EL II: Pregnancy decreases the requirement of inhaled anesthetic agents, Anesthesiology 41:82-83, 1974.

31. Phelan JP and Yurth DA: Severe preeclampsia. I. Peripartum hemodynamic observations, Am J Obstet Gynecol 144:17-22, 1982.

32. Pitkin RM: Nutritional influences during pregnancy, Med Clin North Am 61:3, 1977.

33. Pitkin RM and Witte DL: Platelet and leukocyte counts in pregnancy, JAMA 242:2696-2698, 1979.

34. Pritchard JA: Changes in the blood volume during pregnancy and delivery, Anesthesiology 26:393-399, 1965.

35. Rosen MA et al: Epidural morphine for relief of postoperative pain after cesarean delivery, Anesth Analg 62:666-672, 1983.

36. Rosenberg P and Kirves A: Miscarriages among operating theatre staff, Acta Anaesth Scand 53:S37-S42, 1973.

37. Safra MJ and Oakley GP: Association between cleft lip with or without cleft palate and prenatal exposure to diazepam, Lancet 2:478-480, 1975.

38. Shnider SM: Serum cholinesterase activity during pregnancy, labor and puerperium, Anesthesiology 26:335-339, 1965.

39. Snider SM et al: Uterine blood flow and plasma norepinephrine changes during maternal stress in the pregnant ewe, Anesthesiology 50:524-527, 1979.

40. Strauss RG et al: Hemodynamic monitoring of cardiogenic pulmonary edema complicating toxemia of pregnancy, Obstet Gynecol 55:170-174, 1980.

41. Tomkins J et al: Report on confidential enquiries into maternal deaths in England and Wales 1976-1978. London, 1982, Department of Health and Social Security, Her Majesty's Stationery Office.

42. Ueland K: Maternal cardiovascular dynamics. VII. Intrapartum blood volume changes, Am J Obstet Gynecol 126:671-677, 1976.

43. Ueland K and Hansen JM: Maternal cardiovascular dynamics. III. Labor and delivery under local and caudal analgesia, Am J Obstet Gynecol 103:8-18, 1969.

44. Ueland K, Novy MJ, and Peterson EN: Maternal cardiovascular dynamics. IV. The influence of gestational age on the maternal cardiovascular response to posture and exercise, Am J Obstet Gynecol 104:856-864, 1969.

CHAPTER **23**

Renal Failure

CLAIR F. MILLER

Perioperative management of patients requiring
  dialysis
  Perioperative risks
  Perioperative management

Perioperative acute renal failure: prevention and
  management
  Incidence and outcome
  Causes and pathogenesis
  Preventive management
  Management of acute perioperative renal
    failure

Patients with preexisting renal disease and those who develop renal dysfunction after anesthesia and surgery have greater than normal perioperative morbidity and mortality. Management goals designed to improve outcome vary with the extent of preexisting renal dysfunction. This chapter addresses two distinctly different management issues: (1) perioperative management of patients with established renal failure and (2) management strategies designed to minimize the risk for developing acute renal failure, a common perioperative complication. The chapter first discusses specific problems unique to patients with severely impaired renal function and identifies how these disturbances require alterations in perioperative management. The second part of the chapter examines mechanisms responsible for development of perioperative renal failure and reviews therapeutic options designed to decrease the incidence of this severe complication.

PERIOPERATIVE MANAGEMENT OF PATIENTS REQUIRING DIALYSIS

The population of functionally anephric patients who require regular dialytic care for survival is growing. These patients probably require more operative interventions in their lifetimes than any other group of patients. Pinson et al[102] reported the following statistics: per patient per year, dialysis patients undergo 1.1 vascular access and 0.28 nonaccess surgical procedures. Of all operations performed on these patients, 86% are procedures to establish vascular access for dialysis. Thus an expanding population of high-risk patients requires frequent operative interventions.

Perioperative Risks

Factors that increase morbidity and mortality of dialysis patients undergoing anesthesia and surgery include the following: (1) underlying diseases that

TABLE 23-1. Causes of end-stage renal failure in 16,000 patients

	Percent of cases
Glomerulonephritis	28.3
Pyelo/interstitial nephritis	20.4
Unknown	12.8
Hereditary/congenital	11.6
Diabetes	10.2
Miscellaneous known	8.6
Vascular/hypertensive	8.1

Adapted from Broyer M et al: Demography of dialysis and transplantation in Europe, 1984, Nephrology Dialysis Transplantation 1:1-8, 1986.

Abnormalities of End-stage Renal Failure That May Alter Perioperative Management

Acid base balance
Electrolyte disturbances
Impaired nutrition
Defective immune responses
Anemia
Bleeding disorders
Cardiovascular abnormalities
Impaired drug elimination

---

cause renal failure, (2) interactions of physiologic abnormalities of renal failure with the stresses of the perioperative time, and (3) the type of surgical procedure performed.

Diseases that cause renal failure. The primary causes of renal failure in 16,000 patients who began regular dialysis therapy in Europe during 1984 are listed in Table 23-1.[17] Diseases such as hypertension and diabetes may themselves adversely influence outcome and require special perioperative management. Management of these diseases is discussed in other chapters in this book. The goal of this section is to assess the impact of renal failure itself on the clinical course and management of dialysis patients.

Physiologic complications of renal failure. End-stage renal disease results in many physiologic abnormalities, which are outlined in the box above, right. These abnormalities occur regularly and predictably regardless of the immediate cause of renal disease. Despite intuitive assumptions that such derangements adversely affect outcome, few reports detail the impact of these abnormalities on the perioperative course of patients with renal failure.

Before dialysis techniques were established as standard renal replacement therapy, the perioperative outcome of patients with the uremic syndrome was dismal. Schreiner et al[108] reviewed the clinical course of 24 nondialyzed patients with chronic renal failure (BUN, mean value = 124; range = 41-300 mg/dl) having unidentified "major surgical procedures" under general anesthesia; operative mortality was 12.5%. Two patients died intraoperatively of cardiac arrest and another patient died in the early postop-

erative period of uncontrolled hypotension. Patients in whom BUN levels exceeded 100 mg/dl had a 50% incidence of significant perioperative bleeding, whereas patients with BUN values below 100 mg/dl had a 12% incidence of bleeding. Schreiner suggested that perioperative dialysis therapy may decrease the high morbidity and mortality observed in uremic patients.[108] Since controlled studies to evaluate the effect of dialysis on perioperative outcome will never be done, it is remarkable that few institutions have reported their experience with dialysis patients undergoing surgical procedures. The collective results of five such studies are reviewed below.[16,50,51,77,102]

The 585 surgical procedures performed on 334 patients are summarized chronologically in Figure 23-1. These procedures do not include vascular access operations, renal transplantation, or radiographic or diagnostic procedures except endoscopy. Procedures directly related to pathologic conditions of the kidney predominated in the early years of dialysis, but operations in recent years include a greater percentage of elective hernia, endoscopic, breast, gynecologic, and orthopedic procedures. The declining percentage of nephrectomies reflects both increased numbers of other elective procedures and elimination of pretransplant nephrectomy as a routine procedure.[110]

The preoperative characteristics of these patients are shown in Table 23-2. All patients required regular maintenance dialysis for more than 1.5 months before surgery. Preoperative hematocrit values averaged 23% to 29% and blood transfusions were infrequently given before surgery. Serum potassium, BUN, and creatinine concentrations were well controlled because 68% of patients underwent dialysis

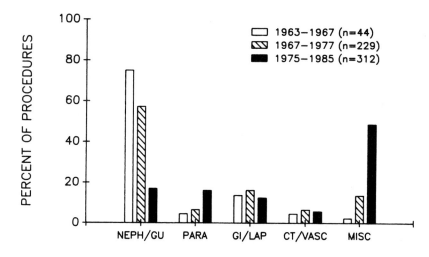

FIGURE 23-1. Chronologic distribution of 585 surgical procedures performed on 334 dialysis patients from 1963 through 1985. NEPH/GU, nephrectomy/other genitourinary; PARA, parathyroidectomy; GI/LAP, gastrointestinal/other laparotomy; CT/VASC, cardiothoracic/major vascular; MISC, miscellaneous.

From Brenowitz JB, Williams CD, and Edwards WS: Am J Surg 134:765-769, 1977; Haimov M et al: Ann Surg 179:863-867, 1974; Hampers CL et al: Am J Surg 115:747-754, 1968; Lissoos I et al: Br J Urol 45:359-365, 1973; and Pinson CW et al: Am J Surg 151:567-571, 1986.

TABLE 23-2. Preoperative data for dialysis patients undergoing surgical procedures

REF	N	Laboratory values				Preop dialysis		
		HCT	K+	BUN	CREAT	<24	24-48	>48
51	44	28	4.8	54	9.0	30	9	5
77	113	23	<6.0	50	4.3	61	41	3
50	67	24	NA	50	4.3	NA	NA	NA
16	49	26	<5.0	NA	NA	43	5	1
102	312	29	4.7	64	NA	[181]		10

Mean preoperative laboratory values for HCT, hematocrit (%); K+, serum potassium (mEq/L); BUN, blood urea nitrogen (mg/dl); and CREAT, serum creatinine (mg/dl). Timing of last preoperative dialysis in hours. N, number of procedures; REF, reference number of study; NA, not available.

less than 24 hours before surgery. Only 13 procedures were clearly identified as emergencies. No intraoperative information was reported, except that general anesthesia was used in 66%, spinal or epidural techniques in 8%, and local agents with intravenous sedation were employed in 26% of procedures.

Postoperative complications occurred often in these patients; the incidence of each is listed in Table 23-3. While the accuracy of such listings may be flawed by imprecise definitions and interobserver variations in identifying problems, qualitative trends that are relevant to the postoperative course can be observed.[102] Hyperkalemia tended to occur in the early postoperative hours and was the primary reason for which 36% of cases required dialysis within the first 24 hours after surgery. Complications related to intravascular volume status were reflected by arterial blood pressure fluctuations during the first and second postoperative days. Shunt thrombosis caused by

TABLE 23-3. Postoperative complications for dialysis patients undergoing surgical procedures

	Number of occurrences	Percent of occurrences
Hyperkalemia	138	29.4
Shunt thrombosis	55	11.2
Pneumonia	52	11.1
Wound complications (including infection)	45	9.6
Hypotension	41	8.7
Hypertension	36	7.7
Hemorrhage	25	5.3
Hypoventilation	17	3.6
Sepsis	12	2.6
Miscellaneous	49	10.3

Complications observed after 585 surgical procedures on 334 dialysis patients. Some patients had more than one complication. Data compiled from Brenowitz JB, Williams CD, and Edwards WS: Am J Surg 134:765-769, 1977; Haimov M et al: Ann Surg 179:863-867, 1974; Hampers CL et al: Am J Surg 115:747-754, 1968; Lissoos I et al: Br J Urol 45:359-365, 1973; and Pinson CW et al: Am J Surg 151:567-571, 1986.

either malpositioning of the extremities during operation or by perioperative hypotensive episodes was discovered at intervals throughout the first postoperative week. Infectious complications (wound, sepsis, pneumonia, and intraabdominal) were common and occurred late in the postoperative course. Myocardial ischemic events and congestive heart failure were not listed as postoperative complications.

Sixteen deaths occurred in these patients, resulting in an operative mortality of 4.8% of patients (2.7% of procedures). All deaths occurred in patients having major surgical procedures under general anesthesia, and 63% of deaths occurred in patients having emergency procedures. The majority of deaths occurred after the first postoperative day and were caused by hyperkalemia in 25%, protracted sepsis in 25%, and myocardial failure in 12.5%. (The two patients who died of myocardial failure had emergency valve replacement for acute endocarditis.) One remaining patient had fulminant hepatic failure, and the other died as a result of refractory and unexplained hypotension. The authors considered that two deaths could have been prevented if uncorrected hyperkalemia (6.5 mEq/L preoperatively in one and 8.5 mEq/L postoperatively in another) had been more aggressively treated.

Type of surgical procedure. In addition to underlying disease states and the untoward effects of physiologic abnormalities in renal failure, perioperative outcome is also related to the type and invasiveness of the surgical procedure performed. Operations to establish vascular access for dialysis are usually performed under local or regional anesthesia and are generally well tolerated with few complications reported.[73,101] In contrast, studies of large series of dialysis patients undergoing pretransplant nephrectomy report operative mortality rates as high as 4% and note a high incidence of postoperative bleeding, infection, and fluid and electrolyte abnormalities.[81,121,127]

Zamora et al[129] reviewed the clinical course of dialysis patients undergoing cardiac surgical procedures between 1966 and 1984. Of 85 patients, 45 (53%) had coronary revascularization, 37 (43.5%) had valvular procedures, and 3 (3.5%) had combined procedures. Emergency valve replacement for acute endocarditis was the most common cardiac procedure performed in the early years of dialysis; it had an associated mortality rate of 57%. In recent years, elective aortocoronary bypass procedures predominate and have a mortality rate of 4%. Significant postoperative bleeding was observed in 10.6% of these patients and contributed to a fatal outcome in two. Of the seven deaths in this series (12% of patients), sepsis was listed as the cause in two and myocardial failure in two. Ventricular fibrillation, cerebrovascular accident, and insulin overdose each accounted for one death. Myocardial infarction probably contributed to the death of one septic patient.

Summary of perioperative risks. Despite continuation of dialysis therapy in the perioperative time, the rate of complications and death remain high. Mortality rates are greatest in patients having invasive surgical procedures and in patients requiring emergency operations. Whether perioperative outcome has improved in recent years cannot be determined from the existing literature. Nevertheless, optimal management of dialysis patients undergoing anesthesia and surgery must account for all the physiologic abnormalities of the anephric state to minimize perioperative complications.

Perioperative Management

The dialysis records of patients with end-stage renal disease should be reviewed for information that can guide perioperative management. General medical condition and drug requirements should be ascertained before surgical intervention. Correlation of body weight with arterial blood pressure and heart rate before and after dialysis provides a noninvasive index by which to gauge the adequacy of intravascular volume status. Knowledge of the levels of hyperkalemia, anemia, and hypertension the patient normally tolerates without untoward sequelae may assist in determining the need for postoperative dialysis, transfusion, and fluid therapy.

Timing of dialysis therapy. Dialysis therapy must be continued in the perioperative time to remove toxic substances, to manage hyperkalemia, to control metabolic acidosis, and to remove excess sodium and body water. While intraoperative hemodialysis has been successfully accomplished,[96] dialysis-dependent patients should be routinely dialyzed within 24 hours of the planned surgical intervention. Hyperkalemia is the most common indication for early postoperative dialysis in most series. Of various strategies to lower plasma potassium in hyperkalemic emergencies, Blumberg et al[13] recently found hemodialysis to be the most rapidly effective. Insulin in glucose by intravenous infusion was also a fast and reliable form of therapy. In contrast, bicarbonate administration was ineffective, and epinephrine infusion lowered plasma potassium in only 50% of patients.[13] Ion-exchange resins are commonly used to treat postoperative hyperkalemia,[104] but Lillimoe et al[75] warn that enemas of sodium polystyrene sulfonate (Kayexalate, in sorbitol) may cause extensive ischemic colitis and death in uremic patients. Modification of standard dialysis techniques may be required to prevent problems such as bleeding, hypotension, and hypoventilation, which are particularly troublesome to the postoperative patient. Regional anticoagulation during dialysis with heparin or citrate may reduce bleeding complications.[59] Maynard et al[86] reported that increasing the dialysate concentration of calcium protected against hypotension during normovolemic dialysis without causing hypercalcemia or metastatic calcifications. Use of bicarbonate-containing dialysate solutions should avoid the hypoxemia and hypoventilation observed after dialysis with acetate solutions.[33] A review of the principles and complications of various renal replacement techniques (hemodialysis, peritoneal dialysis, and continuous arteriovenous hemofiltration) available for use in the perioperative time was recently presented by Prough.[104]

Management of anemia and bleeding abnor-malities. Anemia is a regular and predictable consequence of end-stage renal failure that is generally well tolerated. Lundin et al[80] studied the response to treadmill exercise of dialysis patients with hematocrits averaging 25%. Exhaustive exercise increased arterial blood pressure and heart rate by 30% and 100% above resting values, respectively, but resulted in minimal changes in arterial pH, lactate, and serum electrolyte levels.[80] These data suggest that the compensatory limits of cardiac output, oxygen delivery, and tissue oxygen extraction[5] were not exceeded at levels of hemodynamic stress that frequently occur in the perioperative time. Routine preoperative transfusion to normal hematocrits is not indicated, but blood administration should not be withheld when needed for fear of sensitization to histocompatibility antigens.[99] Erythropoietin deficiency is the primary cause of the normochromic-normocytic anemia of end-stage renal failure.[41,43] Eschbach et al[41] recently demonstrated that administration of human recombinant erythropoietin to dialysis patients caused a dose-dependent increase in hematocrit to normal values. The major complication of increased hematocrit in erythropoietin-treated patients was the new appearance or exacerbation of hypertension in some patients. Since dialysis patients with normal hematocrit values have better appetites and an improved sense of well-being, widespread use of erythropoietin may increase both dialysis requirements and the need for antihypertensive therapy in some patients.[40] Of note, Livio et al[78] suggest that the rheologic properties of blood at hematocrits above 30% may shorten bleeding time and decrease bleeding tendencies of dialysis patients.

The cause of increased bleeding in dialysis patients is incompletely understood, but prolongation of bleeding time is frequently observed. While total platelet count and indicators of thrombopoietic activity may be lower in these patients than in nonuremic controls,[44] abnormal platelet function appears to be primarily responsible for the prolonged bleeding time. Recent evidence suggests that Factor VIII/ von Willebrand antigen is decreased in uremia and that perioperative infusion of either cryoprecipitate or 1-desamino-8-D-arginine vasopressin (desmopressin) shortens bleeding time, increases circulating levels of Factor VIII/von Willebrand antigen, and decreases blood loss in dialysis patients undergoing surgical procedures.[61,83] Similar effects are also observed in hematologically normal patients undergoing Harrington rod spinal fusion[67] and cardiac surgical procedures.[107] Thus the hematologic effects of desmopressin are not specific to uremia, and this drug can be effectively used to shorten bleeding time in many coagulation disorders. Canavese et al[20] caution that repeated doses of desmopressin to uremic patients postoperatively may lead to a decreased response over time and may actually increase the baseline bleeding time between treatments. Desmopressin may be most effectively used in patients undergoing procedures in which a large blood loss is anticipated, or in patients who develop unexpected perioperative bleeding. Alternatively, recent evidence suggests that conjugated estrogens shorten the bleeding time of dialysis patients, have a longer duration of action than desmopressin, and have no identified side effects.[79] Neither the mechanism of action nor the indications for estrogen use in surgical patients has been defined. Bleeding tendencies in uremia are only minimally improved by dialysis therapy.[27,105]

Gastrointestinal bleeding is common in anephric patients,[84] and these patients should receive prophylactic therapy for stress ulcer bleeding in the perioperative time. Cimetidine, antacids, and sucralfate are equally effective in preventing stress ulcer bleeding.[15,113,118] Driks et al[36] suggest that patients treated with sucralfate have less gastric colonization with gram-negative bacteria and a lower incidence of nosocomial pneumonia than patients treated with either antacids or histamine type 2 blockers. Sucralfate may, therefore, be the prophylactic agent of choice in renal failure unless concerns about aluminum intoxication preclude its use.[100]

Infectious and metabolic problems. Infectious complications occur commonly in patients with chronic renal failure and are often responsible for perioperative morbidity and mortality (see Table 23-3). Cutaneous anergy,[6] protein-calorie malnutrition,[128] and abnormalities of neutrophil and monocyte function[74] contribute to increased susceptibility to infection, and the postoperative catabolic state may accentuate these abnormalities. Cutaneous anergy in surgical patients has been linked to increased risk for sepsis and mortality.[90] Perioperative nutritional support may reverse the anergic status and improve operative outcome in anephric patients.[95] Frequent instrumentation of the vascular tree provides a portal for inoculation with infectious agents. Frequent blood transfusions have made infectious hepatitis (hepatitis B, non-A and non-B) a major

problem for dialysis patients and for the staff who care for them.[114]

Recent evidence indicates that subcutaneous oxygen tension falls markedly and in parallel with decreases in body weight during routine hemodialysis.[62] Subcutaneous oxygen tension is similarly reduced in nonuremic surgical patients during periods of hypovolemia.[22,64] Reduced oxygen tensions promptly increase with volume repletion but are unaffected by increased concentrations of inspired oxygen.[62,64] While no attempt was made to correlate low subcutaneous oxygen tension with impaired wound healing in these studies, perioperative hypovolemia in the dialysis patient may contribute both to the high incidence of this problem and to the increased overall susceptibility to infection observed in patients with end-state renal disease. Prudent management of uremic surgical patients should, therefore, include both maintenance of effective intravascular volume and strict adherence to aseptic techniques. Reflexly limiting fluid therapy in patients with anuric renal disease may be detrimental since large fluctuations of intravascular volume occur in the perioperative time.[110]

Cardiovascular and fluid management. Ischemic myocardial disease is the most common cause of death in patients with end-stage renal disease.[17] The high incidence of coronary artery disease in this population probably reflects the presence of multiple risk factors for ischemic disease[106] rather than accelerated atherosclerotic processes peculiar to uremia.[76] Despite the high incidence of coronary artery disease, ischemic complications in the perioperative time are rarely reported in dialysis patients (see Table 23-3). While myocardial failure is a common cause of postoperative death, most of these deaths were in patients who had acute endocarditis with valvular disruption, rather than ventricular failure from ischemic disease. However, cardiovascular complications referable to intravascular volume status such as hypertension, hypotension, and shunt thrombosis are frequently observed (see Table 23-3). Uremic patients exhibit a wide range of hemodynamic abnormalities when studied during hemodialysis.[39,66] The striking feature of these studies is that the peripheral vasculature responds abnormally to hypovolemia induced by dialysis. Hypovolemia decreases arterial blood pressure without increasing heart rate. Peripheral vascular resistance is unchanged or decreased because cardiac output tends to increase. Thus the cardiovascular management of dialysis patients can be difficult because of existing myocardial dysfunction, coronary artery disease, presence of arteriovenous shunts, autonomic dysfunction, and the unpredictable effects of uremia, acidosis, and adrenergic stimuli on the peripheral circulation.[39,66] Patients undergoing major surgical procedures probably should be monitored with central venous or pulmonary capillary wedge pressure measurements to guide perioperative fluid management. Continued careful observation is required throughout the first postoperative week because resorption of "third space" fluid into the intravascular compartment occurs during this time. Increased intravascular volume is often manifested initially by progressively elevated arterial blood pressure in anephric patients. If dialysis therapy is promptly instituted, the consequences of severe volume overload such as pulmonary edema, respiratory failure, congestive heart failure, and precipitation of myocardial ischemia in susceptible patients can be avoided.

Pharmacologic management. Dialysis-dependent patients require many medications for treatment of both underlying and intercurrent diseases. Since drug usage increases unavoidably in the perioperative time, surgical patients are at risk of adverse drug reactions regardless of preexisting renal function.[85] To minimize the effects of drug reactions, pharmacologic management of anephric surgical patients must account for the loss of renal mechanisms for drug elimination, the biochemical derangements of uremia that alter drug bioavailability, the altered volume of distribution, and the effect of dialysis on drug removal. Comprehensive reviews of recommended dosage schedules for patients with renal failure are published regularly.[11,120] The specific concerns of end-stage renal failure affecting intraoperative administration of anesthetic agents have been discussed in recent reviews.[123,126] This discussion briefly summarizes the effects of drugs commonly used in the perioperative time to illustrate several pharmacologic principles affecting drug therapy in renal failure.

Analgesic therapy is required throughout the perioperative time, but prolonged narcosis and ventilatory depression are reported after standard dosages of morphine in surgical patients with renal failure.[34] Chauvin et al[23] demonstrated that high levels of pharmacologically active glucuronide metabolites of morphine, but not unchanged morphine, accumulated in plasma of renal failure patients. Thus hepatic metabolism appears to be normal, but loss of renal mechanisms for elimination of morphine metabolites accounts for the untoward effects. Titration of small doses of morphine under close observation will achieve the desired analgesic effect without causing respiratory depression.

Dundee et al[37] noted that standard anesthetic induction doses of short-acting barbiturates have prolonged sedative effects in uremic patients. Ghoneim et al[47] later demonstrated that approximately 60% of a standard dose of thiopental remained free and unbound to plasma proteins in uremic patients compared to 28% in normal patients. Thus the bioavailability of barbiturates in uremia is dramatically increased as a result of impaired serum protein binding. As with morphine, careful titration of small doses of barbiturates to obtain the desired effect will avoid prolonged postoperative somnolence and respiratory depression.

The recent introduction of non–renally excreted muscle relaxants should decrease the incidence of residual neuromuscular blockade as a cause of postoperative ventilatory failure in uremic patients. Although traditional nondepolarizing blocking agents (gallamine, metocurine, pancuronium, and d-tubocurarine) can be safely used with careful neuromuscular monitoring in anephric patients; these agents depend 50% to 100% on the kidney for their elimination. The newer and shorter-acting nondepolarizing agents (vecuronium and atacurium) are eliminated from the body virtually independent of renal function. Vecuronium is 80% to 90% excreted in the bile,[119] and atacurium is nonenzymatically eliminated by Hoffmann degradation.[42] Succinylcholine, a depolarizing relaxant often used to facilitate endotracheal intubation, is hydrolyzed within minutes of administration by plasma pseudo-cholinesterases independent of renal function. However, succinylcholine predictably increases serum potassium levels by approximately 0.5 mEq/L in all patients and thus should be avoided in patients with elevated preoperative potassium levels.[68]

In summary, surgical procedures are increasingly common in a growing population of patients with end-stage renal failure who require dialysis for survival. Compared with patients with normal kidneys, the perioperative course of these patients is complicated by a high incidence of untoward events that may result in death. Since these complications reflect the abnormal physiology of the anephric state, they are predictable and can be minimized by careful perioperative supportive management. Recent advances in understanding and treatment of the hematologic, metabolic, cardiovascular, and pharmacologic abnormalities of renal failure may result in improved perioperative outcome for dialysis patients in the future.

PERIOPERATIVE ACUTE RENAL FAILURE: PREVENTION AND MANAGEMENT

Prevention of renal injury is the perioperative goal for management of patients with functioning kidneys. Regardless of the level of preoperative function, renal impairment that develops after anesthesia and surgery is associated with increased mortality. However, the factors responsible for mediating renal dysfunction are incompletely defined, and identification of high-risk patients is difficult. This section reviews the prognosis, suspected causes, and pathogenesis of acute perioperative renal deterioration so that management strategies that may improve outcome can be developed.

Incidence and Outcome

The prognosis for patients who develop acute renal failure after anesthesia and surgery depends on the level to which renal function deteriorates. Acute perioperative renal failure requiring dialysis has a worse prognosis than renal deterioration not requiring dialysis.

The incidence of acute perioperative renal failure requiring dialysis is not known for the overall population of patients undergoing anesthesia and surgery, because most studies are confined to specific and almost always high-risk operative procedures. Acute renal failure develops in 1.5% to 2.5% of patients having cardiac surgical procedures,[45,58,69] and in 2.0% to 2.5% of patients having aortic reconstructive procedures.[31,89] It is interesting that the incidence of acute renal failure in patients with functional renal allografts having cardiac or aortic procedures is similar to that of patients with native kidneys undergoing the same procedures, but the number of reported cases is small.[14,48,54,70,72]

The outcome of patients who develop acute perioperative renal failure requiring dialysis is listed in Table 23-4.[2,12,24,89,91] The extraordinarily high mortality is not related to the type of surgical procedure,

and the outcome of postoperative renal failure has not improved in recent years despite advances in management. To account for these disappointing statistics, Abreo et al[2] suggest that a higher incidence of nephrotoxin exposure, sepsis, and hypotension occurs in patients with more severe underlying diseases than was encountered in previous decades.

The incidence of developing less severe impairment of renal function following surgery has not been vigorously studied, but it appears to be fairly high and is also associated with increased mortality.[60,115] Hou et al[60] observed that renal insufficiency developed in 4.9% of 2216 consecutive admissions to the general medical and surgical wards of a large university hospital. (Renal insufficiency was defined as an increase in creatinine of 0.5 mg/dl or more for patients with an admission creatinine level of 1.9 mg/dl or less, an increase of 1.0 mg/dl or more for patients with a baseline level of 2.0 to 4.9 mg/dl, and an increase of 1.5 mg/dl for patients with a baseline creatinine level of 5.0 mg/dl or greater.) Of patients who developed renal insufficiency, those in whom serum creatinine increased less than 3.0 mg/dl above admission values had a 15% mortality rate, in contrast to 64% mortality in patients in whom serum creatinine increased more than 3.0 mg/dl. In a comparable study, Shusterman et al[115] documented a 2% incidence of hospital-acquired renal insufficiency in 1,819 consecutive medical and surgical hospital admissions. (Renal insufficiency was defined as an increase of serum creatinine level of at least 0.9 mg/dl when admission creatinine level was less than 2.0 mg/dl, and an increase of at least 1.5 mg/dl when the baseline level was greater than 2.0 mg/dl.) The mortality of patients who developed renal insufficiency was 35.3%, in contrast to 3.5% of the control subjects. While neither study permits separation of medical and surgical patients, the results suggest that perioperative renal deterioration is more common and more lethal than is generally appreciated.

Causes and Pathogenesis

To prevent renal injury and improve outcome, investigators have attempted to identify factors that increase the risk for perioperative renal deterioration. The reported causes of acute renal failure range from broad etiologic categories (surgery, trauma, and anesthesia) over which the clinician has little or no control, to listings of specific etiologic factors (see

TABLE 23-4. Outcome of acute postoperative renal failure requiring dialysis

Ref	Date	Number of patients	Type of procedure		Deaths number (%)		Series mortality
12	1968-71	18	GS/T	11	8	(73)	67%
			VASC	7	4	(57)	
91	1968-74	125	GS/T	76	48	(63)	69%
			VASC	49	38	(78)	
89	1970-77	17	AAA	17	8	(47)	47%
24	1973-80	65	GS/T	38	30	(79)	81%
			AAA	14	14	(100)	
			CARD	13	9	(69)	
2	1962-69	40	GS/T	33	17	(52)	53%
			AAA	3	3	(100)	
			CARD	4	1	(25)	
2	1979-81	26	GS/T	19	12	(63)	65%
			AAA	6	4	(67)	
			CARD	1	1	(100)	

Outcome of postoperative renal failure analyzed by date and type of surgical procedure. GS/T, general surgical/trauma; VASC, major vascular; AAA, abdominal aortic aneurysm; CARD, cardiac surgical procedure.

the box at right) to which management strategies may be effectively directed.[115] In a careful case-controlled study of hospital-acquired renal insufficiency, Shusterman et al[115] identified five risk factors (sepsis, intravascular volume depletion, congestive heart failure, aminoglycoside, and radiocontrast exposure) that independently increased the risk of renal deterioration regardless of the medical or surgical status of the patient. In comparison with control subjects in this study, the presence of either volume depletion or myocardial failure increased the risk of developing renal impairment tenfold, while the nephrotoxic effects of aminoglycoside or radiocontrast agents each increased the risk approximately fivefold. These results support the conclusions of other investigators that renal perfusion defects caused by hypotension, myocardial failure, dehydration, cardiopulmonary bypass, or aortic cross-clamping account for the majority of cases of perioperative renal deterioration.[18,56,60,125]

It is common in the perioperative time for several of these risk factors to occur simultaneously, and the interaction of one variable with another may increase the risk for renal deterioration in some patients. Aminoglycoside nephrotoxicity, for example, may be enhanced in the presence of either intravascular volume depletion or arterial hypotension.[92,93] In addition, the interaction of other diseases with known

---

Causes of perioperative renal failure

Decreased renal perfusion

Intravascular volume contraction
Congestive heart failure
Sepsis
Anesthetic effects on renal blood flow
Cardiopulmonary bypass
Aortic cross-clamping

Nephrotoxin exposure

Aminoglycosides
Radiocontrast agents
Anesthetic agents

---

risk factors may increase perioperative risks. Diabetic patients are particularly vulnerable to the nephrotoxic effects of radiocontrast agents,[52,53] and Shusterman et al[115] noted that diabetes enhances the effect of volume depletion more than tenfold.

A conceptual model to describe the pathogenesis and clinical course of hemodynamically mediated acute renal insufficiency was recently presented by Myers and Moran.[94,97] Based on detailed clinical studies and a mathematical assessment of creatinine kinetics, this model also illustrates the interactive effects of known risk factors in the perioperative time. Patients exposed to renal ischemia during cardiopulmonary bypass often develop an abbreviated form of renal failure characterized by transient elevation of serum creatinine level and decreased creatinine clearance rate. Other patients, in whom myocardial dysfunction complicates the postoperative course, develop a more protracted form of overt renal failure, which improves over several weeks as myocardial function returns to normal. In contrast to the relatively benign course of renal dysfunction in these two groups, severe protracted and irreversible renal failure develops in patients in whom either myocardial function fails to improve or in whom the development of other nephrotoxic insults, such as sepsis, interfere with recovery of either myocardial or renal function or both.[97]

While decreased renal perfusion and nephrotoxic exposures probably account for most cases of renal insufficiency, other factors such as preexisting renal disease and anesthetic agents may also contribute to perioperative risk. Patients with normal kidneys are quite resistant to renal ischemic insults and can withstand up to 50 minutes of total renal ischemia during suprarenal aortic cross-camping and up to 150 minutes of partial renal ischemia during cardiopulmonary bypass before the incidence of irreversible renal damage markedly increases. Although it has not been clearly established that preexisting renal disease increases risk for perioperative deterioration of renal function, renal insufficiency has been shown to increase susceptibility to additional nephrotoxic insults in nonsurgical settings. For example, the nephrotoxic effects of radiocontrast agents used for pyelography and cardiac angiography are significantly enhanced in patients with renal dysfunction.[109,115] Both renal plasma flow and glomerular filtration rate decrease sharply in patients with renovascular hypertension and mild azotemia (serum creatinine values averaging 2.4 mg/dl) as arterial blood pressure is decreased with sodium nitroprusside infusion,[117] suggesting an increased susceptibility to ischemic injury. In support of this hypothesis, animal studies demonstrate that the deterioration of renal function that accompanies reduction of arterial blood pressure is proportional to the degree of preexisting renal dysfunction.[98] Finally, Abel et al[1] observed in cardiac surgical patients who developed postoperative renal impairment that the preoperative creatinine value was predictive of the level to which serum creatinine increased in the perioperative time, and

noted that mortality increased progressively with the level to which creatinine increased. However, this study does not specifically imply that the incidence of acute renal failure is higher in patients with preexisting renal disease. The risk of postoperative renal dysfunction in patients with functioning renal allografts having subsequent anesthesia and surgery is not known. Similarly, many living kidney donors have proteinuria and mildly elevated serum creatinine values,[4,10] but perioperative risk for this population of patients has not been reported.

The role of anesthetic agents in mediating perioperative renal injury is unclear despite a variety of functional abnormalities associated with their use. Direct nephrotoxicity caused by accumulation of inorganic fluoride ion is rarely encountered in modern anesthetic practice because practitioners have abandoned the use of methoxyflurane. Depending on the dose and length of exposure, serum fluoride levels may enter a toxic range (50 to 80 μmol/L) during postoperative metabolism of methoxyflurane and result in a polyuric, vasopressin-resistant acute renal failure, which is often irreversible.[25] Of the volatile anesthetic agents in common use today (enflurane, halothane, and isoflurane), only enflurane undergoes appreciable metabolic defluorination,[25,87] which does not appear to be inducible by long-term ingestion of alcohol, barbiturates, or phenytoin.[35] Serum fluoride levels of 20 to 30 μmol/L are commonly encountered after enflurane anesthesia,[26] but renal deterioration has not been observed at this level in either normal patients or in patients with renal insufficiency.[88] In addition, enflurane has been used without untoward sequelae in a large series of patients having renal transplantation.[28] However, acute renal failure has been reported in a patient with preexisting renal disease (serum creatinine of 1.4 mg/dl) at serum fluoride concentration of 93 μmol/L after prolonged enflurane exposure.[38] The exact reasons for such a high fluoride level were unclear, but the authors were unable to specifically incriminate the preexisting renal dysfunction as causative.

In contrast to fluoride nephrotoxicity, the role of anesthetic agents in mediating other renal abnormalities in the perioperative time is not known. Bastron et al[9] demonstrated that halothane does not interfere with autoregulation of renal blood flow over a range of arterial blood pressures between 70 and 150 mm Hg in isolated perfused dog kidney. Priano[103] made similar observations during hemorrhagic hypotension in intact halothane-anesthetized dogs, suggesting that the kidney is well protected against common intraoperative events such as hypotension and hypovolemia despite the presence of anesthetic agents. However, decreased urine output has been observed during administration of a wide variety of anesthetic agents in humans, and simultaneous measurements by clearance techniques suggest decreased renal blood flow (30% to 40% from baseline) and decreased glomerular filtration rate (10% to 20% from baseline). These changes return promptly to normal values early in the postanesthesia time.[26,29,30] Whether these changes in renal blood flow and glomerular filtration rate reflect direct anesthetic effects on the kidney, indirect effects of sympathetic and neurohumoral activation, or artifacts of the clearance techniques used to measure them in settings of low urine volume has not been determined. The significance of these changes, if present, to either intraoperative management or to the development of perioperative renal dysfunction has not been defined. Spinal and epidural anesthetics interfere with renal function only to the extent to which blockade of the sympathetic nervous system results in arterial hypotension and renal hypoperfusion.[25]

Preventive Management

The poor outcome associated with development of acute perioperative renal dysfunction highlights the importance of maintaining preexisting renal function in all patients undergoing anesthesia and surgery. Many routine perioperative events and procedures result in periods of partial or complete renal ischemia, and nephrotoxic agents are commonly needed for diagnostic and therapeutic purposes in surgical patients. Improved perioperative outcome may be possible through careful preventive management that attempts to avoid or attenuate the effects of known nephrotoxic insults.

The general medical condition of every patient should be optimal before elective surgery. Continuation of inotropic and antiarrhythmic drugs and normalization of intravascular volume status will help prevent renal perfusion abnormalities in the operative time. Nephrotoxic drugs such as aminoglycosides, methicillin, and nonsteroidal anti-inflammatory agents should be discontinued when possible, but in accord with the pharmacokinetic characteristics of each drug to assure complete preoperative elimina-

tion.[11] If renal impairment develops in patients who require preoperative radiocontrast studies, surgery should probably be delayed until renal function returns to baseline levels. Since diabetic patients are particularly vulnerable to the nephrotoxic effects of contrast agents,[52,53] consideration should be given to limiting the dose or using a low-osmolality agent to reduce the risk of renal injury.[71] Anesthetic management is directed to meeting the physiologic requirements of the patient rather than to avoiding one or another anesthetic drug or technique.

The importance of maintaining effective left ventricular preload in preventing renal impairment in the perioperative time cannot be overstated. Improved outcome of hospitalized soldiers wounded in Vietnam compared with Korean War casualties is largely attributed to prompt and vigorous fluid, blood, and electrolyte resuscitation, which prevented the development of oliguric renal failure.[124] Similarly, civilian trauma patients in whom maintenance of optimal blood volume was a primary perioperative goal had fewer episodes of oliguric renal failure and lower mortality rates than patients whose fluids were restricted.[112] While overt exsanguination is often the primary cause of acute intravascular volume depletion in trauma patients, more insidious but equally dangerous fluid losses occur during controlled elective surgical trauma. Extravascular sequestration of fluid at the operative site and evaporative losses from exposed serosal surfaces accentuate the dehydrating effects of preoperative fluid restriction, vomiting, diarrhea, contrast studies, and bowel preparations. The beneficial effects of adequate intravascular repletion in maintaining renal perfusion and decreasing the incidence of perioperative renal insufficiency have been demonstrated in animals.[63] Clinical studies document that optimal volume loading in patients having a variety of surgical procedures results in higher urine flow rates and a lower incidence of perioperative renal insufficiency as determined by elevation of creatinine levels.[7,19,21,55] Assessment of the adequacy of intravascular volume repletion in high-risk patients may be most effectively accomplished by invasive central venous or pulmonary arterial catheterization since urinary output may not be a very sensitive indicator of renal perfusion.[3] Careful monitoring of volume status is necessary throughout the postoperative period. Extravascular sequestration of fluid often continues for 12 to 24 hours postoperatively and may contribute to intravascular dehydration and decreased renal perfusion. Mobilization of this fluid occurs over the first postoperative week, and care must be taken to avoid volume overload and congestive heart failure in susceptible patients. Shin et al[111] suggest that serial determinations of creatinine clearance rates based on 1-hour urine collections provide the most reliable early warning of impending renal dysfunction. Early detection of renal failure should prompt immediate adjustment of aminoglycoside and other nephrotoxic drug dosages to prevent additional renal injury.

In contrast to the benefits of volume expansion, the renal protective effects of mannitol, furosemide, and dopamine are not as clearly defined, and the clinical indications for their use are not absolute. Nevertheless, the use of mannitol to prevent acute renal failure during surgical procedures on the heart and aorta is almost universal. Since renal blood flow is decreased during infra-renal aortic cross-clamping, renal protection is routinely used in this situation as well.[46] Mann et al[82] recently presented a thorough review of the existing experimental and clinical literature that critically examines the renal protective abilities of mannitol and other agents. The experimental literature consistently reports a protective effect of mannitol in a variety of renal ischemic models in animals. Mannitol increases renal blood flow and restores glomerular filtration rate by decreasing preglomerular vascular resistance in severely hypotensive rats, and these effects are not seen during volume expansion at the same low blood pressure with isotonic saline alone.[63] The clinical literature consistently documents increased urine output in patients treated with mannitol when compared to untreated controls[82]; however, a decreased incidence of postoperative acute renal failure caused by mannitol therapy has not been documented in man. Untoward effects of mannitol are rarely observed, but a recent case report suggests that mannitol can actually cause renal failure.[122] Although the mechanism is unknown, the authors caution against the use of this drug in patients with renal insufficiency and in patients simultaneously treated with furosemide.[122]

As with mannitol, the renal protective effects of dopamine and furosemide are more clearly evident in well-controlled animal studies than in clinical trials, and both agents are also widely used clinically in settings where renal ischemia is anticipated. Of interest, the diuretic effects of dopamine may result from a renal tubular effect resembling that of furosemide, which is independent of any inotropic or renal vasodilating effects mediated by dopamine.[57] Although the use of mannitol, dopamine, furosemide, and other vasodilating substances does not clearly alter the incidence or outcome of acute perioperative renal failure, use of these agents is likely to continue based on the salutary effects observed in experimental animals. Better information regarding optimal timing and dosage schedules for each drug is needed.

Management of Acute Perioperative Renal Failure

Management of acute renal failure has been comprehensively reviewed by others.[32,82,104,125] Special management considerations for patients who are unfortunate enough to develop postoperative renal failure are discussed below. Timing of initial dialysis after diagnosis, attempts to convert oliguric to nonoliguric renal failure, and controversial strategies to maintain renal perfusion pressure in the early stages of acute renal failure are management issues over which the clinician has control, and each therapy has been suggested to alter survival.

Using multivariate regression techniques, Cioffi et al[24] noted that a shorter time interval from diagnosis of acute renal failure to first dialysis was predictive of improved survival. Gillum et al[49] recently tested this hypothesis in two groups of patients with acute renal failure. In the first group, intensive dialysis treatment was begun 5 days after the onset of renal failure, and the mean predialysis BUN was maintained at 60 mg/dl throughout the treatment course. The noninvasive group first underwent dialysis at 7 days after diagnosis, and the mean predialysis BUN was maintained at 101 mg/dl throughout treatment. The intensive dialysis group received 16 dialyses in contrast to 8 in the nonintensive group. Mortality rates were similar in both groups, but hemorrhagic complications were significantly more common in the nonintensive group. Whether undergoing intensive or nonintensive dialysis, patients who were oliguric before dialysis had a 71% mortality in contrast to the 20% mortality in patients who were nonoliguric before dialysis.[49] Thus early and intensive dialysis may reduce bleeding complications without improving survival.

While it may be correct to conclude that oliguric renal failure is more lethal than nonoliguric disease, it may be equally true that oliguric disease simply reflects a more severe initiating insult. Attempts to convert established oliguric renal failure with diuretic or vasodilator therapy to the nonoliguric type are occasionally successful, but there are no controlled studies to demonstrate that conversion to the nonoliguric state results in improved survival.[32] Despite these uncertainties, it seems reasonable to try to establish a nonoliguric state if for no other reason than to simplify postoperative management.

Autoregulation of renal blood flow is lost in the early stages of acute ischemic renal failure,[65] and renal blood flow becomes dependent on perfusion pressure alone. To prevent further ischemic injury, efforts must be made to avoid hypotensive episodes. Unfortunately, life-saving dialysis therapy at this time is probably the most common cause for significant hypotension in these patients. Hemodialysis should therefore proceed cautiously to maintain effective intravascular volume. Animal studies indicate that the renal vasculature is unresponsive to the vasoconstrictor effects of catecholamines during the first week of acute ischemic renal failure.[65] It has been suggested that norepinephrine may be the agent of choice to treat dialysis-related hypotension during this time in humans.[97] Alternatively, continuous arteriovenous hemofiltration may provide more hemodynamic stability than hemodialysis in acute renal failure. Although survival was not improved, Bartlett et al[8] found that continuous arteriovenous hemofiltration facilitated parenteral feeding and allowed for significantly better nutritional status than that of control patients who were treated with hemodialysis.

In summary, deterioration of renal function in surgical patients occurs commonly and is associated with high mortality. The precipitating causes are incompletely defined, but decreased renal perfusion is the most consistently identified risk factor for developing postoperative renal insufficiency. Nephrotoxic exposures to aminoglycosides, contrast agents, and septic events frequently complicate the course of renal impairment in the perioperative time and may precipitate protracted and irreversible renal injury after an ischemic insult. Surgical patients with preexisting renal dysfunction are more vulnerable to these perioperative insults than are patients with normal kidneys. Since treatment of established acute postoperative renal failure is largely unsuccessful, prevention of the disease is the goal of perioperative management.

REFERENCES

1. Abel RM et al: Etiology, incidence, and prognosis of renal failure following cardiac operations: results of a prospective analysis of 500 consecutive patients, J Thorac Cardiovasc Surg 71:323-333, 1976.
2. Abreo K, Moorthy AV, and Osborne M: Changing patterns and outcome of acute renal failure requiring hemodialysis, Arch Intern Med 146:1338-1341, 1986.
3. Alpert RA et al: Intraoperative urinary output does not predict postoperative renal function in patients undergoing abdominal aortic revascularization, Surgery 95:707-711, 1984.
4. Anderson CF et al: The risks of unilateral nephrectomy: status of kidney donors 10 to 20 years postoperatively, Mayo Clin Proc 60:367-374, 1985.
5. Ando R, Saito H, and Takeuchi J: Factors that affect oxygen affinity of hemoglobin in chronic hemodialysis patients, Nephron 46:268-272, 1987.
6. Bansal VK et al: Protein-calorie malnutrition and cutaneous anergy in hemodialysis maintained patients, Am J Clin Nutr 33:1608-1611, 1980.
7. Barry KG, Mazze RI, and Schwartz FD: Prevention of surgical oliguria and renal-hemodynamic suppression by sustained hydration, N Engl J Med 270:1371-1377, 1964.
8. Bartlett RH et al: Continuous arteriovenous hemofiltration: improved survival in surgical acute renal failure? Surgery 100:400-408, 1986.
9. Bastron RD et al: Autoregulation of renal blood flow during halothane anesthesia, Anesthesiology 46:142-147, 1977.
10. Bay WH and Hebert LA: The living donor in kidney transplantation, Ann Intern Med 106:719-727, 1987.
11. Bennett WM et al: Drug prescribing in renal failure: dosing guidelines for adults, Philadelphia, 1987, American College of Physicians.
12. Berne TV and Barbour BH: Acute renal failure in general surgical patients, Arch Surg 102:594-597, 1971.
13. Blumberg A et al: Effect of various therapeutic approaches on plasma potassium and major regulating factors in terminal renal failure, Am J Med 85:507-512, 1988.
14. Bolman RM et al: Cardiac operations in patients with functioning renal allografts, J Thorac Cardiovasc Surg 88:537-543, 1984.
15. Borrero E et al: Comparison of antacid and sucralfate in the prevention of gastrointestinal bleeding in patients who are critically ill, Am J Med 79 (suppl 2C):62-64, 1985.
16. Brenowitz JB, Williams CD, and Edwards WS: Major surgery in patients with chronic renal failure, Am J Surg 134:765-769, 1977.

17. Broyer M et al: Demography of dialysis and transplantation in Europe, 1984, Nephrol Dial Transplant 1:1-8, 1986.

18. Bullock ML et al: The assessment of risk factors in 462 patients with acute renal failure, Am J Kidney Dis 5:97-103, 1985.

19. Bush HL et al: Prevention of renal insufficiency after abdominal aortic aneurysm resection by optimal volume loading, Arch Surg 116:1517-1524, 1981.

20. Canavese C et al: Reduced response of uraemic bleeding time to repeated doses of desmopressin, Lancet 1:867-868, 1985.

21. Carlier M et al: Maximal hydration during anesthesia increases pulmonary arterial pressures and improves early function of human renal transplants, Transplantation 34:201-204, 1982.

22. Chang N et al: Direct measurement of wound and tissue oxygen tension in postoperative patients, Ann Surg 197:470-478, 1983.

23. Chauvin M et al: Morphine pharmacokinetics in renal failure, Anesthesiology 66:327-331, 1987.

24. Cioffi WG, Ashikaga T, and Gamelli RL: Probability of surviving postoperative acute renal failure: development of a prognostic index, Ann Surg 200:205-211, 1984.

25. Cousins MJ, Skowronski G, and Plummer JL: Anaesthesia and the kidney, Anaesth Intensive Care 2:292-320, 1983.

26. Cousins MJ et al: Metabolism and renal effects of enflurane in man, Anesthesiology 44:44-52, 1976.

27. DeMinno G et al: Platelet dysfunction in uremia: multifaceted defect partially corrected by dialysis, Am J Med 79:552-559, 1985.

28. DeTremmerman P and Gribomont B: Enflurane in renal transplantation: report of 375 cases, Acta Anaesthesiol Scand 71(suppl):24-31, 1979.

29. Deutsch S et al: The effects of anaesthesia with thiopentone, nitrous oxide, narcotics and neuromuscular blocking drugs on renal function in normal man, Br J Anaesth 41:807-814, 1969.

30. Deutsch S et al: Effects of halothane anesthesia on renal function in normal man, Anesthesiology 27:793-804, 1966.

31. Diehl JT et al: Complications of abdominal aortic reconstruction: an analysis of perioperative risk factors in 557 patients, Ann Surg 197:49-56, 1983.

32. Dixon BS and Anderson RJ: Nonoliguric renal failure, Am J Kidney Dis 6:71-80, 1985.

33. Dolan MJ et al: Hypopnea associated with acetate hemodialysis: carbon dioxide-flow-dependent ventilation, N Engl J Med 305:72-75, 1981.

34. Don HF, Dieppa RA, and Taylor P: Narcotic analgesics in anuric patients, Anesthesiology 42:745-747, 1975.

35. Dooley JR et al: Is enflurane defluorination inducible in man? Anesthesiology 50:213-217, 1979.

36. Driks MR et al: Nosocomial pneumonia in intubated patients given sucralfate as compared with antacids or histamine type 2 blockers: the role of gastric colonization, N Engl J Med 317:1376-1382, 1987.

37. Dundee JW and Richards R: Effect of azotemia upon the action of intravenous barbiturate anesthesia, Anesthesiology 15:333-346, 1954.

38. Eichhorn JH et al: Renal failure following enflurane anesthesia, Anesthesiology 45:557-559, 1976.

39. Endou K et al: Hemodynamic changes during hemodialysis, Cardiology 63:175-187, 1978.

40. Erslev A: Erythropoietin coming of age, N Engl J Med 316:101-103, 1987.

41. Eschbach JW et al: Correction of the anemia of end-stage renal disease with recombinant erythropoietin: results of a combined phase I and II clinical trial, N Engl J Med 316:73-78, 1987.

42. Fahey MR et al: The pharmacokinetics and pharmacodynamics of atacurium in patients with and without renal failure, Anesthesiology 61:699-702, 1984.

43. Fisher JW: Mechanisms of the anemia of chronic renal failure, Nephron 25:106-111, 1980.

44. Gafter U et al: Platelet count and thrombopoietic activity in patients with chronic renal failure, Nephron 45:207-210, 1987.

45. Gailiunas P et al: Acute renal failure following cardiac operations, J Thorac Cardiovasc Surg 79:241-243, 1980.

46. Gamulin Z et al: Effects of infrarenal aortic cross-clamping on renal hemodynamics in humans, Anesthesiology 61:394-399, 1984.

47. Ghoneim MM and Pandya H: Plasma protein binding of thiopental in patients with impaired renal or hepatic function, Anesthesiology 42:545-549, 1975.

48. Gibbons GW et al: Aortoiliac reconstruction following renal transplantation, Surgery 91:435-437, 1982.

49. Gillum DM et al: The role of intensive dialysis in acute renal failure, Clin Nephrol 25:249-255, 1986.

50. Haimov M et al: General surgery in patients on maintenance hemodialysis, Ann Surg 179:863-867, 1974.

51. Hampers CL et al: Major surgery in patients on maintenance hemodialysis, Am J Surg 115:747-754, 1968.

52. Harkonen S and Kjellstrand CM: Exacerbation of diabetic renal failure following intravenous pyelography, Am J Med 63:939-946, 1977.

53. Harkonen S and Kjellstrand CJ: Contrast nephropathy, Am J Nephrol 1:66-77, 1981.

54. Harris JP and May J: Successful aortic surgery after renal transplantation without protection of the transplanted kidney, J Vasc Surg 5:457-461, 1987.

55. Hesdorffer CS et al: The value of Swan-Ganz catheterization and volume loading in preventing renal failure in patients undergoing abdominal aneurysmectomy, Clin Nephrol 28:272-276, 1987.

56. Hilberman M et al: Sequential pathophysiological changes characterizing the progression from renal dysfunction to acute renal failure following cardiac operations, J Thorac Cardiovasc Surg 79:838-844, 1980.

57. Hilberman M et al: The diuretic properties of dopamine in patients after open-heart operation, Anesthesiology 61:489-494, 1984.

58. Hilberman M et al: Acute renal failure following cardiac surgery, J Thorac Cardiovasc Surg 77:880-888, 1979.

59. Hocken AG and Hurst PL: Citrate regional anticoagulation in haemodialysis, Nephron 46:7-10, 1987.

60. Hou SH et al: Hospital-acquired renal insufficiency: a prospective study, Am J Med 74:243-248, 1983.

61. Janson PA et al: Treatment of the bleeding tendency in uremia with cryoprecipitate, N Engl J Med 303:1318-1322, 1980.

62. Jensen JA et al: Subcutaneous tissue oxygen tension falls during hemodialysis, Surgery 101:416-421, 1987.

63. Johnston PA et al: Effect of volume expansion on hemodynamics of the hypoperfused rat kidney, J Clin Invest 64:550-558, 1979.

64. Jonsson K et al: Assessment of perfusion in postoperative patients using tissue oxygen measurements, Br J Surg 74:263-267, 1987.

65. Kelleher SP, Robinette JB, and Conger JD: Sympathetic nervous system in the loss of autoregulation in acute renal failure, Am J Physiol (Renal Fluid Electrolyte Physiol)15:F379-F386, 1984.

66. Kinet J et al: Hemodynamic study of hypotension during hemodialysis, Kidney Int 21:868-876, 1982.

67. Kobrinsky NL et al: 1-desamino-8-D-arginine vasopressin (desmopressin) decreases operative blood loss in patients having Harrington rod spinal fusion surgery: a randomized, double-blinded, controlled study, Ann Int Med 107:446-450, 1987.

68. Koide M and Waud BE: Serum potassium concentrations after succinylcholine in patients with renal failure, Anesthesiology 36:142-145, 1972.

69. Kron IL, Joob AW, and Van Meter C: Acute renal failure in the cardiovascular surgical patient, Ann Thorac Surg 39:590-598, 1985.

70. Lacombe M: Abdominal aortic aneurysmectomy in renal transplant patients, Ann Surg 203:62-68, 1986.

71. Lasser EC et al: Pretreatment with corticosteroids to alleviate reactions to intravenous contrast material, N Engl J Med 317:845-849, 1987.

72. Laws KH et al: Cardiac surgery in patients with chronic renal disease, Ann Thorac Surg 42:152-157, 1986.

73. Lawton RL, Gulesserian HP, and Rossi NP: Surgical problems in patients on maintenance dialysis, Arch Surg 97:283-290, 1968.

74. Lewis SL and Van Epps DE: Neutrophil and monocyte alterations in chronic dialysis patients, Am J Kidney Dis 9:381-395, 1987.

75. Lillemoe KD et al: Intestinal necrosis due to sodium polystyrene (Kayexalate) in sorbitol enemas: clinical and experimental support for the hypothesis, Surgery 101:267-272, 1987.

76. Linder A et al: Accelerated atherosclerosis in prolonged maintenance hemodialysis, N Engl J Med 290:697-701, 1974.

77. Lissoos I et al: Surgical procedures on patients in end-stage renal failure, Br J Urol 45:359-365, 1973.

78. Livio M et al: Uraemic bleeding: role of anaemia and beneficial effect of red cell transfusions, Lancet 2:1013-1015, 1982.

79. Livio M et al: Conjugated estrogens for the management of bleeding associated with renal failure, N Engl J Med 315:731-735, 1986.

80. Lundin AP et al: Fatigue, acid-base and electrolyte changes with exhaustive treadmill exercise in hemodialysis patients, Nephron 46:57-62, 1987.

81. Malek GH, Kisken WA, and Taylor CA: The management of patients undergoing bilateral nephrectomy, Surg Gynecol Obstet 131:973-976, 1970.

82. Mann HJ, Fuhs DW, and Hemstrom CA: Acute renal failure, Drug Intell Clin Pharm 20:421-437, 1986.

83. Mannucci PM et al: Desamino-8-D-arginine vasopressin shortens the bleeding time in uremia, N Engl J Med 308:8-12, 1983.

84. Margolis DM et al: Upper gastrointestinal disease in chronic renal failure: a prospective evaluation, Arch Intern Med 138:1214-1217, 1978.

85. May JR, DiPiro JT, and Sisley JF: Drug interactions in surgical patients, Am J Surg 153:327-335, 1987.

86. Maynard JC et al: Blood pressure response to changes in serum ionized calcium during hemodialysis, Ann Intern Med 104:358-361, 1986.

87. Mazze RI, Calverley RK, and Smith NT: Inorganic fluoride nephrotoxicity: prolonged enflurane and halothane anesthesia in volunteers, Anesthesiology 46:265-271, 1977.

88. Mazze RI, Sievenpiper TS, and Stevenson J: Renal effects of enflurane and halothane in patients with abnormal renal function, Anesthesiology 60:161-163, 1984.

89. McCombs PR and Roberts B: Acute renal failure following resection of abdominal aortic aneurysm, Surg Gynecol Obstet 148:175-178, 1979.

90. Meakins JL et al: Delayed hypersensitivity: indicator of acquired failure of host defenses in sepsis and trauma, Ann Surg 186:241-250, 1977.

91. Merino GE, Buselmeier TJ, and Kjellstrand CM: Postoperative chronic renal failure: a new syndrome? Ann Surg 182:37-44, 1975.

92. Meyer RD: Risk factors and comparison of clinical nephrotoxicity of aminoglycosides, Am J Med 80 (suppl 6B):119-125, 1986.

93. Moore RD et al: Risk factors for nephrotoxicity in patients treated with aminoglycosides, Ann Intern Med 100:352-357, 1984.

94. Moran SM and Myers BD: Pathophysiology of protracted acute renal failure in man, J Clin Invest 76:1440-1448, 1985.

95. Mullen JL et al: Reduction of operative morbidity and mortality by combined preoperative and postoperative nutritional support, Ann Surg 192:604-613, 1980.

96. Murkin JM et al: Hemodialysis during cardiopulmonary bypass: report of twelve cases, Anesth Analg 66:899-901, 1987.

97. Myers BD and Moran SM: Hemodynamically mediated acute renal failure, N Engl J Med 314:97-105, 1986.

98. Okuda S et al: Effects of acute reduction in blood pressure on the renal function of rats with diseased kidneys, Nephron 45:311-315, 1987.

99. Opelz G: Blood transfusion: current relevance of the transfusion effect in renal transplantation, Transplant Proc 27:1015-1022, 1985.

100. Pai S et al: Elevation of serum aluminum in humans on a two-day sucralfate regimen, Clin Pharmacol 27:213-215, 1987.

101. Palder SB et al: Vascular access for hemodialysis: patency rates and results of revision, Ann Surg 202:235-239, 1985.

102. Pinson CW et al: Surgery in long-term dialysis patients: experience with more than 300 cases, Am J Surg 151:567-571, 1986.

103. Priano LL: Effect of halothane on renal hemodynamics during normovolemia and acute hemorrhagic hypovolemia, Anesthesiology 63:357-363, 1985.

104. Prough PS: Perioperative management of acute renal failure, Adv Anesth 5:129-172, 1988.

105. Remuzzi G et al: Bleeding in renal failure: altered platelet function in chronic uraemia only partially corrected by haemodialysis, Nephron 22:347-353, 1978.

106. Rostand SG et al: Ischemic heart disease in patients with uremia undergoing maintenance hemodialysis, Kidney Int 16:600-611, 1979.

107. Salzman EW et al: Treatment with desmopressin acetate to reduce blood loss after cardiac surgery: a double-blind randomized trial, N Engl J Med 314:1402-1406, 1986.

108. Schreiner GE and Maher JF: The patient with chronic renal failure and surgery, Am J Cardiol 12:317-323, 1963.

109. Shafi T et al: Infusion intravenous pyelography and renal function: effect in patients with chronic renal insufficiency, Arch Intern Med 138:1218-1221, 1978.

110. Sheinfeld J et al: Selective pretransplant nephrectomy: indications and perioperative management, J Urol 133:379-382, 1985.

111. Shin B, Mackenzie CF, and Helrich M: Creatinine clearance for early detection of posttraumatic renal dysfunction, Anesthesiology 64:605-609, 1986.

112. Shin B et al: Postoperative renal failure in trauma patients, Anesthesiology 51:218-221, 1979.

113. Shuman RB, Schuster DP, and Zuckerman GR: Prophylactic therapy for stress ulcer bleeding: a reappraisal, Ann Intern Med 106:562-567, 1987.

114. Shusterman N and Singer I: Infectious hepatitis in dialysis patients, Am J Kidney Dis 9:447-455, 1987.

115. Shusterman N et al: Risk factors and outcome of hospital-acquired acute renal failure: clinical epidemiologic study, Am J Med 83:65-71, 1987.

116. Taliercio CP et al: Risks for renal dysfunction with cardiac angiography, Ann Intern Med 104:501-504, 1986.

117. Textor SC et al: Critical perfusion pressure for renal function in patients with bilateral atherosclerotic renal vascular disease, Ann Intern Med 102:308-314, 1985.

118. Tryba M et al: Prevention of acute stress bleeding with sucralfate, antacids, or cimetidine: a controlled study with pirenzepine as a basic medication, Am J Med 79 (suppl 2C):55-61, 1985.

119. Upton RA et al: Renal and biliary elimination of vecuronium (ORG NC 45) and pancuronium in rats, Anesth Analg 61:313-316, 1982.

120. Van Scoy RE and Wilson WR: Antimicrobial agents in adult patients with renal insufficiency: initial dosage and general recommendations, Mayo Clin Proc 62:1142-1145, 1987.

121. Viner NA et al: Bilateral nephrectomy: an analysis of 100 consecutive cases, J Urol 113:291-294, 1975.

122. Weaver A and Sica DA: Mannitol-induced acute renal failure, Nephron 45:233-235, 1987.

123. Weir PHC and Chung FF: Anesthesia for patients with chronic renal disease, Can Anaesth Soc J 31:468-480, 1984.

124. Whelton A, and Donadio JV: Post-traumatic acute renal failure in Vietnam: a comparison with the Korean War experience, Johns Hopkins Med J 124:95-105, 1969.

125. Wilkes M and Mailloux LU: Acute renal failure: pathogenesis and prevention, Am J Med 80:1129-1136, 1986.

126. Wong KC, and Liu WS: Anesthesia for urologic surgery, Adv Anesthesiology 3:349-392, 1986.

127. Yarmimizu SN, et al: Mortality and morbidity in pretransplant bilateral nephrectomy: analysis of 305 cases, Urology 12:55-58, 1978.

128. Young GA et al: Anthropometry and plasma valine, amino acids, and proteins in the nutritional assessment of hemodialysis patients, Kidney Int 21:492-499, 1982.

129. Zamora JL et al: Cardiac surgery in patients with end-stage renal disease, Ann Thorac Surg 42:113-117, 1986.

CHAPTER **24**

Hematologic Disorders

MICHAEL J. SENDAK
BARRY BRASFIELD
CHARLES L. SCHLEIEN
CLIFFORD S. DEUTSCHMAN

This chapter addresses implications of hematologic disorders on perioperative outcome and discusses management strategies. Disorders of red blood cells and coagulation have received the greatest attention. Although perioperative changes in in vitro white cell function have been described, their effect on perioperative outcome is unknown, and no data exist on interventions to modify these abnormalities. Pulmonary embolism is discussed in detail in this chapter since it is primarily the result of excessive coagulation.

DISORDERS OF RED BLOOD CELLS

This section reviews physiologic alterations and management considerations for surgical patients with preexisting disorders of red blood cells including anemia, sickle cell disease, and polycythemia.

Chronic Anemia

Normal tissue oxygen delivery. Transport of oxygen to tissues is required for survival of aerobic organisms. Oxygen transport depends on convection, chemical reactions, and diffusion processes that occur along a path of decreasing oxygen tensions from 100 mm Hg in the alveolus to approximately 1 mm Hg in the mitochondria. In spite of its complexity, this system ensures an adequate oxygen supply to even the most remotely situated cells. Tissue hypoxia and cell death can occur as a result of (1) inadequate tissue perfusion, (2) low arterial oxygen tensions caused by impaired pulmonary gas exchange, (3) disturbances of cellular respiration, or (4) reduced oxygen carrying capacity of blood. This section addresses the latter mechanism.

When a gas that contains oxygen interfaces with plasma, the plasma oxygen concentration rises to a constant value. The quantity of dissolved oxygen is determined by the atmospheric pressure, the proportion of oxygen in the gas, and the solubility coefficient of oxygen for plasma (Henry's Law):

$$\text{Dissolved } O_2 = C \times PO_2 / PATM$$

where C is the solubility coefficient for oxygen in the plasma (0.023 ml O_2 per ml of blood at 38° C), PATM is atmospheric pressure, and PO_2 is the partial pressure of O_2 in plasma. When the above equation is rewritten to express dissolved oxygen in milliliters of oxygen at STP per 100 ml of blood:

$$\text{Dissolved } O_2 = 0.0031 \times PO_2$$

Regardless of how high the oxygen tension rises, the amount of dissolved oxygen contained within blood is extremely small and cannot meet metabolic requirements.

Hemoproteins within red blood cells significantly augment the oxygen carrying capacity of blood. Ninety-five percent of red blood cell intracellular protein is hemoglobin that binds and transports oxygen.[29] Each mole of hemoglobin (molecular weight 64,458) binds 4 moles of oxygen (22,400 ml/mole).[122] Thus one gram of hemoglobin binds:

$$(4 \times 22,400 \text{ ml})/64,458 = 1.39 \text{ ml } O_2$$

The actual value is somewhere between 1.34 and 1.39 because of uncertainty in determining the molecular weight of hemoglobin[84] and because the theoretical maximum binding of oxygen to hemoglobin is rarely achieved in the clinical setting. The total content of oxygen in blood (CaO_2) is described in the equation below:

$$CaO_2 = (1.39 \times Hb \times SaO_2) + 0.0031 \times PaO_2$$

and is affected by the degree to which hemoglobin is saturated with oxygen (SaO_2), the total amount of hemoglobin (Hb) contained in the blood, and the partial pressure of oxygen.

Maintenance of adequate blood oxygen content (primarily determined by the amount of hemoglobin present) is a major goal in management of the anemic surgical patient. Chronic reduction of circulating red cell mass is most often a result of bleeding, but may also result from decreased production or increased destruction of red blood cells. Abnormal hemoglobin production such as occurs in sickle cell anemia is often associated with reduced red blood cell mass. Regardless of how it develops, chronic anemia results in compensatory mechanisms that are designed to prevent cellular hypoxia and death.

Adaptations to anemia. Compensatory mechanisms in chronic anemia include increased P50, microvascular redistribution of blood flow, increased plasma volume, decreased blood viscosity, and increased cardiac output.

Anemia results in a rightward shift of the oxyhemoglobin dissociation curve because of increased levels of red cell 2,3-DPG.[13,32] Alveolar oxygen tensions are high enough so that the elevated P50 does not significantly affect O_2 uptake by erythrocytes in the pulmonary capillaries. At increased P50, tissue O_2 delivery is facilitated in the presence of low capillary O_2 tensions[35,159,213] and 2,3-DPG-mediated alterations in P5O may compensate for as much as 50% of the expected O_2 deficit in chronic anemia.[159] The net result is that O_2 extraction increases and adequate tissue O_2 tensions are maintained. During exercise, trauma, or major surgery, increased tissue O_2 extraction can occur at less cardiac work than would otherwise be the case at an equivalent level of O_2 consumption.[159]

The microcirculation increases oxygenation in anemia by selectively dilating precapillary sphincters in metabolically active tissues to increase blood flow and oxygen delivery.[63,222] Studies have documented lower regional vascular resistances and increased blood flows in cerebral,[90,222] cardiac,[56] and skeletal muscle[2] with reduction in cutaneous blood flow in anemia.[2] In dogs with severe, chronic anemia, basal mesenteric and renal blood flows also increase.[12] Mechanisms to account for regional vasodilation are not known, but input from the autonomic nervous system, release of endogenous vasoactive substances, and decreased tissue pH appear to play a role. Anemia also results in local release of adenosine that dilates precapillary sphincters, increases the density of capillaries, and decreases the distance that oxygen must diffuse to reach the most remote cells.* The benefit of redistributing blood flow is to ensure that those organ systems with the greatest oxygen needs are unaffected by mild to moderate reductions in oxygen-carrying capacity.

With chronic reduction in circulating red cell

*Referencs 44, 46, 84, 96, 114, 147, 187.

mass, total intravascular volume remains at normal values as a result of compensatory expansion of the plasma volume.[5,83,97,227] Increased plasma volume is the main reason for the decreased viscosity observed in chronic anemia. Red blood cells are the main contributors to blood viscosity. As hematocrit drops from 40%, blood viscosity rapidly declines and eventually approaches that of plasma alone (only 1.5 times greater than water).[85] It has been demonstrated that a 15% reduction in hemoglobin results in a 30% decrease in blood viscosity and a 50% increase in cerebral blood flow.[209]

Cardiac output is usually increased in anemia.[23,192] In mild, chronic anemia, increased cardiac output is often the result of tachycardia with unchanged stroke volume.[83] In severe, chronic anemia (hemoglobin <10 gm/dl), heart rate is usually normal and increased cardiac output is a consequence of increased stroke volume.[23,180,181] As the hemoglobin further decreases from 7 to 2 gm/dl, cardiac output increases linearly[222] at normal left ventricular end-diastolic pressure and increased left ventricular end-diastolic volume.[83,178] In a study of asymptomatic chronically anemic patients (mean hemoglobin of 1.2 gm/dl) with no evidence of heart disease, stroke volume was elevated 36% at rest with no associated increase in heart rate.[200] Exercise in these patients increased oxygen consumption and cardiac output by an amount equivalent to that observed in nonanemic control subjects. These data suggest that anemia may improve coronary blood flow by either reducing blood viscosity or by recruitment of coronary collateral vessels.[58,229] Thus anemia results in changes in blood viscosity, peripheral vascular tone, preload, and afterload that create a favorable advantage for maintaining high stroke volume, increased cardiac output, and normal oxygen delivery.[137,169,173]

Minimal acceptable hemoglobin value. Despite attempts to define a minimally acceptable hemoglobin or optimal hemoglobin level for patients undergoing anesthesia and surgery, no single value has ever been defined that clearly minimizes perioperative morbidity and mortality. Two large retrospective clinical studies were unable to show that the presence of anemia (independent of its etiologic cause and other coexisting diseases) conferred an increased risk of complications during or after surgery.[24,172] The adequacy of wound healing appears to be normal in anemic patients if malnutrition and hypovolemia are corrected.* Hematocrits of 30% do not adversely affect wound oxygenation, collagen production, or bone graft healing in animals.[89,214] Nevertheless, the finding that 88% of 1,249 hospitals surveyed require a preoperative hemoglobin of greater than 9 gm/dl, and 44% require a value of greater than 10 gm/dl, suggests that most practitioners intuitively believe that higher hemoglobin values are associated with fewer perioperative complications.†

The impact of preexisting anemia on individual surgical patients is far more important than globally applied standards for minimally acceptable hemoglobin levels. Patients with chronic renal failure routinely undergo anesthesia and surgery uneventfully at hemoglobin levels of 6 to 8 gm/dl,[154] and hemoglobin levels of 2 to 3 gm/dl are capable of sustaining life in normal patients in the perioperative time.[80,157] However, preoperative assessment of the interaction of anemia with coexisting diseases such as coronary artery disease, and the ability of a given patient to safely withstand surgical stresses such as bleeding, must be determined to guide preoperative transfusion therapy and judgements regarding whether or not to proceed with surgery.

During isovolemic anemia in animals, coronary blood flow progressively rises as hematocrit is reduced to levels as low as 5%.[107] Myocardial oxygen delivery and consumption remain at maximum baseline values until the hematocrit is reduced below 20%. Despite extreme reductions in hematocrit, the myocardial oxygen extraction ratio remains remarkably constant. Exercise-induced stress in animals at hematocrits of 18% does not alter the distribution of myocardial blood flow and does not produce ventricular dysfunction.[1] While these myocardial adaptations to anemia may not be representative of systemic oxygen supply and demand relationships in other organs,[72,107] a patient who is free of heart disease and has an adequate blood volume should have normal cardiovascular function with hematocrit reductions as low as 20%. After short-term coronary artery occlusion in the presence of anemia (hematocrit of 20%), reactive hyperemia is compromised in animals. Despite this decreased coronary flow reserve, myocardial blood flow remains sufficient to prevent myocardial infarction and ventricular dysfunction.[72] However, patients with fixed occlusive disease of the coronary arteries would probably ben-

---

*References 3, 131, 132, 136, 172, 185.

†References 76, 80, 116, 172, 175, 198.

efit from a greater circulating red cell mass and increased myocardial oxygen delivery to prevent ischemia.[73,176]

The ability of a patient to tolerate massive blood loss must also be evaluated preoperatively. Studies investigating the relationship between hematocrit and survival in canine hemorrhagic shock have shown that between hematocrits of 10% to 60%, the greatest resistance to the development of irreversible shock occurred at a prehemorrhage hematocrit of 37%.[42,43] Animals with initial hematocrits of greater or lesser magnitude tolerated the shock state for shorter periods of time. A hematocrit of 37% allowed a survival time during shock (systolic blood pressure of 30 mm Hg) that was 5 times longer than if the initial hematocrit was 12%. However, if only those animals with natural hematocrit variations are analyzed, survival time appears to be similar for animals with initial hematocrits between 25% and 45%. Thus, in the presence of mild to moderate chronic anemia where blood volume is normal and compensatory mechanisms are functioning, there may be a wide range of hematocrits that provide equal protection against hemorrhagic shock.

Regardless of the minimal acceptable hemoglobin value that one is guided by, it is critically important that an anemic surgical patient maintain normal circulating blood volume. Hypovolemia is far more deleterious than isovolemic anemia.* An adequate circulating intravascular volume is more important than either the effects of decreased blood viscosity or increased red cell mass in delivery of oxygen to tissues.[156] Reduced intravascular volume compromises tissue perfusion in normal as well as anemic patients.

Management of anemia

General considerations. It is important to assess the integrity and functional reserve of all major organ systems in anemic patients. Most chronically anemic patients adequately compensate for their anemia, but it is necessary to determine if these compensatory mechanisms will provide enough reserve to undergo the stresses of major surgery and anesthesia, including changes in temperature, pH, catecholamine levels, and intravascular volume. Critically narrowed coronary, carotid, or cerebral arteries may pose no problem in a resting patient, but these abnormalities may precipitate end-organ ischemia or

*References 5, 64, 106, 126, 156.

infarction during periods of stress. In the case of coronary disease, a history of activity tolerance alone may supply enough information to assess the adequacy of oxygen delivery in the face of increased demand. When the history is insufficient for such an assessment, treadmill stress testing may provide insight into the amount of hemodynamic stress that can be tolerated by an anemic patient. Patients with compromised exercise capabilities can then be given appropriate pharmacologic and/or transfusion therapy preoperatively.

Anemic patients who smoke cigarettes should quit smoking before surgical intervention. Smoking results in the formation of carbon-monoxy-hemoglobin (COHb), and smokers may have COHb levels as high as 15%.[78,121] COHb reduces the amount of functional hemoglobin and diminishes the oxygen-carrying capacity of blood. COHb also lowers the P50 of the remaining oxyhemoglobin and produces a more hyperbolic oxyhemoglobin dissociation curve.[66,179] Further, COHb inhibits red blood cell glycolysis and ultimately results in reduced 2,3-DPG formation.[8] Because the half-life of COHb in blood is at least 4 hours,[121] patients should stop smoking for a minimum of 24 hours before surgery.

Despite the importance of compensatory increases in cardiac output in anemia, the negative inotropic effects of general inhalational anesthetics are offset by simultaneous reductions in systemic and myocardial oxygen requirements under anesthesia even in the presence of anemia.[127,191,207,208] Coronary blood flow reserve remains present at hematocrits as low as 13% under inhalation anesthesia,[206] and there is no redistribution of myocardial blood flow suggestive of ischemia.[127] Thus, potent inhalational anesthetics appear to be safe in the presence of well-compensated isovolemic anemia.

Regional anesthesia (epidural or spinal techniques) is associated with significantly lower intraoperative blood loss than general anesthesia in patients undergoing prostatectomy and other pelvic and lower extremity procedures. Several randomized, prospective, controlled studies in patients having total hip replacement under regional anesthesia have demonstrated a reduction of 30% to 40% in blood loss compared to patients receiving general anesthesia.[112,141,177,219] Modig and Karlstrom compared blood loss during epidural anesthesia, general anesthesia with spontaneous ventilation, and general anesthesia with positive-pressure ventilation and found a strong correlation between central and peripheral venous pressures and the amount of blood loss.[144] They postulated that positive-pressure ventilation (with a lesser contribution from general anesthesia) increases venous pressures sufficiently to explain their observations that spontaneously breathing, awake patients under regional anesthesia tend to have less perioperative blood loss than patients under general anesthesia. Coupled with the frequent reports of a decreased incidence of postoperative thromboembolism in patients submitted to regional anesthesia,[146,211] regional anesthesia may be preferred over general techniques in anemic patients as often as surgical procedures and patient cooperation will allow.

Transfusion therapy. If there were no risks associated with blood transfusion, it would be a simple matter to transfuse all anemic patients to a level of hemoglobin or hematocrit that seemed optimal. However, increasing public and professional concern regarding transfusion-related Autoimmune Deficiency Syndrome (AIDS) and non A-non B hepatitis has mandated a more rational approach to perioperative transfusion therapy. Despite voluntary donations and widespread screening for infectious agents, it is estimated that 5 of every 1 million units of blood may be infected with the AIDS virus.[21,163] This estimate has been recently increased to 26 per 1 million units.[104,224] The incidence of transfusion-associated hepatitis is 7% to 12%.[21] Therefore the risks of transfusion therapy must be carefully weighed against the potential benefits.[74]

Consideration of the need for perioperative transfusion should be initiated, when possible, weeks before the planned procedure. The safest technique that the surgeon can offer the patient is procurement of autologous blood donations. Patients with coronary disease, extremes of age, and pregnancy have made autologous donations without significant morbidity.[129,133] Currently, autologous donations are permitted every 7 to 10 days, with the average donation before planned elective procedures being 2.2 units per patient.[117,133] In the future, use of recombinant human erythropoietin (r-HUEPO) may stimulate red cell production sufficiently to allow more frequent donation. A recent study in baboons given iron and r-HUEPO resulted in 10 units of autologous blood over a 5-week period.[125] Many patients donate up to 48 hours before the planned procedure, a time sufficient to allow reequilibration of intravascular volume.

If a patient needs more units than can be collected

within the shelf lif of the first collected unit, autologous blood can be frozen.[4,50] Freezing autologous blood may be most important to patients with rare blood types or with unusual antibodies. While new adenosine-based additive solutions have made liquid storage possible for up to 42 days, the Food and Drug Administration allows frozen red blood cell storage for up to 3 years. Should this time be extended (some feel 10 to 11 years may be possible), it is conceivable that private citizens could store their own blood for personal use at a later time if needed. Currently, the availability of both autologous and frozen red blood cell storage may be limited, depending on the geographic area and the willingness of local blood centers to participate in such programs. Other blood components including plasma and platelets may also be collected for autologous use.

Transfusion of banked blood carries several important risks to anemic patients. Blood products are stored at 2° to 6° C and should be warmed to body temperature before infusion. Even moderate volumes of blood at room temperature may decrease core body temperature, shift the oxyhemoglobin dissociation curve, and contribute to thermogenic shivering with attendant increase in oxygen consumption. Depending on its age and volume, banked blood contains lower than normal levels of 2,3-DPG. The advantage gained in blood oxygen content (increased hemoglobin concentration) after infusion of banked blood can be temporarily offset by decreased P50.[221] The 2,3-DPG concentration gradually increases over several hours after small volume transfusions,[15] but P50 may not normalize for up to 24 hours after infusion of large volumes of blood.[221]

Requests from patients for avoidance of homologous blood transfusions can occasionally be accommodated with direct (recipient-designated) donations from family members or close friends with compatible blood groups. As pressure to allow directed donations increased in 1983 with the advent of the AIDS crisis, the American Red Cross, American Association of Blood Banks, and Council of Community Blood Centers issued a joint statement that strongly discouraged directed donations.[7] This reluctance was based on the absence of scientific evidence that directed donations were safer than volunteer donations and also on concerns for the increased burden placed on blood collection centers by such programs. Nevertheless, a few centers that permitted directed donations have reported that up to 47% of directed donors have entered the general volunteer donor pool and increased blood bank supplies.[65] While directed donations do not entirely avoid the risk of homologous transfusions, they may reduce the anxiety associated with requirements for perioperative transfusion in some patients.

Perioperative hemodilution. Hemodilution may be an important component of a perioperative blood conservation program in some patients. Replacement of collected fresh whole blood with cell-free substitutes (lactated Ringer's at 3 ml/ml or hetastarch at 1 ml/ml of whole blood) can be performed in the operating room before induction of anesthesia. This technique requires careful monitoring of arterial and central venous pressures especially when the target hematocrit is less than 26% to 28%. The collected whole blood can then be used as replacement for blood shed during the procedure. The lowest hematocrit unit is usually transfused first and the highest hematocrit unit (the first unit collected) is reinfused after completion of the major blood loss. Concomitant diuresis may be necessary because red cell mass is increased at the end of the procedure. Patients undergoing spinal fusion procedures require fewer homologous transfusions if they are hemodiluted.[108] Hemodilution is used routinely during cardiopulmonary bypass and has been shown to improve patency of bypass grafts.[124] Lower hematocrits correlate highly with increased free flap survival in plastic surgical patients. Other studies have reported increased platelet counts and improved hemostasis in patients who undergo preoperative hemodilution.[111,193] Reported complications are rare in spite of concerns about tissue hypoxia. Patients with right coronary artery disease who were hemodiluted to 11 gm/dl did not demonstrate any signs of ischemia or right ventricular dysfunction.[19] In animals hemodiluted to hematocrits of 10%, oxygen consumption did not decrease and increases in myocardial blood flow appear to have prevented increases in coronary sinus lactate concentration.[47] Before intraoperative hemodilution can be more widely employed, selection of appropriate patients with regard to type of procedure, general state of health, and optimal anesthetic and monitoring protocols must be established. However, hemodilution may be a promising technique for avoiding homologous transfusions in many patients.

Deliberate hypotension. Deliberate hypotension as an adjunct to general anesthesia has been reported to reduce intraoperative blood loss during surgery for scoliosis, hip arthroplasty, major head and neck explorations, thoracoabdominal dissections, radical cystectomy, and middle ear surgery. Hypotension is usually defined as reduction of systolic blood pressure to 80 to 90 mm Hg (mean blood pressure of 50 to 75 mm Hg). The benefits of deliberate hypotension have been most clearly documented during total hip replacement with reduction of approximately 50% in surgical blood loss and decreased transfusion requirements of 20% to 83%.[47,67,82] Many hypotensive agents have been used including trimethaphan, sodium nitroprusside, inhalational anesthetic agents, beta-blockers, labetalol, nitroglycerin, and various combinations of these agents. No particular agent has proven to be superior or more effective than another. Sivarajan observed no difference in the patient's blood loss between use of trimethaphan and sodium nitroprusside when each agent was titrated to achieve the same target blood pressure.[195] Complications associated with deliberate hypotension have been surprisingly few. This finding probably reflects an avoidance of the technique in patients with vascular disease, hypertension, and other conditions that may increase the risk of organ ischemia. Careful monitoring of intraarterial and central venous pressures is generally recommended when deliberate hypotension is used. Somatosensory evoked potentials or EEG monitoring may be particularly useful during procedures in which neurologic injury may be precipitated.

Intraoperative blood salvage. Devices to salvage autologous red blood cells from the surgical field have recently been refined and marketed. The semicontinuous flow cell-washing centrifuge has now reached a stage of development that makes it practical and cost effective for salvage of as little as 2 to 3 units of red blood cells. Widespread use of autotransfusion devices without significant complications has been reported for patients undergoing cardiac, vascular, orthopedic, and liver transplant procedures.[168] Theoretical contraindications to its use include surgery in the area of malignant tumors and surgery in possibly contaminated fields such as large bowel procedures. Washing of the cells in 0.9% normal saline before transfusion effectively removes fat, bone chips, and other particulate matter. Washing may also remove platelets and plasma, and these products may need to be given to promote hemostasis after more than 6 to 8 units have been reinfused. Defibrination and fibrin degradation products may be present in salvaged blood, but induction of disseminated intravascular coagulation has not been reported in humans. Careful monitoring of coagulation profiles and appropriate replacement of indicated factors is required for effective management of patients receiving salvaged blood.

Summary

Chronic anemia is a significant problem requiring thorough consideration in the perioperative time. Proper management of anemia requires an understanding of the processes normally involved in oxygen delivery and consumption and an appreciation of the physiologic adaptations occurring with anemia. It is unlikely that there are ideal concentrations for minimally acceptable or optimal hemoglobin that are universally applicable to surgical patients. Hemoglobin values need to be individualized and based on coexisting disease and functional reserve. The chronically anemic surgical patient will receive the highest quality of care only if the etiologic causes of commonly occurring intraoperative and postoperative problems are understood and anticipated. High quality of care necessitates thorough and repeated patient evaluations before, during, and after a surgical blood loss and variations in systemic and regional oxygen consumption.

Sickle Cell Disease

The incidence of sickle cell trait in American blacks is 8% to 14% and the frequency of sickle cell disease is estimated at 0.15% in this population.[152] Sickling of red blood cells is uncommon in patients with sickle trait, except under severe conditions of deoxygenation, and most individuals are asymptomatic. In contrast, patients with sickle disease, in whom the concentration of hemoglobin S is 85% to 95%, usually have severe disease with frequent vasoocclusive crises, which manifest as infarctive events. Other crises causing severe anemia are caused by hemolysis, sequestration, or acute aplasia, and are seen less often. Achieving optimal perioperative management of patients with sickle cell disease requires an appreciation of the end-organ effects of chronic sickle disease and a management plan designed to avoid those events that precipitate acute crises.

Chronic clinical problems. The clinical problems commonly seen in patients with sickle disease are secondary to repetition of crises and include problems secondary to repeated vasoocclusive events, chronic anemia, and hemolysis.[115] (Table 24-

TABLE 24-1. Chronic problems in patients with sickle cell disease

Crises	Vasoocclusive
	Hemolytic
	Sequestration
Pulmonary	Infarction
	Infection
	Pulmonary hypertension
	Hypoxemia and $\dot{V}/\dot{Q}$ mismatching
Cardiac	Biventricular enlargement
	Flow murmur
	LVH/RVH
	Cor pulmonale
	Congestive heart failure caused by high output
	Myocardial ischemia/infarction
Renal	Hyposthenuria
	Hematuria
	Nephrotic syndrome
	Chronic renal failure
Immunologic	Asplenic
	Infarcted tissue—infection
Neurologic	Cerebral infarcts
	Cerebral hemorrhage
	Altered mental status
	Sensory/motor disturbance
	Seizures
	Meningeal signs
Airway	Maxillary overgrowth
Gastrointestinal	Hepatomegaly
	Elevated LFTs
	Gallstones

1.) The lung is a common site of infarction and, if infarction is recurrent, patients can develop pulmonary hypertension and, rarely, cor pulmonale.[105] Mild hypoxemia caused by $\dot{V}/\dot{Q}$ mismatching is common. Biventricular enlargement is often seen as a result of chronic anemia and flow murmurs are often present. Left ventricular hypertrophy occurs in 50% of patients and right ventricular hypertrophy is seen in 10% to 15%. High output congestive heart failure occurs occasionally. Although cardiac output is usually increased above normal levels, recent data suggest that ventricular function is often impaired. Rarely, coronary microthrombi can cause myocardial ischemia and infarction. Most patients with sickle cell disease (and trait) have an impaired ability to concentrate their urine, which can result in intravascular volume depletion if fluid intake is inadequate.[28] Hematuria caused by papillary necrosis, nephrotic syndrome, and renal failure secondary to multiple thrombotic episodes also occur. Hepatomegaly is common and liver function tests are often abnormal. Hepatitis from blood transfusions and pigmented gallstones after repeated episodes of hemolysis are also seen. Most patients with sickle disease are functionally asplenic.[161] Asplenism, abnormalities of opsonization and white cell killing, and the frequent presence of infarcted tissue, all predispose sickle patients to infectious complications. Cerebral infarcts also occur in patients with sickle cell disease secondary to vasoocclusive crisis or hemorrhage associated with congenital aneurysm or hypoxic necrosis of a cerebral vessel. Altered consciousness, sensory and motor disturbance, meningeal signs, and seizures may also be seen as part of the spectrum of central nervous system disease.

Physiology. Many factors, including the percentage of hemoglobin S, interactions with other hemoglobins, the state of cellular hydration, temperature, and pH, affect the extent to which red blood cells sickle. The clinical severity of the various hemoglobinopathies correlate well with viscosity; SS > SD > SC > SF > AS.[33] Hemoglobin S levels in excess of 50% are usually required for sickling to occur. Hemoglobin F, which has no beta chain and therefore cannot interact with Hb S, is protective in infants with sickle disease. Under normal conditions, in patients with sickle disease, red blood cells traverse the capillary bed but do not actually sickle until after leaving the capillary, because there is a delay period below polymerization of the abnormal hemoglobin.[228] These cells then unsickle in the lung when oxygen levels increase. Clinical problems occur when the delay in polymerization is decreased as a result of acidosis, hypothermia, or hyperthermia, or intravascular volume depletion.[57] Under these conditions cells may sickle while still in the capillary causing thrombosis, and a vasoocclusive crisis ensues. Similarly, arterial hypoxemia prevents desickling of cells and can also precipitate a crisis. Unfortunately, abnormalities of oxygenation and hydration state, extremes of temperature, and acid-base disturbances occur in the perioperative period. As a result, anesthesia and surgery represent a major threat to patients with sickle disease.

Outcome. Although there are several published studies examining perioperative outcome in patients with sickle hemoglobinopathies, evaluation of risk is complicated because many of these studies consist of only a few patients, establishing the contribution

of sickle disease to outcome is often difficult, and often severe medical emergencies, which are independently associated with poor outcome, brought these patients to the operating room. Table 24-2 shows results from a number of studies of inpatients with sickle or associated diseases. There were 11 deaths among 144 patients undergoing anesthesia for various procedures.[188] Patients had both intraoperative and postoperative complications, with most related to the pulmonary system. Data on perioperative outcome of patients with sickle trait come mostly from retrospective studies and include data from patients receiving both general and regional anesthetic techniques.[94] Most reported deaths were related to patients' underlying diseases and complications were not often secondary to sickle trait. One study, though, did report 5 children with sickle trait who died in the perioperative period after undergoing general anesthesia.[130] Four of these deaths occurred in patients with undiagnosed sickle trait. The cause of death is not known. Use of a specific anesthetic agent is not critical as all agents and techniques have

TABLE 24-2. Series in which general anesthesia was administered to patients suffering from sickle cell anemia, hemoglobin C disease, and sickle cell B-thalassemia

Series	Genotype*	Number of cases	Number of deaths
Shapiro and Poe (1955)	SS	15	0
Rosenbaum (1965)	SC	1	1
Browne (1965)	SS	9	0
Gilbertson (1965)	SS	3	2
Holzmann (1969)	SS	43	1
	SC	3	0
	SBT	1	0
Oduro (1969)	SS	8	
	SC	7	6
	SF	1	
Oduntan and Isaacs (1971)	SS	6	0
	SC	6	0
Oduro and Searle (1972)	SS	17	0
	SC	21	1
	SF	1	0
	SBT	2	0
TOTALS		144	11

Reprinted from Searle JF: Anesthesia is sickle cell states, a review, Anesthesia 28:48-58, 1973.
*S, C, and F = hemoglobins S, C, and fetal, respectively.
SBT = sickle cell B-thalassemia.

been used successfully in patients with sickle cell disease. One in vitro study showed that at a hematocrit of 20%, viscosity of deoxygenated hemoglobin S blood is increased with the use of halothane.[12] However, no changes in viscosity were observed at higher hematocrits or with oxygenated hemoglobin S.

Perioperative management. As discussed previously, a full preoperative examination should be performed to assess the chronic problems that the patients with sickle cell disease may have, including pulmonary, cardiac, renal, infectious, and neurologic complications. The anesthesiologist and intensivist should closely assess the upper airway for the syndrome of maxillary overgrowth, which is commonly seen in these patients, particularly those with sickle beta-thalassemia syndrome, which may make laryngoscopy and intubation of the tracheal difficult. Preoperative consultation with the hematologist regarding chronic care of the patient and possible exchange transfusion is also highly recommended.

The management of patients with sickle cell disease in the perioperative period is primarily focused on avoiding known precipitants of sickling: hypoxemia, acidosis, dehydration, low blood flow states, and extremes of temperature. In addition to routine monitoring devices, more invasive procedures should be used in those patients with severe chronic organ system problems secondary to their sickle cell disease. Normothermia should be maintained by using warming techniques such as overhead radiant warmers, heating blankets, and wrapping of the extremities and the head by infusing warmed intravenous fluids and by humidifying inspired gases. Positioning of the patient in the operating room and in the recovery room or intensive care unit is critical in these patients to avoid intravascular stasis so that localized sickling does not occur. Most of the complications that occur in the perioperative period occur postoperatively and are usually caused by airway problems, improper fluid management, acid base disturbances, and abnormalities of temperature regulation.

Role of exchange transfusion. Blood transfusion is common therapy for a number of complications associated with sickle cell disease and for preparation of these patients for surgery. The goals of transfusion in sickle cell disease are to reduce viscosity, prevent venous thrombosis and vasoocclusive crises in the microcirculation, and to remove irreversibly sickled cells. By transfusing, the concentration of hemoglobin S is decreased both by dilution and direct removal. When hemoglobin S levels are reduced to less than 40% in well-oxygenated in vitro preparations, resistance to blood flow is significantly reduced, and this is the goal of exchange transfusion therapy.[123] Other studies also indicate that viscosity increases greatly at low shear rates when the hemoglobin S concentration is greater than 40% in deoxygenated blood.[155] Current clinical indications for blood transfusion include the following: (1) to prepare patients for surgery, (2) to decrease pregnancy related morbidity, (3) to prevent repetitive cerebrovascular accidents, and (4) to treat otherwise intractable vasoocclusive or other crises, chronic leg ulcers, priapism, and acute lung syndrome secondary to infarction or embolism. Blood transfusion in children suffering from cerebrovascular accidents prevented further stroke episodes and reversed arteriographic abnormalities.[183] In another study of children with central nervous system symptoms, maintenance of hemoglobin S concentrations under 20% for 2 years resulted in stable symptoms during the period of transfusion therapy. However, 7 of 12 children had recurrence of central nervous system symptoms after stopping transfusion therapy. All types of transfusion methods have been used including partial exchange, multiple exchange, and simple transfusion. For emergency surgery, the partial exchange transfusion has been used most often. For chronic preparation for surgery, both simple transfusions and multiple exchange transfusions have been performed with the goal to indicate reduction of hemoglobin S below 10 g/dl. One retrospective analysis of the three types of preoperative blood transfusion found no difference in total hemoglobin level or hemoglobin S level.[69] Another study reported an increase in perioperative complications when blood transfusion was performed but these patients were more critically ill than patients not undergoing transfusion.[95] At this time, no good randomized study has been performed reviewing the morbidity and mortality from sickle cell disease in the perioperative period in patients undergoing blood transfusion.

Polycythemia

Polycythemia may be defined as the presence of a spun hematocrit of greater than 40% in females or of greater than 52% in males. Relative polycythemia is characterized by normal or decreased total red blood cell mass accompanied by a low plasma volume and is often associated with chronic fluid loss, hypertension, obesity, smoking, or stress. Absolute erythrocytosis may result from one of many hemoglobinopathies that have an increased affinity for oxygen, but more commonly is caused by excessive erythropoietin production (secondary polycythemia). Secondary polycythemia can be further divided into cases in which there is a reasonable physiologic cause for increased erythropoietin production and into those in which there is autonomous production of excessive erythropoietin in the absence of detectable tissue hypoxia. The most commonly reported causes of these entities are shown in the box below. Inappropriate polycythemia has been reported to occur in up to 20% of cerebellar hemangiomas and in 5% to 10% of hepatomas.[210]

Perioperative evaluation and management of polycythemia include determination of the cause and consideration of the physiologic effects of erythrocytosis. In cyanotic patients with low cardiac output, the elevated hematocrit may represent an important physiologic adaptation for preservation of oxygen delivery to the tissues. In contrast, the patient with

an erythopoietin-producing tumor who is experiencing headache, tinnitus, and hypertension may benefit from preoperative phlebotomy. Reduction in levels of cerebral blood flow are associated with hematocrits greater than 60%,[84] a level also reported to be associated with decreased tissue oxygen delivery caused by hyperviscosity in animals.[13] If elective surgery can be postponed, underlying factors such as smoking, hypertension, and obesity should be treated. If phlebotomy is necessary, replacement with 0.9% normal saline may be necessary to avoid hemodynamic fluctuations. Polycythemic patients are good candidates for perioperative hemodilution techniques.

Bleeding and thrombosis in the perioperative period are increased in patients with polycythemia. In 68 patients undergoing 81 major operations, Wasserman and Gilbert[32] reported that those with poor control (HCT > 52%) at the time of operation had a 79% complication rate, a 43% morbidity, and a 36% mortality. In contrast, the control group (HCT < 52%) had a 23% morbidity and a 5% mortality. Subsequently, Pearson and Wetherly-Mein[35] demonstrated a positive correlation between the incidence of vascular occlusive episodes and the hematocrit in polycythemia vera patients. Hematocrit levels of greater than 60% were associated with 7.5 episodes of thrombosis per 10 patient-years compared with 0.2 episodes per 10 patient-years in patients with hematocrits of 40% to 44%. It is not entirely clear whether the increased incidence of thrombosis is caused by increased red cell mass alone or to an accompanying thrombocytosis or hypercoagulable state. It seems prudent, however, to consider these patients at high risk for perioperative deep vein thrombosis and pulmonary embolism and to use prophylactic heparin therapy when indicated.

COAGULATION DISORDERS

This section discusses potential ways in which coagulation abnormalities affect perioperative outcome and reviews management techniques. Coagulation abnormalities which increase risk of bleeding are discussed in detail. Also included in this section is a discussion of perioperative changes in coagulation and their potential to cause thromboembolic phenomena. The last section addresses the incidence of pulmonary embolism and examines the efficacy of different management strategies.

Causes of relative and absolute polycythemia

Relative polycythemia
Chronic fluid loss
Hypertension
Obesity
Smoking
Stress

Absolute polycythemia
Appropriate
High Altitude
Chronic CO poisoning (e.g. heavy smoking)
Hypoxemia
  Right to left shunts
  Pulmonary disease

Inappropriate
Polycythemia vera
Renal vascular disease
Renal cysts
Hydronephrosis
Renal tumors
Uterine myomas
Cerebellar hemangiomas
Hepatomas

Bleeding Disorders

Abnormalities of the clotting system have the potential to cause excessive perioperative bleeding and often require specific interventions. This section addresses evaluation of hemostasis and discusses management of patients presenting for surgery with congenital or acquired coagulation disorders. Problems covered include thrombocytopenia, functional platelet disorders, clotting factor dificencies, and clotting abnormalities caused by circulating anticoagulants and fibrinolytic agents (Table 24-3). Bleeding problems secondary to massive transfusion are discussed elsewhere (see Chapter 10).

Rarely do patients have unrecognized but clinically significant coagulation abnormalities, and routine preoperative screening of the protime (PT), partial thromboplastin time (PTT), platelet count, and bleeding time are not indicated (see Chapter 1). A careful history searching for prior bleeding problems, an inquiry into possible problems encountered during prior surgeries, knowledge of other health problems, and a review of recent drug usage should detect most patients with bleeding disorders. Further evaluation of these patients is often indicated and may require the assistance of a hematologist.

Thrombocytopenia. Patients with thrombocytopenia may develop problems unrelated to their hematologic disorder which bring them to the operating room or may present for surgery as a result of this problem (for example, splenectomy for treatment of idiopathic thrombocytopenia purpura, mesocaval shunt for treatment of variceal bleeding in patients with cirrhosis and hypersplenism). Most available data correlating bleeding with platelet count come from patients with spontaneous hemorrhagic complications in a nonoperative setting or from previously normal individuals who develop acute thrombocytopenia secondary to massive blood loss and transfusion. Spontaneous bleeding, other than petechiae, purpura, or mild epistaxis, rarely occurs unless platelet counts fall below 10,000. Field studies during wartime suggest that the incidence of "nonsurgical" bleeding increases when the platelet count falls below 100,000. These latter data justify the current approach to platelet transfusion therapy during massive blood volume resuscitation but are less helpful in patients with longstanding thrombocytopenia. Often these latter patients have increased destruction of platelets, either as a result of their

underlying disease or secondary to development of antiplatelet antibodies from prior platelet transfusions. Accordingly, correction of thrombocytopenia in these patients may not be possible. In these patients selective destruction of older platelets frequently leaves a population of younger platelets with superior hemostatic capacity, and they may not develop bleeding despite being thrombocytopenic. The use of HLA-matched platelets should be reserved for those who demonstrate alloimmunization with rapid platelet destruction. This is manifest by a significantly reduced increment in platelet count after platelet transfusion.

The nature of the surgical procedure is also a determinant of the likelihood of developing perioperative bleeding. Splenectomy, for example, usually does not involve much trauma to serosal surfaces, and ligation of the vessels supplying the spleen provides excellent hemostasis. Multiple studies have demonstrated that even in patients with severe coagulopathies secondary to myeloproliferative diseases, hypersplenism, or ITP, the incidence of significant bleeding complications after splenectomy ranges from 0% to 5% in spite of platelet counts of 25,000 to 50,000.[61,79] In contrast, open heart surgery is often complicated by postoperative bleeding from small vessels, and patients undergoing these pro-

TABLE 24-3. Coagulation disorders

Thrombocytopenia	ITP
	Hypersplenism
	Drug-induced disorders, including decreased production caused by chemotherapeutic agents or ethanol and increased destruction caused by PCN and heparin
Qualitative defects	Congenital (rare)
	Drug-induced defects, including ASA and nitroprusside as causative agents
	Uremia
	Hypothermia (?)
Clotting deficiencies	Hemophilia A and B
	von Willebrand's disease
	Coumadin therapy
Circulating anticoagulants and fibrinolytic disorders	Heparin therapy
	Lupus anticoagulant
	DIC
	Primary fibrinolysis

cedures probably require higher platelet counts. If platelets are to be given preoperatively, they should be administered immediately before incision to maximize intraoperative levels. When a decision is reached to administer platelets to a patient with a quantitative or qualitative platelet defect, attention should be given not only to measuring an increment in the platelet count done immediately after transfusion (normal increase is approximately 10,000/ul/ unit of platelets transfused, or 50% of the transfused number of platelets) but platelet counts should also be checked 1 hour, 4 hours and daily after transfusion. The initial platelet increment correlates most closely with the immediate clinical response while survival measurements determine the required frequency of transfusion. Causes of reduced increments include hypersplenism, alloimmunization, fever, and infection. In a study of 28 patients receiving 131 transfusions, the increment was 39% in afebrile patients and 21% if the temperature was greater than 38.5° C; platelet survival at 24 hours was 60% for noninfected, afebrile patients, 25% in those with fever greater than 38.5° C, and 12% in septic patients.[62] Evaluation of function after transfusion may be more difficult, and is most simply done by repeat measurements of the template bleeding time. While the in vivo integrity of stored platelets has been an area of major dispute, most researchers agree that platelets stored at 4° C are dysfunctional within 24 hours after use. Frequently, decisions regarding need for additonal platelet transfusions are based on evidence of bleeding.

Qualitative platelet disorders. Inherited platelet disorders are rare and most functional platelet abnormalities result from either drugs or uremia. The box above, right lists commonly encountered drugs which can alter platelet function. Aspirin, because it is a component of so many over-the-counter drugs, is a very common cause of perioperative platelet dysfunction. In one survey, 52% of patients presenting for emergency surgery had ingested some aspirin-containing compound within the previous 8 to 10 days.[62] By inducing irreversible acetylation and inactivation of the platelet cyclooxygenase enzyme, aspirin decreases platelet thromboxane levels. This can result in a prolonged bleeding time, although not necessarily in a dose-dependent fashion. Preoperative aspirin use has been shown to increase perioperative blood loss in patients having cardiac surgical procedures.[138] Two studies, one a case-control

---

> **Commonly used drugs that may affect platelet function**
>
> Aspirin
> Non-steroidal anti-inflammatory drugs (NSAID'S)
> Dipyridamole
> Methylxanthines (caffeine, aminophylline, theophylline)
> Penicillins (pen G, carbenicillin, ticarcillin, ampicillin)
> Cephalosporins (especially moxalactam)
> Nitrofurantoin
> Tricyclic antidepressants (amitriptyline, nortryptriline, imipramine)
> Phenothiazines (chlorpromazine, promethazine, trifluoperazine)
> General anesthetics (halothane)
> Dextrans
> Propranolol
> Furosemide
> Nitroprusside
> Nitroglycerin
> Ethanol
> Heparin

---

and another a randomized, nonblind study, have demonstrated significantly more mediastinal bleeding in the postoperative period, particularly the first 6 hours.[113] Similarly, peripartum bleeding has also been shown to be increased by aspirin ingestion.[202] Decisions regarding postponement of elective surgical procedures as a result of aspirin use should be based on the nature of the surgical procedure and on actual bleeding time results. In practice, there exists considerable institutional variability concerning the importance of aspirin-induced platelet dysfunction, and only cardiac and neurosurgical procedures tend to be delayed. Because aspirin irreversibly inactivates the cyclooxygenase enzyme, platelet function does not return to normal for 7 to 10 days, the effective lifespan of the platelet.

Less data exist on the perioperative implications of platelet abnormalities induced by other drugs. Several studies examining perioperative use of nonsteroidal antiinflammatory agents have shown no effect on blood loss.[204,230] Despite this, several texts recommend that they be discontinued 2 to 4 weeks before surgery. Halogenated anesthetic agents have been demonstrated to alter in vitro platelet aggregation but have never been associated with increased bleeding.[203] Intraoperative use of sodium nitroprusside, a potent vasodilator used commonly in the perioperative period, has been reported to be associated with increased blood loss when used for postoperative blood pressure control in cardiac surgical patients[81]; a subsequent study using low doses found no effect on perioperative blood loss.[91] This effect of nitroprusside has been shown to result from guanylate cyclase-induced decreases in platelet aggregation, perhaps mediated through endothelium-derived relaxation factor.

Hypothermia, long felt to be associated with increased bleeding, has recently been shown to reduce platelet thromboxane production.[220] These biochemical changes are accompanied by a reversible increase in bleeding time from 2.4 ± 0.8 to 5.8 ± 1.5 minutes when skin temperature is reduced from $34°$ to $27°$ C.[220] These temperature-dependent changes in platelet function contribute to platelet dysfunction during cardiopulmonary bypass. In addition, depletion of the von Willebrand factor, hemodilution, and red blood cell transfusions are felt to be contributory. Platelet function abnormalities in uremia and their management are discussed in Chapter 23.

Clotting factor abnormalities Hemophilia A, or factor VIII deficiency, is a sex-linked hereditary disorder with a frequency of approximately 1 in 10,000 U.S. males; hemophilia B, or factor IX deficiency, has a reported incidence of .25 per 10,000 males. Approximately 30% of hemophilia A cases arise spontaneously. The frequency and severity of bleeding in most hemophilias corresponds with the biological assay of the missing plasma factor.

Before the advent of cryoprecopitate by Pool et al in 1964,[167] the mortality of surgical procedures in hemophiliacs ranged from 13% to 67%.[41,164] Once specific commercial concentrates of factors VIII and IX become available, the criteria for operating on hemophiliacs broadened and mortality declined dramatically. Brown et al[27] presented in 1986 the results of 23 operations in 22 patients with hemophilia (18 A and 4 B) including AAA repair, liver transplantation and vagotomy/pyloroplasty. Factor levels were maintained at or above 1.0 U/ml intraoperatively and at 0.5 U/ml for 7 to 14 days postoperatively by administration of factor concentrates, fresh frozen plasma (FFP) or cryoprecipitate. No patient died from coagulopathy; there were two deaths in

the series, both in patients with severe hepatitis. Neither had a clinically apparent coagulopathy.

Preoperative preparation of the hemophiliac presenting for surgery requires, in addition to standard coagulation testing (PT/PTT/template bleeding time), assaying for factor activity, evaluating for circulating inhibitors, and correcting these abnormalities with a variety of factor-containing materials. In severe factor III deficient patients, circulating inhibitors may make elective surgical procedures impossible. Inhibitors have been reported in 4% to 6% of factor VIII deficient patients, with the incidence reportedly as high as 20% in those with activity of less than 1% of normal.[110] Replacement therapy for hemophilia includes fresh frozen plasma, cryoprecipitate, and specific factor concentrates. Use of FFP can result in hypervolemia as a result of the large amounts required to achieve 50% of normal factor activity. FFP has a relatively low risk of infectious complications since each unit comes from a single donor. Cryoprecipitate also comes from single donors and is considerably smaller volume load, but has the disadvantage of possessing variable amounts of factor VIII activity. Lyophilized antihemophilic factor, while providing the most reliable and lowest volume titer of factor activity, carries the highest risk of infectious disease transmission resulting from its pooled origin. In a longitudinal study of 42 hemophiliacs in Ohio followed for 3 years 31 had lymph nodal enlargement and or splenomegaly, 4 died from opportunistic infections, 3 of chronic hepatitis, 1 of Burkitt's lymphoma, 1 of non-Hodgkins lymphoma, and 1 of primary pulmonary hypertension.[171] While screening tests for HIV infectivity in blood products has hopefully minimized the risk of HIV infection in hemophiliacs, a recent study in New Orleans reported that 18 of 37 (49%) hemophiliacs were seropositive and 11 (30%) had generalized lymphadenopathy. It seems prudent at this time to recommend blood and body fluid precautions in the perioperative period for the routine management of the patient with hemophilia.

Von Willebrand Factor (vWF) deficiency is an autosomal dominant disorder, which usually presents as a prolonged bleeding time in a patient with a history of epistaxis, easy bruising, or excessive bleeding after tooth extraction.[17] Because there are mild forms of the disorder which escape clinical detection, the incidence of the condition is difficult to identify; it may be as common as 7 per 100,000.

Von Willebrand Factor is a component of factor VIII and one of the few coagulation factors not made in the liver; it is synthesized by vascular endothelium. There is a twofold role of vWF in hemostasis. One is to bind with factor VIII and maintain its presence in the circulation; the other is to facilitate the binding of platelets to collagen. There can be considerable variability in the amount of clinical bleeding with vWF deficiency, not only between patients but at varying times in the same patient. The following different types of vWF deficiency have been identified: type I, with vWF antigen of 15% to 60% of normal; type III, with undetectable levels of antigen, and types IIa and IIb, in which there is a selective deficiency of the larger (bioactive) multimers of plasma vWF. There is also a pseudo-von Willebrand's disease, in which there is an abnormal affinity of platelets for vWF.

Preoperative evaluation of patients with von Willebrand's disease should include performing a bleeding time (preferable Duke), a PT and PTT, and, ideally, determination of the specific type of deficiency. Platelet-active substances such as aspirin should be avoided for 10 to 14 days before elective procedures. Cryoprecipitate (1 to 3 bags/10kg body weight/day) is used to improve bleeding time when it is prolonged. A target of 5 minutes is commonly aimed for if patients are scheduled for large surgical procedures. For small procedures, such as dental extractions or hernia repair in type I patients, the use of the von Willebrand factor stimulating agent desmopressin acetate (DDAVP) may be adequate, especially when combined with a fibrinolysis inhibitor such as epsilonaminocaproic acid (EACA). In a report of 5 patients given a single dose of DDAVP (0.3 ug/kg) along with EACA, excellent dental hemostasis was achieved; in another report, 4 patients underwent surgery (tonsillectomy, cystectomy, carpal tunnel release, and salpingo-oophorectomy) with DDAVP alone.[48] These drugs provide the advantage of avoiding the infectious and immunologic risks of cryoprecipitate transfusion. It should be pointed out, however, that this therapy is only reportedly useful for type I patients; type III patients may not have enough endogenous vWF factor production to stimulate, and the vWF produced by type II patients may not be effective. DDAVP administration has been associated with mild thrombocytopenia and thus could theoretically cause worse bleeding in patients with pseudo-von Willebrand's disease.[205]

Patients on chronic coumadin therapy because of prior embolic or thrombotic problems or as prophylaxis against embolic complications following valve replacement have decreased levels of factors II, VII, IX, and X. Restoration of normal clotting function occurs several days after discontinuation of the drug; however, this often is not desirable since these patients are then at risk from thrombotic complications for a considerable period of time. To minimize the duration of normal coagulability, these individuals are commonly switched to heparin for preoperative anticoagulation. Discontinuation of heparin 4 to 6 hours before surgery usually results in adequate intraoperative hemostasis. Heparin is then resumed postoperatively and patients are later switched back to coumadin for more long-term anticoagulation. Little data exist on the efficacy of this practice, either as regards the incidence of bleeding complications or thrombotic complications, and the optimal time to resume heparin postoperatively is unknown. Obviously, the nature of the surgical procedure will affect this latter decision.

Circulating anticoagulants and fibrinolytic agents

Heparin. Heparin is a glycosaminoglycan whose principal biological effect is to interact with antithrombin III and thus interfere with the intrinsic clotting factors IX, X and thrombin. A secondary effect is interference with platelet-thrombin and platelet-endothelial interaction. Although naturally occurring in human mast cells as well as vascular endothelium, commercial heparin is derived from porcine or bovine intestines (the porcine reportedly being more antigenic in humans). Indications for heparin in the perioperative period include: prevention of venous thromboembolism, "treatment" (actually, the prevention of propagation of) of deep venous thrombosis and pulmonary embolism, and anticoagulation during vascular surgery. Bleeding complications during heparin therapy are associated with increased dose (the dose that achieves a PTT > 2.0 X control), length of administration (greatest on the third day), and concomitant or recent aspirin or heavy ethanol ingestion.[223] Another infrequent complication of heparin therapy is thrombocytopenia, which may be accompanied by thrombosis.[120] Neutralization of heparin can be achieved on a unit per unit basis with protamine sulfate, which may itself be antigenic or cause perioperative bleeding when given in excess.

Lupus anticoagulant. Circulating coagulants are uncommon, however between 5% and 10% of patients with systemic lupus erythematosus have a blood coagulation disorder characterized by a prolonged whole blood clotting time and a prolonged PT.[60] A similar syndrome is also described in up to one third of psychotic patients on long-term, high dose phenothiazine therapy.[31] Two reports of 34 patients with lupus anticoagulants undergoing a total of 39 surgical procedures did not demonstrate increased perioperative bleeding[22,59]; however, recent reports have found an increased risk of venous and arterial thromboses in these patients. Speculation is that prostacyclin release is inhibited in these patients,[18,59] leading to increased platelet aggregation. The lupus anticoagulant usually persists in the untreated patient, but may diminish or disappear with treatment. Lubbe and coworkers recently reported the delivery of 5 live infants after six women with lupus anticoagulant were treated with prednisone and aspirin. All had a prior history of fetal demise.[128]

Disseminated intravascular coagulation (DIC). DIC or consumptive coagulopathy, is a complex sequence of pathophysiological events which manifests itself as diffuse bleeding, usually from mucous membranes, puncture sites, and the gastrointestinal tract. Laboratory studies demonstrate increased PT, PTT, and fibrin degradation products as well as decreased fibrinogen. It is almost always secondary to some underlying insult such as sepsis or amniotic fluid embolism. Treatment of DIC centers around resolution of the triggering agent; other therapies such as heparin, cryoprecipitate and fresh frozen plasma are controversial.

Primary fibrinolysis. The increasing use of the fibrinolytic agents streptokinase, urokinase, and tissue plasminogen activator in the last few years are only now becoming important in the perioperative period; patients taking these drugs usually present for surgery because of failure of arterial clot lysis and continuing ischemic symptoms, or as a result of a complication of the invasive procedure itself. When ongoing fibrinolysis is considered present, the use of epsilon-aminocaproic acid (EACA) may be indicated to halt the fibrinolytic process. Because urokinase is normally present in urine, bleeding after prostatectomy has been attributed to plasminogen activation and the dissolution of clots in the operative bed. Studies of patients undergoing perineal or suprapubic prostatectomy have demonstrated EACA to be efficacious in reducing perioperative blood loss when hemorrhage is severe.[184]

Perioperative Thrombotic Disorders

The preceding section addresses a number of disorders of coagulation that can result in significant perioperative bleeding. Abnormalities of the coagulation system that result in an increased tendency to form clot can also result in perioperative complications. These latter disorders are less well characterized than those which result in bleeding, and laboratory detection of hypercoagulability is considerably more difficult. Recognized conditions associated with hypercogulability include antithrombin 3 deficiency, certain malignancies (especially adenocarcinomas), DIC, and thrombocytosis and polycythemia (particularly when associated with myeloproliferative disorders). The greater preponderance of perioperative thromboembolic complications, however, occurs in patients without prior thrombotic tendencies. Recent data suggest that surgery itself results in significant changes in the coagulation and fibrinolytic systems which lead to a hypercoagulable state.

While the development of a hypercoagulable state postoperatively can be viewed as beneficial for hemostasis, it can predispose to developing deep venous thrombosis (DVT), myocardial infarction (MI), and peripheral vascular arterial occlusions. This is particularly true in patients with coronary artery disease and peripheral artery disease who are at risk for developing arterial thrombosis and for elderly patients and patients having orthopedic gynecological and urologic procedures who are at increased risk for development of DVT.

The stimulus for the development of increased perioperative coagulant activity is not known, but tissue factors released from surgically damaged vascular and perivascular tissues probably directly initiate the coagulation cascade.[153] This results in elevated levels of the coagulation proteins factor 8, prothrombin, and fibrinogen, and decreased levels of antithrombin 3.[25,174] Additionally, decreases in fibrinolytic activity and altered rheologic properties increase thrombotic potential.[54] Decreases in fibrinolysis can be demonstrated directly and also indirectly by depressed levels of plasminogen activators and increased antiplasmin globulin levels.[142,153] Interestingly, the decrease in fibrinolysis peaks on postoperative days 2 to 3,[142] which is coincident with a peak in postoperative myocardial infarction.[9,170] The postoperative rheologic changes involve an increase in plasma viscosity and a decrease in red blood cell (RBC) deformability.[54,153] The increase in viscosity is caused by an elevation of postoperative acute phase reactants (fibrinogen and globulins) and the cause of the decrease in RBC deformability is unknown. Because of a lower incidence of DVT in patients whose sugery was performed with regional as opposed to general anesthesia[143] surgically induced neurohumoral responses have been hypothesized to contribute to perioperative hypercoagulability. However, coagulation and fibrinolysis studies appear to be similar in patients having regional and general anesthesia except for a lower level of activated factor 8 in the epidural anesthesia group.[25,142] This isolated difference is probably not responsible for the decrease in DVTs, and increased lower extremity blood flow with regional techniques may be the explanation.[145] Further studies in this area are needed and should prove interesting.

Pulmonary Embolism

Pulmonary embolism is often cited as a major cause of mortality and morbidity in hospitalized patients. Despite this, pulmonary embolus is infrequently listed as a cause of death in surgical patients and perioperative prophylaxis against pulmonary embolism and deep venous thrombosis (DVT) is not routine in most institutions. This section we will attempt to answer the following questions: (1) What is the incidence of pulmonary embolism in surgical patients? (2) What strategies are available to deal with the problem of perioperative pulmonary embolism? and (3) Are the approaches to deal with this problem effective?

Incidence of fatal pulmonary embolism in surgical patients. Because prospective studies of the incidence of pulmonary embolism are difficult and expensive, most data come from autopsy studies. These studies, in a variety of different patient populations, report pulmonary embolism as the cause of death in 5% to 25% of patients.* Most report figures of approximately 15%. To put this data in

perspective, approximately 26,000 surgical procedures are performed yearly at Johns Hopkins Hospital. Overall surgical mortality is approximately 1% (260 patients). Assuming that pulmonary embolism accounts for 15% of these deaths, then 40 patients die each year of pulmonary emboli at our hospital. Data from Bell and Zuidema[10] suggest that other institutions have similar incidences of overall surgical mortality (1.3%), and thus death caused by pulmonary embolism occurs in 0.2% of surgical patients. Thus even in a very busy surgical practice, death caused by pulmonary embolism is a rare event.

Approaches to the problem of perioperative pulmonary embolism. Given the low overall incidence of fatal pulmonary emboli in surgical patients, is the cost and potential morbidity of prophylaxis justified? Substitution of a "wait and treat" approach for routine prophylaxis, however, requires that pulmonary emboli can be accurately diagnosed and effectively treated; unfortunately, neither assumption appears to be correct. A considerable number of patients who die from pulmonary embolism die within 50 minutes of the onset of problems, leaving little time for effective intervention.* Furthermore, pulmonary embolism is a difficult diagnosis to make. Autopsy data indicate that fatal pulmonary emboli are often unsuspected†; in pooling data from a number of studies, pulmonary emboli were not suspected in 70% of patients found to have pulmonary emboli on post mortem exam. This high rate of misdiagnosis reflects the fact that clinical diagnosis is difficult. Bell et al[11] found that the classic triad of shortness of breath, chest pain, and hemoptysis is present in less than 20% of patients with documented pulmonary emboli. In the study of Coon and Willis,[38] the diagnosis was made less than 3% of the time. The most common symptoms (pleuritic pain, dyspnea, cough, and apprehension) are nonspecific and often go unnoticed in the absence of pulmonary hemorrhage or pulmonary infarction.[38,51] In a trial evaluating urokinase/streptokinase as treatment for pulmonary embolism,[217,218] only 327 of 6,213 patients entered into the trial (based on classic clinical criteria or suspicion of ongoing pulmonary embolism) had angiographically demonstrable pulmonary emboli, an incidence of 5.3%

The "gold standard" for diagnosis remains the

---

*References 14, 37, 49, 68, 77, 148, 189, 216.

*References 38, 53, 75, 88, 150, 199.
†References 38, 39, 53, 68, 77, 189, 216.

pulmonary angiogram. Angiographic findings correlate well with autopsy results. In the urokinase/streptokinase pulmonary embolism trial, of 906 patients with pulmonary angiograms there were only two false positives.[217,218] However, pulmonary angiogram is expensive, invasive, and requires special personnel. While in the past pulmonary angiography was avoided because of suspected mortality and morbidity, the results in the urokinase/streptokinase pulmonary embolism trial indicate that the morbidity is under 1% and the mortality is under .001%.[217,218] Recent reports suggest that even in patients with pulmonary hypertension, previously considered a high-risk group, angiography is relatively safe.[139,158,162] Most complications of pulmonary angiography relate to catheterization (arrhythmias, bleeding, and pulmonary artery rupture) or to the use of contrast dye (seizures, anaphylaxis, hypotension, and renal insufficiency).[139,158,162] Alternate diagnostic tests include (1) routine chest X-rays, which are neither adequately sensitive nor specific,[16,38,102] (2) perfusion scans, which have a high rate of false positives,[102,135,217,218] and false negatives,[102,135,217,218] and (3) combined ventilation/perfusion scans, which although more specific, still have a high rate of both false positives and false negatives especially in patients felt to be at low risk for pulomanary embolism.[16,102,103] A recent report suggests that digital angiography correlates well with pulmonary angiography,[166] and, if these findings are confirmed, it may offer a valuable alternative.

Finally, even with accurate diagnosis, death from pulmonary embolism occurs despite institution of seemingly appropriate treatment.* Most large studies report an 8% to 11% incidence of recurrent pulmonary emboli in patients receiving adequate treatment. It appears, therefore, that some form of prophylaxis is warranted.

Who should receive prophylaxis? The first question that arises is to whom prophylaxis should be offered. Given the large number of patients having surgery and the overall low incidence of pulmonary embolism, it is impractical and not cost effective to provide prophylaxis for all surgical patients. What, then, are risk factors which define high-risk populations? The risk factor that has been most heavily studied is lower extremity DVT. Thromboses of the veins of the lower extremities give rise to 70%

to 90% of all pulmonary emboli. Autopsy data confirm that virtually all patients with pulmonary emboli have DVT* and similar findings come from study of patients who survive pulmonary embolism.† When examined prospectively, approximately 25% of patients with DVT develop pulmonary emboli.[38,103] When the thrombosis occurs in the proximal veins of the leg or the veins of the pelvis the risk is even higher, in the neighborhood of 50%.[102,151]

Problems with using lower extremity DVT to initiate anticoagulant therapy are threefold; often DVT is difficult to diagnose,[38,149,189,226] DVT may first present with a pulmonary embolism,[30,190] and not all pulmonary emboli arise from this source.[134] The "gold standard" for diagnosis remains venography, which is expensive, invasive, painful, and requires a grest deal of contrast. Furthermore, the entire venous system is not always visualized and flow defects are not always caused by thrombosis.[226] Alternatives to contrast venography include the following: 1. Iodine-125-labelled fibrinogen uptake. This test correlates well with venography for thrombosis below the level of the knee[92,226] but not for lesions above the knee,[26,86,109] and it is from these regions that pulmonary emboli are most likely to arise. 2. Doppler ultrasonic blood flow studies. This test is inexpensive, noninvasive, and can be done at the bedside and in outpatients, but it requires an experienced observer. It is 80% to 90% accurate.[194,201] 3. Impedance plethysmography. This test looks at pressure/volume relationships in the calf after inflation and deflation of a thigh cuff, using electrical impedence to estimate blood volume, run-off is slow in the presence of obstruction. This test is very accurate, particularly for proximal thrombi and has a low false positive rate.[98,99,225] It is, however, technically difficult, and considerably less accurate in cold, apprehensive, or hypovolemic patients.

There are additional problems with waiting for DVT to occur before instituting therapy. Treatment for DVT is not always successful. Dalen et al found a lysis rate of less than 20% in patients with large clots treated with heparin,[52] while Doyle et al and Gallus et al[71] had 10 of 96 and 4.1%, respectively, of heparin-treated patients develop pulmonary embolism. Finally, DVT can recur,[100,191] requires long-term anticoagulant therapy which is associated

---

*References 6, 149, 165, 217, 218.

*References 6, 14, 53, 87, 190.
†References 26, 70, 102, 103, 160.

bleeding complications,[100,101] and can result in venous insufficiency.

A number of randomized prospective studies have focused on risk factors associated with the occurrence of DVT in an attempt to identify a high-risk population for selective prophylactic therapy. A consistent finding in these studies is that the risk of DVT and pulmonary embolism is very low in patients under the age of 40, and progressively increases with advancing age. In addiiton, the risk is low following surgical procedures lasting less than 1 hour. The type of surgery also influences the incidence of DVT. In a study examining pooled data from a large number of randomized, prospective trials investigating the efficacy of subcutaneous heparin in preventing DVT and pulmonary embolism, Collins et al[40] determined that, in the control population, the incidence of DVT was 15.6%, fatal pulmonary embolism 0.46%, and nonfatal pulmonary embolism 1.8%. In patients having lower extremity orthopedic procedures, however, the incidence of DVT was 35.8%, fatal pulmonary embolism 1.6%, and nonfatal pulmonary embolism 7.1%. In patients undergoing urologic surgery, the incidence of DVT was 40%, fatal PE .75% and a nonfatal PE 1.5%. Other types of elective surgery, including gynecologic surgery, do not appear to be associated with an increased incidence of DVT.[12,20,182] An extensive literature has focused on emergent surgical repair of hip fractures. In data pooled from Collins et al,[40] the incidence of DVT in these patients was 47%, and fatal pulmonary emboli occurred in almost 3%. These findings have been confirmed in numerous other studies. Few data exist for other types of emergent surgery including trauma surgery. Sevitt and Gallagher reported in 1959 that the incidence of DVT was 66%[190]; no more recent data are available. Other risk factors include; obesity, the presence of malignancy, prolonged periods of immobility, and a prior history of either DVT or pulmonary embolism.

Options for prophylaxis against DVT and pulmonary embolism. The above discussion suggests that patients having lower extremity orthopedic procedures or repair of hip fracture should receive prophylactic therapy. In addition, elderly patients and patients with other risk factors who undergo extensive procedures, especially urologic operations, should also receive prophylaxis. The following techniques have received the greatest attention:

Compression methods. The use of pneumatic compression stockings in patients with intracranial disease,[196,215] those undergoing orthopedic procedures, those with gynecologic cancer[34] and those undergoing procedures related to trauma[93] has been shown to reduce the incidence of DVT by approximately 50%. In the urologic patient population, in which this device has been most widely used, the reduction is in the neighborhood of 75% to 95%.[36]

Subcutaneous or minidose heparin. The previously mentioned study by Collins et al,[40] in which multiple prior reports were subjected to meta-analysis, provides the most convincing data on the efficacy of subcutaneous heparin for prophylaxis against DVT and pulmonary embolism. In the general surgical population, the incidence of DVT was 22.4% in the untreated group and 8.9% in those patients receiving heparin, for a percent odds reduction of 71 ± 8%. In elective orthopedic procedures the incidence of DVT was reduced from 46% to 21%, for an odds reduction of 70 ± 9%; while in orthopedic trauma (for example, hip fractures) the incidence of DVT was reduced form 49% to 27.6% (odds reduction = 64 ± 12%). Similar reductions were also seen in patients undergoing urological surgery (13.9% versus 41%). The overall incidence of fatal pulmonary embolism (all patient groups) was 0.26% in patients receiving heparin and 0.81% in patients not receiving prophylaxis, for a percent odds reduction of 64 ± 15%. Approximately 1.3% of patients receiving heparin and 2% of patients not receiving heparin had nonfatal pulmonary emboli, for an odds reduction of 41 ± 11%. Mini-heparin has also been used in conjunction with dihydroergotamine, a drug that constricts veins and venules and accelerates venous return. Combined data from several studies indicate that this regimen offers no advantage over mini-heparin alone. Data from the report of Collins et al[40] suggest that minidose heparin is not associated with an increased risk of perioperative bleeding.

Regional anesthesia. Several studies have focused on the use of regional anesthesia as a means for preventing DVT and pulmonary embolism. Modig et al[141] found that patients having total hip replacement who had an epidural anesthetic which was maintained for 24 hours postoperatively had a decreased incidence of DVT (40% versus 66%) when compared to patients having the same procedure but who received a general anesthetic (N_2O, narcotic, relaxant) and parenteral narcotics for postoperative analgesia. The incidence of proximal DVTs, those most likely to embolize, was reduced from 67% to 13%, and pulmonary embolism (diagnosed by ventilation perfusion scanning) occurred in 3 of 30 patients receiving epidural anesthesia (10%) versus 10 of 30 patients receiving general anesthesia (33%). In another study comparing spinal and general anesthesia in patients undergoing total hip replacements,[211] the incidence of DVT was 30% in the spinal anesthesia group and 55% in the general anesthesia group.

Conclusions and recommendations. Pulmonary emboli account for about 15% of surgical deaths. Based on unsatisfactory outcome data when treatment is instituted after DVT and/or pulmonary embolism and the efficacy and low morbidity of prophylaxis, prophylactic therapy of high-risk patients appears to be indicated. At present the greatest amount of data exist for the use of subcutaneous heparin. This is probably also the least expensive prophylactic technique. It must be noted that subcutaneous heparin is not 100% effective in preventing DVT and pulmonary embolism, and few data exist concerning the appropriate duration of treatment. Most clinicians continue treatment until patients are no longer bedridden and/or immobilized. Whether some combination of regional anesthesia, compression stockings, and subcutaneous heparin will further reduce the incidence of these complications (and is cost effective) is unknown.

REFERENCES

1. Abendschein DR et al: Myocardial blood flow during accute isovolumic anemia and treadmill exercise in dogs, J Appl Physiol 53:203, 1982.
2. Abramson DE et al: Resting peripheral blood flow in the anemic state, Am Heat J 25:609, 1943.
3. Alexander JC and Prudden JF: The causes of abdominal wound disruption, Surg Gynecol Obstet 122:1223, 1966.
4. Allen C and Tasswell HF: Case history number 67: frozen storage of autologous blood, Anesth Analg 51:287, 1972.
5. Allen JB and Allen FB: The minimum acceptable level of hemoglobin. In Stehling LC (editor): Techniques of blood transfusion. Stehling LC (editor). Int Anesthesiol Clin 20(4):1, 1982.
6. Alpert, et al: Mortality in patients treated for pulmonary embolism, JAMA 236:1477-1480, 1976.
7. American Association of Blood Banks and Council of Community Blood Centers, American Red Cross blood services letter 83-43: joint statement on directed donations, Washington, DC, 1983, American Red Cross.
8. Asakura T et al: Effect of deoxygenation of intracellular hemoglobin on red cell glycolysis, J Biochem (Tokyo) 59:524g, 1966.
9. Becket RC and Underwood DA: Myocardial infarction in patients undergoing noncardiac surgery, Cleve Clin J Med 54:25-28, 1987.
10. Bell WR and Zuiudema GD: Low-dose heparin—concern and perspective, Surgery 85:469-471, 1979.
11. Bell WR et al: The clinical features of submassive and massive pulmonary emboli, Am J Med 62:355-360, 1977.
12. Bellord RM et al: Low doses of subcutaneous heparin in the prevention of deep vein thrombosis after gynaecologic surgery, Br J Obstet and Gynaecol 80:469-472, 1973.
13. Benesch R and Benesch RE: Intracellular organic phosphates as regulators of oxygen release by hemoglobin, Nature 221:618, 1969.
14. Bergqvist D and Lindbled B: A 30-year survey of pulmonary embolism verified at autopsy: an analysis of 1274 surgical patients, Br J Surg 72:105-108, 1985.
15. Beutler E and Wood L: The in vivo regeneration of red cell 2, 3-diphosphoglyceric acid (DPG) after transfusion of stored blood, J Lab Clin Med 74:300, 1969.
16. Biello DR: Radiological evaluation of patients with suspected pulmonary thrombo-embolism, JAMA 257:3257-3259, 1987.
17. Bloom AL: The von Willebrand syndrome, Semin Hematol 17:215, 1980.
18. Boey ML et al: Thrombosis in systemic lupus erythematosus: striking association with the presence of circulating lupus anticoagulant, Br Med J 287:1021, 1983.
19. Boldt J et al: Influence of acute preoperative hemodiluation on right ventricular function, J Cardiothor Anesth 2:765, 1988.
20. Bonner J and Welsh J: Prevention of thrombosis after pelvic surgery by British dextran 70, Lancet 614-616, 1972.
21. Bove JR: Transfusion-associated hepatitis and AIDS: What is the risk? N Engl J Med 317:242, 1987.
22. Boxer M, Ellman L, and Carualho A: The lupus anticoagulant, Arthritis Rheum 19:1244, 1976.
23. Brannon ES et al: The cardiac output in patients with chronic anemia as measured by the technique of right atrial catheterization, J Clin Invest 24:332, 1945.
24. Brazier J: The adequacy of myocardial oxygen delivery in acute normovolemic anemia, Surgery 75:508, 1974.
25. Bredbacka S et al: Pre- and postoperative changes in coagulation and fibrinolytic variables during ab-

dominal hysterectomy under epidural or general anesthesia, Acta Anaesthesiol Scand 30:204-210,
1986.

26. Browse NL and Lea M: Source of non-lethal pulmonary emboli, Lancet 258-259, 1974.

27. Brown B et al: General surgery in adult hemophiliacs, Surgery 99:154, 1986.

28. Buckalew VM and Someren A: Renal manifestation
of sickle cell disease, Arch Intern Med 133:660-669,
1974.

29. Bunn HF, Forget BG, and Ranney HM: Human hemoglobins, Philadelphia, 1977, WB Saunders Co.

30. Byrne JJ: Phlebitis and pulmonary embolism, N Engl
J Med 827-838.

31. Canoso RT and Hutton RA: A chlorpromazine-in-
duced inhibitor of blood coagulation, Am J Hematol
2:183, 1977.

32. Chanutin A and Curnish RR: Effect of organic and
inorganic phosphates on the oxygen equilibrium of
human erythrocytes, Arch Biochem Biophys 121:96,
1967.

33. Charache S and Conley CL: Rate of sickling of red
cells during deoxygenation of blood from persons
with various sickling disorders, Blood 24:25-48,
1964.

34. Clark-Pearson DL et al: Prevention of venous thromboembolism by external calf compression in patients with gynecologic malignancy, Obstet Gynecol
63:92-98, 1984.

35. Clocke RA: Oxygen transport and 2, 3-diphospho-
glycerate, Chest 62:7951, 1972.

36. Coe NP et al: Prevention of deep vein thrombosis in
urological patients: a controlled randomized trial of
low dose heparin and external pneumatic boots, Surgery 83:230A, 1978.

37. Coon WV: Risk factors in pulmonary embolism surgery, Gynecol Obstet 143:385-390, 1976.

38. Coon WW and Willis PW: Deep venous thrombosis
and pulmonary embolism, Am J Cardiol 4:611-621,
1959.

39. Coon WW and Collier FA: Cliniopathologic correlation in thromboembolism, Surg Gynecol Obstet
109:259-269, 1959.

40. Collins R et al: Reduction in fatal pulmonary embolism and venous thrombosis by perioperative administration of subcutaneous heparin, N Engl J Med
109:259-269, 1959.

41. Craddock C, Fenninger L, and Simmons B: Hemophilia. Problem of surgical intervention for accompanying disease. Review of the literature and
report of a case, Ann Surg 128:888, 1948.

42. Crowell JW, Ford RG, and Lewis VM: Oxygen
transport in hemorrhagic shock is a function of the
hematocrit ratio, Am J Physiol 196:1033, 1959.

43. Crowell JW, Bounds SH, and Johnson WW: Effect

of varying the hematocrit ratio on the susceptibility
to hemorrhagic shock, Am J Physiol 192:171, 1958.

44. Crystal GJ and Weiss HR: Vo$_2$ of resting muscle
during arterial hypoxia: role of reflex vasoconstriction, Microvasc Res 20:30, 1980.

45. Daul CB, DeShazo RD, and Andes WA: Human
immunodeficiency virus infection in hemophiliac patients, Am J Med 84:801, 1988.

46. Davidson D and Stalcup SA: Systemic circulatory
adjustments to acute hypoxia and reoxygenation in
unanesthetized sheep, J Clin Invest 73:317, 1984.

47. Davis NJ, Jennings JJ, and Harris WH: Induced
hypotensive anesthesia for total hip replacement,
General Orthopedics, 101:93, 1974.

48. De La Fuenta B et al: Response of patients with mild
and moderate hemophilia A and von Willebrand's
disease to treatment with desmopressin, Ann Int Med
103:6, 1985.

49. Dismulke SE and Wagner EH: Pulmonary embolism
as a cause of death, JAMA 255:2039-2042, 1986.

50. Doane TA, Valeri CR, and Barton RK: Autotrans-
fusions of previously frozen blood in elective gynecologic surgery, Am J Obstet Gynecol 105:394,
1969.

51. Dolen JE et al: Pulmonary embolism, pulmonary
hemorrhage and pulmonary infarction, N Engl J Med
296:1431-1435, 1977.

52. Dolen JE et al: Venous thromboembolism: scope of
the problem, Chest 3705-3735, 1986.

53. Donaldson GA et al: A re-appraisal of the application
of the Trendelenberg operation to total invasive pulmonary embolism, N Engl J Med 268:171-174,
1963.

54. Doods AJ et al: Changes in red cell deformability
following surgery, Thrombosis Res 18:561-566,
1981.

55. Doyle DJ et al: Adjusted subcutaneous heparin or
continuous intravenous heparin in patients with acute
deep vein thrombosis, Ann Int Med 107:441-447,
1987.

56. Duke M and Abelmann WH: The hemodynamic response to chronic anemia, Circulation 39:503, 1969.

57. Eaton WA et al: Delay time in gelatin: a possible
determinant of clinical severity in sickle cell disease,
Blood 47:621-627, 1976.

58. Eckstein RW: Development of interarterial coronary
anastomoses by chronic anemia. Disappearance following correction anemia, Circ Res 3:306, 1955.

59. Elias M and Eldor A: Thromboembolism in patients
with the "lupus"-type circulating anticoagulant,
Arch Int Med 144:510, 1984.

60. Feinstein DI and Rapaport SI: Acquired inhibitors
of blood coagulation, Prog Hemost Thromb 1:75,
1972.

61. Ferguson CM: Splenectomy for ITP related to human

immunodeficiency virus, Surg Gynecol Obstet 135:300, 1988.

62. Ferraris VA and Swanson E: Aspirin usage and perioperative blood loss in patients undergoing unexpected operations, Surg Gynecol Obstet 156:439, 1983.

63. Finch CA and Lenfant C: Oxygen transport in man, N Engl J Med 286:407, 1972.

64. Fine JH: Fluid therapy before and after operation, Anesthesiology 3:65, 1942.

65. Fischer A et al: Safety and effectiveness of directed blood donation in a large teaching hospital, Transfusion 26:600, 1986.

66. Forster RE: Carbon monoxide and the partial pressure of oxygen in tissue, Ann NY Acad Sci 174:233, 1970.

67. Fredin H, Gustoffson C, and Rosberg B: Hypotensive anesthesia, thrombophylaxis and postoperative thromboembolism in total hip arthroplasty, Acta Anaesthesiol Scand 28:503, 1984.

68. Freiman DG et al: Frequency of pulmonary thromboembolism in man, N Engl J Med 1278-1280, 1963.

69. Fullerton MV et al: Preoperative exchange transfusion in sickle cell anemia, J Pediatr Surg 16:297-300, 1981.

70. Gallus AS and Hirsh J: Preventions of venous thromboembolism, Thromb Haemostasis 2:232-290, 1970.

71. Gallus A et al: Safety and efficacy of warfarin studied early after submassive venous thrombosis or pulmonary embolism, Lancet 1293-1296, 1986.

72. Geha AS: Coronary and cardiovascular dynamics and oxygen availability during acute normovolemic anemia, Surgery 80:47, 1976.

73. Geha AS and Baue A: Graded coronary stenosis and coronary flow during acute normovolemic anemia, World J Surg 2:645, 1978.

74. George CD and Morello PJ: Immunologic effects of blood transfusion upon renal transplantation, tumor operations and bacterial infections, Am J Surg 152:329, 1986.

75. Gifford RW and Grores LK: Limitations in the feasibility of pulmonary embolectomy: a cliniopathologic study of 101 cases of massive pulmonary embolism, Circulation 39:523-530, 1969.

76. Gillies IDS: Anaemia in anaesthesia, Br J Anaesth 46:589, 1974.

77. Goldhober SZ et al: Factors associated with correct antemortem diagnosis of major pulmonary embolism, Am J Med 73:822-826, 1982.

78. Goldsmith JR: Contribution of motor vehicle exhaust, industry, and cigarette smoking to community carbon monoxide exposures, Ann NY Acad Sci 174:122, 1970.

79. Grant IR et al: Elective splenectomy in hematological disorders, 1987.

80. Graves CL and Allen RM: Anesthesia in the presence of severe anemia, Rocky Mt Med J 67:35, 1970.

81. Graybar G, Lober D, and Jones J: Comparison of nitroprusside and nitroglycerin in perioperative blood loss with open heart surgery, Crit Care Med 2:240, 1980.

82. Gross HP: Hypotensive anesthesia in total hip replacement. Orthop Surg 30:27.

83. Grossman W and Braunwald E: High-cardiac output states. In Braunwold E (editor): Heart disease, a textbook of cardiovascular medicine, ed 3, Philadelphia, 1988, WB Saunders Co.

84. Gutierrez G: Peripheral delivery and utilization of oxygen. In Dantzler, DR (editor): Cardiopulmonary critical care, Orlando, Fla, Grune & Stratton.

85. Guyton AC: Physics of blood, blood flow, and pressure: Hemodynamics. In Guyton AC (editor): Textbook of medical physiology, ed 6, Philadelphia, 1981, WB Saunders Co.

86. Harris WH et al: Comparison of I^{125} fibrinogen count scanning with phlebography for detection of venous thrombi after elective hip surgery, N Engl J Med 292:665-667, 1975.

87. Havig O: Source of pulmonary emboli, Acta Chir Scan 478(Suppl):42-47, 1977.

88. Hermann RE, et al: Pulmonary embolism: a clinical and pathologic study with emphasis on the effects of prophylactic therapy with anticoagulants, Am J Surg 102:19-28, 1961.

89. Heughan C et al: The effect of anemia on wound healing, 179:163, 1974.

90. Heyman A et al: Cerebral circulation and metabolism in sickle cell and other chronic anemias with observations on the effects of oxygen inhalation, J Clin Invest 31:824, 1952.

91. Hines R and Barash PG: Infusion of sodium nitroprusside induces platelet dysfunction in vitro, Anesthesiology 70:611, 1989.

92. Hirsh J and Gallus AS: ^{125}I labeled frininogen scanning: use in the diagnosis of venous thrombosis, JAMA 233:970-977, 1975.

93. Holford CP: Graded compression for preventing deep venous thrombosis, Brit Med J 2:969-970, 1970.

94. Holzmann L, Finn H, Lichtman HC, et al: Anesthesia in patients with sickle cell disease: A review of 112 cases. Anesth Analg 48:566-572, 1969.

95. Homi J, Reynolds J, Skinner A, et al: General anesthesia in sickle cell disease. Br Med J 1:1599-1601, 1979.

96. Honig CR and Frierson JL: Role of adenosine in exercise vasodilatation in dog gracilis muscle, Am J Physiol 238:H703, 1980.

97. Huber H, Lewis SM, and Szur L. The influence of anemia, polycythemia and splenomegaly on the relationship between venous hematocrit and red-cell volume, Br J Haematol 10:567, 1964.

98. Huisman MV et al: Serial impedence plethyangiography for suspected deep venous thrombosis in outpatients, N Engl J Med 314:823-828, 1986.

99. Hull R et al: Impedence phethysmography: the relationship between venous filling and sensitivity and specifity for proximal vein thrombosis, Circulation 898-902, 1978.

100. Hull R et al: Warfarin sodium vs low-dose heparin in the long term treatment of venous thrombosis, N Engl J Med 301:855-858, 1979.

101. Hull R et al: Different intuisities of oral anticoagulant therapy in the treatment of proximal-vein thrombosis. N Engl J Med 307:1676-1681, 1982.

102. Hull RD et al: Pulmonary angiograph, ventilation lung scanning and venography for clinically suspected pulmonary embolism with abnormal perfusion lung scan, Ann Int Med 98:891-899, 1983.

103. Hull RD et al: Prophylaxia for venous thromboembolism: an overview, Chest 89:3745-3835, 1986.

104. Human immunodeficiency virus infection in the United States, MMWR 36:801, 1987.

105. Hutchinson RM, Merrick MV, and White JM: Fat embolism in sickle cell disease, Arch Intern Med 133:660-669, 1974.

106. Jacoby JJ: A review of the present status of preoperative hemoglobin requirements - comment, Anesth Analg 51:77, 1982.

107. Jan KM and Chien S: Effect of hematocrit variations on coronary hemodynamics and oxygen utilization, Am J Physiol 233:H106, 1977.

108. Kafer ER et al: Automated acute normovolemic hemodilution reduces homologous blood transfusion requirements for spinal fusion, Anesth Analg 65:576, 1986.

109. Kakkar VV: ^{125}Iodine-fibrinogen uptake test, Semin Nucl Med 7:229-244, 1977.

110. Kasper CK: Incidence and course of inhibitors among patients with classic hemophilia, Thromb Diath Haemorrh 30:264, 1973.

111. Kauy SV et al: The pathogenesis and control of the hemorrhagic defect in open-heart surgery, Surg Gynecol Obster 123:313, 1966.

112. Keith I: Anaesthesia and blood loss in total hip replacement, Anaesthesia 32:444, 1977.

113. Kennedy BM: Aspirin and surgery - a review, Ir Med J 77:363, 1984.

114. Kille JM and Klabunde RE: Adenosine as a mediator of postcontraction hyperthermia in dog gracilis muscle, Am J Physiol 246:H274, 1984.

115. Konotey-Ahulu FI: The sickle cell diseases: clinical manifestations including the "sickle crisis," Arch Intern Med 133:611-619, 1974.

116. Kowalyshyn TJ, Prager D, and Young J: A review of the present status of preoperative hemoglobin requirements, Anesth Analg 51:75, 1972.

117. Kruskall MS et al: Utilization and effectiveness of hospital autologous preoperative blood donor program, Transfusion 26:335, 1984.

118. Laasberg LH and Hedley-Whyte J: Viscosity of sickle disease and trait blood: changes with anesthesia, J Appl Physiol 35:837-843, 1973.

119. Lagerstedt CI et al: Need for long-term anticoagulant treatment in symptomatic calf-vein thrombosis, Lancet 515-518, 1985.

120. Laster J et al: The heparin-induced thrombocytopenia syndrome: an update, surgery 102:163, 1987.

121. Lawther PJ and Commins BT: Cigarette smoking and exposure to carbon monoxide, Ann NY Acad Sci 174:122, 1970.

122. Lehninger A: Biochemistry: the molecular basis of cell structure and function, New York, 1975, Worth Publishers, Inc.

123. Lessin LS, Kuranstin-Mills J, and Klug PP et al: Determination of rheologically optimal mixtures of AA and SS erythrocytes for transfusion. In Liss AR: Erythrocyte membranes: recent clinical and experimental advances Prog Clin Biol Res 20:123-134, 1978.

124. Leveen HH: Normovolemic hemodilution and autotransfusion in surgry. In: Mauer JM, Thurer RL, Dawson RB, (editors): Autotransfusion New York, 1981, Elsevier Science Publishing Co, Inc.

125. Levine EA et al: Recombinant human erytheopoletin and autologous blood donation, Surgery 104:365, 1988.

126. Linman JW: Physiological and pathophysiologic effects of anemia, N Engl J Med 279:812, 1968.

127. Loarie DJ et al: The hemodynamic effects of halothane in anemic dogs, Anesth Analg 58:195, 1979.

128. Lubbe WF et al: Lupus anticoagulant in pregnancy, Br J Obstet Gynaecol 91:357, 1984.

129. Lubin J et al: The use of autologous blood in open heart surgery, Transfusion 14:602, 1974.

130. McGarry P and Duncan C: Anesthetic risks in sickle cell trait, Pediatrics 51:507-512, 1973.

131. Macon WL and Pries WJ: The effect of iron deficiency anemia on wound healing, Surgery 69:792, 1971.

132. Mann LS et al: Disruption of abdominal wounds, JAMA 180:1021, 1962.

133. Mann M, Sacks HJ, and Goldfinger D: Safety of autologous blood donations prior to elective surgery for a variety of potentially "high-risk" patients, Transfusion 23:229, 1983.

134. Marks J et al: Treatment of venous thrombosis with anticoagulants: Review of 1135 cases, Lancet 1:611-624, 1954.

135. Marsh JD et al: Pulmonary angiography. Applica-

tions to a new spectrum of patients, Am J Med 75:763-770, 1983.

136. Marsh RC et al: Factors involved in wound dehiscence survey of 1,000 cases JAMA 155:1197, 1954.

137. Messmer K: Compensatory mechanisms for acute dilutional anemia, Bibl Haematologica 47:31, 1987.

138. Michelson EL et al: Relationship of preoperative use of aspirin to increased mediastinal blood loss after coronary artery bypass graft surgery, J Thor Cardiovasc Surg 78:694, 1978.

139. Mills SR et al: The incidence, etiologies and avoidance of complications of pulmonary angiography in a large series, Radiology 136:295-299, 1980.

140. Modig J et al: Anesth Analg

141. Modig J et al: Thromboembolism after total hip replacement. Role of epidural and general anesthesia, Eur J Anaesthsiol 4:345, 1987.

142. Modig J et al: Role of extradural and of general anesthesia in fibrinolysis and coagulation after total hip replacement, Br J Anaesth 55:625-629, 1983.

143. Modig J et al: Comparative influences of epidural and general anesthesia in deep venous thrombosis and pulomonary embolism after total hip replacement, Acta Chir Scand 147:125-130, 1981.

144. Modig J and Karlstrom G: Intra- and postoperative blood loss and hemodynamics in total hip replacement when performed under lumbar epidural versus general anesthesia, Eur J Anaesthiol 4:345, 1987.

145. Modig J, Malmberg P, and Saldeen T: Effects of epidural versus general anesthesia on calf blood flow, Acta Anaesthesiol Scand 24:305-309, 1980.

146. Modig J, Maripuu E, and Sahlstedt B: Thromboembolism following total hip replacement. A prospective Investigation of 94 patients with emphasis on the efficacy of lumbar epidural anesthesia in prophylaxis, Reg Anaesth 11:72, 1986.

147. Morff RJ and Granger HJ: Contribution of adenosine to arteriorlar autoregulation in striated muscle, Am J Physiol 244:H567, 1983.

148. Morrell MT and Dunnhill MS: The post-mortem incidence of pulmonary embolism in a hospital population, Brit J Surg 55:347-352, 1968.

149. Morris GK and Mitchell JRA: Clinical management of venous thromboembolism, Br Med Bull 34:169-175, 1978.

150. Morrison MCT: Is pulmonary embolectomy obsolete? Br J Dis Chest 57:187, 1963.

151. Moser KM and Lemoine JR: Is embolic risk conditioned by locations of deep venous thrombosis, Ann Int Med 94:439-444, 1981.

152. Motulsky AG: Frequency of sickling disorders in U.S. blacks, N Engl J Med 288:31-33, 1973.

153. Muller R and Musikic P: Hemorheology in surgery — a review, Angiology 38:518-592, 1987.

154. Muller MC: Anesthesia for the patient with renal dysfunction. In Priebe HJ (editor): The kidney in anesthesia, Int Anaesthesiol Clin 22:169, 1984.

155. Murphy JR, Wengard M, and Brereton W: Rheological studies of the HbSS blood: Influence of hematocrit, hypertonicity, separation of cells, deoxygenation, and mixture with normal cells, J Lab Clin Med 87:475-486, 1976.

156. Murray JF, Gold P, and Johnson BL: The circulatory effects of hematocrit variations in normovolemic and hypervolemic dogs, J Clin Invest 42:1150, 1963.

157. Nearman HS and Eckhauser ML: Postoperative management of a severely anemic Jehovah's Witness, Crit Care Med 2:142, 1983.

158. Nicod P et al: Pulmonary angiography in severe chronic pulmonary hypertension, Ann Int Med 107:565-568, 1987.

159. Oski FA et al: Red-cell 2, 3-diphosphoglycerate levels in subjects with chronic hypoxemia, N Engl J Med 280:1165, 1969.

160. Parker BM and Smith JR: Pulmonary embolism and infarction, Am J Med 23:402-427, 1950.

161. Pearson HA, Spencer RP, and Cornelius EA: Functional asplenia in sickle cell anemia, E Engl J Med 281:923-926, 1969.

162. Perlmutt LM et al: Pulmonary angiography in the high-risk patients, Radiology 162:187-189, 1987.

163. Peterman TA et al: Estimating the risks of transfusion-associated acquired immunodeficiency syndrome and human immunodeficiency virus infection, Transfusion 27:371, 1987.

164. Pieper G, Perry S, and Burrought J: Surgical intervention in hemophilia. Reviews of the literature and report of two cases, JAMA 170:33, 1957.

165. Pollock CW et al: Pulmonary embolism: An approsal of therapy in 516 cases. Arch Surg 107:66, 1973.

166. Pond CD et al: Comparison of conventional pulmonary angiography with intravenous digital subtraction angiography for pulmonary embolism: An appraisal of therapy in 516 cases, Arch Surg 107:66, 1973.

167. Pool JG, Hershgold EJ, and Pappenhagen AR: High-potency antihaemophilic factor concentrate prepared from cryoglubulin precipitate, Nature 203:312, 1964.

168. Popovsky MA, Davine PA, and Taswell HF: Intraoperative autotransfusion, Mayo Clinic Proc 60:125, 1985.

169. Quinones MA, Gaesch WH, and Alexander JK: Influence of acute changes in preload, afterload, contractile state and heart rate on ejection and isovolemic indices of myocardial contractility in man, Circulation 53:293, 1976.

170. Rao TLK, Jacobs KH, and El-Etr AA: Reinfarction following anesthesia in patients with myocardial infarction, Anesthesiology 59:25-28, 1987.

171. Ratnoff OD: Some complications of the therapy of classic hemophilia, J Lab Clin Med 103:653, 1984.

172. Rawstron RE: Anaemia and surgery: a retrospective clinical study, Aust NZ J Surg 39:425, 1970.

173. Reichek N et al: Non-invasive determination of left ventricular and systolic stress: validation of the method and initial application, Circulation 65:99, 1982.

174. Rem J et al: Postoperative changes in coagulation and fibrinolysis independent of neurogenic stimuli and adrenal hormones, Br J Surg 68:229-233, 1981.

175. Rigor BM: Questions and answers, Anesth Analg 51:399, 1972.

176. Rosberg B and Wulff K: Hemodynamics following normovolemic hemodilution in elderly patients, Acta Anaesthesiol Scand 25:402, 1981.

177. Rosberg B, Fredin H, and Gustafson C: Anesthetic techniques and surgical blood loss in total hip arthroplasty, Acta Anaesthesiol Scand 26:189, 1982.

178. Rosenthal DS and Braunwald E: Hematological oncological disorders and heart disease. In Braunwald E (editor): Heart disease, a textbook of cardiovascular medicine, ed 3, Philadelphia, 1988, WB Saunders Co.

179. Roughton FJW and Darling RC: The effect of carbon monoxide on the oxyhemoglobin association curve, Am J Physiol 141:17, 1944.

180. Roy SB et al: Hemodynamic effects of chronic severe anemia, Circulation 28:346, 1963.

181. Roy SB et al: Determinants and distribution of high cardiac output in chronic severe anemia, Indian Heart J 18:325, 1966.

182. Ruckley CV: Heparin vs dextran in the prevention of deep vein thrombosis, Lancet 2:118-121, 1974.

183. Russell MO et al: Transfusion therapy for cerebrovascular abnormalities in sickle cell disease, J Pediatr 88:382-387, 1976.

184. Sack E et al: Reduction of postprostatectomy bleeding by epsilonamino caproic acid, N Engl J Med 266:541, 1962.

185. Sandberg N and Zederfeldt B: Influence of acute hemorrhage on wound healing in the rabbit, Acta Chir Scand 118:367, 1960.

186. Sandler SG et al: Autologous blood transfusions and pregnancy, Obstet Gynecol 53 (Suppl 3):62s, 1979.

187. Schantz P: Capillary supply in heavy-resistance trained non-postural human skeletal muscle, Acta Physiol Scand 117:153, 1983.

188. Searle JF: Anesthesia in sickle cell states, a review, Anaesthesia 28:48-58, 1973.

189. Savitt S: Venous thrombosis and pulmonary embolism, Am J Med 33:703-716, 1962.

190. Sevitt S and Gallagher N: Venous thrombosis and pulmonary embolism. A clinico-pathologic study in injured and burned patients, Brit J Surg

191. Shackman R, Graber GI, and Redwood C: Oxygen consumption and anesthesia, Clin Sci 10:219, 1951.

192. Sharpey-Schafer EP: Cardiac output in severe anemia, Clin Sci 5:125, 1944.

193. Sherman MM et al: Autologous blood transfusion during cardiopulmonary bypass, Chest 70:592, 1976.

194. Siegel B et al: Risk assessment of pulmonary embolism by multivariate analysis, Arch Surg 114:188-192, 1979.

195. Sivarajan M et al: Blood pressure, not cardiac output, determines blood loss during induced hypotension, Anesth Analg 59:203, 1980.

196. Skillman JJ et al: Prevention of deep vein thrombosis in neurological patients: a controlled randomized trial of external pneumatic compression boots, Surgery 83:354-358, 1978.

197. Slichter SJ: Controversies in platelet transfusion therapy, Ann Rev Med 31:509,

198. Smith RM: Questions and answers, Anesth Analg 51:399, 1972.

199. Soloff LA and Rodman T: Acute pulmonary embolism II. Clinical. Am Heart J 74:829-847, 1967.

200. Sproule BJ, Mitchell JH, and Miller WF: Cardiopulmonary physiological responses to heavy exercise in patients with anemia, J Clin Invest 39:378, 1960.

201. Stranchess DE et al: Ultrasound flow detection: a useful technique in the evaluation of peripheral vascular disease, Am J Surg 1132:311-320, 1967.

202. Stuart MJ et al: Effects of acetylsalicylic-acid ingestion on maternal and neonatal hemostasis, N Engl J Med 909, 1982.

203. Sweeney D and William V: The effect of halothane general anesthesia on function, Anaesth Intensive Care 15:278, 1987.

204. Taivainen T et al: The effect of continuous intravenous indomethacin infusion on bleeding time and postoperative pain in patients undergoing emergency surgery of the lower extremities, Acta Anaesthesiol Scand 33:58, 1989.

205. Takahashi TT et al: Platelet aggregation induced by DDAVP in platelet type von Willebrand's disease, N Engl J Med 310:722, 1984.

206. Tarnow J et al: Hemodynamic interactions of hemodilution, anesthesia, propranolol pretreatment and hypovolemia II: coronary circulation, Basic Res Cardiol 74:123, 1979.

207. Theye RA and Michenfelder JD: Whole body and organ VO_2 changes with enflurane, isoflurane and halothane, Br J Anaesth 47:813, 1975.

208. Theye RA: The contributions of individual organ systems to the decrease in whole-body VO_2 with halothane, Anesthesiology 37:367, 1972.

209. Thomas DJ et al: Effect of hematocrit on cerebral blood flow in man, Lancet II:941, 1977.

210. Thorhng EB: Paraneoplastic erythrocytosis and inappropriate erythropoietin: a review, Sand J Haematol 17 (Suppl 17):1,

211. Thornburn S, Londen JR, and Vallance R: Spinal and general anaesthesia in total hip replacement: frequency of deep vein thrombosis, Br J Anaesth 52:1117, 1980.

212. Thornburn et al: Br J Anaesth

213. Torrance J et al: Intra-erythrocytic adaptation to anemia, N Engl J Med 283:165, 1970.

214. Triplett RG, Branham GB, and Gregory EW: The effect of chronic red cell mass depletion on healing of bone graphs, J Oral Maxillofac Surg 41:592, 1983.

215. Turpie AGG et al: A randomized controlled trial of low molecular weight heparin to prevent deep vein thrombosis in patients undergoing elective hip surgery, N Engl J Med 315:925-929, 1986.

216. Uhland H and Goldberg LM: Pulmonary embolism: a commonly missed clinical entity, Chest 45:533-536, 1964.

217. Urokinase-Streptokinase: Pulmonary embolism trial phase II results, JAMA 229-1606, 1974.

218. Urokinase-Streptokinase: Pulmonary embolism: a commonly missed clinical entity, Chest 45:533-536, 1964.

219. Valentin N et al: Spinal or general anaesthesia for surgery of the fractured hip? A prospective study of mortality in 578 patients, Br J Anaesth

220. Valeri R et al: Hypothermia induced reversible platelet dysfunction, Ann Surg 205:175, 1987.

221. Valtis DJ and Kennedy AC: Defective gas-transport of stored red blood cells, Lancet 1:119, 1954.

222. Varet MA, Adolph RJ, and Fowler NO: Cardiovascular effects of anemia, Am Heart J 83:415, 1972.

223. Walker AM and Siek H: Predictors of bleeding during heparin therapy, JAMA 244:1209, 1980.

224. Ward JW et al: Transmission of human immunodeficiency virum (HIV) by blood transfusions screened as negative for HIV antibody, N Engl J Med 318:473, 1988.

225. Wheeler HB et al: Impedence phlebography-techniques, interpretations and results, Arch Surg 104:164-169, 1972.

226. Wheeler HB and Anderson FA: Diagnostic approaches for deep vein thrombosis, Chest 85:4075-4125, 1986.

227. Wintrobe MM: The approach to the patient with anemia. In Wintrobe MM (editor): Clinical hematology, Philadelphia, 1981, Lea & Febiger.

228. Zarbowsky HS and Hochmuth RM: Sickling times of individual erthrocytes at zero PO_2, J Clin Invest 56:1023-1034, 1976.

229. Zoll F, Wessler S and Schlesinger MJ: Interarterial anastomeses in the human heart with particular reference to anemia and relative cardiac anoxia, Circulation 4:794, 1951.

230. Zucker MB and Peterson J: Effect of acetylsalicylic acid, other non-steroidal anti-inflammatory agents and dipyridamole on human blood platelets, J Lab Clin Med 76:66, 1970.

CHAPTER 25

Obesity

LINDA S. HUMPHREY

In our wealthy, industrialized society, excessive body fat is the primary nutritional problem. Obesity has been statistically associated with a large number of chronic diseases, such as diabetes, heart disease and cholelithiasis. Significant derangements in baseline physiology are also common in obese persons, and there are social and psychologic consequences of body weight significantly greater than the norm. Each of these factors makes the obese patient a high-risk consumer of anesthetic and surgical services.

The problem of how best to care for these patients is not trivial; some experts have suggested that as much as 25% to 45% of the American adult population can be considered obese,[92] with 5% to 7% considered severely or massively obese.[39] Massively obese patients are appearing on the surgical schedule with increasing frequency, particularly because of the advent of procedures designed to treat obesity itself.[22] The high incidence of moderate obesity ensures that moderately obese patients are also well represented on operative schedules. This chapter re- views various aspects of dealing with the obese patient in the perioperative period.

DEFINITION

Many of us think of obesity in the same terms that one of our Supreme Court justices did pornography: we cannot precisely define it, but we know it when we see it. Unfortunately, our personal aesthetic values are probably not the best way to identify the obese. One need only spend a few hours in an art museum admiring the works of Rubens and other artists to realize that preoccupation with extreme thinness is a relatively recent phenomenon. Even today, some primitive cultures are said to prize excessive weight highly; a massively obese woman is clearly a credit to her husband's ability as a provider. In underdeveloped countries, the ruling classes are often obese.[46] Finally, it appears that optimal body fat may not be a fixed number, but rather a conditional one.[73] Mann has pointed out that thinness can be detrimental in situations ranging from a popula-

368

TABLE 25-1. 1983 Metropolitan height and weight tables for men and women according to frame, ages 25-59

Height (in shoes)†		Weight in pounds (in indoor clothing)*		
Feet	Inches	Small frame	Medium frame	Large frame
		Men		
5	2	128-134	131-141	138-150
5	3	130-136	133-143	140-153
5	4	132-138	135-145	142-156
5	5	143-140	137-148	144-160
5	6	136-142	139-151	146-164
5	7	138-145	142-154	149-168
5	8	140-148	145-157	152-172
5	9	142-151	148-160	155-176
5	10	144-154	151-163	158-180
5	11	146-157	154-166	161-184
6	0	149-160	157-170	164-188
6	1	152-164	160-174	168-192
6	2	155-168	164-178	172-197
6	3	158-172	167-182	176-202
6	4	162-176	171-187	181-207
		Women		
4	10	102-111	109-121	118-131
4	11	103-113	111-123	120-134
5	0	104-115	113-126	122-137
5	1	106-118	115-129	125-140
5	2	108-121	118-132	128-143
5	3	111-124	121-135	131-147
5	4	114-127	124-138	134-151
5	5	117-130	127-141	137-155
5	6	120-133	130-144	140-159
5	7	123-136	133-147	143-163
5	8	126-139	136-150	146-167
5	9	129-142	139-153	149-170
5	10	132-145	142-156	152-173
5	11	135-148	145-159	155-176
6	0	138-151	148-162	158-179

*Indoor clothing weighing 5 pounds for men and 3 pounds for women.
†Shoes with 1-inch heels.
Source of basic data: *Build Study, 1979,* Society of Actuaries and Association of Life Insurance Medical Directors of America, 1980.
Copyright 1983 Metropolitan Life Insurance Company.

tion in a period of famine to a child with a febrile illness. In the early twentieth century, thinness was often associated with chronic diseases such as tuberculosis and therefore did not suggest optimal health.[16] Consequently, it seems that a more precise definition of obesity is necessary.

One of the first groups to attempt to define obesity in an orderly fashion was the insurance industry. Since excessive mortality in a particular subset of the population increases the likelihood of an early claim against the insurance company for a member of that subset, the industry is eager to identify such groups. However, insurance company lists of desirable weights corresponding to particular heights (Table 25-1)[82,83] have been criticized because of the very select population they analyze: primarily white, middle-class males who have been screened for insurability.[16,73] At best, relative mortality is underestimated by the inclusion of only the more favorable risk individuals in a given category.[16,41] Data from a longitudinal Veterans Administration study support the contention that early mortality among the obese is actually much higher than insurance statistics would suggest (Figure 25-1).[41] In addition, the data may be skewed if individuals are covered by more than one policy.[16] Despite these drawbacks, insurance data are widely quoted. Tables of "ideal" weight for height have arisen from data suggesting that mortality is lowest in individuals at particular weights.[82,83]

On the basis of insurance industry height-weight tables, various levels of obesity can be defined. "Overweight" individuals are those whose body weight is less than 20% above predicted ideal weight; those who weigh more than 20% above ideal weight are said to be *obese*.[92] *Morbid obesity* is defined as body weight either two times predicted ideal weight or greater than 100 pounds above ideal weight.[17,22]

Since excessive body fat is a more important concern than overall body weight, investigators have sought a means of isolating this factor. Two general approaches have been used: those which attempt to measure fat content directly and those which approximate it through manipulation of more readily available measures such as height and weight.

The most common measurement techniques are body density measurements and skin fold thickness measurements. Body density measurements recently have become popular among the physically fit because low-percent body fat has been associated with

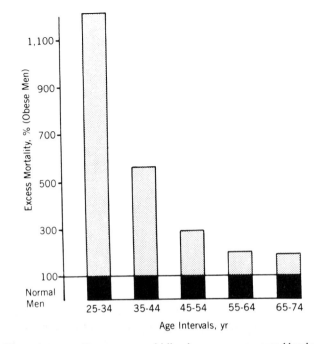

FIGURE 25-1. Excessive mortality among morbidly obese men, computed by decade, as compared with overall mortality for American men. From Drenick EJ et al: Excessive mortality and causes of death in morbidly obese men, JAMA 243:443-445, 1980.

world-class athletic performance; this popularity has led to an increased availability of the procedure. The technique involves total immersion in a tub of water and exhalation to residual volume. Since body fat is less dense than other tissues, lower body density is associated with higher body fat.[73] Obtaining body density measurements on a routine basis is obviously impractical. Skin fold thickness measurements are performed with special calipers at specific body sites. The primary limitations of this technique are its relative imprecision, variability between investigators, and the fact that only subcutaneous fat is sampled.

To avoid the need for exotic measurements, various indices based on height and weight have been devised. Optimally, the contribution of height to weight should be eliminated by the calculations.[15,66,73,84,106] Typical indices include the weight-to-height ratio (W/H), the ponderal index, written as either $\sqrt[3]{W}/H$ or $H/\sqrt[3]{W}$, and the Quetelets' index or body mass index (BMI), W/H^2.[39,67,73,84,106] Billewicz found that obesity as measured by den-

sitometry correlates most highly with BMI.[15] Obesity was overestimated among shorter individuals and underestimated among taller ones by the ponderal index, whereas the weight-to-height ratio produced the opposite effect. Similarly, Keyes et al[66] found that BMI correlates most closely with both body density and skin fold thickness measurements. Thus many investigators have adopted BMI as the most useful index for quantifying obesity on a regular basis.* BMI in kilograms per square meter ranges from less than 25 in those of normal weight to greater than 30 in the obese, with those between considered overweight but at minimal risk of morbidity or mortality on the basis of their weight.[19,22,106] A BMI above 40 kg/m^2 is found in persons described as morbidly obese.[19]

It is important to note that morbidly obese individuals may be subdivided between those with simple obesity and those with obesity-hypoventilation syndrome (OHS) or Pickwickian syndrome.[22,93,106]

*References 19, 22, 39, 66, 84, 106.

The latter group, described originally by Siecker et al.[98] and Burwell et al.,[25] are distinguished from the remainder of the obese population by the presence of hypercarbia caused by alveolar hypoventilation. The extensive physiologic derangements in OHS are described further on p. 382.

PHYSIOLOGIC CHANGES ASSOCIATED WITH OBESITY
Pulmonary

It has been known for many years that obesity is typically accompanied by hypoxemia. Several mechanisms underlie this hypoxemia, but they can be grouped into three general categories: (1) increased work and energy cost of breathing, (2) higher minute ventilation at rest to handle the metabolic needs of the increased tissue mass, and (3) changes in lung volumes, which result in closure of small airways and V/Q mismatch during normal breathing.

Work done in the 1950s by Fritts et al[49] demonstrated that the efficiency of the respiratory muscles in the obese is well below normal. Five obese patients complaining of dyspnea on exertion were compared with seven normal controls. The amount of work performed on the lungs was estimated from the area under the transpulmonary pressure-volume curve. Mechanical work performed on the lungs was slightly above normal in two of the obese patients, whereas it was normal in the other three. On the other hand, the energy expended to perform that work was greatly enhanced. As a result, percent efficiency, defined as work performed on the lungs divided by total energy used for breathing, was reduced. Moreover, as work load increased, excessive amounts of energy were expended by the obese, which could not be explained on the basis of work done on the lungs; it was presumed that the excess energy was used to move extrapulmonary structures. However, later work by Cherniak and Guenter[27] suggested that work of breathing is not significantly different for normal and obese subjects, even when differences in elastic resistance of the chest wall are considered. Thus the apparent inefficiency of respiratory muscles in the obese is not caused by additional workload but is a real inefficiency. Interestingly, a similar inefficiency has been produced in normal subjects by banding the chest wall to simulate reduced compliance. This suggests that low chest wall compliance itself or breathing at abnormally low lung volumes may alter respiratory muscle ef-

ficiency. On the other hand, Sharp et al[97] found mechanical work to be 30% above normal in obese patients, suggesting that efficiency may not always be as low as was previously thought.

Although pulmonary compliance is normal in some obese patients,[65] others have reduced compliance, particularly individuals with obesity-hypoventilation syndrome.[22,93] The mechanism is not entirely clear, although increased pulmonary blood volume, increased extravascular lung water, and abnormal closure of prealveolar airways have all been proposed. Abnormal chest wall compliance is usual in the obese but does not seem to be directly proportional to weight.[93] This may result in part from varying distribution of weight among the obese, with excessive weight overlying the abdomen and chest wall more likely to influence respiratory mechanics detrimentally than weight in the buttocks or extremities.[22,106]

Oxygen consumption at various levels of ventilation was studied by Kaufman et al.[65] Eighteen of 25 obese subjects increased oxygen consumption with increasing ventilation considerably more than nonobese control subjects. The discrepancy became progressively greater at the higher ventilatory levels (Figure 25-2). There was a tendency for the patients with the highest cost of increased ventilation to have the lowest resting PaO_2s and highest $PaCO_2$s. Both airway resistance and lung compliance were normal in two patients with the highest cost of ventilation and $PaCO_2$. The authors suggested (citing the hypothesis of Cain and Otis) that hypoventilation might represent an adaptive mechanism. Varying degrees of hypoxemia and hypercapnia might be tolerated to spare the inordinant energy expenditure that would be required to normalize ventilation. They also pointed out that an individual with an increased cost of breathing at rest is on the brink of disaster; any further need for increased ventilation as a result of concurrent pulmonary disease could so greatly increase the metabolic cost of breathing that decompensation could result.

Despite much work, efforts to find a metabolic defect with an etiologic role in obesity have been unsuccessful.[39,73] The basal metabolic rate of the obese individual is normal.[22] Nonetheless, the large mass of adipose tissue is metabolically active to some degree, and both oxygen consumption and carbon dioxide production are linearly increased with increasing weight.[4] As a result, minute ventilation

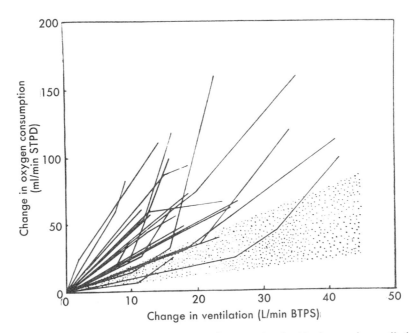

FIGURE 25-2. The changes in oxygen consumption associated with changes in ventilation in 25 obese subjects. The stippled area represents the range found in normal subjects. From Kaufman BJ et al: Hypoventilation in obesity, J Clin Invest 38:500-507, 1959.

must increase even at rest. An increase in metabolic demand as, for example, occurs with exercise or fever will again strain an already stressed system. Some obese individuals may have little tolerance for any additional stress.

The final mechanism underlying hypoxemia in the obese is abnormal resting lung volumes as compared with nonobese subjects. Functional residual capacity (FRC), vital capacity, and total lung capacity are all reduced in the obese subject as a result of lower respiratory compliance.[17,22,56,93,106] FRC is less primarily because expiratory reserve volume (ERV) is less, but residual volume is unchanged (Figure 25-3). Loss of ERV adversely affects the relationship between FRC and closing capacity (CC), the lung volume at which small airways begin to close. Since CC is unchanged in obesity, a lower FRC can result in lung volume dipping below CC in the course of normal tidal ventilation.[56] As perfusion of the no-longer-ventilated distal alveoli continues, V/Q mismatch and venous admixture develop.[33,36-38,94,106] Such V/Q mismatch has been documented by both Barrera et al.[8] and Holley et al.[59] They found that

distribution of ventilation to various lung regions in the obese does not differ significantly from normal unless ERV is drastically reduced, but overperfusion of underventilated areas or perfusion of completely unventilated areas occurs. Premature airway closure is most likely to occur in dependent regions,[32] and these regions, as in normal weight individuals, are better perfused.[59]

Assumption of the supine position, which is necessary in most operative procedures, further aggravates the lung volume changes (Figure 25-4). Paul et al[88] found a clinically significant increase in both intrapulmonary shunting and oxygen consumption as a group of obese patients changed position from sitting to supine. The supine position is known to reduce FRC in normal individuals,[33,37,38] since abdominal pressure increases more rapidly per centimeter of tissue height than thoracic pressure, causing the diaphragm to shift cephalad.[50] It is presumed that this effect is exaggerated in the obese, resulting in further decreased FRC, closure of more small airways, and increased work of breathing. It should be noted that general anesthesia is also known to de-

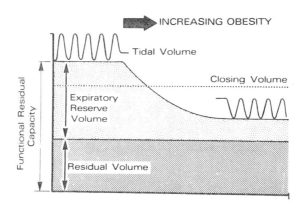

FIGURE 25-3. The progressive decrement in functional residual capacity that occurs with increasing weight results in tidal ventilation occurring at or below closing volume. From Fox GS: Anaesthesia for intestinal short circuiting in the morbidly obese with reference to the pathophysiology of gross obesity, Can Anaesth Soc J 22:307-315, 1975.

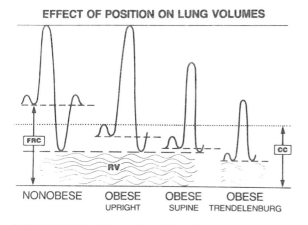

FIGURE 25-4. Effect of position change on lung volumes in obese subjects. Further decline in functional residual capacity *(FRC)* worsens the relationship between FRC and closing volume or capacity *(CC)*. *(RV,* residual volume) From Vaughan RW: Pulmonary and cardiovascular derangements in the obese patient. In Brown BR, (editor): Anesthesia and the obese patient, Philadelphia, 1982, FA Davis Co.

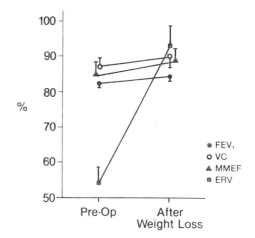

FIGURE 25-5. Pulmonary function tests (PFTs) measured in 37 obese patients before and after weight loss averaging 52 kg. (FEV$_1$, forced expiratory volume in one second; VC, vital capacity; MMEF, maximum mid-expiratory flow rate; ERV, expiratory reserve volume.) From Vaughan RW et al: The effect of massive weight loss on arterial oxygenation and pulmonary function tests, Anesthesiology 54:325-328, 1981.

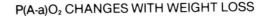

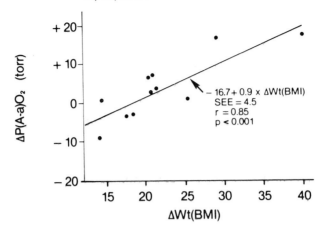

FIGURE 25-6. Change in alveolar to arterial oxygen tension difference (P(A-a)O₂) as a function of weight loss, expressed in units of body mass index (BMI). A change in BMI of > 20 results in improved oxygenation. From Vaughan RW et al: The effect of massive weight loss on arterial oxygenation and pulmonary function tests, Anesthesiology 54:325-328, 1981.

crease FRC.[36,37,56,70] Thus a supine, anesthetized obese individual is at significant risk of hypoxemia.[22,56]

Weight loss can reverse some of these effects of obesity. A group of 37 obese patients studied by Vaughan et al were found to increase their ERV significantly after an average weight loss of 52 kg (Figure 25-5).[107] Mean PaO₂ increased from 83 to 87 torr (p = 0.053) in the eleven patients in which it was measured. The increase in PaO₂ and the decrease in alveolar-arterial oxygen tension difference (P(A-a)O₂) both correlated with the increase in ERV (Figure 25-6). Sugerman and Fairman[100] suggested in response to this report that oxygenation improves even more significantly following weight loss in patients with obesity-hypoventilation syndrome.

Cardiovascular

The relationship between obesity and cardiovascular disease has been elucidated through longitudinal studies of large populations. The Framingham Study, for example, has been following a segment of the adult population of Framingham, Massachusetts, since 1948.[60,64] After 12 years of follow-up, an association was found between angina pectoris and initial weight in both sexes and between sudden death and initial weight in men.[64] These relationships

persisted in men but not in women after controlling for elevated blood pressure and serum cholesterol, both frequently associated with obesity. The combination of obesity and either or both of the other factors resulted in potentiation of risk beyond that seen for the other factors alone or in combination. Interestingly, no association between obesity and myocardial infarction was demonstrated.

On the other hand, several studies have suggested that increased risk of cardiovascular disease among the obese can be accounted for solely on the basis of coexisting risk factors. Keys et al[66,67] have suggested that failure to account for weight gain with age results in those individuals classified as obese being older and thus more likely to suffer from "ill health." The consensus of these investigators, summarized by Mann[73] in 1974, is that the contribution of obesity to coronary heart disease is either small or nonexistent in the absence of other risk factors.

In contrast, follow-up of the Framingham population at 26 years again showed obesity to be an important predictor of cardiovascular disease, particularly in individuals younger than 50 years.[60] Risk of coronary artery disease, myocardial infarction, and sudden death was higher among the obese of both sexes. Risk of congestive heart failure was enhanced in men, but in women it was greater only in the heaviest subgroup; risk of atherothrombotic stroke was enhanced primarily in women. Once again, the effect of obesity on risk could be demonstrated in individuals without other risk factors, although only a small percentage of obese individuals were free of these other factors. Differing results between the Framingham study and others might be due to different levels of obesity between the populations or to different lengths of follow-up.[60] Bray has pointed out that the issue of obesity as an independent risk factor may be irrelevant; in a particular obese patient, the risk of cardiovascular disease is enhanced regardless of mechanism.[19]

The association of hypertension with obesity is well known, although cause and effect have not been established.[73,79] While it is obviously critical to use a blood pressure cuff of appropriate size to avoid artifactual elevation of the measurement,[19,24,74] it is also clear that hypertension in the obese is not solely a technical artifact.[73,79,92] Hypertension developed 10 times more often in the subset of the Framingham population that was 20% or more above ideal weight. Mann has suggested that while the relationship between obesity and hypertension is clear, there is little to support the idea that obesity causes hypertension and therefore weight loss would be unlikely to ameliorate it,[73] while Messerli, Bray, and others have stated that weight reduction is commonly associated with a fall in arterial pressure.[4,19,39,79,92]

The mechanism underlying the development of hypertension is not entirely clear. Both Alexander[3,4] and de Divitiis[34] found normal systemic vascular resistance in a group of morbidly obese patients. Blood volume was increased in direct proportion to weight, suggesting a hydraulic basis for the elevation in blood pressure. Similarly, Messerli has pointed out that greater blood volume in the obese results in greater cardiac output and thus lower calculated systemic vascular resistance (SVR) for the same level of arterial pressure.[79,80] Hypertension and obesity could then coexist with a normal peripheral resistance.[79] SVR might increase over time in the presence of chronically elevated cardiac output and blood volume. The combination of obesity, with its consequent high preload, and hypertension associated with high SVR can lead to early left ventricular dysfunction and congestive heart failure (Figure 25-7).[80]

Regardless of the level of blood pressure, increasing blood volume has been noted as weight increases

above ideal (Figure 25-8).* Excess body mass increases total body oxygen consumption, and hence cardiac output must be increased to meet the demand.† In patients whose weight is 100 kg above ideal both blood volume and cardiac output are twice the values predicted for ideal weight.[2,4,6,17] Despite this, cardiac output indexed for body surface area is generally normal[4] or slightly below normal.[79] Organ blood flow does not change appreciably with increasing weight; thus the additional cardiac output must be perfusing primarily adipose tissue.[4,6,17,93,106] Elevated cardiac output is caused by increased stroke volume, and left ventricular stroke work is therefore consistently increased.[2,34,79]

Since the distribution of the extra blood volume between the peripheral and central circulations is the same in obese and nonobese persons, both the right and left ventricles are distended at end-diastole in the obese, which results in the observed increase in stroke volume.[80,93,106] Chronically elevated preload results in both dilation and hypertrophy of the left ventricle, a phenomenon known as eccentric hypertrophy (Figure 25-9).[79] Workload increases correspondingly and both systolic performance and compliance suffer. The combination of elevated left-ventricular end-diastolic volume and reduced compliance leads to abnormally high left ventricular end-diastolic pressure (LVEDP) and therefore pulmonary artery occluded pressure (PAOP).

Alexander has proposed that grossly obese patients with congestive signs and symptoms may be subdivided into two categories.[4] The first group consists of those patients in whom the hypertrophic response has been sufficient to normalize wall stress, left-ventricular systolic function is maintained, and congestive symptoms develop because of the inappropriately elevated central blood volume and altered left ventricular compliance. In the second group are patients with dilated left ventricular chambers, "inadequate" hypertrophy, and chronically elevated wall stress. These patients are predisposed to depressed systolic function and myocardial decompensation, with pulmonary congestion developing as a consequence.

Pulmonary hypertension, either at rest or during exercise, is also a common finding.[4,34] Most of 40

---

*References 4, 5, 6, 61, 79, 93, 106.
†References 6, 17, 19, 34, 79, 80, 92, 106.

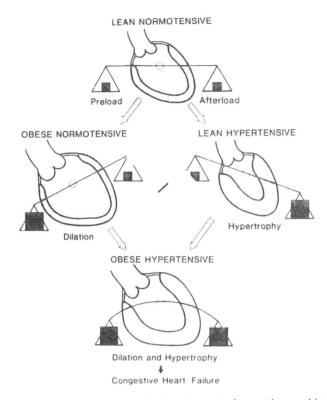

FIGURE 25-7. Adaptation of the heart to obesity, hypertension, and a combination of the two. While hypertension produces concentric hypertrophy only, obesity plus hypertension produces hypertrophy and dilation (eccentric hypertrophy), which is associated with a high incidence of congestive heart failure. From Messerli FH: Cardiovascular effects of obesity and hypertension, Lancet 1:1165-1168, 1982.

obese patients studied by Alexander et al. had pulmonary hypertension accompanied by elevated PAOP, suggesting high LVEDP as the source of the pulmonary hypertension.[2,5] On the other hand, patients with OHS often suffer from both right-sided and left-sided heart failure.[2,4,93] The right-sided signs and symptoms, presumably caused by hypoxia-induced pulmonary hypertension, are often the predominant clinical problem.

The highly significant association between obesity and sudden death led Messerli et al to investigate the incidence of arrhythmias in obese subjects.[81] Holter monitoring of 15 obese hypertensive persons without other cardiac disease revealed an incidence of premature ventricular contraction 10 times higher than control. A second group of obese subjects with eccentric left ventricular hypertrophy (N = 14) had

30 times more ventricular ectopy, including asymptomatic runs of trigeminy, quadrigeminy, and ventricular tachycardia. Left-ventricular mass and end-systolic wall stress were elevated in all obese subjects but to the greatest extent in those with eccentric hypertrophy. Although ventricular ectopy has not been proven to result in sudden death, the findings were nonetheless felt to be ominous.

Significant changes in cardiovascular parameters with postural changes were reported by Paul et al.[88] Both PAOP and cardiac output increased significantly when the supine position was assumed by the obese subjects. Oxygen consumption, which increased significantly in the supine position as a result of increased work of breathing, may have contributed to the elevated cardiac output. The authors felt that the ability of the heart to respond to increased

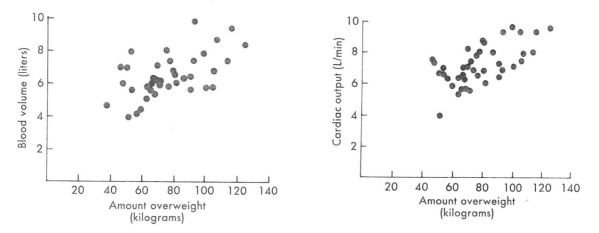

FIGURE 25-8. Relationships between excessive weight, blood volume and cardiac output in 40 obese subjects. From Alexander JK: The cardiomyopathy of obesity, Prog Cardiovasc Dis 27:325-334, 1985.

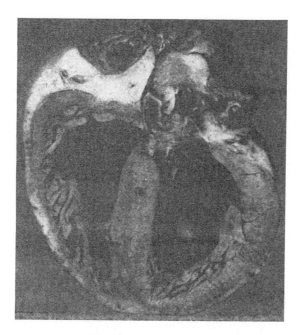

FIGURE 25-9. Gross appearance of the heart of postmortem examination of an obese man dying of cardiac failure at age 42 (body weight 225 kg). Biventricular hypertrophy with chamber dilation is demonstrated. From Alexander JK: The cardiomyopathy of obesity, Prog Cardiovasc Dis 27:325-334, 1985.

preload by increasing cardiac output minimized the elevation in both the left side of the heart and pulmonary artery pressure. Pulmonary congestion or edema might be expected in individuals unable to tolerate the higher venous return and further elevated central blood volume.

Gastrointestinal/Metabolic Changes

The gastrointestinal physiology of obese persons differs from normal in two primary respects: high gastric volume and low pH in the fasting state and abnormalities of hepatic function. Alterations in drug metabolism, both qualitative and quantitative, are common in obese patients. Diabetes mellitus, which will not be discussed further in this chapter, is also common; the severity of glucose intolerance increases with age, duration of obesity, and degree of overweight.[39,40]

Vaughan et al,[104] observing that obese patients are similar to obstetrical patients in abdominal bulk, discovered that the obese are likewise at risk for aspiration during the induction of anesthesia. Fifty-six healthy obese patients were compared to a similar number of nonobese controls. Eight-six percent of the obese patients had a gastric fluid volume exceeding 25 ml (mean 42.3 ml), the volume beyond which aspiration increases in frequency. Eighty-eight percent had gastric pH levels below 2.5 (mean 1.7), a level associated with pulmonary parenchymal damage should aspiration occur, and 75% had a combination of both factors and were considered to be at high risk for aspiration. The authors speculated that gastric emptying was delayed by the abdominal mass, leading to antral distention, gastrin release, and lowering of pH by parietal cell secretion.

Subsequently, other authors have confirmed the high volume and low pH of gastric contents in the fasting obese,[69,72,116] but gastric emptying time was shown to be normal.[28,69] Thus the mechanism underlying abnormal fluid volumes remains obscure. The incidence of hiatal hernia is very high in the obese and intraabdominal pressure is certainly greater than normal, but what role these factors play is unknown. Stress reflux of gastric contents into the esophagus with increased intraabdominal pressure has been demonstrated[35]; this might contribute to the risk of aspiration.

More recent work focuses on the possibility of preoperative pharmacologic correction of the problem. Cimetidine, administered orally in two 300 mg doses or intravenously (300 to 600 mg) at least 60 minutes preoperatively, increases pH above the danger level but does not consistently decrease gastric volume.[69,116] Potential problems associated with the use of cimetidine include reduced hepatic blood flow and inhibition of microsomal enzyme activity.[69] In addition, administration of cimetidine by the intravenous route has been associated with bradycardia and asystole. Ranitidine, which is also an H_2 antagonist but does not have the aforementioned side effects, may be a preferable agent. Ranitidine, 150 to 300 mg given orally the night before and the morning of surgery, elevated pH in all 40 patients studied by Manchikanti et al and decreased the incidence of elevated gastric volume somewhat.[72] The addition of metoclopromide, 10 to 20 mg orally, on the morning of surgery decreased gastric volume to less than 25 ml in all patients. The combination of metoclopromide and ranitidine appears to provide the best protection against aspiration in the obese patient.

The liver of the obese patient is often abnormal.[22,110] Fatty infiltration occurs in the majority of massively obese individuals, and a multitude of other histopathologic changes have been reported. These include inflammation, focal necrosis, and cirrhosis. Mortality from cirrhosis among obese men was 250% of the expected rate in one study, although a causal relationship between fatty infiltration and the development of cirrhosis has not been established[110] and others dispute this figure.[41] Hepatic enzymes may be slightly elevated in obese individuals, perhaps as a result of disruption of hepatocytes and/or obstruction of cannuliculi by extravasated lipid.[22,110] Additional pathologic conditions can result from cholelithiasis, common among obese persons.[106]

Biotransformation of volatile anesthetic agents differs both qualitatively and quantitatively in obese from in nonobese subjects. Quantitative differences were first noted by Young et al,[118] who showed significantly greater biotransformation of methoxyflurane by obese patients than previously reported values obtained in nonobese patients (Figure 25-10). Cousins et al,[31] while investigating the biotransformation of enflurane to free fluoride ion (F^-), found an unexpectedly high peak concentration of F^- in one obese patient after 4 MAC-hours (52 μmol/L versus a mean of 22 μmol/L for the entire group). Bentley et al[9] measured F^- levels in a group of 24 markedly obese patients during and after an enflurane anesthetic of less than 2 MAC-hours (Figure

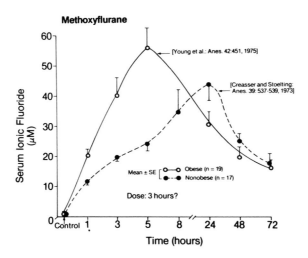

FIGURE 25-10. Serum ionic fluoride concentration with time following approximately 3 hours of methoxyflurane anesthesia in obese (N = 19) and nonobese (N = 17) patients from two nonconcurrent studies. From Vaughan RW: Biochemical and biotransformation alterations in obesity. In Brown BR, (editor): Anesthesia and the obese patient, Philadelphia, 1982, FA Davis Co.

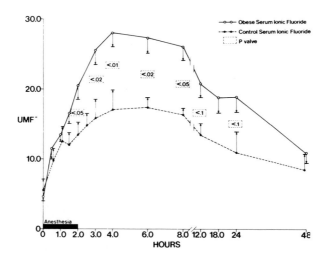

FIGURE 25-11. Serum ionic fluoride concentration with time during and following 2 hours of enflurane anesthesia in obese (N = 24) and nonobese (N = 7) patients. From Bentley JB et al: Serum inorganic fluoride levels in obese patients during and after enflurane anesthesia, Anesth Analg 58:409, 1979.

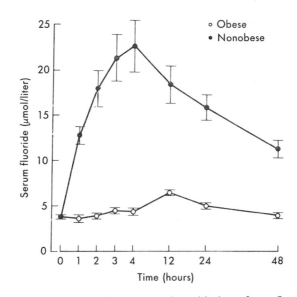

FIGURE 25-12. Serum inorganic fluoride concentration with time after enflurane (closed circles, N = 5) and isoflurane (open circles, N = 5) anesthesia in obese patients. From Strube PJ et al: Serum flroride levels in morbidly obese patients: enflurane compared with isoflurane anaesthesia, Anaesthesia 42:685-689, 1987.

25-11). They found a more rapid rate of rise, higher peak concentration, and more prolonged elevation of F^- in the obese group than in seven nonobese controls, suggesting enhanced biotransformation of enflurane by the obese. While clinical nephrotoxicity was not seen after this brief anesthetic exposure, the authors speculated that prolonged exposure to enflurane might result in concentration of F^- within the range associated with subclinical renal dysfunction (30 μmol/L)[31.75] or even frank nephrotoxicity (90 μmol/L).[43.76] Biotransformation of isoflurane by the obese results in F^- concentrations that are not clinically significant (Figure 25-12).[99]

The mechanism of enhanced biotransformation of volatile anesthetics by the obese is unknown. Increased hepatic uptake of lipid-soluble anesthetic resulting from higher-than-normal hepatic lipid could lead to enhanced exposure of microsomal enzymes to anesthetic. Alternatively, increased uptake of agent into adipose tissue could result in subsequent prolonged delivery of drug to the liver.[9.118] Other speculative mechanisms include increased splanchnic blood flow, with a greater fraction of cardiac output and volatile agent thereby delivered to the liver[9.118] and higher-than-normal levels of cytochrome P-450 enzymes.[85.110] In the case of enflurane,

a decreased blood-gas partition coefficient has been found in the obese, which results in more rapid uptake of anesthetic.[18.85] Lower affinity of enflurane for blood might result in greater tissue-blood partitioning, increasing the volume of distribution for enflurane.[85]

The study of Young et al.,[118] mentioned above, included a control group of obese patients anesthetized with halothane. Interestingly, serum F^- concentrations increased in the control group to a peak of 10.4 μmol/L, whereas a previous study of nonobese subjects receiving halothane had shown no change in F^- concentration.[75] Bentley et al[10.12] confirmed this finding, attributing it to reductive metabolism of halothane (Figure 25-13). They cited data associating reductive metabolism of halothane with hepatic injury in animals, suggesting that obese individuals might be at increased risk of such injury. Reductive metabolism is no longer felt to be a primary etiologic factor in "halothane hepatitis," so this concern may or may not be warranted. It remains a fact that 38% of patients with unexplained jaundice following anesthetization with halothane in one large investigation were obese.[115]

Elevation of bromide ion following halothane anesthesia was also found in the obese.[12] In fact, serum

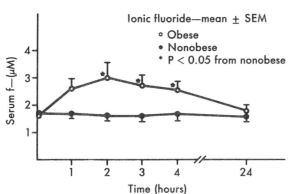

FIGURE 25-13. Serum ionic fluoride concentration with time after halothane anesthesia in obese (N = 17) and nonobese (N = 8) patients. From Bentley JB et al: Halothane biotransformation in obese and nonobese patients, Anesthesiology 57:94-97, 1982.

concentration of bromide ion in the obese was approximately double that measured in the nonobese. Although sedative levels of bromide ion were not reached, the occurrence of such levels following prolonged exposure to halothane remains a possibility. In addition, peak concentrations of bromide ion did not occur until the third postoperative day in the obese patients, suggesting the theoretical potential for prolonged postoperative sedation.

Excess adipose tissue can also affect the serum half-life of fixed agents. Serum concentration and half-life are affected by two pharmacokinetic parameters, volume of distribution and clearance. If an agent is lipid soluble, its steady-state volume of distribution will be larger in an obese person, the serum concentration resulting from a given dose will be lower and the terminal elimination half-life will be greater (assuming the same clearance). Midazolam, a commonly used benzodiazepine for control of preoperative or intraoperative anxiety, is a perfect example. The elimination half-life of midazolam, which is highly lipophilic, is markedly longer in obese subjects than in normal weight controls (8.4 versus 2.7 hours).[55] This occurs because of a significantly greater volume of distribution; clearance is unchanged. Thus although midazolam is generally considered to be a short-acting sedative, it has the potential to produce prolonged sedation in obese patients, particularly because higher loading doses (based on body weight) are required to achieve adequate serum concentrations.

In contrast, fentanyl, a lipophilic narcotic anesthetic, has been found to have similar pharmacokinetic parameters in obese and nonobese subjects and should be administered on the basis of lean body weight.[11] This result is surprising; a larger volume of distribution in the obese had been anticipated for such a lipid-soluble agent. On the other hand, alfentanil, a newer synthetic narcotic, has a longer terminal elimination half-life in the obese as a result of decreased clearance.[14] The unpredictability of these pharmacokinetics highlights the need for careful studies in obese patients. In the absence of such studies, it is critical that data obtained in lean individuals not be assumed to apply to the obese.

Unfortunately, few drugs have undergone pharmacokinetic investigation in the obese. A few that have are digoxin, thiopental, theophylline, and the neuromuscular blockers. Digoxin half-life is unchanged following weight reduction, suggesting that its dosage should be calculated on the basis of lean body weight.[44] The commonly used induction agent thiopental, like midazolam, has a larger volume of distribution in the obese and repeated doses can lead to accumulation and prolonged somnolence.[63] In contrast, theophylline loading doses are best based on total body weight, since the volume of distribution is similar in obese and normal weight subjects.[52] Theophylline clearance is reduced if total body weight is used in its calculation, so maintenance doses should be given on the basis of ideal body weight.

Despite its low fat solubility, requirements for pancuronium, a nondepolarizing neuromuscular blocker, are significantly higher in the obese.[101] However, once a correction is made for body surface area, the same dosage may be used in obese and nonobese patients. Tsueda et al[101] postulated that the additional requirement is accounted for by the increased extracellular fluid space into which the drug is distributed, although this explanation has been questioned.[45] Pseudocholinesterase activity increases linearly with increasing weight; this factor, coupled with the larger extracellular fluid compartment, means that a larger dose of succinylcholine is required in the obese individual.[45] Dosage on the basis of total body weight results in appropriate twitch depression and a recovery time equivalent to that seen in nonobese patients dosed on a similar milligram-per-kilogram schedule. Since adequate relaxation can be critical to both surgical exposure and wound closure in the obese, monitoring of neuromuscular function is recommended. Excessive subcutaneous adipose tissue can overlie peripheral nerves; Vaughan has recommended the use of needle electrodes for neuromuscular junction monitoring in obese patients.[22]

OBESITY-HYPOVENTILATION SYNDROME

Patients suffering from obesity-hypoventilation syndrome (OHS), or Pickwickian syndrome, constitute approximately 50% of the obese population and thus represent a small but interesting group.[22,40] The term *Pickwickian* was coined by Burwell to describe an obese, somnolent patient reminiscent of Dickens's "Joe the fat boy" from *The Posthumous Papers of the Pickwick Club*.[25] Although the syndrome is not directly correlated with weight, all of its sufferers are massively obese and improve greatly with even minor weight loss. The cardinal sign of OHS is hypercarbia; since CO_2 retention is not a feature of simple obesity, patients with OHS are easily diagnosed. Other characteristics include severe hypoxemia, somnolence, periodic breathing, pulmonary hypertension, enlargement of both ventricles but particularly the right, dependent edema, polycythemia, rales, and pulmonary edema.[25,40,92] Where total pulmonary compliance is decreased by 20% in simple obesity, it is reduced by 60% in OHS.[93,97] The work of breathing is dramatically elevated, approximating three times the normal level, as opposed to 0% to 30% above normal in the simple obese.[93,97] Oxygen cost of breathing is high, respiratory muscle efficiency is reduced and weakness of inspiratory muscles has been identified. Rochester and Enson[93] envisioned a viscious cycle of transient

hypercapnia with an inadequate ventilatory response and worsening hypoxia leading to pulmonary hypertension and transudation of fluid into the lung. Lung compliance is thereby reduced, work of breathing increased, and deterioration in ventilation-perfusion matching occurs. In some patients, pulmonary hypertension may be worsened by left-ventricular dysfunction, but in general, a drop in pressure across the pulmonary circuit (i.e., between pulmonary artery diastolic and LVEDP or PAOP) is noted. If this condition is untreated, the end result of this cycle is extreme hypoxemia and cyanosis, hypercapnia, pulmonary edema, and cor pulmonale.

The characteristic somnolence is ascribed to intermittent nocturnal upper airway obstruction leading to apnea, followed by arousal and resumption of respiration. Daytime somnolence then results from sleep deprivation.[68,114]

Clearly, patients with OHS represent an extremely high anesthetic and surgical risk. Simply assuming the supine position can prove fatal for these patients. A history of sleeping in the sitting position should be taken very seriously.[102] Since even relatively minor weight loss can improve the physiologic state of these patients significantly,[25,93] weight loss should be strongly encouraged before elective surgery. Where this is impossible or the surgery is urgent, aggressive cardiopulmonary management, including early endotracheal intubation, has been recommended.[86]

PERIOPERATIVE MANAGEMENT
Preoperative Concerns

In addition to the usual preoperative evaluation, certain issues unique to the obese patient must be addressed. Cardiorespiratory status requires more thorough evaluation than would normally be warranted by age, the appropriateness of outpatient surgery should be considered, and suitable preoperative medication must be determined.

A thorough cardiopulmonary review of symptoms is clearly indicated, with particular attention paid to tolerance of both activity and position changes. A chest x-ray examination, electrocardiogram, serum electrolyte panel (including glucose), and possibly liver function tests should be obtained before surgery in addition to the usual urinalysis and hematologic assessment. Finally, and perhaps most importantly, determination of arterial blood gas levels will rule out OHS and establish a baseline level of oxygenation.[22] Pulmonary function tests are advisable in older individuals and those with concurrent pulmonary disease, OHS, or an addiction to cigarettes.

The current push for cost containment has led to progressively older and sicker patients undergoing surgery as outpatients. Federal government requirements for outpatient surgery were developed with the complexity of the surgical procedure in mind; little or no attention was paid to concurrent disease or potential anesthetic difficulties. Thus ASA III and IV patients are now occasionally treated without hospital admission. Several experts have questioned the wisdom of handling the morbidly obese in this fashion. Apfelbaum and Conahan[7] have suggested that the likelihood of cardiopulmonary pathology and the potential for intraoperative problems make not only morbidly obese but also some moderately obese individuals unsuitable candidates for ambulatory surgery. They have proposed that active morbidly obese persons (an unusual combination), who are highly motivated can be considered for surgery as outpatients.

Lastly, the issue of appropriate preoperative medication must be considered. The tenuous respiratory status of many obese individuals makes excessive sedation hazardous.[17] Some experts recommend avoidance of narcotics, whereas others eliminate premedication entirely.[7,22] Small doses of oral benzodiazepines are generally well tolerated. Prolonged respiratory depression from long-acting agents such as lorazepam or scopolamine can delay weaning and extubation postoperatively. The route of administration is also of concern. Intramuscular injections in obese individuals may in fact be deposited into adipose tissue, making uptake and distribution unpredictable.[7,22,29] There is evidence that uptake and distribution of diazepam is more predictable by the oral route in the obese, but intramuscular diazepam is notoriously variable in action regardless of weight. As mentioned earlier, the combination of metoclopromide and ranitidine appears to provide the optimum defense against aspiration.[72]

Intraoperative Management

Intraoperative care of the morbidly obese patient is complicated by an assortment of technical difficulties. Assurance of adequate oxygenation during the procedure is a major concern, as are hemodynamic changes unique to this population. Finally, the issue of regional versus general anesthesia must be resolved.

The technical difficulties begin with transport of the patient to the operating room and transfer to the operating room table. The table width is often inadequate to accommodate both the patient's body and his or her upper extremities comfortably. In extreme cases, two tables pushed together may be required.[17] If the arms must be tucked, careful padding of the ulnar nerves is important, with or without the addition of a metal "sled" to protect the limb (Figure 25-14). If the arms remain extended on arm boards, extreme abduction to accommodate the operating team must be avoided.

Establishing vascular access is the next hurdle, a procedure which is occasionally so difficult that venous cut-down is required.[17,22,26] Arterial, central venous, and pulmonary artery catheters are similarly difficult because landmarks and arterial pulses can be obscured by subcutaneous fat.

Blood pressure measurements will be artifactually elevated if a cuff too small for the arm is used.[19,73,74] This can be avoided by using cuffs with bladders that encircle a minimum of 75% of the upper arm circumference or, preferably, the entire arm.[22,73] In some instances, this might mean using a cuff ordinarily intended for use on the thigh. On the other hand, an excessively large cuff may artifactually lower blood pressure, so some experts have suggested that 50% of arm circumference is the ideal bladder size; others feel that the width rather than the length of the cuff is the key feature.[24] Even with an appropriately sized cuff, Korotkoff sounds can be difficult to hear. In view of these problems and the fact that measurement of arterial blood gases might be required during surgery, the use of intra-arterial pressure monitoring is recommended.

Airway management is notoriously difficult in the morbidly obese individual. Inadequate mask fit, airway obstruction by soft tissue, and laryngospasm can complicate airway management by mask. In addition, the stomach can become inflated with air as a result of the high pressures required for controlled or assisted mask ventilation, increasing the risk of regurgitation.[46] Endotracheal intubation is far from straightforward,[23] yet must be accomplished expediently to ensure protection of the airway from aspiration of gastric contents. A "rapid sequence" induction is recommended by Apfelbaum and Conahan[7] and has been our practice, but the increasingly frequent horror stories of obese patients who prove to be neither intubatable nor ventilatable have made

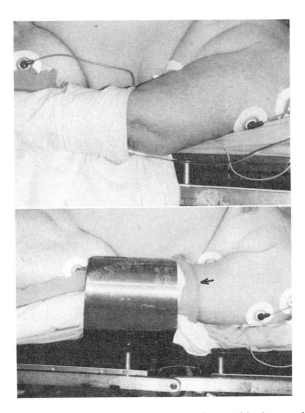

FIGURE 25-14. A, Demonstration of the difficulty in safely positioning an obese patient's arms by his side. The potential for ulnar nerve injury is great when the elbow dangles off the mattress in this fashion. **B,** Use of a foam pad *(arrow)* and metal slide protects the extremity from harm.

many of us more conservative. The obese patient's small FRC results in rapid desaturation in the absence of ventilation,[23] and tracheotomy can be technically difficult.[54] A "rapid sequence" induction might be appropriate for the moderately obese and has been recommended when one is "sure" the patient can be intubated. (Innumerable lawsuits raise the question of whether this is ever the case.) The alternative is awake intubation, with or without fiberoptic laryngoscopy, which, in experienced hands, need not be traumatic.

Chronic physiologic abnormalities in obese patients can deteriorate further during surgery. Unexplained deaths occurring during and immediately after surgery are reported in older literature. In fact, as recently as 1972, mortality following abdominal operations in obese patients was said to be 2½ times that in nonobese patients.[90] Part of this morbidity

and mortality may occur as a result of inadequate appreciation of the tenuous cardiopulmonary status of the obese patient.

Intraoperative respiratory problems can be significant. As described above, obese patients have reduced FRC, which deteriorates further in the supine position and still further with the induction of general anesthesia.[22,37,56] Subsequent tidal ventilation occurs at a lung volume that can be below the closing capacity throughout its cycle, resulting in worsened hypoxemia.[22,36,38] Adequate oxygenation is not guaranteed with an FIO_2 of 0.4 or less.[113] Additional decrements in FRC occur with the head down 15 degrees (Trendelenburg positioning) or placement of an abdominal pack beneath the diaphragm. In the latter instance, PaO_2 less than 65 mm Hg has been reported in 100% of a group of patients receiving 40% inspired oxygen.[113]

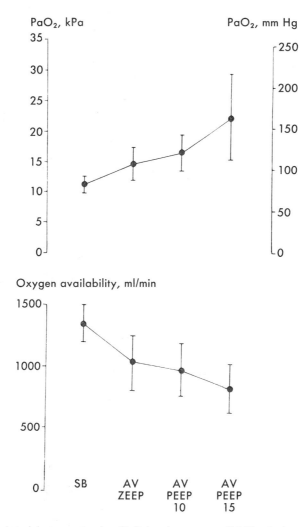

FIGURE 25-15. Arterial oxygen tension (PaO_2) and oxygen availability during spontaneous breathing (SB), and artificial ventilation (AV) with zero end-expiratory pressure (ZEEP) and positive end-expiratory pressure (PEEP) of 10 and 15 cm H_2O. From Santesson J: oxygen transport and venous admixture in the extremely obese. Influence of anaesthesia and artificial ventilation with and without positive end-expiratory pressure, Acta Anaesth Scand 20:387-394, 1976.

It might be supposed that positive end-expiratory pressure (PEEP) would be useful to reverse the decrease in FRC. Santesson[96] found improved PaO_2 and decreased $P(A-a)O_2$ in a group of extremely obese patients receiving 10 to 15 cm H_2O PEEP. Unfortunately, cardiac output fell progressively with increasing PEEP, and oxygen delivery was thereby reduced despite improved O_2 content (Figure 25-15).

Salem et al[95] found improved PaO_2 and decreased $P(A-a)O_2$ after PEEP was discontinued (Figure 25-16). So, although disagreeing on mechanism, both authors found PEEP is detrimental to oxygen delivery in the obese. Current recommendations are for high inspired oxygen concentration and a large tidal volume, administered by mechanical ventilation. The use of PEEP remains a controversial issue, but

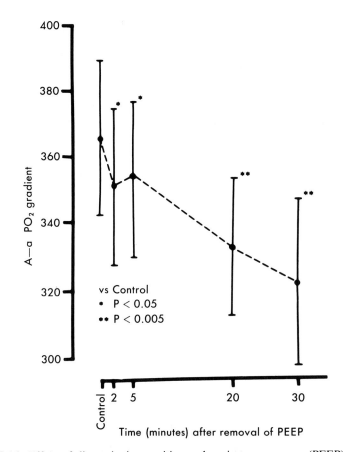

FIGURE 25-16. Effect of discontinuing positive end-expiratory pressure (PEEP) on alveolar to arterial oxygen tension (A-a PO_2) gradient. From Salem MR et al: Does PEEP improve intraoperative arterial oxygenation in grossly obese patients? Anesthesiology 48:280-281, 1978.

certainly if its use is anticipated, the response in terms of oxygen delivery should be documented. A more novel approach to increasing FRC is hydraulic suspension of the abdominal panniculus, relieving the high transdiaphragmatic pressure (Figure 25-17).[117] This maneuver is reportedly quite successful at increasing arterial oxygen tension.

Even with a mechanical ventilator, ensuring adequate alveolar ventilation can be complicated. Generally, high peak inspiratory pressures are required, which may be beyond the range of the average volume ventilator. Administration of large tidal volumes to prevent airway closure and atelectasis, a commonly recommended practice,[22] conflicts with data supporting the calculation of tidal volumes on the basis of ideal body weight to avoid hyperventilation.[51] High intrathoracic pressure can also increase pulmonary vascular resistance and right ventricular afterload.

Lateral thoracotomy in conjunction with one-lung anesthesia can be associated with hypoxemia in normal-weight individuals. The same procedure in a morbidly obese individual might be cause for concern. Data on 22 morbidly obese patients undergoing transthoracic gastric stapling revealed marked shunting during collapse of the nondependent lung but adequate oxygenation in all patients.[21,87] This result may be caused in part by the decrease in abdominal pressure resulting from lateral displacement of the panniculus in this position. Patients undergoing tho-

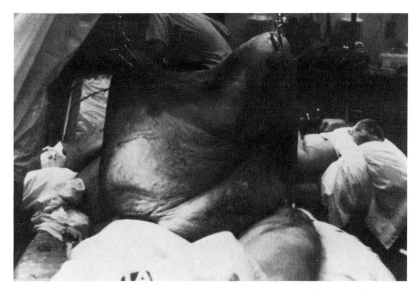

FIGURE 25-17. Mechanical suspension of the abdominal panniculus in a morbidly obese patient. Marked improvement in arterial oxygen tension resulted. From Wyner J et al: Massive obesity and arterial oxygenation, Anesth Analg 60:691-693, 1981.

racic procedures were not different from those undergoing upper abdominal procedures postoperatively. Not addressed by the authors is the problem of positioning a double-lumen tube in a massively obese individual while protecting the airway against aspiration.

Abnormal hemodynamic responses to anesthesia and surgery were reported by Agarwal et al.[1] Throughout the course of gastric stapling procedures, obese patients had higher filling pressures than either their own preoperative values or values in nonobese patients undergoing abdominal surgery. Cardiac index and right ventricular stroke work were significantly lower than the values obtained in nonobese patients; left ventricular stroke work was reduced by 40% (not significant). Left-ventricular stroke work remained depressed postoperatively.

Both regional and general anesthesia have been advocated for obese patients, and several groups promote a combination of the two. The primary advantage of general anesthesia is the assurance of adequate oxygenation and ventilation while simultaneously protecting the airway. A high regional anesthetic could theoretically impair accessory respiratory muscle function in a patient who required all available ventilatory capability. On the other hand, there are several undesirable features of general anesthesia in this population. High concentration of volatile anesthetic might be required since the obligate high FIO_2 restricts N_2O administration; as noted earlier, increased metabolism of these agents is a concern. Hemodynamic instability and arrhythmias have been reported during induction of anesthesia in the obese.[47] Prolonged recovery from both fixed (intravenous) and volatile anesthetic agents is also a possibility, with respiratory depression and sedation potentially persisting into the postoperative period.

Recovery from general anesthesia by morbidly obese individuals was assessed by Cork et al.[30] Despite theoretic concerns based on lipid solubility and biotransformation of volatile anesthetics, neither delayed awakening nor excessive recovery room stay was found. In addition, there was no difference in recovery time between patients receiving halothane, enflurane, or fentanyl anesthesia. However, fentanyl dosages were low (average 2.6 μg/kg), and thiopental was the only other intravenous agent. The effect of higher doses or other agents on awakening is unknown.

Finally, the decision of when to extubate must be made. In some series of obese patients, few of the patients were ventilated postoperatively,[78,91,103] but this must certainly be determined on an individual basis. Even when early extubation is planned, the best method of transporting the patient to the recovery room or intensive care unit should be carefully considered. As with any difficult intubation, the endotracheal tube should be left in place until there is no question that the patient no longer requires it, as determined from alertness and measurements of inspiratory force, vital capacity, and reversal of neuromuscular blockade. Obese patients extubated in the operating room should receive oxygen during transport, regardless of distance, because hypoxia can develop extremely rapidly. The head of the bed should be elevated as soon as possible.

Many of the problems associated with general anesthesia can be avoided, in principle, with a carefully administered regional anesthetic. The patient remains awake and can protect his or her own airway. At least one group has data to suggest that arterial blood gases are not compromised by even a high spinal anesthetic.[89] Complete relaxation of abdominal musculature is provided, which otherwise might be accomplished only with deep general anesthesia and large doses of neuromuscular blockers. Metabolism of volatile and / or fixed agents is not a concern. Finally, postoperative pain relief can be provided, avoiding the need for narcotics with their associated respiratory depression.

Undoubtedly the biggest drawback to regional anesthesia is its technical difficulty. Vertebral spines and iliac crests may not be palpable at all. One ingenious solution to this problem is the placement of two 26-gauge needles to mark the spinous processes above and below the desired interspace.[71] Usual spinal and epidural needles may or may not be long enough; specially designed equipment may decrease the problem of holding the hub indented far enough into the skin to permit administration of agent or passage of an epidural catheter.[23,47]

Another problem is the unpredictability of anesthetic levels during spinal or epidural anesthesia.[26,42,77,89] Levels may be higher than expected[77] and can creep up slowly over at least 30 minutes.[26,57] This fact might explain the sudden deaths reported during spinal anesthesia.[26] The sitting position, maintained for 5 minutes after administration of an epidural block, limited the spread of anesthesia in a group of 250 obese parturients.[58] Epidural anesthesia might be preferable to spinal, since anesthetic levels are somewhat more titratable,[71] although continuous spinal anesthesia has a few proponents.[26,62] Precipitous hypotension can follow sympathetic blockade in the obese.[26,47]

The combination of epidural and general anesthesia has been used by several groups. The use of lumbar epidural combined with general anesthesia was reported by Fox.[47] Sixteen patients undergoing intestinal bypass surgery received epidural lidocaine combined with a balanced (nitrous-narcotic) general anesthetic. None of the patients required postoperative mechanical ventilation, and postoperative narcotics were avoided. The suggestion was made that respiratory status was improved by the absence of abdominal "splinting," although subsequent data in 110 patients from the same group revealed no difference in blood gas tensions between patients receiving epidural analgesia and those receiving narcotics postoperatively.[48] Pneumonia was slightly less common in the epidural group (2.9% versus 5% in the narcotic group).

Thoracic epidural was compared with "balanced" anesthesia by Gelman et al.[53] All patients were intubated and ventilated with nitrous oxide and oxygen. Patients receiving epidural anesthesia continued to be treated with epidural bupivicaine postoperatively for pain relief, and patients receiving balanced anesthesia were treated with morphine sulfate intravenously. Interestingly, the epidural space could not be identified in 5 of the first 12 patients, and subsequent epidurals were performed under fluoroscopic control.

Although no particular advantage to epidural anesthesia was demonstrated intraoperatively, the patients in this group were extubated at the end of the surgical procedure, whereas 12 of 17 of the patients in the balanced anesthesia group were too sedated to permit immediate extubation. Epidural analgesia postoperatively provided more predictable pain relief resulting in significantly less sympathetically mediated hemodynamic responses. With adequate pain relief, restoration of vital capacity did not differ between the groups. In a similar study (although not prospective or randomized), Buckley et al[23] found a greater number of postoperative pulmonary complications in patients receiving general anesthesia than

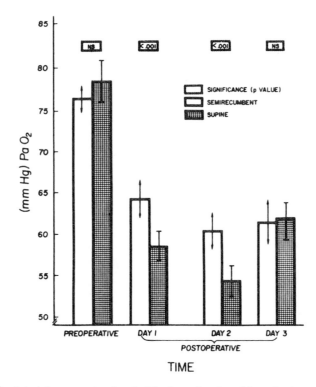

FIGURE 25-18. Arterial oxygen tension in 22 obese female subjects in the semirecumbent and supine positions preoperatively and on days 1 through 3 postoperatively. On postoperative days 1 and 2 a significant effect on PaO$_2$ resulted from changing to the supine position. From Vaughan RW et al: Postoperative arterial blood gas measurement in obese patients: effect of position on gas exchange, Ann Surg 182:705-709, 1975.

in those receiving epidural plus general anesthesia, although the operative procedures were significantly shorter in the latter group.

Postoperative Management

Issues to be considered in the postoperative care of the obese patient include assurance of adequate oxygenation, management of pain, and prevention of thrombophlebitis and pulmonary embolism.

Obese patients are significantly at risk for postoperative hypoxemia.[108] Room air PaO$_2$ remains depressed for up to 4 days (Figure 25-18). Hypoxemia is worse when surgery is performed through a vertical incision.[109,111] More importantly, care of the patient in the supine position during the early postoperative period results in a significant deterioration in oxygenation.[105,112] Keeping the patient in a semire-

cumbent position during this time is highly recommended.

As with other postoperative patients, various options exist for pain control. Aside from epidural local anesthetics, discussed previously, narcotics are the mainstay of therapy, given either intravenously, intramuscularly, or into the epidural space.[20,91] A randomized, double-blind study by Rawal et al[91] compared intramuscular with epidural morphine. Patients receiving epidural morphine were more likely to sit, stand, and walk unassisted during the first postoperative 24 hours than were patients receiving morphine intramuscularly. Pulmonary complications were less common in the epidural group, and hospitalization of those patients was significantly shorter. These investigators provide the most compelling evidence supporting the superiority of a regional anesthetic technique in the obese, at least for postoperative management.

Although all postsurgical patients are at increased risk of thrombophlebitis, obese patients may be especially likely to develop this complication.[46] Early ambulation is therefore desirable. In this regard, investigators whose patients ambulate sooner after a particular technique often suggest that this represents a significant advantage to the technique. For example, Fox found that continuous epidural analgesia permitted the patients to perform "vigorous leg exercises," which he felt to be important in the prevention of deep venous thrombosis.[48] Nevertheless, the percentage of patients having pulmonary embolism was higher in the group that received epidural analgesia than in the group that received narcotics (5.7% versus 2.5%). In addition, Rawal et al[91] were unable to document a difference in the incidence of thrombophlebitis, using a radioisotopic technique, in their patients who did or did not receive epidural anesthesia. Regardless of technique, postoperative pain control should be adequate to permit early transfer of the patient to a bedside chair and subsequent ambulation. There is little question that prolonged bed rest increases the risk of thrombophlebitis.

Caring for the obese patient is a significant challenge to all concerned when a surgical procedure becomes necessary. The temptation to proceed in the routine fashion employed for nonobese individuals must be resisted. Careful attention to the details of the preoperative evaluation, intraoperative management, and postoperative care will ensure a safe and uneventful operative experience.

REFERENCES

1. Agarwal N et al: Hemodynamic and respiratory changes in surgery of the morbidly obese, Surgery 92:226-234, 1982.
2. Alexander JK: Obesity and cardiac performance, Am J Cardiol 14:860-865, 1964.
3. Alexander JK: Chronic heart disease due to obesity, J Chron Dis 18:895-898, 1965.
4. Alexander JK: The cardiomyopathy of obesity, Prog Cardiovasc Dis 27:325-334, 1985.
5. Alexander JK and Dennis EW: Circulatory dynamics in extreme obesity, Circulation 20:662, 1959.
6. Alexander JK et al: Blood volume, cardiac output, and distribution of systemic blood flow in extreme obesity, Cardiovasc Res Cent Bull 1:39-44, 1962–1963.
7. Apfelbaum JL and Conahan TJ: An approach to the management of a patient with morbid obesity scheduled for outpatient surgery, Society for Ambulatory Anesthesia Newsletter 1:3-8, 1986.
8. Barrera F et al: Ventilation-perfusion relationships in the obese patient, J Appl Physiol 26:420-426, 1969.
9. Bentley JB et al: Serum inorganic fluoride levels in obese patients during and after enflurane anesthesia, Anesth Analg 58:409-412, 1979.
10. Bentley JB et al: Does evidence of reductive halothane biotransformation correlate with hepatic binding of metabolites in obese patients? Anesth Analg 60:548-551, 1981.
11. Bentley JB et al: Fentanyl pharmacokinetics in obese and nonobese patients, Anesthesiology 55:A177, 1981.
12. Bentley JB et al: Halothane biotransformation in obese and nonobese patients, Anesthesiology 57:94-97, 1982.
13. Bentley JB et al: Weight, pseudocholinesterase activity, and succinylcholine requirement, Anesthesiology 57:48-49, 1982.
14. Bentley JB et al: Obesity and alfentanil pharmacokinetics, Anesth Analg 62:245-251, 1983.
15. Billewicz WZ, Kemsley WFF, and Thomson AM: Indices of adiposity, Br J Prev Soc Med 16:183-188, 1962.
16. Blackburn H and Parlin RW: Antecedents of disease. Insurance mortality experience, Ann NY Acad Sci 134:965-977, 1966.
17. Blass NH: Morbid obesity and other nutritional disorders. In Katz J, Benumof J, and Kadis LB (editors): Anesthesia and uncommon diseases, Philadelphia, 1981, WB Saunders Co.
18. Borel JD et al: Enflurane blood-gas solubility: influence of weight and hemoglobin, Anesth Analg 61:1006-1009, 1982.
19. Bray GA: Obesity and the heart, Mod Conc Cardiovasc Dis 56:67-71, 1987.
20. Brodsky JB, Shulman MS, and Kim SK: Epidural morphine following abdominoplasty, Plast Reconstr Surg 78:125-126, 1986.
21. Brodsky JB et al: One-lung anesthesia in morbidly obese patients, Anesthesiology 57:132-134, 1982.
22. Brown BR et al, editors: Anesthesia and the obese patient, Philadelphia, 1982, FA Davis Co.
23. Buckley FP et al: Anaesthesia in the morbidly obese, Anaesthesia 38:840-851, 1983.
24. Burch GE and Shewey L: Sphygmomanometric cuff size and blood pressure recordings, JAMA 225:1215-1218, 1973.
25. Burwell CS et al: Extreme obesity associated with alveolar hypoventilation—a Pickwickian syndrome, Am J Med 21:811-818, 1956.
26. Catenacci AJ, Anderson JD, and Boersma D: Anesthetic hazards of obesity, JAMA 175:657-665, 1961.

27. Cherniack RM and Guenter CA: The efficiency of the respiratory muscles in obesity, Can J Biochem Physiol 39:1215-1222, 1961.

28. Christian PE, Datz FL, and Moore JG: Gastric emptying studies in the morbidly obese before and after gastroplasty, J Nucl Med 27:1686-1690, 1986.

29. Cockshott WP et al: Intramuscular or intralipomatous injections? N Engl J Med 307:356-358, 1982.

30. Cork RC, Vaughan RW, and Bentley JB: General anesthesia for morbidly obese patients—an examination of postoperative outcomes, Anesthesiology 54:310-313, 1981.

31. Cousins MJ et al: Metabolism and renal effects of enflurane in man, Anesthesiology 44:44-53, 1976.

32. Couture J et al: Airway closure in normal, obese, and anesthetized supine subjects, Fed Proc 29:269A, 1970.

33. Craig DB et al: "Closing volume" and its relationship to gas exchange in seated and supine positions, J Appl Physiol 31:717-721, 1971.

33a. Creasser CW and Stoelting RK: Serum inorganic fluoride concentrations during and after halothane, fluroxene, and methoxyflurane anesthesia in man, Anesthesiology 39:537-540, 1973.

34. de Divitiis O, Fazio S, and Petitto M: Obesity and cardiac function, Circulation 64:477-482, 1981.

35. Dodds WJ et al: Mechanisms of gastroesophageal reflux in patients with reflux esophagitis, N Engl J Med 307:1547-1552, 1982.

36. Don HF, Wahba WM, and Craig DB: Airway closure, gas trapping, and the functional residual capacity during anesthesia, Anesthesiology 36:533-539, 1972.

37. Don HF et al: The effects of anesthesia and 100 per cent oxygen on the functional residual capacity of the lungs, Anesthesiology 32:521-529, 1970.

38. Don HF et al: The measurement of gas trapped in the lungs at functional residual capacity and the effects of posture, Anesthesiology 35:582-590, 1971.

39. Drenick EJ: Definition and health consequences of morbid obesity, Surg Clin North Am 59:963-976, 1979.

40. Drenick EJ: Risk of obesity and surgical indications, Int J Obesity 5:387-398, 1980.

41. Drenick EJ et al: Excessive mortality and causes of death in morbidly obese men, JAMA 243:443-445, 1980.

42. Edelist G: Extreme obesity, Anesthesiology 29:846-847, 1968.

43. Eichhorn JH et al: Renal failure following enflurane anesthesia, Anesthesiology 45:557-560, 1976.

44. Ewy GA, Groves BM, and Ball MF: Digoxin metabolism in obesity, Circulation 44:810-814, 1971.

45. Feingold A: Pancuronium requirements of the morbidly obese, Anesthesiology 50:269-270, 1979.

46. Fisher A, Waterhouse TD, and Adams AP: Obesity: its relation to anaesthesia, Anaesthesia 30:633-647, 1975.

47. Fox GS: Anaesthesia for intestinal short circuiting in the morbidly obese with reference to the pathophysiology of gross obesity, Can Anaesthesiol Soc J 22:307-315, 1975.

48. Fox GS, Whalley DG, and Bevan DR: Anaesthesia for the morbidly obese. Experience with 110 patients, Br J Anaesth 53:811-816, 1981.

49. Fritts HW et al: The efficiency of ventilation during voluntary hyperpnea: studies in normal subjects and in dyspneic patients with either chronic pulmonary emphysema or obesity, J Clin Invest 38:1339-1348, 1959.

50. Froese AB and Bryan AC: Effects of anesthesia and paralysis on diaphragmatic mechanics in man, Anesthesiology 41:242-255, 1974.

51. Furgerson CL, Sivashankaran S, and Dauchot PJ: Ventilator settings to mitigate hypocarbia in the obese patient, Anesth Analg 65:S53, 1986.

52. Gal P et al: Theophylline disposition in obesity, Clin Pharmacol Ther 23:438-444, 1978.

53. Gelman S et al: Thoracic epidural vs. balanced anesthesia in morbid obesity: an intraoperative and postoperative hemodynamic study, Anesth Analg 59:902-908, 1980.

54. Ghorayeb BY: Tracheotomy in the morbidly obese patient, Arch Otolaryngol Head Neck Surg 113:556-558, 1987.

55. Greenblatt DJ et al: Effect of age, gender, and obesity on midazolam kinetics, Anesthesiology 61:27-35, 1984.

56. Hedenstierna G, Santesson J, and Norlander O: Airway closure and distribution of inspired gas in the extremely obese, breathing spontaneously and during anesthesia with intermittent positive pressure ventilation, Acta Anaesthesiol Scand 20:334-342, 1976.

57. Hodgkinson R and Husain FJ: Obesity and the cephalad spread of analgesia following epidural administration of bupivacaine for cesarean section, Anesth Analg 59:89-92, 1980.

58. Hodgkinson R and Husain FJ: Obesity, gravity, and spread of epidural anesthesia, Anesth Analg 60:421-424, 1981.

59. Holley HS et al: Regional distribution of pulmonary ventilation and perfusion in obesity, J Clin Invest 46:475-481, 1967.

60. Hubert HB et al: Obesity as an independent risk factor for cardiovascular disease: a 26-year follow-up of participants in the Framingham Heart Study, Circulation 67:968-977, 1983.

61. Huff RL and Feller DD: Relation of circulating red cell volume to body density and obesity, J Clin Invest 35:1-10, 1956.

62. Jacobs LL, Berger HC, and Fierro FE: Obesity and continuous spinal anesthesia: a case report, Anesth Analg 42:547-549, 1963.

63. Jung D et al: Thiopental disposition in lean and obese patients undergoing surgery, Anesthesiology 56:269-274, 1982.

64. Kannel WB et al: Relation of body weight to development of coronary heart disease, Circulation 35:734-744, 1967.

65. Kaufman BJ, Ferguson MH, and Cherniack RM: Hypoventilation in obesity, J Clin Invest 38:500-507, 1959.

66. Keys A, Aravanis C, and Blackburn H: Coronary heart disease: overweight and obesity as risk factors, Ann Intern Med 77:15-27, 1972.

67. Keys A et al: Indices of relative weight and obesity, J Chron Dis 25:329-343, 1972.

68. Kryger M et al: The sleep deprivation syndrome of the obese patient. A problem of periodic nocturnal upper airway obstruction, Am J Med 56:531-539, 1974.

69. Lam AM et al: Prophylactic intravenous cimetidine reduces the risk of acid aspiration in morbidly obese patients, Anesthesiology 65:684-687, 1986.

70. Laws AK: Effects of induction of anaesthesia and muscle paralysis on functional residual capacity of the lungs, Can Anaesthesiol Soc J 15:325-331, 1968.

71. Maitra AM et al: Continuous epidural analgesia for cesarean section in a patient with morbid obesity, Anesth Analg 58:348-349, 1979.

72. Manchikanti L, Roush JR, and Colliver JA: Effect of preanesthetic ranitidine and metoclopramide on gastric contents in morbidly obese patients, Anesth Analg 65:195-199, 1986.

73. Mann GV: The influence of obesity on health, New Engl J Med 291:178-185 (part I), 226-232 (part II), 1974.

74. Maxwell MH et al: Error in blood pressure measurement due to incorrect cuff size in obese patients, Lancet 2:33-36, 1982.

75. Mazze RI, Calverley RK, and Smith NT: Inorganic fluoride nephrotoxicity: prolonged enflurane and halothane anesthesia in volunteers, Anesthesiology 46:265-271, 1977.

76. Mazze RI, Trudell JR, and Cousins MJ: Methoxyflurane metabolism and renal dysfunction: clinical correlation in man, Anesthesiology 35:247-252, 1971.

77. McCulloch WJD and Littlewood DG: Influence of obesity on spinal analgesia with isobaric 0.5% bupivacaine, Br J Anaesth 58:610-614, 1986.

78. McKenzie R et al: Anesthesia for jejunoileal shunt: review of 88 cases, Anesth Analg 54:65-70, 1975.

79. Messerli FH: Cardiovascular effects of obesity and hypertension, Lancet 1:1165-1168, 1982.

80. Messerli FH: Cardiopathy of obesity—a not-so-victorian disease, New Engl J Med 314:378-380, 1986.

81. Messerli FH et al: Overweight and sudden death. Increased ventricular ectopy in cardiopathy of obesity, Arch Intern Med 147:1725-1728, 1987.

82. Metropolitan Life Insurance Company: New weight standards for men and women, Statistical Bulletin 40:1-4, 1959.

83. Metropolitan Life Insurance Company: 1983 Metropolitan height and weight tables, Statistical Bulletin 64:1-9, 1983.

84. Metropolitan Life Insurance Company: Measurement of overweight, Statistical Bulletin 65:20-23, 1984.

85. Miller MS et al: Disposition of enflurane in obese patients, J Pharmacol Exp Ther 215:292-296, 1980.

86. Neuman GG, Baldwin CC, and Petrini AJ: Perioperative management of a 430 kilogram (946 pound) patient with pickwickian syndrome, Anesth Analg 65:985-987, 1986.

87. Oakes DD et al: Lateral thoracotomy and one-lung anesthesia in patients with morbid obesity, Ann Thorac Surg 34:572-580, 1982.

88. Paul DR, Hoyt JL, and Boutros AR: Cardiovascular and respiratory changes in response to change of posture in the very obese, Anesthesiology 45:73-78, 1976.

89. Pitkanen MT: Body mass and spread of spinal anesthesia with bupivacaine, Anesth Analg 66:127-131, 1987.

90. Postlethwait RW and Johnson WD: Complications following surgery for duodenal ulcer in obese patients, Arch Surg 105:438-440, 1972.

91. Rawal N et al: Comparison of intramuscular and epidural morphine for postoperative analgesia in the grossly obese: influence on postoperative ambulation and pulmonary function, Anesth Analg 63:583-592, 1984.

92. Reisin E and Frohlich ED: Obesity. Cardiovascular and respiratory pathophysiological alterations, Arch Intern Med 141:431-434, 1981.

93. Rochester DF and Enson Y: Current concepts in the pathogenesis of the obesity-hypoventilation syndrome, Am J Med 57:402-420, 1974.

94. Said SI: Abnormalities of pulmonary gas exchange in obesity, Ann Intern Med 53:1121-1129, 1960.

95. Salem MR et al: Does PEEP improve intraoperative arterial oxygenation in grossly obese patients? Anesthesiology 48:280-281, 1978.

96. Santesson J: Oxygen transport and venous admixture in the extremely obese. Influence of anaesthesia and artificial ventilation with and without positive end-expiratory pressure, Acta Anaesthesiol Scand 20:387-394, 1976.

97. Sharp JT et al: The total work of breathing in normal and obese men, J Clin Invest 43:728-739, 1964.

98. Sieker HO et al: A cardiopulmonary syndrome associated with extreme obesity, J Clin Invest 34:916, 1955.

99. Strube PJ, Hulands GH, and Halsey MJ: Serum fluoride levels in morbidly obese patients: enflurane compared with isoflurane anaesthesia, Anaesthesia 42:685-689, 1987.

100. Sugerman HJ and Fairman RP: Massive weight loss with improve arterial oxygenation in selected patients, Anesthesiology 55:604-605, 1981.

101. Tsueda K et al: Pancuronium bromide requirement during anesthesia for the morbidly obese, Anesthesiology 48:438-439, 1978.

102. Tsueda K et al: Obesity supine death syndrome: reports of two morbidly obese patients, Anesth Analg 58:345-347, 1979.

103. Vaughan RW: Anesthetic considerations in jejunoileal small bowel bypass for morbid obesity, Anesth Analg 53:421-429, 1974.

104. Vaughan RW, Bauer S, and Wise L: Volume and pH of gastric juice in obese patients, Anesthesiology 43:686-689, 1975.

105. Vaughan RW, Bauer S, and Wise L: Effect of position (semirecumbent versus supine) on postoperative oxygenation in markedly obese subjects, Anesth Analg 55:37-41, 1976.

106. Vaughan RW and Conahan TJ: Cardiopulmonary consequences of morbid obesity, Life Sciences 26:2119-2127, 1980.

107. Vaughan RW, Cork RC, and Hollander D: The effect of massive weight loss on arterial oxygenation and pulmonary function tests, Anesthesiology 54:325-328, 1981.

108. Vaughan RW, Engelhardt RC, and Wise L: Postoperative hypoxemia in obese patients, Ann Surg 180:877-882, 1974.

109. Vaughan RW, Engelhardt RC, and Wise L: Postoperative alveolar-arterial oxygen tension difference: its relation to the operative incision in obese patients, Anesth Analg 54:433-437, 1975.

110. Vaughan RW, Gandolfi AJ, and Bentley JB: Biochemical considerations of morbid obesity, Life Sciences 26:2215-2221, 1980.

111. Vaughan RW and Wise L: Choice of abdominal operative incision in the obese patient: a study using blood gas measurements, Ann Surg 181:829-835, 1975.

112. Vaughan RW and Wise L: Postoperative arterial blood gas measurement in obese patients: effect of position on gas exchange, Ann Surg 182:705-709, 1975.

113. Vaughan RW and Wise L: Intraoperative arterial oxygenation in obese patients, Ann Surg 184:35-42, 1976.

114. Walsh RE et al: Upper airway obstruction in obese patients with sleep disturbances and somnolence, Ann Intern Med 76:185-192, 1972.

115. Walton B et al: Unexplained hepatitis following halothane, Br Med J 1:1171-1176, 1976.

116. Wilson SL, Mantena NR, and Halverson JD: Effects of atropine, glycopyrrolate, and cimetidine on gastric secretions in morbidly obese patients, Anesth Analg 60:37-40, 1981.

117. Wyner J, Brodsky JB, and Merrell RC: Massive obesity and arterial oxygenation, Anesth Analg 60:691-693, 1981.

118. Young SR et al: Anesthetic biotransformation and renal function in obese patients during and after methoxyflurane or halothane anesthesia, Anesthesiology 42:451-457, 1975.

CHAPTER 26

Malignant Hyperthermia

THOMAS J. J. BLANCK
MICHAEL HUMPHREY

A 21-year-old male with compound fractures of his tibia and fibula agreed to general anesthesia with halothane for repair of his fractures. This serious but normal set of circumstances was complicated by the fact that 10 of 24 of the patient's relatives who had undergone general anesthesia had died either during or shortly after receiving anesthesia. All had received ether anesthesia; therefore the propositus was given the newer, safer anesthetic, halothane. Within 10 minutes of exposure to halothane he became pale, cyanotic, hot, and sweaty. He was tachycardiac to 160 per minute; the anesthetic was stopped, the patient was packed in ice, and, fortunately, recovered. This series of events was reported by Denborough and Lovell in the *Lancet* in 1960.[12] The authors were uncertain of the cause but requested that any of the readers of their letter who were aware of a similar history or possible cause contact them.

The letter in the *Lancet* was the first suggestion that a genetic disorder existed, that it was related to anesthesia and surgery, and that it could be fatal. Since that time our understanding of malignant hyperthermia (MH) has increased considerably.

MALIGNANT HYPERTHERMIA CRISIS

The typical series of events surrounding a crisis can be exemplified by the following scenario. A young, healthy patient who has been adequately premedicated is given halothane for induction and maintenance of anesthesia and, subsequently, succinylcholine to facilitate endotracheal intubation. Within 5 to 10 minutes a sudden tachycardia develops, along with mottling of the skin and cyanosis. The ensuing events occur in rapid succession. The patient, if he or she was breathing spontaneously, is noted to hyperventilate. Muscle tone, particularly in the limbs, gradually increases despite the use of a muscle relaxant. The patient's core temperature begins to rise rapidly. This combination of signs and symptoms should indicate to the anesthesiologist that an MH episode has begun. The anesthesiologist will also note that the end-tidal CO_2 is markedly elevated and that the arterial blood gas shows a decreased pH and marked base deficit. The increase in end-tidal CO_2 was probably the first abnormal sign to appear.

If this series of events goes unnoticed, the syndrome progresses to its inevitable end, including marked temperature elevation to over 105° F, marked acidosis, extraordinary muscle rigidity, and ultimately cardiovascular collapse. This progression was not unusual 15 or more years ago when the MH syndrome had not been adequately described and the anesthesia community was unaware of its proper treatment. At that time the mortality rate was approximately 80%. Fortunately, now it is unusual that the syndrome progresses to this fatal ending; it is more likely that the initial events are recognized as premonitory for MH and proper treatment ensues. The mortality rate today is less than 20%.[5]

Despite the fact that the MH syndrome is most often apparent soon after induction of anesthesia, this is not the only time MH appears. Some reports have indicated 1 or 2 hours of normal responses to anesthesia and surgery, followed by a sudden tachycardia and subsequent progression of acidosis, muscle rigidity, and hyperthermia. No obvious reasons for the delay in the appearance of the syndrome or the sudden onset in the midst of what appeared to be a normal procedure have been evident. Two possible mechanisms have been postulated. Other drugs may act as modifying agents in preventing the appearance of the syndrome. This has been demonstrated in the MH swine model, where Gronert et al[21] have shown that paralysis with pancuronium has prolonged the onset of the syndrome. An alternative explanation is that MH is not a single genetic entity but can result from one of several genetic defects that differ in such manifestations as the rate of development of the syndrome and its virulence.

Despite the varied appearance of MH, there is a consensus on its incidence. It is believed that among anesthetized patients 1 in 50,000 adults and 1 in 15,000 children will develop the syndrome. The source of these figures is currently uncertain, but they have appeared in most reviews of MH.[20] Recent muscle biopsies of patients who have had masseter spasm following induction of anesthesia with halo-

thane and succinylcholine have confounded our estimates of the incidence of MH and will be discussed in more detail below.

VARIANT PRESENTATION

As indicated, the classic features of MH are rigidity, fever, and acidosis. However, many presentations of the syndrome are not complete and may consist of fever and acidosis, or rigidity in the absence of fever. However, if fever never develops, the diagnosis of MH cannot be made with certainty. Only a few years after Denborough's initial report,[12] Saidman[47] described a case in which rigidity never developed, yet the fever and acidosis were dramatic. Retrospective review suggests MH without rigidity occurs in about 25% of cases.[7] Rigidity is only slightly more common when succinylcholine is used.

Masseter muscle spasm is also an atypical presentation of MH. It occurs in about 1% of pediatric patients receiving halothane and succinylcholine and may or may not be a harbinger of a fulminant hyperthermic crisis.[45] When masseter spasm occurs, the anesthetic is usually discontinued, so the percentge of cases that would have progressed to hyperthermic crisis is unknown. Some patients with masseter spasm who do not become hyperthemic will nevertheless develop tachycardia, myoglobinuria, and elevated creatine kinase (CK).[4] Muscle destruction associated with anesthesia in the absence of fever may be part of the MH spectrum or it may be caused by the presence of an unrelated myopathy. Rosenberg[46] and others[16] have found that the diagnostically examined muscle of about 50% of patients who have had masseter spasm following induction of anesthesia responds positively to in vitro halothane and caffeine contracture tests. However, the contracture test may not be specific enough for MH to exclude other myopathies. This is discussed in more detail below.

These data suggest a much higher incidence of MH susceptibility than is currently apparent. When masseter spasm occurs, the anesthetic should be discontinued, the patient observed in the intensive care unit for 24 hours, and multiple determinations made of serum potassium, CPK, and urinary myoglobin. Dantrolene (see "Treatment of an acute episode") should not be administered unless a fever develops. Because of recent reports of the high rate of positive results from muscle biopsies in patients with masseter spasm, all patients with masseter spasm must be informed that they may have MH. The decision to obtain a muscle biopsy should be based on the entire clinical presentation and not on the occurrence of masseter spasm alone. In any case, the patient and family should be kept well informed so they can relate all the information to subsequent physicians.

There are case reports of "MH" without fever,[4,10,29] but the patients either had muscular dystrophy or the muscle contracture was confined to the masseter muscle. Gronert has published a case report suggesting that awake episodes of fever associated with a positive caffeine contracture test might be MH.[22] Several of the conventional features of MH are absent in this case, however, and very little of the medical workup is presented.

RISK FACTORS

Other than the history of a classic presentation, the only risk factor reliably associated with MH susceptibility is the occurrence of generalized muscular rigidity during a previous anesthetic.[33]

The inheritance pattern of MH susceptibility is very erratic, poorly understood, and of only some small value in assessing the risk to family members. There are certainly susceptible families in whom transmission is autosomal dominant,[8] but there are also families in whom only a single member appears susceptible. Triggering agents (succinylcholine and inhalation agents) should be avoided in patients with a close family member who has had a clinically convincing episode of MH.

Some populations are slightly more likely to have an MH episode, but these tendencies are of no value in assessing the risk for an individual patient. The incidence of MH may be slightly higher in children, males, and patients with other musculoskeletal abnormalities. King and Denborough[30] have described a syndrome occurring only in boys characterized by short stature, lordosis, cryptorchidism, crowned lower teeth, and a very high susceptibility to MH.

Another puzzling feature of this disease is its occurrence in patients who have had no adverse reaction when previously exposed to triggering agents. Almost half the episodes of MH occur in patients who have previously had an unremarkable anesthetic.[6] Consequently, there is no low-risk category, and temperature and end-tidal CO_2 monitoring is necessary during every administration of general anesthesia.

DIAGNOSIS

The diagnosis of MH is not simple and carries with it serious implications for the rest of the patient's life and for the lives of family members. The patient who has had severe acidosis, muscle rigidity, and hyperthermia during anesthesia and who also has marked postoperative increases in creatine kinase (CK) can be certain that he or she has MH. There is little benefit to the patient to subsequently verify this diagnosis with a muscle biopsy. However, now that the anesthesia community is highly sensitized to the early signs of MH, it is infrequent that a patient will express the full-blown MH syndrome; the consequence is that the diagnosis of MH is often based on a more uncertain clinical history. The patient with such a history would benefit from a diagnostic evaluation for MH. What diagnostic procedures give reliable results?

One of the unfortunate aspects of the history of MH is the number of invalidated assays that have been used to "diagnose" MH. These include the adenosine triphosphate (ATP) depletion of muscle samples, ATP, adenosine diphosphate (ADP) content of platelets, hemolysis of red blood cells, phosphorylase activity of muscle samples, and calcium uptake by thin sections of muscle.[9,19,31,40,50] Each of these assays had a brief period of popularity, and it is probable that many patients still believe they have or do not have MH based on the results of these unvalidated or invalidated assays. The halothane and caffeine contracture test of excised muscle is the only diagnostic test currently available that appears to have some validity. However, this test itself carries with it many uncertainties. For example, the criteria for diagnosis of MH in the United States have never been published. The test requires that a fresh muscle biopsy be performed, which means that the biopsy must be done and taken to the laboratory within 1 hour. The laboratory personnel performing the test must be experienced with the handling of muscle and must have performed a sufficient number of normal biopsies so that they can distinguish normal from diseased muscle. The biopsy procedure requires extreme care in the handling of the muscle specimen and requires performance by an experienced and careful surgeon. The muscle should not be stretched or traumatized, because this could increase sensitivity to both caffeine and halothane. The specimen is divided into small bundles; several bundles, usually three or more, are attached to a force transducer and then exposed to increasing doses of halothane or caffeine. MH-susceptible muscle has been shown to generate greater contracture force at lower drug concentrations.

The European MH group has presented their diagnostic criteria, and as of 1986 they had performed 70 control biopsies.[43] From the examination of control muscle and suspected MH muscle they determined that MH susceptibility could be defined by a threshold (that is, an increase in tension >0.2 g) at 2% or less halothane or at 2 mM caffeine. Normal patients were defined by the absence of tension >0.2 g when exposed to either 2% halothane or 2 mM caffeine. A separate group, called MH equivocal, were found to have a response to *either* halothane or caffeine, but not both. Of 971 patients studied by the European MH group, 14.1% were classified as MH equivocal. The European MH group has set down a specific protocol for examination of muscle and arrived at specific criteria for the diagnosis of MH susceptibility; despite this, 14% of their patients could not be diagnosed because of the equivocal status of the results.

In the United States, there are approximately 12 MH biopsy centers, and, unfortunately, the methodology and diagnostic criteria for MH biopsy are not as uniform as those for the European MH group. Therefore, it is relatively impossible to write down exact criteria used overall in the United States for determining MH susceptibility on the basis of a muscle biopsy. It is apparent that MH susceptibility is diagnosed on the basis of an increased sensitivity to halothane and/or caffeine, but beyond that each laboratory appears to have their own specific criteria.

Currently, the caffeine and halothane contracture test appears to be the only diagnostic test that gives reliable and believable results. Other investigators had undertaken the examination of "skinned" muscle fibers to determine MH susceptibility.[49,54] The term *skinned fiber* refers to a single muscle fiber whose outer membrane has been either removed mechanically or chemically and modified such that it no longer acts as a permeability barrier to small molecules. This type of assay held great promise in that it depended on the response of the membrane system in muscle, the sarcoplasmic reticulum, which is believed to be defective in MH. Unfortunately, extensive use of this technique has not occurred because

it is extremely tedious and requires the expertise of a very subspecialized muscle physiologist, few of whom are available for screening procedures. The data initially generated by this method appeared quite promising but, similar to contracture testing, left many uncertainties about the necessary criteria for declaring a patient MH positive. A single fiber is a small sample of the total number of fibers in a muscle bundle. How many need to be studied? What percent of the number studied need to be abnormal to classify the muscle specimen positive and the patient MH? Takagi said he required 50% of the fibers to have increased caffeine sensitivity to classify a patient as MH susceptible. Woods, however, declared a biopsy positive if 2 out of 20 fibers were found to have a caffeine response outside the range of 1000 control fibers. He first examined 10 fibers; if 1 was found to be positive, a second set of 10 was examined. If no others were positive, then the patient was not classified MH susceptible; if 1 or more of the second set were positive the patient was classified MH susceptible (personal communication). At this time we do not know how many fibers must be abnormal before an MH crisis will result from exposure to triggering drugs.

TRIGGERING EVENTS

The total number of the drugs and conditions that trigger MH are unknown. However, it is known that all volatile anesthetics are triggering agents, and, furthermore, that depolarizing muscle relaxants (succinylcholine) are potent triggering agents. Other drugs have been implicated as triggering agents in MH including N_2O and curare. Little positive evidence exists, however, that they are in fact MH triggers, and both have been used safely in MH patients.

Which drugs can be administered safely to MH patients? It appears that the nondepolarizing muscle relaxants pancuronium, vecuronium, and atracurium can be used safely. Anesthetics that can be administered safely to the MH patient include fentanyl and sufentanil, diazepam, lorazepam, midazolam, and ketamine. We have used N_2O extensively as an anesthetic adjunct for MH patients. Much inconvenience and discomfort to MH patients has arisen from the recommendation that amide local anesthetics should be avoided and are dangerous. As indicated in a recent letter to *Anesthesiology*, there have been few experimental or clinical data to support this recommendation.[37] Furthermore, lidocaine, an amide anesthetic, has been found *not* to trigger MH in MH swine.[54] Several investigators have used amide local anesthetics for nerve blocks for muscle biopsies in MH patients.

The mechanism of triggering has not been clarified, but it appears that preoperative stress resulting from inadequate sedation[36] and intraoperative stress resulting from light anesthesia might be important in initiating the disastrous metabolic events.[23] It has also been shown that the onset of MH can be slowed by the addition of certain drugs; this has been documented for both pancuronium and thiopental in the porcine model of MH.

Progress in MH treatment and research can in large part be attributed to the occurrence of a syndrome in pigs that is quite similar to MH. The porcine stress syndrome (PSS), which occurs in both awake-stressed pigs and anesthetized pigs, mimics MH in most of its manifestations. In 1966 Hall reported the triggering of MH by halothane and succinylcholine in PSS pigs.[25] It was later noted that specific strains of pigs were MH-susceptible and others were not. The availability of the MH-susceptible pig led to the discovery that intravenous dantrolene could effectively stop the otherwise lethal progress of MH.[26]

TREATMENT OF THE ACUTE EPISODE

The following is the suggested therapy for an MH emergency as published by the Malignant Hyperthermia Association of the United States:

1. All inhalation anesthetics should be discontinued and hyperventilation with 100% oxygen begun.
2. In the absence of blood gas analysis, bicarbonate 1 to 2 mg/kg should be administered.
3. Dantrolene sodium (20 mg/vial) should be obtained, mixed with 60 ml of distilled water, and 1 mg/kg administered intravenously. At present, dantrolene is packaged as a lyophilized preparation that contains 20 mg of dantrolene per vial.
4. Simultaneously, cooling should be started by all routes; surface, nasogastric lavage, intravenous cold solutions, wound, and rectally.
5. Anesthetic tubing, and if possible, soda lime should be replaced.
6. Arrhythmias will respond to treatment of acidosis and hyperkalemia. If they persist and are life threatening, 200 mg of procainamide should

be administered in repeated doses as required.
7. Further doses of dantrolene should be administered as necessary, titrated to the heart rate, muscle rigidity, and temperature. Response to dantrolene should be monitored. Although the average successful dose of dantrolene is about 2 mg/kg, much higher doses may be needed (10 mg/kg and more). Fortunately, dantrolene does not produce significant myocardial depression at these doses.
8. Urine output, serum potassium level, calcium level, arterial blood gas values, and clotting studies should be determined and monitored closely. Hyperkalemia is common in the acute phase of MH and should be treated with intravenous glucose and insulin.
9. The patient should be observed in an ICU setting for at least 24 hours, since recrudescence of MH may occur, particularly following a case that was difficult to treat.
10. CK, calcium, and potassium levels should be observed until they return to normal.
11. ECG should also be obtained and followed postoperatively.
12. Body temperature should be monitored closely, since overvigorous treatment of MH may lead to hypothermia. Temperature instability may persist for several days after the acute episode. Body temperatures of 41° C to 42° C are compatible with survival and normal brain function if treated promptly.
13. Urine output should be greater than 1 ml/kg/hour. CVP monitoring should be considered because fluid shifts may occur.
14. When the patient's condition has stabilized, treatment should be converted from intravenous to oral dantrolene. Although data are not available regarding optimal doses and duration of treatment with dantrolene after an episode, the patient should probably receive a total dose of 4 mg/kg/day in divided doses for 48 hours after surgery.

This protocol may need to be modified in meeting the needs of individual patients.

The key to a successful outcome is the early recognition of the syndrome and an immediate response with intravenous dantrolene and vigorous surface cooling with ice. A complete resuscitation requires the help of several people, so a call for help should go out as soon as the problem is identified. Extra people are needed to mix the dantrolene, draw blood for laboratory analysis, start arterial and additional venous lines, and carry ice for surface cooling. Some institutions keep a rubber raft near the operating room so the patient's torso (or the entire body if the patient is a child) can be placed in the raft and packed in ice. In addition to providing effective cooling, the raft prevents water from draining onto the floor and making walking treacherous.

A supply of dantrolene, a minimum of 1 g, should be immediately available in the operating room suite. Currently, dantrolene is supplied in 20 mg vials that require reconstitution with 60 ml of sterile water. Dantrolene is not very soluble in water, so each vial contains 3 g of mannitol to help dissolve the dantrolene. Dantrolene must be given early in the episode to be successful, and even when given early it is not always effective.

The treatment of MH-associated cardiac arrhythmias is a somewhat controversial subject. Until recently many authorities recommended against the use of lidocaine, an amide, in a MH-susceptible patient.[2,30] Administration of lidocaine during an MH crisis was thought to prolong or exacerbate the pathologic process. However, lidocaine has been used successfully to treat arrhythmias during an episode of MH[28] and has been extensively used without difficulty as a local anesthetic in MH-susceptible patients.[1] Consequently, arrhythmias should be treated in the usual manner; lidocaine will often be the first drug of choice in treating ventricular arrhythmias.

Hyperkalemia often occurs during an episode of MH.[7,20] Injured muscle releases large amounts of potassium, and intracellular potassium is shifted to the extracellular space by acidosis. Hyperkalemia may be first recognized through monitoring of the electrocardiogram, but serial serum potassium determinations should be made as soon as the crisis is recognized. When the potassium exceeds 6.5 mEq/L, the QRS complexes widen; as the serum potassium increases further, the P wave amplitude decreases and the PQ-R interval becomes prolonged. The P wave may disappear, and the QRS complex resembles a sine wave as the serum potassium approaches 8.0 mEq/L.[41] Ventricular fibrillation or cardiac arrest will soon follow. Hyperkalemic cardiac toxicity should be treated by administration of calcium chloride or calcium gluconate. The theoretic concern that calcium may exacerbate the crisis has not been substantiated by any reports of calcium

alone being a triggering agent in humans; in any case, if the widening QRS complex is not treated, the patient is likely to die. The serum potassium level can be decreased by infusing glucose and insulin to increase glycogen and potassium storage. In an adult, 1000 ml of 10% dextrose with 10 units of insulin is given over 1 hour. Correcting metabolic acidosis with bicarbonate will also help lower the serum potassium. Total body potassium can be decreased by normal kidney function, dialysis, or cation-exchange resins, but these methods take several hours to work and can only be employed in the stable patient. The serum potassium should be monitored for at least 2 days following an unequivocal episode.

Serum calcium levels usually decrease during an malignant hyperthermia crises in humans.[7] The cause is not clear, but the hypocalcemia may be the result of calcium salt deposition into the traumatized muscle. Calcium salt formation is stimulated by the release of phosphorus from the damaged muscle and, at least in the case of physical trauma, salt formation and deposition can occur quickly enough to produce acute hypocalcemia.[32] Correcting the hypocalcemia is difficult and, except in the case of cardiac conduction abnormalities, intravenous calcium should not be administered.

Patients who survive the initial episode may develop acute renal failure from the rhabelomyolosis and shock. Producing a brisk diuresis during the episode may help to prevent the problem.

Calcium channel blockers were once thought to be useful in the treatment of MH, because diltiazem prevented abnormal contractures in a caffeine-contracture test of muscle obtained from a patient who had a clinically convincing episode.[24,27] However, subsequent studies in MH-susceptible swine found calcium channel blockers to be of no benefit[18] or even to be dangerous.[48] Unfavorable results in the pig model have prevented wide-scale investigations in humans. Currently, calcium channel blockers should not be used in the treatment of MH.

Dantrolene, the first-line treatment for MH, is a hydantoin derivative whose major site of action is skeletal muscle. Dantrolene acts by reducing myoplasmic calcium concentrations, either by stabilizing the sarcoplasmic reticulum or by uncoupling the signal-carrying T-tubule system from the sarcoplasmic reticulum, or both.[39] Dantrolene has little effect on the heart, although some animal studies suggest an antiarrhythmic action.[11] The only significant adverse action from short-term administration is muscle weakness, which in otherwise healthy patients does not usually extend to the respiratory muscles (in doses up to at least 3 mg/kg).[17] However, in patients with clinically apparent neuromuscular disease, small doses of dantrolene may produce significant respiratory depression.[38,51] Prolonged administration may result in hepatitis; therefore, the drug is now infrequently used to treat spasticity or muscle contractures.

Dantrolene is absorbed well orally. It binds to albumin at two or more sites and was found to cross the placenta in two patients taking the drug for MH prophylaxis. Dantrolene is primarily metabolized in the liver by hydroxylation and, although there is substantial individual variation, the mean elimination half-life is about 12 hours.[51]

ANESTHESIA FOR THE ELECTIVE PATIENT WITH MH TENDENCY

Anesthetic agents for patients predisposed to MH should not include inhalation agents or succinylcholine. The anesthesia machine should be flushed with 100% oxygen for several hours before the planned anesthetic and the soda lime replaced so the patient will not be exposed to even trace levels of inhalation agents. Anesthesia should consist of only those "safe agents" discussed earlier. The usual scenario includes induction with thiopental, paralysis with a nondepolarizing neuromuscular blocker, and maintenance of anesthesia with narcotics and nitrous oxide; additional hypnosis can be provided with thiopental, midazolam, or other intravenous hypnotic agents. Regional anesthesia can certainly be used when possible.

The use of prophylactic dantrolene is somewhat controversial because the effective dose is unknown. At least two case reports[14,15] suggest the occurrence of MH after the administration of dantrolene, but although both patients were acidotic, neither was febrile. Flewellen and Nelson[15] speculate that the optimal prophylactic dose is one that produces maximal skeletal muscle twitch depression, usually about 2.5 mg/kg intravenously over 10 to 15 minutes immediately before induction of anesthesia. This dose produces higher levels than probably occurred in either of the patients just cited. Regardless of the route or dosage, dantrolene may prolong the action of the nondepolarizing neuromuscular blockers,[13] and patients should be monitored for adequacy of

respiration, as well as for signs of MH. But which patients, if any, should be given dantrolene prophylaxis? The prime concern in anesthetizing any MH patient is avoiding triggering agents and verifying that dantrolene is *immediately* available. Factors considered in a decision to give prophylaxis should include the complexity of the surgery and anesthesia, surgical skill, whether the patient has had a real MH crisis before and whether there is uncertainty about the MH diagnosis itself. Most anesthetics for MH patients can be safely administered without the need for prophylaxis. However, since muscle weakness is the only side-effect of dantrolene administration, its prophylactic use can be undertaken without other serious concern.

MECHANISM OF MALIGNANT HYPERTHERMIA

Studies of the porcine model of MH have indicated that the major defect of this disorder lies in skeletal muscle.[3] Because of the similarities between porcine and human MH, it is believed that an abnormality of skeletal muscle is also the seat of the primary defect in human MH. The increased sensitivity of MH muscle strips to caffeine has suggested that sarcoplasmic reticulum (SR) function and Ca^{2+} regulation may be abnormal in MH muscle. Recent data from several independent investigators[35,40a,42] have given direct evidence that the SR is abnormal and Ca^{2+} levels in muscle are elevated.

Skeletal muscle contraction depends on the interaction of Ca^{2+} with the myofibrils. A neural stimulus at the neuromuscular junction results in depolarization of the outer membrane, the sarcolemma, of the muscle; this event leads to transmission of an as yet undefined signal from the sarcolemma across the T-tubular system to the sarcoplasmic reticulum. The sarcoplasmic reticulum releases its stored Ca^{2+}, resulting in a 1000-fold increase in the myoplasmic Ca^{2+} concentration. At this elevated concentration of Ca^{2+}, Ca^{2+} binds to troponin, leading to a conformational change in protein, the cycling of actin-myosin crossbridges, and tension development. As the sarcolemma is repolarized, the sarcoplasmic reticulum, which contains an ATP-dependent Ca^{2+} pump, removes Ca^{2+} from the myoplasm, sequestering it in the membranous space of the sarcoplasmic reticulum. The Ca^{2+} pump of the sarcoplasmic reticulum is able to decrease the myoplasmic Ca^{2+} concentration to approximately 10^{-7}M, resulting in muscle relaxation.

Although it had been hypothesized for many years that a defect existed in sarcoplasmic reticulum from MH muscle and that during an MH crisis intracellular Ca^{2+} was elevated, it is only in the past 5 years that direct experimental evidence has proven this to be true. In 1983 both Ohnishi et al and Nelson, working independently, demonstrated an abnormality in the Ca^{2+} release mechanism of sarcoplasmic reticulum from MH-susceptible swine. Ohnishi[42] isolated a heavy fraction of sarcoplasmic reticulm and, using a metallochromic dye, Arsenazo III, demonstrated that both halothane and calcium could induce larger amounts of Ca^{2+}-release from sarcoplasmic reticulum from MH-susceptible swine than from normal sarcoplasmic reticulum. Nelson, using a similar preparation and method, noted that the threshold, i.e., Ca^{2+} load, for Ca^{2+} release was much lower in the sarcoplasmic reticulum of MH-susceptible swine than in that of normal swine.[40a] These reports have definitely confirmed an abnormality of the sarcoplasmic reticulum. Whether the defect in release is directly related to the pharmacologically induced series of events that occur in a triggered MH episode is uncertain.

Another exciting series of experiments has measured the intracellular Ca^{2+} concentration in muscle of MH swine and humans.[35] Lopez has used an intracellular Ca^{2+} electrode to measure the free myoplasmic Ca^{2+} concentration in vivo in MH and normal swine. He noted that intracellular Ca^{2+} concentration was four times higher in MH swine than in normal swine; furthermore, remarkably, administration of halothane increased Ca^{2+} by a factor of approximately 20. Subsequent infusion of dantrolene resulted in the decrease of Ca^{2+} to levels equivalent to the nontriggered state. These data verified that the regulation of intracellular Ca^{2+} is an abnormality of MH muscle.[35] Lopez has demonstrated that Ca^{2+} in human MH muscle is also elevated to levels greater than those found in normal human muscle. He has also demonstrated that the treatment of MH-susceptible patients with dantrolene results in a lowering of Ca^{2+} as measured in diagnostically examined intercostal muscle.[34]

These studies, although a major contribution to the understanding of malignant hyperthermia, leave several important questions unanswered. We are still uncertain about the molecular events by which the volatile anesthetics and depolarizing muscle relaxants alter Ca^{2+} concentration. Is there a modification in the protein composition of the Ca^{2+} release channel of sarcoplasmic reticulum or is the lipid composition of the membrane surrounding the release channel altered? Further investigations into molecular interactions or anesthetics, membrane constituents, and dantrolene are required to complete our understanding of the pathophysiology of MH.

REFERENCES

1. Adragna MG: Medical protocol by habit—the avoidance of amide local anesthetics in malignant hyperthermia susceptible patients, Anesthesiology 62:99-100, 1985.
2. American Society of Anesthesiology: Technical bulletin for malignant hyperthermia, Newsletter 46:5, 1982.
3. Berman MC et al: Changes underlying halothane-induced malignant hyperyrexia in landrace pigs, Nature 225:653-655, 1970.
4. Bloom BA, Fonkalsrud EW, and Reynolds RC: Malignant hyperpyrexia during anesthesia in childhood, J Pediatr Surg 11:185-190, 1976.
5. Britt BA: Preanesthetic diagnosis of malignant hyperthermia, Int Anes Clin 17(4):63-96, 1979.
6. Britt BA: Malignant hyperthermia, Can Anaesth Soc J 32:666-677, 1985.
7. Britt BA and Kalow W: Malignant hyperthermia: a statistical review, Can Anaesth Soc J 17:293-315, 1970.
8. Britt BA, Locher WG, and Kalow W: Hereditary aspects of malignant hyperthermia, Can Anaesth Soc J 16:88-98, 1969.
9. Britt BA and Scott EA: Failure of the platelet-Halothane nucleotide depletion test as a diagnostic or screening test for malignant hyperthermia, Anesth Analg 65:171-175, 1986.
10. Brownell AKW et al: Malignant hyperthermia in Duchenne muscular dystrophy, Anesthesiology 58:180-182, 1983.
11. Butterfield JL et al: Antiarrhythmic activity of dantrolene sodium, Abstract Pharmacologist 25:246, 1983.
12. Denborough MA and Lovell RRH: Anaesthetic deaths in a family, Lancet 2:45, 1960.
13. Driessen JJ, Wuis EW, and Gielen MJM: Prolonged vecuronium neuromuscular blockade in a patient receiving orally administered dantrolene, Anesthesiology 62:523-524 1985.
14. Fitzgibbons DC: Malignant hyperthermia following preoperative oral administration of dantrolene, Anesthesiology 54:73-75, 1981.
15. Flewellen EH and Nelson TE: Dantrolene dose response in malignant hyperthermia susceptible (MHS)

swine method to obtain prophylaxis and therapeusis, Anesthesiology 52:303-308, 1980.

16. Flewellen EH and Nelson TE: Masseter spasm induced by succinylcholine in children: contracture testing for malignant hyperthermia: report of six cases, Can Anaesth Soc J 29:42-49, 1982.

17. Flewellen EH et al: Dantrolene dose response in awake man: implications for management of malignant hyperthermia, Anesthesiology 59:275-280, 1983.

18. Gallant EM et al: Verapamil is not a therapeutic adjunct to dantrolene in porcine malignant hyperthermia, Anesth Analg 64:601-606, 1985.

19. Gronert GA: Muscle contractures and ATP depletion in porcine malignant hyperthermia, Anesth Analg 58:367-371, 1979.

20. Gronert GA: Malignant hyperthermia, Anesthesiology 53:395-423, 1980.

21. Gronert GA and Milde JH: Variations in onset of porcine malignant hyperthermia, Anesth Analg 60:499-503, 1981.

22. Gronert GA, Thompson RL, and Onofrio BM: Human malignant hyperthermia: awake episodes and correction by dantrolene, Anesth Analg 59:377-378, 1980.

23. Gronert GA and Thye RA: Suxamethonium-induced porcine malignant hyperthermia, Br J Anaesth 48:513-517, 1976.

24. Gruener R and Blanck TJJ: Volatile anesthetics and skeletal muscle: evidence for sarcolemmal involvement in malignant hyperthermia. In Fink BR, editor: Molecular mechanisms of anesthesia, Progress in Anesthesiology, vol 2, New York, 1980, Raven Press.

25. Hall LW et al: Unusual reaction to suxamethonium chloride, Br Med J 2:1305, 1966.

26. Harrison GG: Control of malignant hyperpyrexic syndrome in MHS swine by dantrolene sodium, Br J Anaesth 47:62-65, 1975.

27. Iwatsuki N, Koga Y, and Amaha K: Calcium channel blocker for treatment of malignant hyperthermia, Anesth Analg 62:861-862, 1983 (letter).

28. Katz D: Recurrent malignant hyperthermia during anesthesia, Anesth Analg 49:225-230, 1970.

29. Kelfer HM, Singer WD, and Reynolds RN: Malignant hyperthermia in a child with Duchenne muscular dystrophy, Pediatrics 71:118-119, 1983.

30. King JO and Denborough MA: Anesthetic-induced malignant hyperpyrexia in children, J Pediatr 83:37-40, 1973.

31. Kistler P, Fletcher JE, and Rosenberg H: Erythrocyte fragility is not a tool for diagnosis of human malignant hyperthermia, Anesth Analg 66:1004-1007, 1987.

32. Knochel JP: Serum calcium derangements in rhabdomyolysis, N Engl J Med 305:161-163, 1981.

33. Larach MG et al: Prediction of malignant hyperthermia susceptibility by clinical signs, Anesthesiology 66:547-550, 1987.

34. Lopez JR, Medine P, and Alamo L: Dantrolene sodium is able to reduce the resting ionic $[Ca^{2+}]$ in muscle from humans with malignant hyperthermia, Muscle Nerve 10:77-79, 1987.

35. Lopez JR et al: Myoplasmic free $[Ca^{2+}]$ during a malignant hyperthermic episode in swine, Muscle Nerve 11:82-88, 1988.

36. Mogensen JV, Misfeldt BB, and Hanel HK: Preoperative excitement and malignant hyperthermia, Lancet 1:461, 1974.

37. Moore DC: Ester or amide local anesthetics in malignant hyperthermia—who knows? Anesthesiology 645:294-296, 1986.

38. Mora CT, Eisenkraft JB, and Papatestas AE: Intravenous dantrolene in patient with myasthenia gravis, Anesthesiology 64:371-373, 1986.

39. Morgan KG and Bryant SH: The mechanism of action of dantrolene sodium, J Pharmacol Exp Ther 201:138-147, 1977.

40. Nagarajam K et al: Calcium uptake in frozen muscle biopsy sections compared with other predictions of malignant hyperthermia susceptibility, Anesthesiology 66:680-685, 1987.

40a. Nelson TE: Abnormality in calcium release from skeletal sarcoplasmic reticulum of pigs susceptible to malignant hyperthermic, J Clin Invest 72:862-870, 1983.

41. Newmark SR and Sluhy RG: Hyperkalemia and hypokalemia, JAMA 231:631-633, 1975.

42. Ohnishi ST, Taylor S, and Gronert GA: Calcium-induced Ca^{2+} release from sarcoplasmic reticulum of pigs susceptible to malignant hyperthermia, FEBS Lett 161:103-107, 1983.

43. Ranklev E: Results from the European MH group, patients and normal controls. Fourth International Malignant Hyperthermia Workshop, York, 1986.

44. Rhuhland G and Hinkle AJ: Malignant hyperthermia after oral and intravenous pretreatment with dantrolene in a patient susceptible to malignant hyperthermia, Anesthesiology 60:159-160, 1984.

45. Rosenberg H: Trismus is not trivial, Anesthesiology 67:453-455, 1987.

46. Rosenberg H and Fletcher JE: Masseter muscle rigidity and malignant hyperthermia susceptibility, Anesth Analg 65:161-164, 1986.

47. Saidman LJ, Harvard ES, and Eger EI: Hyperthermia during anesthesia, JAMA 190:1029-1032, 1964.

48. Salzman LS et al: Hyperkalemia and cardiovascular collapse after verapamil and dantrolene administration in swine, Anesth Analg 63:473-478, 1984.

49. Takagi A: Skinned fiber studies in MH. Proceedings of the Third International Workshop on Malignant Hyperthermia, Canada, 1982.

50. Traynor CA, VanDyke RA, and Gronert GA: Phosphorylase ratio and susceptibility to malignant hyperthermia, Anesth Analg 62:324-326, 1983.

51. Ward A, Chaffman MO, and Sorkin EM: Dantrolene: a review, Drugs 32:130-168, 1986.

52. Watson CB, Reierson N, and Norfleet EA: Clinically significant muscle weakness induced by oral dantrolene sodium prophylaxis for malignant hyperthermia, Anesthesiology 65:312-314.

53. Wingard DW and Bobko S: Failure of lidocaine to trigger porcine malignant hyperthermia, Anesth Analg 58:99-103, 1979.

54. Wood DS, Willner JH, and Salviati G: Malignant hyperthermia: the pathogenesis of abnormal caffeine contracture. In Schotland D, editor: Disorder of the motor unit, New York, 1982, John Wiley & Sons.

CHAPTER 27

Liver Disease, Including Postoperative Hepatic Dysfunction

PATRICIA TEWES

The interactions of liver function with anesthetic agents and other intraoperative stresses are complex. First, patients with preexisting liver dysfunction metabolize many anesthetic drugs abnormally; they are thus susceptible to numerous postoperative complications and a greater risk of perioperative mortality. Secondly, intraoperative stresses such as hypotension and hypoxia may cause or worsen hepatic dysfunction. Transfusion of blood products may cause virally mediated liver disease. Finally, anesthetic agents themselves, particularly halothane, may cause liver dysfunction ranging from asymptomatic increases in liver enzymes to massive hepatic necrosis. This chapter discusses preoperative assessment and preparation and intraoperative management of patients with preexisting liver disease and evaluation and treatment of patients with postoperative hepatic dysfunction.

PREOPERATIVE SCREENING

Preoperative evaluation of all patients undergoing a surgical procedure should include a detailed history and physical examination to screen for previously unrecognized liver disease and to carefully evaluate patients with known hepatic disease. A history of previous liver disease, family history of liver disease, jaundice, heavy alcohol intake, exposure to hepatotoxic chemicals, multiple transfusions, or symptoms of liver disease (including unexplained abdominal pain, indigestion, itching, coagulopathy, or alterations in urine or stool color) should initiate biochemical screening for abnormalities of serum aminotransferases, alkaline phosphatase, bilirubin, albumin, and HbSAg. If these studies are normal, it is generally felt that surgery can proceed without further evaluation of liver function.

On preoperative physical examination, physical

stigmata of liver disease such as jaundice, palmar erythema, spider angiomata, gynecomastia, and ascites should be sought, since patients with relatively advanced cirrhosis may have a normal biochemical screen.[29] The anesthetic plan may be altered, depending on the physical examination. Patients with marked ascites, for example, should be induced in a manner that will minimize the risk of regurgitation of gastric contents. In patients with known liver disease, the preoperative evaluation will depend on the type and severity of disease. Biochemical screening will aid in the initial evaluation of disease. Elevations of aminotransferases, glutamic-oxaloacetic transaminase (SGOT), also referred to as aspartate aminotransferase (AST), and serum glutamic pyruvic transaminase (SGPT), also referred to as alanine aminotransferase (ALT), are caused by the release of intracellular proteins from several different organs including the liver, heart, kidney, skeletal muscle, brain, and adipose tissue. Elevations occur with parenchymal damage to these organs. Acute parenchymal lesions such as hepatitis A or B may produce elevations in the range of 500 to 5000 IU/L. Nonhepatic diseases may generally be distinguished from hepatic disease because elevations of the transaminases are much lower. Patients with elevated transaminases should undergo further investigation before surgery proceeds.

Other tests of liver function, specifically synthetic function, include serum albumin and coagulation factors. Abnormalities of vitamin K absorption caused by obstructive hepatic disease affect synthesis of clotting factors I, II, V, VII, and X and are reflected in the prothrombin time.[62] The severity of the hemostatic defect caused by low vitamin K–dependent factors is proportional to the extent of liver damage.[7,64] Administration of vitamin K may correct the prothrombin time in mild hepatic disease, but failure to correct the abnormality indicates severe disease.[49] Coagulation tests are particularly important because the risk of perioperative bleeding is higher when coagulation defects exist. If possible, anomalies should be corrected before surgery to improve hemostasis. Injection of vitamin K (phytomenadione) 10 mg intramuscularly on 3 consecutive days is recommended; one injection may be sufficient in patients with mild disease.[67] Fresh frozen plasma is also used to correct more severe anomalies, but large quantities are often required, which may cause fluid overload. In such a case, the correction

is short lived.[29] The majority of other clotting factors, including fibrinogen, factors II, VII, IX, and X, as well as factors V, XI, XII, XIII, are also thought to be synthesized by the liver.[62] Prothrombin time, partial thromboplastin time, thrombin time, and platelet count are useful in monitoring the hematologic state of the patient with liver disease, although defects in these tests may not necessarily correlate with the degree of bleeding disorder.[65] Hepatic disease may also be accompanied by thrombocytopenia caused by bone marrow suppression, splenic sequestration, and folate deficiency, and patients may require platelet transfusions preoperatively.

The serum bilirubin reflects the excretory function of the liver. Conjugated bilirubin increases as a result of dysfunction of the liver parenchyma or the bile ducts. Conjugated bilirubin may also be elevated in unconjugated hyperbilirubinemia from acute hemolysis. In this case, however, it will be accompanied by a high unconjugated bilirubin.

Other laboratory evaluations are necessary in patients with liver disease. Serum electrolytes should be measured, since these patients often develop hyponatremia caused by impairment of free water clearance or hypokalemia caused by diuretic therapy or secondary hyperaldosteronism. Blood urea nitrogen (BUN) and serum creatinine should be evaluated, since impaired metabolism of aldosterone stimulates the renin-angiotensin system and may result in vasoconstriction. In patients with evidence of renal involvement, a creatinine clearance should be obtained. Terminal cirrhotic patients may develop hepatorenal syndrome, in which the kidney fails because renal vasodilators are unable to compensate for the vasoconstrictive stimulus.

Patients with unexplained liver disease may require liver biopsy before surgery, and patients with cholestatic jaundice require either endoscopic retrograde or transhepatic cholangiography and biopsy to evaluate their disease. It is essential that the etiology of cholestasis be evaluated, because patients with acute hepatocellular disease (intrahepatic cholestasis) are at greater risk of morbidity and mortality during anesthesia and surgery.[32]

It is debated whether asymptomatic patients without a history of hepatic dysfunction should undergo preoperative biochemical screening.[29,66] Preoperative screening of 7620 asymptomatic healthy patients identified 11 patients with abnormal transaminases.[70]

TABLE 27-1.   Child's classification

	Class A	Class B	Class C
Bilirubin (mg/dl)	<2.0	2.0-3.0	>3.0
Albumin (g/dl)	>3.5	3.0-3.5	<3.0
Ascites	None	Easily controlled	Poorly controlled
Encephalopathy	None	Mild	Advanced
Nutritional status	Excellent	Good	Poor

Adapted from Child GG and Turcotte JG: Surgery and portal hypertension. In Child GG, editor: The liver and portal hypertension, Philadelphia, 1964, WB Saunders Co.

These 11 patients were found to have overt liver pathologic factors by further laboratory testing, but only 3 became clinically jaundiced. None of the other 7609 patients developed jaundice in the year following surgery. It is questionable whether the cost of routine screening in all preoperative patients can be justified when so few patients have abnormal biochemical screens and even fewer develop clinically evident disease. Therefore, routine screening is not generally recommended in healthy patients.[29]

PERIOPERATIVE RISK ASSESSMENT

Assessment of operative risk in patients with liver dysfunction, especially cirrhosis, has been the subject of numerous studies. It is difficult to provide specific estimates based on these studies because of variable patient selection criteria and because it is unclear whether the cause of cirrhosis affects surgical outcome. It is clear, however, that the operative morbidity and mortality of patients with liver disease is high and appears to be related directly to the degree of preoperative hepatic dysfunction.[46]

Child's classification[16] was originally established for preoperative evaluation of patients undergoing esophageal transection for bleeding varices; it has since been used to evaluate other patients with liver disease having other types of surgery. The scale describes three classes based on clinical and biochemical parameters including bilirubin, albumin, presence and degree of ascites and encephalopathy, and nutritional status (Table 27-1). Child's classification has been shown to be a useful predictor of surgical mortality.[6,30] A study of 100 cirrhotic patients undergoing abdominal surgery found Child's classification to be the best predictor of operative mortality among 53 variables examined; mortality rates of 10%, 31%, and 76% were reported for classes A, B, and C, respectively.[30] Pugh et al[63a] (1973) mod-

ified Child's scale by replacing nutritional status with prothrombin time. This scale also predicted operative mortality in patients undergoing esophageal transection for bleeding varices (grade A, 71% 6-month postoperative survival; grade B, 36% 6-month survival; grade C, 0% 6-month survival), but it has not been studied in patients undergoing other operations.

Child's scale also appears to correlate with the degree of other postoperative complications including worsening hepatic encephalopathy, bleeding, infection, sepsis, renal failure, and wound dehiscence.[30,95] The main causes of death in cirrhotics in nonsurgical settings are hepatic coma and variceal bleeding[61]; however, the major cause of perioperative death is sepsis. A report of 100 cirrhotic patients undergoing nonshunt abdominal procedures in which 30 died postoperatively found that 87% of deaths were caused by sepsis with multiple organ system failure.[30] Operative and postoperative factors that predicted mortality included infection (64% mortality), emergency surgery (57% mortality), and Child's classification (76% mortality in class C patients). Perioperative morbidity was also high (30%) in this group of cirrhotic patients, and the majority of complications were caused by infection. Neither the surgical procedure nor the organs operated on influenced morbidity or mortality. Child's classification is thus considered the standard predictor of risk. Class A patients have a relatively low morbidity and mortality and can undergo elective surgery, but patients in classes B and C have an extremely high perioperative risk and should undergo careful preoperative preparation to reduce their risk factors. If the status of these patients cannot be improved preoperatively, elective surgery should not be performed, and emergency surgery should proceed with the knowledge that the operative risk is extremely high.

Extraction of drugs from the blood by the liver	
Efficiently extracted drugs	**Poorly extracted drugs**
Lidocaine	Acetaminophen
Meperidine	Amobarbital
Morphine	Antipyrine
Nortriptyline	Chloramphenicol
Pentazocine	Clindamycin
Propoxyphene	Chlorpromazine
Propranolol	Diazepam
	Digitoxin
	Hexobarbital
	Phenytoin
	Quinidine
	Theophylline
	Tolbutamide
	Warfarin

Adapted from Williams RL and Benet LZ: Hepatic function and pharmacokinetics. In Zakim D and Boyer TD: Hepatology: a textbook of liver disease, Philadelphia, 1982, WB Saunders.

PERIOPERATIVE MANAGEMENT
General Measures

Few studies have reported definitive intraoperative management strategies for patients with severe liver disease, despite the multiple organ system involvement in this disease process. Patients may have disorders of pulmonary function caused by ascites or shunts. Massive ascites increases the risk for regurgitation of gastric contents during anesthetic induction because intragastric pressure is increased. Some suggest that the airway should be secured by rapid-sequence induction or awake intubation; or, alternatively, prophylactic histamine antagonists can be administered to minimize the likelihood of pulmonary injury should aspiration occur. Severe ascites causes cephalad displacement of the diaphragm, and patients may require paracentesis before surgery to improve oxygenation. Ascitic fluid may move into the chest, cause hydrothorax, and increase ventilation-to-perfusion mismatching. Central hyperventilation may lead to respiratory alkalosis in patients with encephalopathy. Systemic and pulmonary arterial-to-venous shunting may develop and contribute to oxygenation defects. Arterial blood gases should be measured preoperatively, and an arterial line is probably indicated for frequent measurements of arterial blood gases intraoperatively.

Because the liver is responsible for the elimination of many drugs, hepatic dysfunction caused either by altered liver blood flow or by changes in hepatocellular function may decrease the ability of the body to metabolize drugs. Drugs that are easily extracted by the liver are generally more affected by changes in delivery to the hepatocytes caused by reduced hepatic blood flow, whereas drugs that are inefficiently extracted are more sensitive to changes in the intrinsic ability of the liver to metabolize them (see box above, left). Sedative agents such as diazepam and narcotics should be used in smaller doses, because slower metabolism may result in prolonged depression of consciousness. Benzodiazopines and opiates frequently precipitate hepatic coma in patients with altered pharmacokinetics or with increased central nervous system sensitivity due to cirrhosis.[61]

Metabolism of muscle relaxants may also be altered in severe hepatic disease. In patients with liver disease, protein binding of muscle relaxants such as pancuronium, d-tubocurarine, and atracurium is increased, causing a relative resistance to the actions of these drugs.[31] Greater volume of distribution also creates a relative resistance to the actions of drugs such as pancuronium. Succinylcholine, however, may have a prolonged duration of action because of deficiency of plasma cholinesterase.[38]

Induction of liver microsomal enzymes by a variety of agents will increase metabolism of substances that are metabolized by the liver microsomal system. Agents that induce these enzymes include barbiturates, alcohol, cigarette smoking, insecticides, organic solvents, and environmental contaminants. Patients exposed to these agents may have increased anesthetic requirements.

Abnormal glycemic control may also complicate the anesthetic management of patients with hepatic disease. The liver contributes to normal glycemic control by a combination of glycogenesis, glycogenolysis, gluconeogenesis, and glycolysis. Patients with cirrhosis most often have glucose intolerance, hyperglycemia, and insulin resistance. However, hypoglycemia is also seen in hepatic disease and is probably caused by decreased hepatic glucose stores and lack of responsiveness of hepatic tissue to glucagon. Intraoperative monitoring should include frequent determinations of blood glucose to guide appropriate treatment.

The adequacy of intravascular volume may be difficult to predict in patients with hepatic failure. Vigorous preoperative treatment of ascites with diuretics or paracentesis may lead to electrolyte abnormalities or hypovolemia. A pulmonary artery catheter may be necessary to monitor the ascitic patient undergoing abdominal surgery because large fluid shifts may occur when the peritoneum is opened.

Encephalopathy should be evaluated and treated preoperatively. Patients with hepatic encephalopathy should be evaluated for precipitating factors such as gastrointestinal bleeding and sepsis. Protein intake should be restricted and lactulose given either orally or rectally to decrease intestinal protein load. If encephalopathy cannot be controlled preoperatively, all except emergency surgery should be avoided because this group has an extremely high risk of developing hepatic coma perioperatively.[16,30] If esophageal varices are suspected, the patient should be examined and treated preoperatively to decrease the risk of hemorrhage. Patients with ascites should have a diagnostic paracentesis if there has been a change in the ascites or a recent fever, to rule out bacterial peritonitis.

Miscellaneous Problems Requiring Special Management

Alcoholism. The alcoholic surgical patient presents several specific problems, including liver disease, withdrawal, and delirium tremens. The alcoholic patient is also prone to trauma and must be examined for intracranial pathologic conditions before surgical interventions. While the alcohol-tolerant patient may require more anesthesia, in the acutely intoxicated patient additive drug effects can occur. Asymptomatic alcoholic fatty liver develops after acute episodes of heavy drinking, resulting in an enlarged liver and elevated transaminases. Liver function is usually preserved, however, and it is probably safe to proceed with elective surgery in these patients after alcohol-induced nutritional deficiencies are corrected. Specific prospective studies concerning the outcome of anesthesia in these patients, however, have not been reported. These patients may have increased anesthetic requirements because of tolerance and microsomal enzyme induction by alcohol.[33,37]

Alcohol withdrawal begins within a few hours after the peak blood alcohol concentration and pre-

sents difficult management problems in the surgical patient. The first signs of withdrawal are tremulousness, hyperreflexia, hypertension, tachycardia, sweating, agitation, and brief visual hallucinations. Patients may have generalized seizures at this time. Patients who develop delirium tremens (DTs) have profound disorientation, hallucinations, tachycardia, tremors, and profuse perspiration, which can lead to dehydration, hyperthermia, cardiovascular collapse, and death. DTs have a mortality rate of 10% to 15%.[27,78] Anesthesia and surgery may increase this risk, and all but urgent surgery should probably be avoided in the patient who exhibits signs of withdrawal. Little has been written about the operative management of patients with DTs, but management suggestions are similar to those for alcohol withdrawal in the nonsurgical setting. Mild withdrawal symptoms may not require treatment with drugs, but sedatives should probably be used to prevent seizures and DTs.[71] Shorter-acting benzodiazepines should be used in patients with liver disease because metabolism may be altered. Clonidine, a centrally acting alpha-adrenergic antagonist, is effective in relieving the sympathetic nervous system manifestations of DTs[47,93]; however, it does not prevent DTs and may cause hypotension. DTs should be treated supportively with airway maintenance, intravenous fluids, thiamine, correction of metabolic abnormalities, and a cooling blanket for hyperthermia.

Cirrhosis. Patients with cirrhosis often require emergency surgery for gastrointestinal bleeding from esophageal varices or peptic ulcer disease. These procedures are associated with high mortality and should be done only in patients whose conditions have failed to respond to other conservative measures such as drug therapy or endoscopic sclerosis. The value of emergency portocaval shunts for variceal hemorrhage has been debated because of the extremely high mortality associated with this procedure. However, recent reports[89] suggest that portocaval shunts have an acceptable long-term survival rate (78% at 1 year) if patients are stabilized hemodynamically before surgery and are classified with mild to moderate liver disease (Child's class A or B).

For the anesthesiologist, the patient with gastrointestinal bleeding presents problems of hypovolemia and high risk for pulmonary aspiration of blood. Profuse bleeding may require awake intubation. Frequent monitoring of arterial blood gases, hematocrit levels, and central venous or pulmonary artery pressures should guide volume and blood replacement.

Liver transplantation. Management of patients undergoing liver transplantation has been discussed in several recent reviews.[14,82] Transplantation can be divided into three distinct phases: the preanhepatic phase, which extends until completion of liver dissection to its vascular pedicle; the anhepatic phase, which begins when blood flow to the liver is disrupted and ends when blood supply is anastomosed to the donor liver; and the postanhepatic phase, which includes the time from reperfusion to the end of the operation. In addition to the problems occurring in any operation in patients with liver failure, liver transplantation presents several special problems. The duration of the surgery (6 to 24 hours) necessitates strict attention to padding of extremities and maintenance of body temperature. Massive fluid shifts and rapid blood loss can occur, and rapid autotransfusion devices are necessary. Massive blood and fluid replacement accentuates preexisting coagulopathy and electrolyte disorders, and successful management requires frequent assessment of hematocrit, coagulation profiles, and electrolytes. Hyperglycemia frequently occurs after perfusion of the donor liver. Decreased urine output and hypotension may be caused by blood loss, myocardial dysfunction, decreased ionized calcium, or surgical manipulation of abdominal vessels that prevent adequate venous return. Constant invasive hemodynamic monitoring is necessary. Veno-venobypass is used to augment venous return and provide cardiovascular stability during the anhepatic phase, but decreased cardiac output and hypotension may require additional therapeutic interventions.

EFFECTS OF ANESTHESIA ON LIVER BLOOD FLOW

Blood flow to the liver is supplied by the hepatic artery (one third) and the portal vein (two thirds). Total liver blood flow is normally between 800 and 1200 ml/min and is affected by a variety of factors that may be dramatically altered during anesthesia and surgery. The hepatic artery and the portal vein have a reciprocal relationship; decreased flow through one circuit generally causes increased flow through the other. However, arterial flow cannot completely compensate for reduced portal vein flow, and disruption of portal flow leads to hepatic necrosis.

Arterial hypoxemia ($PaO_2 < 30$ mm Hg) increases hepatic arterial flow, and hypercarbia and acidosis increase both hepatic arterial and portal flow. Hypocarbia and alkalosis have the opposite effect. Sympathetic stimulation and exogenous administration of epinephrine decrease liver blood flow markedly, but dopamine has little effect. Glucagon causes hepatic arterial vasodilation.

Intraoperative events influence liver blood flow by a variety of mechanisms. Positive pressure ventilation decreases hepatic blood flow by increasing splanchnic vascular resistance, and application of positive end expiratory pressure accentuates these changes. Anesthetic agents change liver blood flow by means of direct effects on the hepatic vasculature or via effects on cardiac output. Halothane and enflurane increase hepatic arterial flow at low concentrations, but decrease flow at higher concentrations by depressing cardiac output. Isoflurane preserves blood flow at clinically effective doses and thus may be the preferred agent in patients with liver disease. Nitrous oxide alone has little effect, but in combination with hyperventilation it decreases hepatic blood flow by one third. Intravenous narcotics have little effect. Spinal and epidural anesthesia decrease liver blood flow in varying degrees, corresponding to the decrease in blood pressure caused by sympathetic blockade.

While intraoperative decreases in blood flow are usually well tolerated in normal subjects,[63] patients with preexisting disease may be more susceptible to hypoxic liver injury.[23,39] Further studies are required to assess the extent of increased risk in patients with portal hypertension who already have decreased portal blood flow. If possible, deliberate hypotensive anesthetic techniques should probably be avoided in advanced cirrhosis. However, Roth and Run[68] reported that deliberate reduction of mean arterial blood pressure (MAP) to 50 mm Hg was not associated with worsening of hepatic function in a patient with portal hypertension who underwent clipping of a cerebral aneurysm. Experiments in animals suggest that increases in oxygen extraction by hepatic tissue can compensate for decreased portal flow, which occurs with MAP reductions to 50 mm Hg. When sodium nitroprusside was used to decrease MAP to 50 mm Hg in dogs, portal venous flow decreased by 20%, but hepatic lactate extraction remained unchanged because of increased oxygen extraction.[42] Other investigators have noted elevations in transaminases following hypotension, but these occurred only at an MAP of 12 to 25 mm Hg.[20]

POSTOPERATIVE LIVER DYSFUNCTION

There are numerous causes of liver dysfunction following anesthesia and surgery, including viral hepatitis (A, B, non-A, non-B, cytomegalovirus), ischemic injury caused by intraoperative hypotension or hypoxemia, sepsis, and drug-induced hepatotoxicity. The precise cause of postoperative hepatic dysfunction is difficult to determine, because patients may have had more than one hepatotoxic exposure. It is likely, for example, that a patient may be exposed to blood transfusion, hypotension, and volatile anesthetics during a single operation. Exposures to multiple etiologic factors have confused studies of postoperative liver dysfunction, and the existence of "halothane hepatitis" as a clinical entity was debated for many years. This section will describe some of the causes of postoperative hepatic dysfunction; however, it should be understood that in many cases the specific cause is not known.

Non-A, non-B hepatitis accounts for 70% to 90% of cases of posttransfusion viral hepatitis.[1,34] Its epidemiologic characteristics resemble that of hepatitis B[19]: The incubation period is 2 weeks to 6 months after exposure, and symptoms, including anorexia, malaise, nausea, and right upper quadrant pain, usually resolve within 12 weeks of onset but may progress to chronic disease. For unknown reasons, some patients develop fulminant liver failure that is difficult to distinguish from halothane hepatitis because the incubation period and clinical presentation are similar. Diagnosis of non-A, non-B hepatitis is suggested by the appropriate clinical syndrome in the absence of hepatitis B surface antigen and hepatitis A antibody, a negative heterophile test result, and the absence of a rising titer to cytomegalovirus.

Few data exist on the contribution of intraoperative events such as hypotension, hypovolemia, and hypoxia to postoperative hepatic dysfunction. However, it is clear that these events may cause liver damage ranging from a mild reversible defect to massive necrosis.

In contrast, the contribution of volatile anesthetics to postoperative liver failure has been researched extensively and is discussed next. Other agents that are occasionally given in the perioperative period may cause either hepatitis-like reactions (methydopa [Aldomet], antituberculous drugs), cholestasis (sul-

fonylurea derivatives), or granulomas (diphenylhydantoin, phenylbutazone), but these agents are uncommon causes for acute perioperative liver dysfunction and will not be discussed.

Hepatitis following halothane anesthesia is now accepted as a distinct clinical entity, but the incidence of the disease is very low. The first case reports appeared 2 years after halothane was introduced in clinical practice,[13,77,90] but the mechanism of halothane hepatitis remains unknown. The National Halothane Study[11,76] retrospectively reviewed 856,515 general anesthetic administrations from 1959 to 1962 and identified 82 cases of fatal hepatic necrosis as defined by review of liver sections by a panel of pathologists with experience in liver disease.[73] Drug-induced hepatic injury was suggested in nine of these cases, because clinical and pathologic features consistent with shock or hypoxia were absent (Table 27-2). Seven of these nine patients had received halothane, and four of them had received it on more than one occasion during the preceding 6 weeks. It was concluded that the incidence of fatal hepatic necrosis following halothane is approximately 1 in 35,000 administrations of the drug and that the incidence is greater in patients who have

TABLE 27-2.   **Cases of massive hepatic necrosis felt to be drug-induced**

Number of operations within 6 weeks	Day of postoperative jaundice	Day of death following operation	Number of previous exposures to halothane
2	No jaundice	2.2	None
1	14	20	None
2	26,3	31,8	1
2	19,9	19,9	1
1	No jaundice	14	None
2	No jaundice	14,5	1
4	30,24,5,1	34,28,9,5	3
1	28	35	None
1	1	1	None

Adapted from Subcommittee on the National Halothane Study of the Committee on Anesthesia, National Academy of Sciences– National Research Council: Summary of the National Halothane Study, JAMA 197(10):120-134, 1966. A case was unexplained if three or more of four examiners were unable to explain the extent of hepatic necrosis based on the patient's underlying disease, surgical procedure, or recognizable postoperative complication.

had repeated exposures. In another retrospective study, the Fulminant Hepatic Failure Surveillance Study group reviewed 318 patients with postoperative liver failure and identified 64 cases of suspected halothane-associated disease. Seventy-seven percent of these patients had multiple exposures to halothane. This study was criticized because of three factors: (1) some patients had received blood transfusion, (2) determination of incidence was not possible, and (3) the voluntary nature of case reporting may have introduced bias.[52] However, these and other studies[8] established with reasonable certainty an association between halothane exposure and the development of postoperative hepatic necrosis and also suggested that the incidence and severity of liver injury is greater after repeated exposures.

Perhaps the most intriguing evidence for an association between halothane exposure and development of hepatitis are reports of patients who, after recovery from suspected halothane hepatitis, are rechallenged with the drug and develop hepatitis.[18,81] There is a celebrated case[40] of an anesthesiologist who had recurring episodes of hepatitis, chills, and fever after repeated exposures to halothane; biopsy revealed histologic features of hepatitis, hepatocellular necrosis, and eventually cirrhosis. While it has been argued that chronic active hepatitis could not be excluded as the cause in this case, because improvement occurred with steroid therapy[74]; halothane rechallenge at low doses (0.1% to 0.2%) resulted in myalgia and fever at 4 to 6 hours after exposure and increased alanine aminotransferase (SGOT) levels from 41 to 700 IU over the next 2 days.

Although the incidence of HHN is low, halothane may cause asymptomatic increases in transaminases in up to 25% of exposed patients,[56,80,94] but other investigators[1] report no changes in either transaminases or other liver function tests after halothane. It is likely that there are two forms of liver dysfunction associated with halothane. The first is mild, asymptomatic, and reversible. The second form, fulminant hepatic failure, is rare and generally occurs in patients who have repeated exposures to halothane.[8,53] Several investigators have attempted to describe typical characteristics of patients who are susceptible to halothane hepatitis. Böttiger et al[8] retrospectively noted that 72% of patients with probable halothane-induced hepatic necrosis had multiple exposures and that the disease occurred more commonly in middle-aged obese females. Sherlock[73] also noted a high

incidence of obesity in a study of 24 patients with halothane-related hepatitis. Asymptomatic increases in transaminases following halothane administration also occur with greater frequency in obese patients[26]; this effect may be caused by increased metabolism of halothane during slow release of large amounts of the drug that had been deposited in fat stores during anesthesia administration. Some authors claim that halothane-induced hepatic necrosis does not occur in children, but five of 56 patients with hepatic necrosis attributed to halothane were children in one study,[56] and other reports of halothane hepatitis in children exist.[92] A familial susceptibility to halothane has been suggested.[35] No correlation has been found between site, duration, or type of surgery and the development of HHN.

The clinical features of halothane hepatitis range from mild liver dysfunction to massive hepatic necrosis with encephalopathy and death.[55,91] Fever, malaise, anorexia, nausea, and nonspecific gastrointestinal symptoms usually develop 8 to 14 days following the first exposure[41,53,73] and 1 to 11 days after subsequent exposures. Peters et al[59] observed that unexplained fever is the most common characteristic of halothane-associated hepatic necrosis.

TABLE 27-3.　Management of fulminant hepatic failure

Complication	Management
Encephalopathy with cerebral edema	Mannitol infusions ?Mechanical ventilation ?Intracranial pressure monitoring
Maldistribution of blood	Correct hypovolaemia ?Prostacyclin
Hypoglycemia	10% dextrose infusion
Gastrointestinal bleeding	H_2 antagonists and/or antacids
Reduced host defenses	?Prophylactic antimicrobials ?Fresh frozen plasma infusions to replace complement deficiency
Renal failure	Hemofiltration/dialysis
Respiratory failure	Mechanical ventilation
Coagulation and platelet abnormalities	No treatment unless bleeding occurs

Adapted from Bihari D: Acute liver failure. In Current topics in intensive care, Clinics in Anesthesiology 3(4):973-997, 1985.

Jaundice usually appears about 1 week after the fever and may be associated with pruritus, palmar erythema, hepatomegaly, liver tenderness, ascites, and hepatic encephalopathy. Of note, jaundice may appear as late as 18 to 20 days after exposure[75] and therefore may not become evident until after the patient is discharged. These clinical features cannot distinguish halothane hepatitis from fulminant hepatic failure of any other cause.

Laboratory studies reveal elevated serum transaminases, bilirubin, alkaline phosphatase, and cholesterol.[53] Eosinophilia was also a feature in seven of 24 patients with halothane-associated hepatic necrosis, and eosinophilic infiltration of the liver may also occur. Histologic studies revealed acute hepatitis with mild to massive degrees of centrilobular necrosis.[53] These pathologic findings cannot be distinguished from viral hepatitis.

The pathogenesis of halothane hepatitis is unknown. Halothane itself probably does not produce hepatic damage,[84] but metabolites of halothane may be responsible for hepatic damage, and this effect may be mediated immunologically. Halothane is metabolized by hepatic monooxygenase enzymes by either an oxidative pathway, which is stimulated by high oxygen tensions and generates trifluoracetate, or by a reductive pathway, which is stimulated by low oxygen tensions and generates fluoride (Figure 27-1). Metabolites generated by both pathways bind covalently to other macromolecules.[83] Normal metabolism occurs preferentially through the oxidative pathway, but increased metabolism by the reductive pathway occurs under hypoxic conditions and may lead to hepatocellular damage. Animals pretreated with enzyme inducers such as phenobarbital and subjected to halothane under hypoxic conditions develop hepatotoxicity.[51] While this was originally proposed as an animal model for halothane hepatitis, the utility is questioned because there is no requirement for multiple exposures, and the clinical entity of halothane hepatitis does not appear to be related to hypoxia.

Many features of the clinical syndrome suggest that immune sensitization to halothane or halothane metabolites plays a role in this disorder. These features include increased incidence after multiple exposures and the presence of rash, arthralgias, eosinophilia, and circulating immune complexes and autoantibodies. Neuberger[56] demonstrated that 80% of patients with probable halothane hepatitis had antibodies that reacted by indirect immunofluorescence and cytotoxicity techniques with halothane-altered liver cell membranes. These antibodies were not present in the sera of other patients with liver damage from other causes, even after exposure to halothane.[57] In addition, lymphocytes from patients with halothane hepatitis are sensitized to antigens present on hepatocyte membranes isolated from rabbits previously exposed to halothane, but not to liver cells from control rabbits.[88]

Farrell[25] developed an in vitro test to assess susceptibility to halothane hepatitis. This test evaluates lymphocyte toxicity from electrophilic drug interactions (Figure 27-2) and implicates both an immune and a metabolic mechanism for halothane-induced hepatic damage as cells appear to become susceptible to immune-mediated interactions only after damaged by electrophilic drug intermediates. While many patients generate reactive metabolites, only a few appear to acquire antibodies and subsequently develop hepatic necrosis on exposure to halothane. Thus, while a clear cause of halothane hepatitis has not been demonstrated, the current consensus is that the syndrome probably involves an autoimmune process occurring in susceptible patients following metabolic activation of halothane and covalent binding of halothane metabolites to liver macromolecules.[10,54]

Recommendations concerning the use of halothane remain controversial. Some authors suggest that halothane be avoided entirely. Both enflurane and isoflurane, although metabolized to a lesser extent than halothane, have also been associated with postoperative hepatic necrosis,[28,44] but the incidence of hepatic injury is so low that some authors doubt that it occurs with either agent.[22,24] Halothane is widely used in underdeveloped countries because it is both inexpensive and preferable to alternatives such as diethyl ether. It is generally recommended that any patient who has had jaundice, fever, or malaise following halothane should not receive repeated administrations. There is no defined interval after which halothane can be safely repeated, and it should be avoided in patients with any possible susceptibility. Residual traces of the drug in anesthetic equipment may produce fever, abnormal liver function tests, or recurrence of hepatitis in susceptible patients,[15,85] and thus a halothane-free system should be used when anesthetizing these patients.

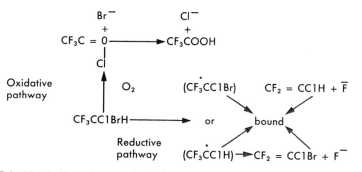

FIGURE 27-1. Metabolic pathways of halothane.

From Van Dyke RA: Metabolism of anesthetic agents: toxic implications, Acta Anaesth Scand 75:7-9, 1982.

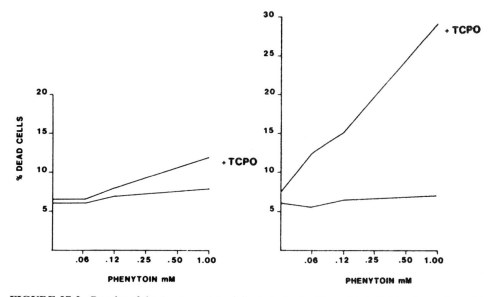

FIGURE 27-2. Results of the *in vivo* cytotoxicity test of a healthy subject *(left)* and a patient with halothane hepatitis *(right)*. The lower lines indicate cytotoxicity toward lymphocytes with increasing concentrations of phenytoin in the presence of a mixed-function oxidase system. The upper lines indicate the cytotoxicity produced when epoxide hydrolase was inhibited by the addition of 1,1,1-trichloropropene oxide (TCPO) to this system.

From Farrell G, Prendergast D, and Murray M: Halothane hepatitis. Detection of a constitutional susceptibility factor, N Engl J Med 313(21):1310-1314, 1985.

Management of acute liver failure in the postoperative period is similar to that of fulminant hepatic failure in other settings and has been the subject of recent reviews.[4] Fulminant hepatic failure is defined as acute impairment of hepatic function with onset of encephalopathy within 8 weeks of the primary illness. The specification of 8 weeks for the onset of encephalopathy is important because it excludes patients with chronic liver disease who develop fulminant failure. The prognosis for this latter group is exceedingly poor[69] because of preexisting liver damage and decreased regenerative potential. Changes in the electroencephalogram, consisting of slow waves with high amplitude and paroxysmal bilateral synchronous delta waves, are helpful in the diagnosis of hepatic encephalopathy and have a good correlation with neuropsychiatric profiles. Complications of fulminant hepatic failure and their supportive management are summarized in Table 27-3.

SUMMARY

Management of patients with either preexisting liver disease or hepatic dysfunction acquired perioperatively requires careful assessment of the extent of hepatic disease and the systemic sequelae of that damage. Liver disease ultimately involves many organ systems including the central nervous system, lungs, cardiovascular system, kidneys, and coagulation system. Thorough evaluation and treatment of problems involving these systems may decrease the high morbidity and mortality associated with anesthesia and surgery in these patients. Cirrhotic patients have a particularly high rate of perioperative mortality, and the risks of any surgical procedure planned for these patients should be carefully weighed against the expected benefit. Fulminant hepatic failure caused by halothane is rare, but this form of perioperative hepatic dysfunction can be eliminated entirely by avoiding halothane exposure in susceptible patients.

REFERENCES

1. Allen PJ and Downing JW: A prospective study of hepatocellular function after repeated exposures to halothane or enflurane in women undergoing radium therapy for cervical cancer, Br J Anaesth 49:1035-1039, 1977.
2. Alter HJ et al: Non-A/non-B hepatitis: a review and interim report of an ongoing prospective study. In Vyas GN, Cohen SN, and Schmid R, editors: Viral hepatitis, Philadelphia, 1978, Franklin Institute Press.
3. Berman N et al: The chronic sequelae of non-A, non-B hepatitis, Ann Intern Med 91(1):1-6, 1979.
4. Bihari D: Acute liver failure. In Current topics in intensive care, Clin Anesth 3(4):973-997, 1985.
5. Blake DA, Barry JQ, and Cascorbi HF: Quantitative analyses of halothane metabolites in man, Anesthesiology 25:270-283, 1964.
6. Bloch RS, Allaben RD, and Walt AJ: Cholecystectomy in patients with cirrhosis: a surgical challenge, Arch Surg 120:669-672, 1985.
7. Bloom AL: Intravascular coagulation in the liver, Br J Haematol 30:1-7, 1975.
8. Böttiger LE, Dalen E, and Hallen B: Halothane-induced liver damage: an analysis of the material reported to the Swedish Adverse Drug Reaction Committee, 1966-1973, Acta Anaesth Scand 20:40-46, 1976.
9. Brown BR: Halothane hepatitis revisited, N Engl J Med 21:1347-1348, 1985.
10. Brown BR and Sipes IG: Biotransformation and hepatotoxicity of halothane, Biochem Pharmacol 22(26):2091-2094, 1977.
11. Bunker JP et al: The national halothane study, Washington, DC, 1969, US Government Printing Office.
12. Burke TR et al: Mechanism of defluorination of enflurane. Identification of an organic metabolite in rat and man, Drug Metab Dispos 9(1):19-244, 1981.
13. Burnap TK, Galla SJ, and Vandam LD: Anesthetic, circulatory and respiratory effects of flurothane, Anesthesiology 19:307-320, 1958.
14. Carmichael FJ, Lindop MJ, and Farman JV: Anesthesia for hepatic transplantation: cardiovascular and metabolic alteration and their management, Anesth Analg 64:108-116, 1985.
15. Chapman BA, Laurenson VG, and Cook HB: Halothane hepatitis: toxicity or hypersensitivity? NZ Med J 98:793-794, 1985.
16. Child CG and Turcotte JG: Surgery and portal hypertension. In Child CG: The liver and portal hypertension, Philadelphia, 1964, WB Saunders.
17. Colombo M et al: A multicenter, prospective study of post-transfusion hepatitis in Milan, Hepatology 7(4):709-712, 1987.
18. Combes B: Halothane-induced liver damage: an entity, New Engl J Med 280:558-559, 1969.
19. Czaja AJ: Hepatitis nonA, nonB. Manifestation and implications of acute and chronic disease, Mayo Clin Proc 57:639-652, 1982.
20. Dong WK, Bledsoe SW, and Eng DY: profound arterial hypotension in dogs: brain electrical activity and organ integrity, Anesthesiology 58:61-71, 1983.
21. Douglas HJ et al: Hepatic necrosis associated with viral infection after enflurane anesthesia, N Engl J Med 296:553-555, 1977.
22. Dykes MHM: Is enflurane hepatotoxic? Anesthesiology 61(3):235-237, 1984.

23. Dykes MHM and Waltzer SG: Preoperative and postoperative hepatic dysfunction, Surg Gynecol Obstet 124:747-751, 1969.

24. Eger EI et al: Is enflurane hepatotoxic? Anesth Analg 65:21-30, 1986.

25. Farrell G, Prendergast D, and Murray M: Halothane hepatitis. Detection of a constitutional susceptibility factor, N Engl J Med 313(21):1310-1314, 1985.

26. Fee JHP et al: A prospective study of liver enzyme and other changes following repeat administration of nalothane and enflurane, Br J Anaesth 51:1133-1139, 1979.

27. Feuerlein W and Reiser E: Parameters affecting the course and result of delerium tremens treatment, Acta Psychiatr Scand (suppl 329)73:120-123, 1986.

28. Fisher NA et al: Hepatic necrosis associated with herpes virus after isoflurane anesthesia, Anesth Analg 64:1131-1133, 1985.

29. Friedman LS and Maddrey WC: Surgery in the patient with liver disease, Med Clin North Am 71(3):453-476, 1987.

30. Garrison RN et al: Clarification of risk factors for abdominal operations in patients with hepatic cirrhosis, Ann Surg 199:648-655, 1984.

31. Gyasi HK and Naguib M: Atracurium and severe hepatic disease: a case report, Can Anaesth Soc J:161-164, 1985.

32. Harville DD and Summerskill WH: Surgery in acute hepatitis. Causes and effects, JAMA 184:257-261, 1963.

33. Han YH: Why do chronic alcoholics require more anesthesia? Anesthesiology 30:341-342, 1969.

34. Hernandez JM et al: Posttransfusion hepatitis in Spain. A prospective study, Vox Sang 44(4):231-237, 1983.

35. Hoft RH et al: Halothane hepatitis in three pairs of closely related women, N Engl J Med 304(17):1023-1024, 1981.

36. Inman WHW and Mushin WW: Jaundice after repeated exposure to halothane: an analysis of reports to the Committee on Safety of Medicines, Br Med J 1:5, 1974.

37. Johnston RE: Effects of acute and chronic ethanol administration on isoflurane requirements in mice under anesthesia, Anesth Analg 54:277-291, 1975.

38. Kaufman K: Serum cholinesterase activity in the normal individual and in people with liver disease, Ann Int Med 41:533-545, 1954.

39. Keeri-Szanto M and Lafleur F: Postanesthetic liver complications in a general hospital: a statistical study, Can Anaesth Soc J 10:531-538, 1963.

40. Klatskin G and Kimberg DV: Recurrent hepatitis attributable to halothane sensitization in an anesthetist, N Engl J Med 280:515-522, 1969.

41. Klion FM, Schaffner F, and Popper H: Hepatitis after exposure to halothane, Ann Intern Med 71:467-477, 1969.

42. Lagerkranser M, Andreen M, and Irestedt L: Central and splanchnic haemodynamics in the dog during controlled hypotension with sodium nitroprusside, Acta Anaesth Scand 28:81-86, 1984.

43. Lamont JT: The liver. In Vandam LD, editor: To make the patient ready for anesthesia: medical care for the surgical patient, Menlo Park, Calif, 1984, Addison-Wesley Publishing Co, Inc.

44. Lewis JH et al: Enflurane hepatotoxicity. A clinicopathologic study of 24 cases, Ann Intern Med 98:984-992, 1983.

45. Lewis RB and Blair M: Halothane hepatitis in a young child, Br J Anaesth 54:349-354, 1982.

46. Lindenmuth WM and Eisenberg MM: The surgical risk in cirrhosis of the liver, Archives of surgery 86:235, 1963.

47. Manhem P et al: Alcohol withdrawal: effects of clonidine sympathetic activity, the renin-aldosterone system, and clinical symptoms. Alcoholism Clin Exp Res 9(3):238-243, 1985.

48. Mathiesen LR et al: Hepatitis type A, B and non-A, non-B in fulminant hepatitis, Gut 21:72-77, 1980.

49. Maze M: Hepatic physiology. In Miller RD (editor): Anesthesia 2. Churchill Livingstone, 1986, New York.

50. McEwan J: Liver function tests following anesthesia, Br J Anaesth 48:1065-1070, 1976.

51. Mclain GE, Sikes IG, and Brown BR: An annual model of halothane hepatotoxicity: roles of enzyme induction and hypoxia, Anesthesiology 35:321, 1979.

52. McPeek B and Gilbert JP: Onset of postoperative jaundice related to anesthetic history, Br Med J 3:615, 1974.

53. Moult PJ and Sherlock S: Halothane-related hepatitis. A clinical study of twenty-six cases, Q J Med NS 44 173:99-114, 1975.

54. Neuberger J and Kenna JG: Halothane hepatitis: a model of immune mediated drug hepatotoxicity, Clin Sci 72:263-270, 1987.

55. Neuberger JM, Kenna JG, and Williams R: Halothane hepatitis: attempt to develop an animal model, Int J Immunopharmacol 9:123-131, 1987.

56. Neuberger J and Williams R: Halothane anaesthesia and liver damage, Br Med J 289:1136-1139, 1984.

57. Neuberger J et al: Specific serological markers in the diagnoses of fulminant hepatic failure associated with halothane anaesthesia, Br J Anaesth 55:15-18, 1983.

58. Parsons-Smith B et al: The electroencephalograph in liver disease, Lancet 2:867-871, 1957.

59. Peters RL et al: Hepatic necrosis associated with halothane anesthesia, Am J Med 47:748-764, 1969.

60. Plummer JL et al: Free radical formation in vivo and hepatotoxicity due to anesthesia with halothane, Anesthesiology 57:160-166, 1982.

61. Podolsky DK and Isselbacher KJ: Derangements of hepatic metabolism. In Braunwald E et al (editors): Harrison's principles of internal medicine, McGraw-Hill, 1987, New York.

62. Prentice CR: Acquired coagulation disorders, Clin Haematol 2:413-442, 1985.

63. Price HL, Deutsch S, and Davidson IA: Can general anesthetic produce splanchnic visceral hypoxia by reducing regional blood flow? Anesthesiology 27:24-32, 1966.

63a. Pugh RNH et al: Transection of the oesophagus for bleeding oesophageal varices, Brit J Surg 60:646-649, 1973.

64. Ratnoff OD: Hemostatic mechanisms in liver disease, Med Clin North Am 47:721-736, 1963.

65. Ratnoff OD: Hemostatic defects in liver and bilary disease and disorders of vitamin K metabolism. In Ratnoff OD and Forbes CD, editors: Disorders of hemostases, Grune & Stratton, 1984, New York.

66. Robbins JA and Mushlin AI: Preoperative evaluation of the healthy patient, Med Clin North Am 63:1145-1156, 1979.

67. Roberts HR and Cederbaum AI: The liver and blood coagulation: physiology and pathology, Gastroenterology 63:297-320, 1972.

68. Roth S and Run S: Safe use of induced hypotension in a patient with cirrhotic liver disease, Can J Anaesth 34(2):186-189, 1987.

69. Rueff B and Benhamou JP: Acute hepatic necroses and fulminant hepatic failure, Gut 14:805-815, 1973.

70. Schemel WH: Unexpected hepatic dysfunction found by multiple laboratory screening, Anesth Analg 55:810-812, 1976.

71. Sellers EM, Naranjo CA, and Harrison M: Oval diazepam loading: simplified treatment of alcohol withdrawal, Clin Pharmacol Ther 34:822-826, 1983.

72. Sherlock S: Progress report. Halothane hepatitis, Gut 12:324-329, 1971.

73. Simpson BR, Strunin L, and Walton B: Halothane hepatitis—fact or fallacy, Proc R Soc Lond (Biol) 66:56-63, 1973.

74. Stock JG and Strunin L: Unexplained hepatitis following halothane, Anesthesiology 63:424-439, 1985.

75. Subcommittee on the national halothane study of the Committee on Anesthesia, National Academy of Sciences National Research Council: Summary of the national halothane study, JAMA 197(10):120-134, 1966.

76. Temple RL, Cote RA, Gorens SW: Massive hepatic necrosis following general anesthesia, Anesth Analg 41:586-592, 1962.

77. Thompson WL: Management of alcohol withdrawal syndrome, Arch Intern Med 138:278-283, 1978.

78. Tornetta FJ and Tamaki HT: Halothane jaundice and hepatotoxicity, JAMA 184(8):658-660, 1963.

79. Trowell J, Peto R, and Snufin AC: Controlled trial of repeated halothane anaesthetics in patients with carcinoma of the uterine cervix treated with radium, Lancet 1:821-823, 1975.

80. Tygstrup N: Halothane hepatitis, Lancet 2:466-467, 1963.

81. Tzakis AG et al: Clinical consideration in orthopedic liver transplantation, Radiol Clin North Am 25(2):289-297, 1987.

82. Van Dyke RA: Metabolism of volatile anesthetics. 3. Induction of microsomal dechlorinating and ether-cleaning enzymes, J Pharmacol Exp Ther 154:364-369, 1966.

83. Van Dyke RA: Metabolism of anesthetic agents: toxic implications, Acta Anaesth Scand 75:7-9, 1982.

84. Varma RR, Whitesell RC, and Iskandarani MM: Halothane hepatitis sans halothane: role of inapparent circuit contamination and its prevention, Hepatology 5(6):1159-1162, 1965.

85. Venning GR: Identification of adverse drug reactions to new drugs. II. How were 18 important adverse reactions discovered and with what delays? Br Med J 286:289-292, 1983.

86. Vergani D et al: Demonstrating of a circulating antibody to halothane altered hepatocytes in patients with hepatitis, Gut 19:A994, 1978.

87. Vergani D et al: Antibodies to the surface of halothane-altered rabbit hepatocytes in patients with severe halothane-associated hepatitis, N Engl J Med 303:66-71, 1980.

88. Villeneuve JP et al: Emergency portacaval shunt for variceal hemorrhage. A prospective study, Ann Surg 206(1):48-52, 1987.

89. Virtue RW and Payne KW: Postoperative death after flurothane, Anesthesiology 19:562-563, 1958.

90. Walton B et al: Unexplained hepatitis following halothane, Br Med J 1:1171-1176, 1976.

91. Whitburn RH and Sumner E: Halothane hepatitis in an 11-month-old child, Anaesthesia 41:611-613, 1986.

92. Wilkins AJ, Jenkins WJ, and Steiner JA: Efficacy of clonidine in treatment of alcohol withdrawal state, Psychopharmacology 81:78-80, 1983.

93. Wright R et al: Controlled prospective study of the effect on liver function of multiple exposures to halothane, Lancet 1:818-819, 1975.

94. Yonemoto RH and Davidson CS: Herniorrhaphy in cirrhosis of the liver with ascites, N Engl J Med 255:733-739, 1956.

CHAPTER **28**

Neuromuscular Disease

CECIL BOREL

Perioperative care of patients with neuromuscular diseases is challenging. These diseases result from a variety of pathologic processes that affect peripheral nerve, neuromuscular junction, or muscle itself. Although these processes are quite dissimilar each can adversely affect respiratory, cardiovascular, and nutritional function. Often acute illness, anesthesia, and surgery often overwhelm the capacity of these diseased organ systems to respond to stress and unmask the severity of the underlying neuromuscular disorder, which may have been underestimated preoperatively. This chapter reviews the common effects of neuromuscular illness on respiratory, cardiovascular, and nutritional physiology. This is followed by a discussion of general perioperative management strategies and a review of neuromuscular effects of anesthetic agents in patients with neuromuscular disease. Finally, detailed recommendations concerning management of patients with

Guillain-Barré syndrome, myasthenia gravis, and muscular dystrophy are included, because these illnesses represent classic examples of diseases of peripheral nerve, neuromuscular junction, and muscle, respectively.

ORGAN SYSTEM DYSFUNCTION IN NEUROMUSCULAR DISEASE
Respiratory

Ventilatory performance depends on effective skeletal muscle activity. Respiratory insufficiency is the major cause of death in patients with neuromuscular disorders.[19,39] Although the extent of respiratory system involvement depends on the type, distribution, and duration of neuromuscular disease, respiratory function does not directly parallel the extent of general muscle weakness.[73] Thus essential respiratory functions such as inspiratory ventilatory effort, forced expiratory effort (cough), and main-

417

tenance of airway patency require careful assessment.[59]

Insidious loss of ventilatory reserve and inability to increase minute ventilation on demand are often the initial effects of impaired respiratory function in neuromuscular disease.[19] Perioperative changes in lung function and increased metabolic rate frequently increase work of breathing and can precipitate respiratory muscle fatigue and ventilatory insufficiency.[8] Early responses to increased inspiratory work include frequent changes in respiratory pattern to alternate work between fatiguing muscles and accessory respiratory muscles[26,67] and increasing respiratory rate. Although increasing respiratory rate allows more efficient use of weakened muscles,[67] it also results in an increase in inspiratory time and in the ratio of dead space to tidal volume.[19] Both these latter responses decrease ventilatory efficiency and can worsen ventilatory failure. Respiratory muscle fatigue is associated with impaired ventilatory responses to carbon dioxide and hypoxia*; these changes are especially problematic in patients who are dependent on central drive mechanisms.[5,61] Some authors have recommended nocturnal assisted ventilation for these patients in nonsurgical settings.[15,19]

Expiratory muscle dysfunction in neuromuscular disease impairs the ability to cough and further exacerbates reductions in forced expiratory capacity observed after abdominal and thoracic procedures.[3,60,71,73] Impaired cough and retained secretions lead to collapse of lung segments and predispose to bacterial contamination and pneumonia. Continued perfusion of these nonventilated lung regions can result in arterial hypoxemia. Microatelectasis has been implicated in the reduced lung compliance, decreased functional residual capacity, and increased work of breathing observed in patients with neuromuscular disease who have respiratory muscle dysfunction.[11,16,23]

Impaired laryngeal and glottic muscle function occurs in patients with neuromuscular disease[39,71] and when severe, results in recurrent aspiration and airflow obstruction.[19] Residual anesthesia and persistent effects of muscle relaxants administered intraoperatively, which can result in postoperative aspiration and positional airway obstruction in normal patients, exacerbate upper airway muscle dysfunction in patients with neuromuscular disease. Pre-

*References 25, 39, 52, 53, 60, 64, 76.

operative assessment of upper airway muscle function is required in these patients. Often, however, problems with upper airway tone are not recognized until after extubation.

Cardiovascular

Cardiovascular dysfunction is the second most common cause of morbidity in patients with neuromuscular illness. Cardiovascular involvement ranges from autonomic dysfunction with neuropathic diseases (see the box on p. 417, top) to myocardial failure with myopathic disease (see the box on p. 417, bottom). During the perioperative period, the cardiovascular response to anesthetics, blood loss, dehydration, and infection will be hindered if the cardiovascular system is impaired by neuromuscular disease. Because of the broad dependence of the cardiovascular system on nerve and muscle function, patients with neuromuscular illness commonly have low cardiac reserve.

The autonomic nervous system regulates heart rate, inotropic state, venous tone, and systemic vascular resistance.[55] Heart rhythm is balanced by sympathetic and parasympathetic influences; cardiac arrhythmias ranging from sinus tachycardia to bradycardia and asystole occur when either system is impaired. Loss of beat-to-beat variability in heart rate is probably the most sensitive indicator of autonomic cardiac involvement.[58] Resting tachycardia and postural hypotension have been associated with intraoperative hemodynamic instability and need for vasopressor therapy, and unexplained cardiorespiratory arrest during anesthesia has been reported in patients with dysautonomia.[34,47] Vasomotor nerve dysfunction may result in postural hypotension from loss of vasoconstriction or in hypertension from a disordered response to peripheral vasomotor paresis. Volume and electrolyte disorders frequently occur in dysautonomic diseases because the autonomic nervous system controls distribution of systemic blood flow, modulates blood volume by sodium retention through aldosterone release, and limits insensible loss of fluids from the sweat glands. Hypovolemia may be relative, the result of venous pooling, or absolute, the result of increased insensible volume losses. Hypovolemia is a potent stimulus for the release of arginine vasopressin from the pituitary gland, which results in water retention and an increase in venous tone. Patients with dysautonomia frequently become hyponatremic in the perioperative

---

Neuropathies associated with dysautonomia

Complete autonomic paralysis

Primary peripheral neuropathies with secondary dysautonomia
Guillain-Barré[1,9,14,19,38,48]
Acute infectious mononucleosis
Acute intermittent porphyria[36]
Heavy metal intoxication and poisoning[37,43]

Systemic diseases with secondary dysautonomia
Diabetes mellitus[34]
Systemic amyloidosis[78]
Uremia
Connective tissue diseases (particularly progressive systemic sclerosis)[28,33]
Leprosy[35]

Neuromuscular diseases associated with cardiac muscle dysfunction[57]

Hereditary neuromyopathic disorders
Myotonic dystrophy
Friedreich's ataxia
Progressive muscular dystrophies
   Duchenne's muscular dystrophy
   Becker's muscular dystrophy
   Limb-girdle dystrophy of Erb[74]
   Facioscapulohumeral muscular dystrophy

Other neuromuscular diseases with occasional association
Peroneal muscular atrophy (Charcot-Marie-Tooth)
Humeroperoneal dystrophy (Emery-Dreifuss)
Myotubular myopathy (centronuclear myopathy)
Oculocraniosomatic syndrome (Kearns-Sayre)[5]
Nemaline myopathy
Guillain-Barré syndrome

Neuromuscular disorders presenting as cardiomyopathy
Poliomyelitis
Periodic paralysis
Alcoholic myopathy

From Tobin MJ, et al: Am Rev Respir Dis 135(6):1320-1328, 1987.

---

period from the combination of hypovolemia, arginine vasopressin release, stress, and volume replacement with hyponatremic solutions.

Diseases of muscle are heterogeneous in expression; when cardiac muscle is affected in myopathic disease congestive heart failure, complex cardiac arrhythmias, or mural thrombus formation can result.

Patients with neuromuscular diseases, particularly those in whom the autonomic nervous system is involved, need careful monitoring of cardiovascular performance, volume replacement, and sodium metabolism during the perioperative period when fever, dehydration, blood loss, and increased gastrointestinal losses place all patients at risk.

Nutritional

Malnutrition commonly accompanies neuromuscular diseases.[60] Appetite, glutition, gastric emptying, intestinal motility, defecation, and metabolic requirements are affected to some degree in most patients with chronic neuromuscular diseases. Patients avoid eating or drinking when swallowing function is impaired. Paralytic ileus results in the loss of nutrient absorption from the intestine when the autonomic enervation to the gut is impaired. Protein energy malnutrition exacerbates ventilatory dysfunction[60] and probably increases the risk of wound dehiscence and infection. The role of preoperative nutritional support is controversial, but repletion therapy is probably beneficial because postoperative return to normal dietary intake is likely to be delayed in patients with neuromuscular disease. Nutrients can be delivered in a predigested or "elemental" form so that enteric absorption of nutrient is possible even when dysautonomia causes ileus. Vagal damage during generalized demyelinating neural disorders may lead to delayed gastric emptying and disordered gastric acid secretion during times of perioperative stress.

GENERAL PERIOPERATIVE MANAGEMENT
Preoperative Assessment

Respiratory. Preoperative assessment of respiratory dysfunction in neuromuscular disease requires assessment of ventilatory muscle function, oxygenation status, and airway integrity. Voluntary measures of inspiratory force or tidal volume are widely used to assess ventilatory muscle function.[23,73] Negative inspired forces of less than 20 cm H_2O and forced vital capacity of less than 15 ml/kg have been associated with a need for ventilatory support in the postoperative period. Arterial PO_2 less than 70 on room air or chest x-ray examination showing atelectasis or decreased lung volume suggests a risk of hypoxemia postoperatively. The clinical examination, supplemented by flow-volume loop measurements, should reveal involvement of bulbar musculature.[71] Clinically detectable upper airway dysfunction often requires prolonged postoperative tracheal intubation.

Cardiovascular. The extent and severity of autonomic dysfunction are difficult to assess noninvasively. Orthostatic hypotension, resting tachycardia, paralytic ileus, anhydrosis, and constricted pupils are all clinical signs of generalized autonomic dysfunction.[40] The presence of clinical signs of dysautonomia may indicate profound hemodynamic instability from adrenergically active anesthetics or blocking drugs. Assessment of peripheral vascular tone with invasive monitoring may be indicated perioperatively.

Cardiomyopathy from myopathic illness is relatively common, and preoperative history, assessment of electrocardiogram, echocardiogram, and chest x-ray examination will identify most individuals with serious involvement.[51] The standard electrocardiogram is the most reliable tool for suspected cardiac involvement; tall right precordial R waves and Q waves in leads 1, aVL, and V5-6 are most characteristic.[57] Conduction system abnormalities and arrhythmias are frequent findings, although the implications of these findings for perioperative care are uncertain.[51] Left ventricular dysfunction and mitral valve prolapse are frequently found on echocardiography.[51,77] Determination of creatine phosphokinase (CPK) has long been used to identify active systemic myopathy, but it may not accurately detect myocardial dystrophy.[57]

Nutritional. A history of weight loss, poor appetite, or difficulty swallowing should be sought in the preoperative period. Laboratory confirmation of hypoalbuminemia, anemia, hypocalcemia, and decreased transferrin levels suggests important preoperative malnutrition that may require repletion therapy to prevent infection and improve wound healing.

Role of Plasma Exchange Therapy

Half of all therapeutic plasma exchanges performed annually in the United States are done in patients with neurologic disorders.[6] Physical separation of plasma from formed elements of the blood and subsequent reinfusion of the formed elements with a plasma replacement permits removal of circulating toxic substances. Plasma exchange is useful in neurologic diseases such as myasthenia gravis and Guillain-Barré syndrome that are mediated by circulating antibodies or other immunologically active substances.[7,24,46]

Preoperative plasma exchange in patients with severe myasthenia gravis undergoing thymectomy reduces the need for postoperative mechanical ventilation, decreases time to extubation, and decreases the length of stay in intensive care.[10,24] Patients with myasthenia gravis who are difficult to wean from mechanical ventilation postoperatively may benefit from plasma exchange. Plasma exchange improves ventilatory function when used early in the course of treatment of patients with Guillain-Barré syndrome.[46] The risks of plasma exchange therapy are probably higher in the perioperative period than at any other time. Bleeding associated with depletion of coagulation factors, regional anticoagulation, citrate-induced hypocalcemia, and activation of either complement or fibrinolytic cascades has been reported.[7] Replacement of coagulation factors with fresh frozen plasma and platelets may reduce the risk of bleeding. Complement activation may result in noncardiogenic pulmonary edema and adult respiratory distress syndrome. Acute changes in plasma volume may aggravate fluid imbalances in the perioperative period and require continuous monitoring of ventricular preload and cardiac output during exchange therapy.

Neuromuscular Effects of Anesthetic Agents

General anesthesia. Inhalational anesthetics (halothane, enflurane, and isoflurane) suppress neuromuscular transmission and, at high concentrations, produce up to 50% diminution in the force of muscle contraction. As blood anesthetic levels decrease in normal patients, clinically important muscle weakness on emergence from anesthesia is not apparent. However, even low concentrations of residual inhalational anesthetics in patients with neuromuscular disease may prolong postoperative return of baseline neuromuscular function.

The perioperative effects of depolarizing and nondepolarizing muscle relaxants depend on the type of neuromuscular disease, and each class of drugs must be used cautiously (Table 28-1). Depolarizing re-

TABLE 28-1. Response to muscle relaxants in neuromuscular disease

Neuromuscular diagnosis	Nondepolarizing	Depolarizing
Muscular denervation from neuropathy	Normal	Hyperkalemia
Myasthenia gravis	Increased	Resistant
Myasthenic syndrome	Increased	Increased
Myotonia	Normal-increased	Increased risk of malignant hyperthermia
Muscular dystrophy	Normal-increased	Increased risk of malignant hyperthermia

From Azar I: Anesthesiology 61:173-187, 1984.

laxants such as succinylcholine may cause pathologic muscle contracture and lethal hyperkalemia in patients with neuropathic muscle denervation.[2,20] Abnormal contracture of facial and respiratory musculature in response to depolarizing agents may make orotracheal intubation impossible and impair mechanical ventilatory efforts. Succinylcholine increases serum potassium concentrations in normal patients, and exaggerated release of intracellular potassium may produce lethal hyperkalemia in patients with denervated muscle.[27] This hyperkalemic response develops approximately 3 weeks after acute denervation injury, and depolarizing relaxants should be avoided in all patients with chronic motor neuropathy. Pretreatment with nondepolarizing relaxants does not prevent succinylcholine-induced hyperkalemia. Nondepolarizing muscle relaxants have normal effects in patients with denervated muscle,[2] but the clinical response may be prolonged.

The intensity and duration of nondepolarizing relaxants is enhanced in patients with myasthenia gravis. Although some anesthesiologists avoid nondepolarizing agents in these patients, other practitioners use small doses while carefully monitoring the extent of relaxation with a neuromuscular blockade monitor.[2] The effect of depolarizing relaxants in patients with defects of neuromuscular transmission is variable. Some patients are resistant to succinylcholine, but others develop prolonged noncompetitive (phase II) block. It is probably wise to avoid depolarizing relaxants in patients with myasthenia gravis.

Muscle relaxants have variable and unpredictable effects in patients with primary muscle diseases. Relaxants have little effect on muscle tone of diseased fibers since the site of disease is distal to the neuromuscular junction. However, the response of normal muscle fibers may be exaggerated, and smaller doses of both depolarizing and nondepolarizing

agents may be required.[2]

Regional anesthesia. Studies to evaluate the effects of regional anesthetic techniques in patients with neuromuscular diseases have not been reported. Major conduction anesthesia relaxes all enervated muscle groups distal to the site of blockade. No data exist to indicate that regional techniques with local anesthetics adversely affect the progression of neuromuscular diseases. Major conduction blockade also produces sympathectomy, but the clinical consequences of this response on preexisting autonomic dysfunction have not been studied.

Postoperative Mechanical Ventilation

Mechanical ventilation must be continued as long as ventilatory drive or muscle strength is inadequate to maintain minute ventilation. Ventilatory support machinery is designed to perform the inspiratory work of breathing by sustaining minute ventilation without patient effort, but disuse atrophy may weaken unused muscles and aggravate ventilatory dysfunction. All weaning strategies involve gradual reduction in the amount of supported minute ventilation to encourage recruitment of ventilatory musculature. Mechanical support can be weaned by a variety of techniques that encourage ventilatory muscle activity, but the muscles should not be allowed to fatigue.[65] When ventilatory drive is normal, pressure-assisted mechanical ventilation offers an excellent approach to weaning neuromuscular patients while supporting spontaneous ventilatory effort.[41] Pressure-assisted ventilation delivers a specified positive end-inspiratory pressure independent of flow and tidal volume, improving patient comfort, reducing ventilatory work, and providing a balanced pressure and volume form of muscle work.[41] These characteristics of work may be important in reconditioning an endurance muscle such as the diaphragm.[4] Ventilatory support should be increased before muscle failure occurs, because recovery from muscle fatigue may prevent further weaning for several days.[25] Tachypnea is an early warning of ventilatory muscle fatigue.[6,67,68] All techniques for weaning the patient from mechanical ventilation are usually effective if muscle fatigue is avoided.[65] Recovery to preoperative ventilatory status requires sufficient support to prevent ventilatory muscle fatigue, but not so much support that ventilatory muscles atrophy.

SPECIFIC NEUROMUSCULAR DISEASES
Guillain-Barré Syndrome

Guillain-Barré syndrome is an inflammatory polyneuropathy that may affect all motor, sensory, autonomic, and cranial nerves. Although this neuropathy most commonly follows acute viral infection, it has been reported in postoperative patients without apparent preceding viral illness. Ascending, symmetrical muscle weakness that evolves over several days is the major clinical manifestation. Motor involvement may include ventilatory and facial musculature. Transient paresthesias are common early in the disease. Loss of deep tendon reflexes suggest the diagnosis. Nerve conduction studies differentiate polyneuropathy from high cervical spinal cord lesions or transverse myelitis.[49] Conduction velocities are slowed early as paralysis develops, and denervation potentials appear later with profound disease. Spinal fluid remains acellular, but protein levels increase to maximum levels 4 to 6 weeks after onset of illness. Other causes of acute polyneuropathy, such as acute intermittent porphyria and heavy metal poisoning, must be excluded.

Respiratory failure in Guillain-Barré syndrome begins with weakness of forced exhalation and impaired cough.[66] Forced vital capacity and negative inspiratory force are markedly decreased. Loss of voluntary abdominal and thoracic muscle contraction result in paradoxical abdominal protrusion during inspiration. Atelectasis or hypoxemia suggest imminent ventilatory failure. Inspiratory muscle weakness develops later in the disease and is manifested by rapid shallow breathing. Abnormal inward motion of the abdomen during inspiration and use of accessory inspiratory muscles are often observed. Minute ventilation decreases and any elevation of carbon dioxide tension portends rapidly progressive ventilatory failure. Abnormal swallowing and glottic

dysfunction may occur at any time in the course of Guillain-Barré syndrome. Inability to handle oral secretions, recurrent aspiration, and positional airway obstruction are ominous signs of imminent ventilatory failure.[54] Tracheostomy is indicated early in the course of ventilatory failure, and airway access may be required for management of bulbar muscle weakness long after ventilatory function returns to normal.

Autonomic dysfunction frequently accompanies motor weakness in patients who progress to ventilatory failure.* Sinus tachycardia and repolarization abnormalities are commonly observed on electrocardiogram.[55] Intermittent bradyarrhythmias have resulted in death in some patients, and continuous electrocardiographic monitoring is indicated early in the course of disease.[29] Episodic hypertension[31,50,79] and profound hypotension regularly occur in patients with severe disease who have quadriparesis and ventilatory failure.[69] Continuous arterial blood pressure monitoring may be indicated for patients with dysautonomia, and pulmonary artery and pulmonary artery occlusion pressure measurements may assist in intravascular volume management.[9,75] Hypotension may require use of vasoconstrictor agents, volume expansion, or inotropic support.

Supportive care is the mainstay of therapy in Guillain-Barré syndrome because recovery is nearly always complete. Maintenance of minute ventilation to keep arterial blood gases normal at respiratory rates less than 30/minute without paradoxical chest and abdominal movements is required to successfully wean the patient from mechanical ventilatory support. Weaning is usually unsuccessful if forced vital capacity is less than 10 ml/kg or negative inspiratory force is less than 20 cm of water. Glucocorticoids may speed recovery or prevent ventilatory failure, but clear indications for steroid therapy do not exist. Plasma exchange decreases the time on mechanical ventilation if started within 2 weeks of the onset of symptoms[46]; this modality is regularly used in seriously ill patients.

Myasthenia Gravis

Myasthenia gravis is a neuromuscular disease that is characterized by weakness and fatigability of skeletal muscles. Autoimmune-mediated reduction of

*References 1, 14, 17, 45, 69, 70.

the number of acetylcholine receptors at the neuromuscular junction[12] results in inability to sustain or repeat muscular contractions. Electromyographically, this abnormality corresponds to "fade" of muscle contraction observed during repetitive nerve stimulation after neuromuscular blockade with nondepolarizing muscle relaxants. Muscle strength improves similarly in both myasthenia gravis and nondepolarizing blockade after administration of anticholinesterase drugs.

Prognosis for patients with myasthenia gravis has improved markedly in recent years.[13] Glucocorticoids and regular plasma exchange are particularly effective in patients with severe disease with ventilatory impairment. Although muscle function may initially deteriorate after beginning steroid therapy, improvement of ventilatory function normally occurs after 2 weeks of therapy. Thymectomy improves symptoms in most patients with severe disease, and, in some patients, results in total remission.[42,56] Median sternotomy for thymectomy initially had a mortality rate of approximately 25%, and nonlethal respiratory complications were common.[42] However, a recent series of 27 patients reported one perioperative death, and 60% of patients were drug-free postoperatively.[21] Improved outcome was attributed to complete resection of thymic tissue and excellent support systems for perioperative care.

Preoperative preparation of patients with myasthenia gravis includes assessment of pulmonary mechanical function such as forced vital capacity and negative inspiratory force, arterial blood gases, chest x-ray, and determination of upper airway competence. If severe abnormalities of these parameters are encountered, surgery should be postponed to allow upward adjustment of anticholinesterase medication or plasma exchange therapy unless the patient is already receiving maximal medical therapy. Preoperative plasma exchange decreases time on mechanical ventilation and shortens intensive care stay following thymectomy.[10] Anticholinesterase medications should be continued until the morning of surgery.

The goals of anesthetic management include support of respiratory function during the operation and return of the patient to preoperative levels of neuromuscular function at the end of the procedure.[39] General anesthesia, endotracheal intubation, and high supplemental oxygen flow usually satisfy the need for respiratory support intraoperatively. Inhalation agents are ideal because they provide both effective anesthesia and adequate muscle relaxation without administration of supplemental muscle relaxant drugs. Muscle relaxants should be avoided when possible because myasthenic patients are 10 to 100 times more sensitive than normal patients to the effects of these medications.[13] If muscle relaxation is required, succinylcholine may be the drug of choice for short-term management, but the onset of "phase II" block occurs at very low doses in these patients.[2] Return to preoperative neuromuscular function is facilitated by resuming anticholinesterase medication before emergence from anesthesia. Intravenous infusion of prostigmine ($\frac{1}{60}$ of the usual daily oral dose of pyridostigmine over 24 hours) should begin during wound closure. Mechanical ventilatory support should continue postoperatively until all criteria for adequate ventilatory function and airway patency are met. After surgery, patients with severe disease may improve muscle strength and ventilatory capacity after plasma exchange, and this therapy may shorten time to tracheal extubation.

Rapid deterioration of neuromuscular and respiratory function (myasthenic crisis) may occur at any time perioperatively as a result of infection, stress, or overdose with anticholinesterase drugs. Endotracheal intubation and mechanical ventilatory support are usually required before the cause of myasthenic crisis can be determined. Although crisis may be the result of inadequate anticholinesterase therapy, satisfactory recovery is not often achieved by increasing the dose of these drugs.[39] Instead, anticholinesterase drugs should probably be withdrawn after ventilatory support is initiated to avoid precipitating a cholinergic crisis with respiratory and bulbar muscle weakness, excessive salivation, and abdominal cramps. Although atropine or glycopyrolate will rapidly ameliorate the vagal symptoms, muscular strength returns slowly as the anticholinesterase drug is metabolized. Plasma exchange effectively increases muscle strength, facilitates weaning from mechanical ventilation, and allows reintroduction of anticholinesterases at lower dosages during cholinergic crisis.

Muscular Dystrophy

Muscular dystrophies are a group of primary muscular disorders of unknown cause that often begin in childhood and pursue a rapid and progressive course to death. Duchenne's muscular dystrophy, the most common and severe, is characterized by degeneration of muscle fibers (including the diaphragm) and increased content of fat and fibrous tissue.[48] Cardiac muscle is also involved in the dystrophic process.[57] Most patients have detectable cardiac abnormalities, but only 10% of patients have clinically significant abnormalities, and most of these occur in the terminal phases of disease.[48] In a series of 36 patients, electrocardiographic abnormalities were present in 92%, decreased diastolic endocardial velocity was observed by echocardiogram in 90%, and ejection fraction was decreased in 21%.[18] Echocardiographic abnormalities did not correlate with the extent of skeletal muscle involvement. Most patients do not have cardiovascular symptoms, and cardiovascular disease is rarely the cause of death.

The incidence of serious perioperative complications in patients with muscular dystrophy is low because most surgical procedures are performed early in the course of these diseases. Nondepolarizing muscle relaxants may have either a normal or prolonged response.[2] The response to depolarizing neuromuscular blockade may be normal, but cardiac arrest possibly caused by hyperkalemia has been reported after administration of succinylcholine.[62] Cardiac arrest during induction with halothane and temperature elevation during halothane anesthesia may reflect the increased susceptibility to malignant hyperthermia in this population.[30,62] Other arrhythmias not caused by drug therapy have precipitated cardiac arrests in the immediate postoperative time in patients with muscular dystrophy,[62] and continuous electrocardiographic monitoring may permit early recognition and treatment of this problem. Regional anesthetic techniques have been successfully used to avoid precipitating malignant hyperthermia.

SUMMARY

The status of patients with neuromuscular disease is often severely compromised in the perioperative period because of the impact of neuromuscular disease on organ system function. Although the causes of peripheral nerve, neuromuscular junction, and muscle diseases are varied, the approach to perioperative care may be simplified by an organ systems approach. Assessment and intervention based on the degree of organ system dysfunction seems more rational than gearing management to the diagnosis alone. Chronically ill patients with neuromuscular diseases provide a challenge to acute care physicians who treat these patients perioperatively; return to baseline status requires the best possible perioperative care.

REFERENCES

1. Appenzekkar O and Marshall J: Vasomotor disturbance in the Landry-Guillain-Barré syndrome, Arch Neurol 9:368-372, 1963.
2. Azar I: The response of patients with neuromuscular disorders to muscle relaxants: a review, Anesthesiology 61:173-187, 1984.
3. Braun N, Arora N, and Rochester D: Respiratory muscle and pulmonary function in polymyositis and other proximal myopathies, Thorax 38(8):616-623, 1983.
4. Braun N et al: When should respiratory muscles be exercised? Chest 84:76-84, 1984.
5. Carroll J et al: Depressed ventilatory response to oculocraniosomatic neuromuscular disease, Neurology 26(2):140-146, 1976.
6. Cohen CA et al: Clinical manifestations of inspiratory muscle fatigue, Am J Med 73(3):308-316, 1983.
7. Consensus Conference: The utility of therapeutic plasmapheresis for neurological disorders, JAMA 256(10):1333-1337, 1986.
8. Covert C, Brodie S, and Zimmerman J: Weaning failure due to acute neuromuscular disease, Crit Care Med 14(4):307-308, 1986.
9. Dalos N, Borel C, and Hanley D: Cardiovascular autonomic dysfunction in Guillain-Barré syndrome: therapeutic implications of Swan-Ganz monitoring, Arch Neurol, 1988 (in press).
10. d'Empaire G et al: Effect of prethymectomy plasma exchange on postoperative respiratory function in myasthenia gravis, J Thorac Cardiovasc Surg 89:592-596, 1985.
11. De Troyer A, Borenstein S, and Cordier R: Analysis of lung volume restriction in patients with respiratory muscle weakness, Thorax 35(8):603-610, 1980.
12. Drachman DB: The biology of myasthenia gravis, Ann Rev Neurosci 4:195-225, 1981.
13. Drachman DB: The present and future treatment of myasthenia gravis, New Engl J Med 316(12):743-745, 1987.
14. Durscher AG et al: Autonomic dysfunction in the Guillain-Barré syndrome: hemodynamic and neurological studies, Intensive Care Med 6:3-6, 1980.
15. Ellis E et al: Treatment of respiratory failure during sleep in patients with neuromuscular disease. Positive-pressure ventilation through a nose mask, Am Rev Respir Dis 135(1):148-152, 1987.
16. Estenne M et al: Chest wall stiffness in patients with chronic respiratory muscle weakness, Am Rev Respir Dis 128(6):1002-1007, 1983.

17. Faguis J and Wallin BG: Microneurographic evidence of excessive sympathetic outflow in the Guillain-Barré syndrome, Brain 106:589-600, 1983.

18. Farah M, Evans E, and Vignos P: Echocardiographic evaluation of left ventricular function in Duchenne's muscular dystrophy, Am J Med 69:248-254, 1980.

19. Ferguson R, Murphy R, and Lascelles R: Ventilatory failure in myasthenia gravis, J Neurol Neurosurg Psychiatry 45:217-222, 1982.

20. Fergusson R et al: Suxamethonium is dangerous in polyneuropathy, Br Med J 282:298-389, 1981.

21. Fischer JE et al: Aggressive surgical approach for drug-free remission from myasthenia gravis, Ann Surg 205(5):496-503, 1987.

22. Fresin JC et al: Heart rate variations in the Guillain-Barré syndrome, Br Med J 281:649, 1980.

23. Gibson G et al: Pulmonary mechanics in patients with respiratory muscle weakness, Am Rev Respir Dis 115(3):389-395, 1977.

24. Gracey DR, Howard FM, Jr and Divertie MB: Plasmapheresis in the treatment of ventilator-dependent myasthenia gravis patients: report of four cases, Chest 85(6):739-743, 1984.

25. Grassino A: Determinants of respiratory muscle failure, Am Rev Respir Dis 134:1091-1093, 1986.

26. Grinman S and Whitelaw W: Pattern of breathing in a case of generalized respiratory muscle weakness, Chest 84(6):770-772, 1983.

27. Gronert G and Theyre R: Pathophysiology of hyperkalemia induced by succinylcholine, Anesthesiology 43(1):89-99, 1975.

28. Gudesblatt M et al: Autonomic neuropathy associated with autoimmune disease, Neurology 35(2):261-264, 1985.

29. Haymaker W and Kernohan J: The Landry-Guillain-Barré syndrome: a clinicopathologic report of fifty fatal cases and a critique of the literature, Medicine 28:59-141, 1949.

30. Heiman-Patterson TD et al: Halothane-caffeine contracture testing in neuromuscular diseases, Muscle Nerve 11(5):453-457, 1988.

31. Hobday J and Baker AJ: Guillain-Barré complicated by hypertension and ileitis, Med J Aust 2:536-539, 1968.

32. Hodson A, Hurwitz BJ, and Albrecht R: Dysautonomia in Guillain-Barré syndrome with dorsal root ganglioneuropathy, Wallerian degeneration, and fatal myocarditis, Ann Neurol 15:88-95, 1984.

33. Hoyle C, Ewing DJ, and Parker AC: Acute autonomic neuropathy in association with systemic lupus erythematosus, Ann Rheum Dis 44(6):420-442, 1985.

34. Kahn JK, Sisson JC, and Vinik AI: Prediction of sudden cardiac death in diabetic autonomic neuropathy, J Nucl Med 29(9):1605-1606, 1988.

35. Kyriakidis MK et al: Autonomic neuropathy in leprosy, Int J Lepr 51(3):331-335, 1983.

36. Laiwah AC et al: Autonomic neuropathy in acute intermittent porphyria, J Neurol Neurosurg Psychiatry 48(10):1025-1030, 1985.

37. Le Quesne PM and Fowler CJ: Quantitative evaluation of toxic neuropathies in man, Electroencephalogr Clin Neurophysiol Suppl 39:347-354, 1987.

38. Lichtenfeld P: Autonomic dysfunction in the Guillain-Barré syndrome, Am J Med 50:772-780, 1971.

39. Loh L: Neurological and neuromuscular disease, Br J Anaesth 58:190-200, 1986.

40. Low P: Autonomic neuropathy, Semin Neurol 7(1):49-57, 1987.

41. MacIntyre NR: Respiratory function during pressure support ventilation, Chest 89:677-683, 1986.

42. Maggi G et al: Thymomas: a review of 169 cases, with particular reference to results of surgical treatment, Cancer 58(3):765-776, 1986.

43. Martyn JB, Wong MJ, and Huang SH: Pulmonary and neuromuscular complications of mixed connective tissue disease: a report and review of the literature, J Rheumatol 15(4):703-705, 1988.

44. Matikainen E and Juntunen J: Autonomic nervous system dysfunction in workers exposed to organic solvents, J Neurol Neurosurg Psychiatry 48(10):1021-1024, 1985.

45. Matsuyama H and Haymaker W: Distribution of lesions in the Landry-Guillain-Barré syndrome, with emphasis on involvement of the sympathetic system, Acta Neuropathol 8:230-241, 1967.

46. McKhann GM et al: Plasmapheresis and Guillain-Barré syndrome: analysis of prognostic factors and the effect of plasmapheresis, Ann Neurol 23(4):347-353, 1988.

47. McLeod ME and Creighton RE: Anesthesia for pediatric neurological and neuromuscular diseases, J Child Neurol 1(3):189-197, 1986.

48. Miller J and Lee C: Muscle diseases. In Katz J, Benumof J, and Kadis L (editors): Anesthesia and uncommon diseases Philadelphia, 1981, WB Saunders Co.

49. Miller R: Guillain-Barré syndrome: current methods of diagnosis and treatment, Postgrad Med 77:57-64, 1985.

50. Mitchell P and Meilman E: The mechanism of hypertension in the Guillain-Barré syundrome, Am J Med 42:986-995, 1967.

51. Moorman JR et al: Cardiac involvement in myotonic muscular dystrophy, Medicine 64(6):371-387, 1985.

52. Newsom-Davis J and Loh L: Alveolar hypoventilation and respiratory muscle weakness, Bull Eur Physiopathol Respir 15:45-51, 1979.

53. Newsom-Davis J et al: Diaphragm function and alveolar hypoventilation, Q J Med 177:87-100, 1976.

54. Newton-John H: Prevention of pulmonary compli-

cations in severe Guillain-Barré syndrome by early assisted ventilation, Med J Aust 142(8):444-445, 1985.

55. Oakley CM: The heart in Guillain-Barré syndrome, Br Med J 288:94, 1984.

56. Paptestas A et al: Effects of thymectomy in myasthenia gravis, Ann Surg 206(1):79-88, 1987.

57. Perloff JK: The heart in neuromuscular disease, Curr Probl Cardiol 11(9):509-557, 1986.

58. Person A and Solders G: R-R variations in Guillain-Barré syndrome: a test of autonomic dysfunction, Acta Neurol Scand 67:294-300, 1983.

59. Rochester D: Malnutriton and the respiratory muscles, Clin Chest Med 7(1):91-99, 1986.

60. Rochester D: Respiratory effects of respiratory muscle weakness and atrophy, Am Rev Respir Dis 134(5):1083-1086, 1986.

61. Serisier D, Mastaglia F, and Gibson G: Respiratory muscle function and ventilatory control. I. In patients with motor neurone disease. II. In patients with myotonic dystrophy, Q J Med 51(202):206-226, 1982.

62. Sethna N et al: Anesthesia related complications in children with Duchenne muscular dystrophy, Anesthesiology 68:462-465, 1988.

63. Sivak E et al: Respiratory insufficiency in adult onset acid maltase deficiency, South Med J 80:205-208, 1987.

64. Smith PE, Calverley PM, and Edwards RH: Hypoxemia during sleep in Duchenne muscular dystrophy, Am Rev Respir Dis 137(4):884-888, 1988.

65. Sporn PH and Morganroth ML: Discontinuation of mechanical ventilation, Clin Chest Med 9(1):113-126, 1988.

66. Sunderrajan EV and Davenport J: The Guillain-Barré syndrome: pulmonary neurologic correlations, Medicine 64(5):333-341, 1985.

67. Tobin M et al: The pattern of breathing during successful and unsuccessful trials of weaning from mechanical ventilation, Am Rev Respir Dis 134(6):1111-1118, 1986.

68. Tobin MJ et al: Konno Mead analysis of ribcage abdominal motion during successful and unsuccessful trials of weaning from mechanical ventilation, Am Rev Respir Dis 135(6):1320-1328, 1987.

69. Truax BT: Autonomic disturbances in the Guillain-Barré syndrome, Semin Neurol 4(4):462-468, 1984.

70. Tuck R and McLead J: Autonomic dysfunction in the Guillain-Barré syndrome, J Neurol Neurosurg Psychiatry 44:983-990, 1981.

71. Vincken W, Elleker G, and Cosio MG: Detection of upper airway muscle involvement in neuromuscular disorders using the flow-volume loop, Chest 90(1):52-57, 1986.

72. Vincken W, Elleker M, and Cosio M: Determinants of respiratory muscle weakness in stable neuromuscular disorders, Am J Med 82(1):53-58, 1987.

73. Vincken W, Elleker M, and Cosio M: Flow-volume loop changes reflecting respiratory muscle weakness in chronic neuromuscular disorders, Am J Med 83(4):673-680, 1987.

74. Vrints C et al: Cardiac manifestations of Becker-type muscular dystrophy, Acta Cardiol (Brux) 38(5):479-486, 1983.

75. Weintraub M: Autonomic failure in Guillain-Barré syndrome—value of Swan-Ganz catheterization, JAMA 242:513-514, 1979.

76. Weng TR et al: Pulmonary function and ventilatory response to chemical stimuli in familial myopathy, Chest 88(4):488-495, 1985.

77. Wintzen AR and Schipperheyn JJ: Cardiac abnormalities in myotonic dystrophy: electrocardiographic and echocardiographic findings in 65 patients and 34 of their unaffected relatives. Relation with age and sex and relevance for gene detection, J Neurol Sci 80(2-3):259-268, 1987.

78. Yamada M, Hatakeyama S, and Tsukagoshi H: Peripheral and autonomic nerve lesions in systemic amyloidosis. Three pathological types of amyloid polyneuropathy, Acta Pathol Jpn 34(6):1251-1266, 1984.

79. Yao H et al: Neurogenic hypertension in Guillain-Barré syndrome, Jpn Heart J 26(4):593-596, 1985.

CHAPTER 29

Protein-energy Malnutrition in the Perioperative Period

CLIFFORD S. DEUTSCHMAN

Availability of hyperalimentation has altered medical practice and stimulated interest in the role that malnutrition plays in the pathogenesis of perioperative complications. Most practitioners believe that malnutrition contributes to poor outcome and favor the use of metabolic support, but nutritional support is often used inappropriately. A series of questions is addressed in this chapter to critically examine malnutrition and the role of metabolic repletion in the perioperative period: (1) What is malnutrition, how does it arise, and how does one assess its presence? (2) What is the incidence of malnutrition in surgical patients? (3) What are the effects of malnutrition on individual organs and can these effects be reversed with therapy? (4) Does malnutrition ad-versely affect outcome and is reversal of preexisting malnutrition beneficial? (5) What are the complications of nutritional repletion?

DEFINITION AND SCOPE OF PROTEIN-ENERGY MALNUTRITION

Most studies focusing on malnutrition investigate the effects of macronutrient (carbohydrate, protein, or fat) deprivation. Insufficiency of these entities is collectively referred to as protein-energy malnutrition (PEM), which causes a reduction in body cell mass and was initially described in children in third-world nations[91,92,176,178] as well as in adults placed on an experimental diet designed to reproduce famine conditions.[145] As PEM became recognized as a common problem in hospitalized patients, a better understanding of the interaction between malnutrition and disease has evolved. Bistrian, Blackburn, and associates were first to advance the hypothesis that PEM in hospitalized adults may take a number of forms arising from the interplay of the different metabolic changes brought about by starvation and "stress" (for example, disease, infection, trauma, or surgery).[27] It is important to differentiate between these two because they present with different clinical pictures and because the treatment of "stressed" individuals with management principles derived for use in pure starvation is ineffective and can lead to complications.[51] To further clarify this issue, starvation and stress metabolism are reviewed in the following paragraphs.

In acute, nonstressed fasting metabolism, metabolic rate decreases to conserve stored nutrients, in particularly nitrogen.[50,63,82,164] Glucose, the predominant fuel in early starvation, continues to be made available to tissues. In the first 24 hours glucose is derived from glycogen but is later mobilized from muscle catabolism, which supplies amino acids as precursors for hepatic and renal gluconeogenesis.[164,204] Because these sources are unable to maintain blood glucose concentration at prestarvation levels, insulin secretion decreases.[164,204] Low insulin levels, in turn, promote lypolysis and ketonemia.[97] Ketonemia inhibits pyruvate dehydrogenase, which prevents glucose metabolites from entering the tricarboxylic acid cycle.[175] The primary fuel source for most tissues becomes acetyl CoA derived from fat and ketones rather than glucose. The change from glucose to fat metabolism is reflected in a decrease in the respiratory quotient (CO_2 production/oxygen consumption).[50,164] Fuel for obligate glucose users (brain, fibroblasts, phagocytes, and red blood cells) continues to be derived from gluconeogenesis from muscle. The brain eventually begins to use ketones in place of glucose, which permits a further decrease in glucose requirements and acts to spare protein.[50,101,205] The system is responsive to exogenous substrate; administration of glucose, for example, raises insulin levels, shuts down ketogenesis and prevents muscle breakdown.[164] When energy demand increases, as in increased skeletal muscle activity, anerobic metabolism of glucose meets this need.[82] In addition, skeletal muscle can, to some degree, use branched chain amino acids as fuel.[51,164] Lactate and other amino acids released by exercising muscle are recycled by the liver to provide glucose for aner-

obic metabolism. In this way metabolic rate is responsive to tissue demand and substrate utilization is determined by substrate availability: this process requires low levels of neuroendocrine modulation.[51,81] Fasting metabolism will eventually result in a clinical picture very similar to a form of childhood PEM referred to as marasmus, which is characterized by loss of fat and muscle mass.[91,176,178] It is important to note that the loss of mass is proportional in all tissues and that water is lost in proportion to nonaqueous mass.[149]

In contrast, acute stress metabolism is best described as driven or mediated.[51] In response to inflammation, surgery, injury, or infection, neuroendocrine and humoral mediators, including monokines, lymphokines, prostanoids, hormones, direct neuronal input, complement, and other endogenous substances, are activated.[46,51,85,208] These mediators "drive" metabolism and increase energy expenditure. After a specific injury such as surgery, this response runs a regulated time course that usually peaks about 3 days after initiation and then gradually abates unless a new activating stimulus is provided.[50,51,66,275] The magnitude of the response is proportional to the magnitude of the activating stimulus; thus greater injury results in a greater response.[50,51,67,85] Substrate for this increased metabolism is generated by the liver in response to the altered neuro-humoral-endocrine milieu. Mediators direct substrate (lactate produced by injured, devascularized tissue, amino acids mobilized from endogenous protein by proteolysis, and free fatty acids and glycerol derived from lipolysis) into gluconeogenic pathways.[26,66,68,78,208] Amino acids also act as precursors to structural and enzymatic proteins, while fat is converted to ketone bodies, which serve as an energy source. Since these metabolic processes occur as a result of the activation of endogenous mediators, they are relatively unresponsive to control by exogenous substrate.[14,61,83,127,168] This pattern of metabolism results in depletion of visceral protein, fat deposits, and somatic muscle and is associated with expansion of the extracellular fluid compartment.[89,149,187,252] The state is characterized by physical findings (edema, hypoalbuminemia, fatty liver) similar to childhood kwashiorkor.[27]

Assessment of the presence and extent of PEM, which is necessary to determine its impact on perioperative outcome, is best accomplished by directly measuring body cell mass. Unfortunately, direct measurement of cell mass requires the use of multiple-isotope techniques[91,133,187] and is often not clinically feasible. Alternatives using indirect parameters which are believed to correlate with body cell mass have been developed. These include anthropometrics, biochemical markers, and tests of immunologic function. All are associated with serious drawbacks.

Most anthropometric measures, which were originally derived for application to childhood PEM, neglect factors of importance in assessing the extent of body cell mass loss in adults (frame size, body build, fat patterning).[28,176,178] Ninety-five percent confidence limits for these parameters have also not been firmly established.* Further, the presence of stress-induced edema makes the interpretation of anthropometrics difficult. Decreases in specific transport proteins, most often albumin and transferrin, clearly accompany stress PEM and reflect the interplay of decreased synthesis, extravasation into extravascular tissues, and expansion of the extracellular water.[89] Serum proteins are often normal or only mildly depleted in pure starvation despite significant loss of body cell mass,[43,138,145,225] yet will decrease in pure stress as a result of the expansion of the intravascular space.[89,102,252] Thus low serum protein levels can reflect the presence of stress without significant PEM. Abnormalities of cell-mediated immunity and lymphopenia have also been used to diagnose PEM, but similar abnormalities occur in other disease states such as cancer, collagen-vascular disease, sepsis, uremia, and cirrhosis and with administration of numerous drugs (including general anesthetics).[134,185,267] Finally, all these measures suffer from lack of specificity and are derived from population studies that may have little bearing on individual patients.[106]

To overcome the limitations of the above-mentioned diagnostic tests, alternative approaches have been advocated. Shizgal and coworkers have used isotopic techniques to measure the ratio of exchangeable potassium to exchangeable sodium and thus estimate lean cell mass.[91,92,244] However, as pointed out by Moore[187] and Hill,[122] there may be variability in exchangeable potassium from tissue to tissue, and normal values (which need to be based on cadaver studies) have yet to be determined. Other investigators have advocated following multiple parameters over time.[32,50,258] Several different prognostic indices composed of multiple unrelated pa-

rameters to classify and assess the extent of PEM have been developed.[48,116] Unfortunately, all lack specificity.[176,178] Some clinicians believe that a thorough history and physical examination, coupled with evidence of weight loss or the presence of a known "stress-inducing" catabolic process can be an equally valid indicator of PEM.[18,72,170,203] Finally, indirect calorimetry, which can directly measure oxygen consumption and carbon dioxide production, has recently gained popularity. While useful, this technique requires further testing.[148]

It is clear that the problem of accurate assessment of PEM is significant. Perhaps the best approach, and the one advocated by the author, is to assess each patient initially for weight loss, evidence of a disease process likely to deplete body cell mass, and anticipation of a future course associated with catabolism, for example, surgery. To follow the patients over time, the use of rapid-turnover serum proteins such as prealbumin or retinol-binding protein offers a more accurate index of day-to-day hepatic protein synthesis than albumin or transferrin, although the latter have significant prognostic value.[136,279] New developments may soon alter the approach. Functional testing of peripheral somatic muscle,[134] direct measurement of the extracellular fluid compartment size,[149] and quantification of T-lymphocyte subpopulations[1] are promising new techniques that may soon become routinely available to delineate the presence and extent of PEM in individual patients.

THE INCIDENCE OF MALNUTRITION IN HOSPITALIZED SURGICAL PATIENTS

Early workers identified malnutrition in hospitalized patients,[39,211] but the observations of Bistrian et al that 50% of general surgical[29] and 44% of medical patients[30] in a large urban hospital had abnormalities of anthropometric and biochemical indices consistent with malnutrition heightened interest in the problem. Subsequent investigators have confirmed these findings in other hospital settings and patient populations.* However, the combined use of anthropometrics, transport proteins, and delayed hypersensitivity for diagnosing malnutrition may overestimate the incidence of this problem. For example, a study of Veteran's Administration (VA) patients found abnormalities of at least one variable in 97% of patients, an unreasonable incidence even in the

*References 28, 47, 62, 91, 108, 134, 136, 176, 218, 275.

*References 92, 163, 189, 190, 274, 278.

VA population.[189] Symreng et al found that 28% of surgical patients had three or more abnormalities suggestive of malnutrition on admission,[258] which may be a more valid estimate, and is similar to data reported elsewhere.[123,190] In another study, 75% of surgical patients admitted with "normal" nutritional indices developed abnormalities over the course of their hospitalization.[271] This suggests that not only is malnutrition common in surgical patients on admission, but it can develop over the course of hospitalization. Thus, while the actual incidence is somewhat uncertain, there is little doubt that malnutrition is common in hospitalized patients and may become worse over the course of hospitalization.

EFFECTS OF PEM AND REPLETION THERAPY ON INDIVIDUAL ORGAN STRUCTURE AND FUNCTION

This section summarizes the effects of PEM and reviews the effects of repletion therapy for each of eight organ systems. Human data are presented when possible; otherwise animal studies are cited. Organ changes associated with starvation PEM are disproportionately represented because few studies of stress PEM have been reported.

Cardiovascular Changes

PEM in the absence of stress is associated with morphologic, functional, and electrical cardiovascular abnormalities. Heart size decreases in proportion to loss of body mass,* and the left ventricular free wall is thinned.[5,106] Myocardial atrophy and interstitial edema are noted histologically.[2,52,99] In addition, left-atrial, aortic-root, and left-ventricular end-systolic and end-diastolic dimensions are less than in normal controls[106] and left-ventricular compliance decreases.[5] Resting heart rate, blood pressure, and pulse pressure decrease[36,144,145] and respond subnormally to stress testing.[104] Cardiac index and ejection fraction, however, remain at prestarvation levels[5,104,119] and increase appropriately with exercise[104] and or beta-receptor stimulation.[5] Diminished ECG amplitude, right-axis deviation, PR and QT prolongation, T-wave inversion or flattening, ST-T segment depression, nodal escape beats, and ventricular tachyarrhythmias have been noted.†

In contrast to starvation, stress metabolism in

cachectic humans is associated with increases in heart rate and indexed ventricular mass per kilogram of body weight.[120] These changes suggest that the stressed heart is "spared" from the effects of PEM on body cell mass and is able to respond normally to increases in myocardial work, even when other tissues are being wasted. This may reflect the fact that the heart can use many different fuels including fat, glucose, and lactate. Severe histologic changes are, however, present when PEM is induced in "hypermetabolic" animals such as rats.[201,206]

Protein and calorie repletion in previously healthy semistarved adult males rapidly increases heart size,[94,104,144,145] while heart rate, blood pressure, and pulse pressure initially increase to above prestarvation baseline values and then gradually return to normal. Ejection fraction and cardiac output may decrease, and congestive failure has been reported. The etiologic causes of these abnormalities of myocardial function associated with refeeding are unknown.[144,145] ECG amplitude and QT interval prolongation persist for variable periods despite repletion.[36,104,144]

In the only study looking at the effect of nutritional repletion on cardiac function in patients with stress-induced PEM, ventricular mass, heart rate, end-diastolic volume, cardiac output, and ejection fraction all increased. However, congestive failure developed in 3 of 5 patients, and a pericardial effusion developed in one.[120] Given the small size of this study, the true frequency of such changes is not known.

Pulmonary Changes

Despite the fact that lung cell mass may be somewhat spared (lung to body weight ratio increases), wet and dry lung weights decrease in animal models of starvation.[69,228,229,272] Changes in morphology resemble those seen with emphysema: distances between alveolar walls are increased, surface area for gas exchange is decreased, air spaces are grossly enlarged, and alveolar septa are disrupted.[143,230,232] These changes are most severe in the lung periphery and are correlated with loss of collagen and elastin.* Starvation also results in depletion of the phospholipoprotein component of surfactant.† Initially, pressure-volume relationships re-

---

*References 5, 6, 36, 144, 145.
†References 8, 104, 132, 247, 265.

*References 114, 143, 228, 229-234.
†References 45, 95, 96, 194, 206, 216, 226, 229, 233, 272.

main normal,[95,216,261] presumably because sufficient surfactant exists to cover alveolar surfaces.[95,261] With prolonged PEM, however, surfactant concentration decreases below the level required to maintain normal functional residual capacity, and surface active forces increase.[45,84,206,216]

In addition to changes in lung parenchyma, diaphragmatic muscle mass decreases in direct proportion to loss of body weight.[11,12,142] This results in marked reduction of developed tension in isolated strips of diaphragmatic muscle. However, mechanical efficiency appears unchanged,[166,219] and observed changes in the time to achieve 50% tension reduction after sustained 20 or 100 Hz stimulation may imply reduced diaphragmatic fatigability.[142] Animal studies have revealed that starvation results in a selective depletion of fast (glycolytic or oxidative) muscle fibers with sparing of slow oxidative fibers, supporting this contention.[142]

After mild acute starvation in otherwise normal adult females, forced vital capacity, forced expiratory capacity, forced expiratory volume, inspiratory pressure, and maximal voluntary ventilation are normal.[25] Severe, prolonged malnutrition in both humans and animals is associated with decreases in lung volumes, maximal pressure generation, and maximal ventilatory effort.[11,114,221] In addition, respiratory rate is decreased, perhaps reflecting decreased carbon dioxide production, hypoxic drive is abnormal (although the response to carbon dioxide is normal),[17,77] and there is a decrease in the number and activity of alveolar macrophages leading to impaired clearance of aerosolized *Staphylococcus aureus*.[109,188,240]

Refeeding of starved rats returns lung weight, lung hydroxyproline, elastin, and surfactant contents to normal.[229,230] However, parenchymal emphysematous changes are incompletely reversed.[231] Diaphragmatic contractile force increases in proportion to gain in body weight,[219] respiratory muscle function and maximal inspiratory pressures improve,[141] and pulmonary phagocytic activity improves.[240] Abnormalities of hypoxic ventilatory drive in malnourished men are not prevented by administration of amino acids sufficient to prevent negative nitrogen balance.[17] Effects of repletion on lung volumes and the response to hypoxia are unknown.

The effects of stress metabolism on pulmonary structure and function are not well characterized. Respiratory rate is usually increased in response to increased oxygen consumption and carbon dioxide

production.[66,208,275] Decreased lung compliance and decreased levels of surfactant have been noted in a rat model of trauma.[15,16] Hyperalimentation in critically-ill patients appears to improve inspiratory muscle strength.[141] Surfactant levels and lung compliance improve in rats if fat is included in the nutritional regimen.[15,16]

Renal Changes

Studies of starvation PEM document many changes in renal structure and function. Renal mass decreases in proportion to loss of body mass, and renal protein content is reduced.* Creatinine clearance, free water clearance, effective renal plasma flow, glomerular filtration rate (GFR), and filtration fraction decrease markedly.† Total renal blood flow is normal.[80] The ability to maximally concentrate urine in response to water deprivation is impaired‡ while the response to exogenous antidiuretic hormone administration appears to be normal.[151-154]

Total body water decreases, but exchangeable sodium is normal.[249] Free-water clearance and sodium excretion increase early in the course of PEM[40,53,237] and progressively decline after 4 or 5 days.[35,37,269] While renin and aldosterone are elevated during the natriuretic period, the role of these hormones in regulating sodium excretion is not known.[53,157,237] Excretion of titratable acid decreases, and serum bicarbonate and urinary ammonia concentrations increase.[98,100] Refeeding during starvation PEM increases GFR, filtration fraction, concentrating ability, and free-water clearance.[38,151,227,263] Sodium and acid excretion increase,[158] and both plasma and extracellular volume increase.[24,58]

During surgical stress, trauma, or sepsis, renal mechanisms to conserve salt and water are activated.[216] These effects are mediated in part by ADH and aldosterone, and may be accompanied by mild alkalosis if plasma volume is contracted. The effects of prolonged stress on renal structure and function are not known, and the effects of repletion therapy have not been reported.

Gastrointestinal Changes

Loss of intestinal mass is proportionately greater than that of body weight in starved rats.[269] Protein, DNA, RNA, and nitrogen contents have all been

---

*References 58, 103, 263, 266, 273.
†References 58, 103, 145, 151-154, 212, 227, 235, 263, 266.
‡References 90, 151-154, 225, 235.

shown to decrease in small intestinal and mucosal cells.* Epithelial cell renewal and migration to the villus tip is reduced,[46] and villus size is decreased.[9] In addition, the number of crypt cells is reduced,[131] and crypt size and mitotic figures per crypt are uniformly decreased throughout the intestine.[60] Gastric motility may be reduced in adults,[148] but overall gastrointestinal transit time is unaffected.[84] The incidences of gastric ulceration, gastric and intestinal atrophy, and mucosal hemorrhage increase in humans,[148] and these changes may reflect mucosal breakdown caused by increased lysosomal acid hydrolase activity.[73] Gastrin concentrations decrease.[173] Mucosal changes may occur only during severe PEM, since Knudsen et al[159] found no histologic abnormalities after short-term fasting (7 days) in obese subjects.

Impaired mucosal transport is suggested by diminished uptake of orally administered mannitol.[83] Activities of sucrase and maltase, but not lactase, are decreased,[9,34,209] especially in the proximal bowel.[82] Mucosal transfer of glucose decreases, but active transport of glucose and histidine from mucosa to serosa is enhanced.[124,196] Peptide hydrolase activity in brush border membranes decreases despite an overall increase in mucosal activity of other gluconeogenic enzymes.[146] Loss of brush border enzymes not only impairs absorption but also promotes bacterial overgrowth.[146]

Healing of mucosal ulcerations in patients with Crohn's disease is associated with institution of total parenteral nutrition, suggesting that refeeding may improve the loss of mucosa associated with this disease. Refeeding has been shown to increase nitrogen retention by the small intestine[139] and to partially restore gastric motility in starved individuals.[145] In contrast, crypt and villus size do not appear to change after refeeding. However, the cell population and mitotic pool both increase throughout the gastrointestinal tract and absorptive capacity improves.[9] Sucrase, maltase, and peptide hydrolase activities in brush border membranes rapidly increase to normal levels[71,146,156] while lysosomal enzyme levels decrease to normal.[71,146]

Enteral refeeding appears to be more effective than intravenous alimentation in restoring gastrointestinal function in postoperative patients.[10,236] Restoration of gastrointestinal mucosal integrity, brush border enzyme levels, and absorptive capacity all occur rapidly in orally repleted animals.[86,165,264] This effect may result from the increased availability of glutamine as substrate for the mucosal cells during enteral refeeding.[251]

Pancreatic Changes

Pancreatic mass decreases in proportion to loss of body weight. Acinar atropy, loss of acinar architecture, fibrosis, and dilation of the exocrine duct are noted.[79,162,164] Electron microscopy reveals decreased rough endoplasmic reticulum and mitochondria.[33] Pancreatic contents of amylase and trypsinogen decrease, but lipase content increases.[162,164,207] Levels of lipase, trypsin, and amylase in duodenal aspirates decrease sequentially with progression of PEM. Aspirate volume and pH are unchanged in children, but bicarbonate secretion decreases in adults.[207] Serum amylase and indices of amylase production increase in patients with anorexia nervosa,[64,199] reflecting loss of structural integrity with spilling of enzyme. Responses of the exocrine pancreas to carbecol stimulation are decreased,[162] and responsiveness of insulin secretion to glucose is diminished during PEM in rats.[76,162] Although the effects of nutritional repletion on the pancreas have not been throughly studied, insulin secretion, exocrine responses to carbecol stimulation, and serum levels of amylase and lipase have been reported to return to normal with refeeding.[162,199]

Hepatic Changes

During simple starvation in humans, the liver loses glycogen and protein but gains periportal fat as a result of defective triglyceride excretion.[3,50,150,158,164] This excess fat is eventually lost if PEM is prolonged. Chronic protein deficiency in rats is associated with decreased liver mass and decreased rough endoplasmic reticulum.[257] Although cellular atrophy and intracellular depletion of protein, RNA, water, and fat have been noted[42,177] hepatocytes are remarkably resistant to loss of structure or number.[164,241] Liver biopsies in patients with up to 55-kilogram weight loss are often histologically normal, although iron and chromolipoid pigment deposits, fatty infiltration, and fibrosis may be present.[164,202] Transaminase enzymes and bilirubin levels may be normal or elevated in pure starvation* and albumin

---

**References 125, 126, 129, 145, 181, 187, 255, 269.

*References 20, 21, 206, 223, 224.

synthesis declines.[150] Urea cycle enzyme activities decrease but enzymes that conserve amino acids are activated and urinary nitrogen excretion decreases.[177] Thus protein is conserved and the catabolic response is attenuated.[150]

Protein deficiency reduces the metabolism of many drugs because activity of hepatic microsomal enzymes is decreased and the cytochrome P-450 system/NADPH-dependent electron transport mechanisms are altered.[22,23,172] In contrast, compounds that are normally biotransformed into toxic substances are better tolerated.[179,180] Standard dosages of drugs that are highly protein-bound may have exaggerated effects during PEM because of low levels of serum proteins and albumin.

Liver size and function return slowly to normal with nutritional repletion. Fatty infiltration and other gross and ultrastructural morphologic abnormalities similarly reverse after several weeks of refeeding.[158,257] Serum levels of hepatocellular enzymes may initially increase with refeeding, but eventually return to normal.[20,161] Although hepatic drug metabolism probably also returns to normal, the effects of repletion therapy have not been reported.

Immunologic Changes

PEM reduces the mass of the thymus gland, spleen, and lymph nodes proportionately more than loss of body mass.[75,111] Tonsils and adenoids appear vestigial.[75] Histologic examination of these structures reveals loss of both small lymphocytes and germinal centers. Total circulating polymorphonuclear leukocyte (PMN) counts are reduced, but the PMN to total white cell ratio is increased. The chemotactic, bacterial engulfment, and intracellular killing abilities of PMNs and macrophages are impaired.[56,75,111] Serum level and activity of complement components C3 and C5 appear to be normal during stress malnutrition, but all other direct and indirect pathway components are decreased.[75,111,208]

Peripheral B cells are reduced in absolute number, but account for an increased percentage of the total lymphocyte count. Serum immunoglobulin levels have been reported as normal, increased, or decreased.[76,115] Impaired antibody binding and lack of antigen specificity is noted.[75,111] Cell-mediated immunity is impaired in PEM.* The absolute number of T cells and the T cell to total white cell ratio are

*References 68, 75, 111, 128, 198.

reduced.[74,111] Total numbers of T cells, and the proportion of T helper and suppressor cells are normal in PEM alone, but are markedly reduced in stress.[1]

Lymphoid tissue mass, cellular population, and germinal centers are restored with nutritional therapy. Phagocytosis and chemotaxis improve,[74,75,111] but the effects of repletion on engulfment and intracellular killing are not known. Delayed skin reactivity,[31,160] levels of fixed and circulating antibodies,[75,159,160] and complement levels[74,75] all return to normal after adequate repletion of protein and calories.[69,159,197,198] Short-term nutritional repletion does not improve T cell abnormalities in patients with either starvation or stress PEM.[1]

Nervous-System Changes

Reduced peripheral nerve conduction velocity and associated sensory abnormalities have been noted in children with PEM.[54] Nerve biopsies show normal myelin density in moderate PEM, but segmental demyelination occurs in severe disease.[222,246] Lethargy, confusion, and impaired initiative have been described in patients with chronic PEM.[145] Cerebral atrophy, ventricular dilation, and diffuse EEG slowing are reported.[50,70,164] Adult rats with protein deprivation have low levels of phosphatidylglycerol and sphingophospholipid fraction, but other components of myelin remain normal.[270] The functional significance of these findings is unclear. Refeeding appears to restore peripheral nerve conduction and ultrastructural characteristics[222,246] and to improve mental status in humans.[145]

EFFECTS OF PERIOPERATIVE PEM ON OUTCOME IN THE SURGICAL PATIENTS
Impact on Mortality

In an early and still highly relevant investigation, Studley noted that loss of more than 20% of premorbid weight was associated with a 33% mortality in patients undergoing surgical treatment for peptic ulcer disease.[256] More recent studies have examined the relationship between alterations in anthropometrics, transport proteins and white cell number and function and outcome following surgery. Reinhardt found that depressed albumin levels (< 3.0) were associated with a 30-day mortality of 24%, and patients with levels below 2.0 g/dl the mortality rate was 62%.[214] In a similar study, Seltzer et al found that albumin levels under 3.5 were associated with fourfold increases in mortality and lymphocyte counts under 1500 with a fourfold increase. Abnormalities of both (albumin and lymphocyte count) were associated with a mortality rate 18 times that of patients in whom both indices were normal.[238] Impaired cell-mediated immunity is clearly a marker for increased mortality.[121] Meakins et al observed a 3.1% mortality in surgical patients with normal preoperative skin tests while anergy was associated with a mortality of 35%; the development of anergy following initially normal testing was invariably fatal.[182] Although several other studies have confirmed the association of anergy with perioperative mortality,* numerous factors besides PEM likely contribute to anergy in these patients, and may increase risk independently.

In an attempt to improve specificity, Harvey and co-workers developed a disciminant function based on delayed hypersensitivity, transferrin and albumin levels and total lymphocyte count, which predicted the development of sepsis and surgical mortality.[116,117] Unfortunately, this index has not been evaluated prospectively. Mullen and co-workers also developed a "prognostic nutritional index" (PNI) based on a series of metabolic markers.[189,190] High-risk patients identified by the PNI had a nearly 60% mortality, as opposed to 3% mortality for low-risk patients. Prospective evaluation of the PNI demonstrated increased postoperative mortality in high-risk patients.[19]

Impact on Complications

Several studies have demonstrated an increased incidence of surgical complications in patients with markers for PEM.* Increased rates of postoperative sepsis have been reported in anergic patients and in patients who became anergic following surgery.[182] Preoperative anergy was associated with doubling of nonseptic complications[171,182] and has also been found to be predictive of a prolonged hospital stay.[57] Rhoads and Alexander observed that hypoproteinemic surgical patients had twice the rate of wound infections and a higher incidence of urinary tract, respiratory, and miscellaneous infections.[217] Impaired collagen synthesis has been found in punch biopsy wounds of starved rats and patients,[254] and Cruse and Foord concluded that malnutrition increased the incidence of clean wound infections from 1.8% to 16.6%.[65] An association has been noted

*References 55, 57, 137, 140, 171, 182.

between dehiscence of bowel anastamoses and abnormalities of total plasma protein and albumin.[133] Starved rats with low serum proteins and albumin have been reported to have decreased colonic collagen content, decreased colonic wall bursting tension, and loss of tensile anastamotic strength and collagen content.[130] However, Temple et al were unable to confirm these last findings.[260]

The uniform association of abnormalities of weight loss, serum proteins, and white cell function with mortality and morbidity in surgical patients is impressive. Further, animal studies in which the presence of PEM is verified demonstrate similar results. However, it must be remembered that all the human studies employ nonspecific markers for PEM, and they do not correct for risk factors other than PEM. Thus the true impact of PEM in surgical outcome is unknown.

Effects of Repletion on Perioperative Outcome

Nutritional repletion reverses many abnormalities that develop in individual organ systems but the effect of perioperative alimentation on outcome is unclear. Most clinical studies are poorly designed; patients are not randomized, investigators are not blinded, and patient populations are not uniform. In addition, most compare different alimentation regimens to one another and thus lack a suitable, untreated control group and do not use objective measures of outcome as end-points. Despite these limitations, some conclusions can be drawn.

Patients with mild to moderate preexisting depletion do not appear to benefit from combined preoperative and postoperative alimentation as opposed to postoperative support alone.

Thompson et al were unable to demonstrate a difference in postoperative mortality or morbidity in unrandomized, mildly depleted patients with gastrointestinal malignancies (versus undepleted controls) receiving preoperative and postoperative total parenteral nutrition.[262] Mullen et al,[192] Heatley et al[118] (in patients with gastric or esophageal cancer and normal preoperative albumin levels), and Smale et al[248] (in unrandomized low-risk patients with cancer) compared preoperative and postoperative TPN to postoperative TPN only and confirmed the absence of difference in mortality or morbidity.

A somewhat different picture emerges when

*References 116, 117, 189, 190, 258.

the population in question is significantly nutritionally depleted preoperatively. Both Mullen[192] and Smale[248] reported reduced mortality (9% versus 47%) and morbidity (23% versus 56%) in patients assigned to receive combined preoperative and postoperative TPN compared with patients receiving postoperative therapy alone. Muller et al[193] confirmed these findings in a randomized study of surgical cancer patients. The duration and efficacy of therapy appear to influence morbidity. Rombeau et al[220] retrospectively studied patients who underwent surgery for inflammatory bowel disease and noted that complications developed in 5% of patients receiving 5 or more days of preoperative TPN and 46% of those receiving less than 5 days. Grimes et al[110] noted a lower incidence of complications in depleted surgical patients who received preoperative support for greater than 5 days. In another study, only 1 of 23 patients (4%) who responded to 1 week of repletion (with a contraction of extracellular fluid) had a perioperative complication 9 of 20 patients (45%) who did not respond had complications. When repletion therapy in nonresponders was continued for an additional 4 to 6 weeks (until a response occurred), the complication rate was 13%. It thus appears that preoperative repletion of appropriate duration (that is, until a response consistent with improved nutritional status is noted) is of benefit in reducing perioperative mortality and morbidity in depleted patients.[253] Questions of methodology in all these studies require that such a conclusion be drawn cautiously. Fortunately, Buzby and others associated with the Veterans Administration Cooperative Trial

have recently published the blueprint for a carefully controlled, randomized, prospective study of the effects of perioperative nutritional support in depleted patients.[49]

Finally, the patient who is initially normal but undergoes either a very stressful or who is unable to eat postoperatively should logically benefit from postoperative ailmentation. Despite the multiplicity of studies assessing perioperative nutritional support, there exists no randomized, prospective trial focusing on this issue with an appropriate control group. Thus while it seems evident that appropriate support of the catatonic patient should improve outcome, this hypothesis has never been properly tested.

COMPLICATIONS OF NUTRITIONAL REPLETION THERAPY
Parenteral Nutrition

Technical complications associated with placement of catheters for parenteral alimentation are listed in the box below, left.[50,87,247] Perhaps the most important is catheter-related sepsis, which usually results from migration of organisms through the dermal tunnel formed during catheter insertion.[259] The incidence of infection increases with the length of time the catheter is in place,[236] and is more common with polyvinyl chloride catheters.[87,236] Uncommonly improperly prepared or contaminated solutions can contain organisms and result in bacteremia.[60,115]

Complications related to infusion of hyperalimentation vary according to amino acid, dextrose, fatty acid, and electrolyte composition. Crystalline amino acid solutions generally have little toxicity. Although Grant et al have implicated a tryptophan breakdown product in the development of abnormal liver function in some patients receiving TPN,[107] this finding has not been substantiated by other investigators and more likely represents an effect of gut rest. Wilmore and co-workers have recently implicated glutamine deficiency in the loss of intestinal mucosal integrity and believe this has implications for the development of septic complications in stressed patients.[276] Deamination of infused amino acids can result in prerenal azotemia.[236]

Administration of pure carbohydrate formulas increases carbon dioxide production more than balanced nutritional regimens, and can result in ventilatory insufficiency in marginally compensated individuals.[13] If glucose is administered in excess of the body's ability to use this substrate, hepatic stea-

---

Technical complications of parenteral nutrition

Pneumothorax	Thoracic duct injury
Air embolism	Brachial plexus injury
Subcutaneous emphysema	Phrenic nerve injury
	Arrhythmias
Arterial laceration	Ventricular perforation
Hemothorax	Cardiac tamponade
Mediastinal hematoma	Venous thrombosis
Hydrothorax	Catheter sepsis

From Cerra FB: Surgery 101:1-14, 1987; Fischer JE and Freund HR: Boston, 1983, little Brown & Co, Inc; and Schlichtig R and Ayres SM: 1988, Year Book Medical Publishers.

tosis and elevated levels of very low density lipoproteins may result.[24,174,183] This complication can usually be avoided by using fat as a partial source of calories.[174,183] Hyperglycemia occurs frequently during glucose administration in stressed patients.[50,87,236] While usually easily reversed with insulin administration, use of insulin during stress metabolism may increase cannibalization of visceral protein.[27] Excess insulin can cause hypoglycemia when TPN infusion is slowed or discontinued.[87]

Infusion of long-chain fatty acids can cause febrile reactions with associated chills, nausea, vomiting, and hypotension.[93] This response, however, is rarely observed during infusions of modern soy and safflower-based formulations.[133] Thrombocytopenia occurs with fat administration, but abnormal bleeding has not been reported. Hypertriglyceridemia can occur, and fat preparations should be avoided in patients with abnormal triglyceride clearance.[50,87,236] Fat-induced reduction of neutrophil chemotaxis and impairment of bacterial clearance have been reported in experimental animals.[88,113,200,250] If fat is not included in TPN formulations, essential fatty acid deficiency may result in dermatitis, alopecia, thrombocytopenia, and impaired wound healing.[87,236] Excess lipid infusions (greater than 3 g/kg/dg) may cause cholestatic jaundice.[7] Rapid lipid infusions can cause the arterial partial pressure of oxygen to fall by a mechanism involving increased prostanoid production from infused arachidonate.[112]

Hypokalemia, hypophosphatemia, hypomagnesemia, and other electrolyte abnormalities can develop early in the course of nutritional repletion and can result in seizures, respiratory and cardiac failure, and death.* These abnormalities are thought to occur secondary to calciuria that is responsive to phosphate administration.[277] Unless elemental trace minerals are replaced, deficiencies may develop during TPN. Selenium deficiency is associated with abnormal PMN and T-cell function secondary to its role in the antioxidant glutathione peroxidase.[19,243] Zinc deficiency can result in diarrhea, mental depression, dermatitis, poor wound healing, platelet cluping, and impaired chemotaxis.[210] Chromium deficiency is associated with glucose intolerance and peripheral neuropathy.[135] Copper deficiency results in hypochromic anemia, leukopenia, and reduced levels of superoxide dismutase, a scavenger of superoxide free radicals.[41,242]

*References 4, 131, 155, 186, 215, 236, 245.

Intravenous hyperalimentation is associated with periportal fat infiltration, canalicular plugging, centrilobular cholestasis, and pigment accumulation within hepatocytes.[147,239] Elevated gamma-glutamyltransferase, alkaline phosphatase, and hyperbilirubinemia generally reflect gallbladder sludge formation and/or cholelithiasis.[184,239] A similar pattern of transient enzyme elevation is occasionally observed when enteral feedings are begun after long periods of gut rest; this probably represents clearance of sludge as cholecystokinin release is stimulated.[73]

Enteral Nutrition

Technical complications of enteral nutrition involving misplacement of feeding tubes are, unfortunately, quite common. Tubes can enter the cranium, the tracheobronchial tree, the pleural space, or the lung parenchyma. They can also cause esophagitis, esophageal ulceration, mediastinal perforation, gastric ulceration, and rupture of varices.[247] Pulmonary aspiration is a frequent complication of intragastric feeding in critically ill patients,[50,173,236] but can usually be avoided if the feeding tube is placed distal to the ligament of Treitz.[50,105,236] Diarrhea resulting from either hyperosmolor formulae or malabsortion secondary to depleted brush border enzymes can usually be controlled with bulking agents or substitution of a more dilute formula. Malabsorption caused by villus atrophy and loss of brush border enzymes in stressed states or following prolonged gut rest may necessitate use of elemental feedings.[236] Elemental feedings have occasionally been associated with elevated transaminase enzymes and hyperbilirubinemia.[195,280] As with TPN, high-caloric enteral formulas can increase carbon dioxide production and adversely affect ventilatory function.[268]

SUMMARY

Perioperative protein energy malnutrition is not a single disease entity. Preoperative PEM appears to reflect the metabolic effects of both starvation and stress, but the effects of stress predominate postoperatively. Precise clinical classification and objective assessment of the extent and course of PEM remain elusive. Starvation clearly alters the structure and function of most organ systems and these abnormalities can be reversed with appropriate refeeding. The effects of stress metabolism and refeeding on organ function are less well documented. PEM, when severe, significantly increases perioperative morbidity and mortality. Accordingly, severely depleted surgical patients should receive perioperative alimentation.

REFERENCES

1. Abbott WC et al: The effect of nutritional support on t-lymphocyte subpopulations in protein calorie malnutrition, J Am Coll Nutr 5:577-584, 1986.
2. Abel RM et al: Adverse hemodynamic and ultrastructural changes in dog hearts subjected to protein calorie malnutrition, Am Heart J 97:733-744, 1979.
3. Addis T, Poo JL, and Lew W: The quantities of protein lost by various organs and tissues of the body during a fast, J Biol Chem 115:111-116, 1936.
4. Agusti ASGN et al: Hypophosphatemia as a cause of failed weaning: the importance of metabolic factors, Crit Care Med 12:142-143, 1984.
5. Alden PB et al: Left ventricular function in malnutrition, Am J Physiol 253:H380-H387, 1987.
6. Alexander JK and Peterson KL: Cardiovascular effects of weight reduction, Circulation 45:310-318, 1972.
7. Allerdyce DB: Cholestasis caused by lipid emulsions, Surg Gynecol Obstet 154:641-647, 1982.
8. Alleyne GAO: Cardiac function in severely malnourished Jamaican children, Clin Sci 30:553-562, 1966.
9. Altmann GG: Influence of starvation and refeeding on mucosal size and epithelial renewal in the rat small intestine, Am J Anat 133:391-400, 1972.
10. Alverdy J, Chi HS, and Sheldon GF: The effect of parenteral nutrition on gastrointestinal immunity: the importance of enteral stimulation, Ann Surg 202:681-684, 1985.
11. Arora NS and Rochester DF: Effect of body weight and muscularity on human diaphragm muscle mass, thickness and area, J Appl Physiol 52:64-70, 1982.
12. Arora NS and Rochester DF: Respiratory muscle strength and maximal voluntary ventilation in undernourished patients, Am Rev Respir Dis 126:5-8, 1982.
13. Askanazi J, Rosenbaum SH, and Hyman AI: Respiratory changes induced by the large glucose loads of total parenteral nutrition, JAMA 243:1444-1447, 1980.
14. Asknazi J et al: Influence of total parenteral nutrition on fuel utilization in injury and sepsis, Ann Surg 191:40-46, 1989.
15. Bahrami S et al: Influence of parenteral nutrition on phospholipid metabolism in post-traumatic rat lungs, JPEN 10:617-621, 1986.
16. Bahrami S et al: Mechanical properties of the lungs of post-traumatic rats are improved by including fat in total parenteral nutrition, JPEN 11:560-565, 1987.
17. Baier H and Somani P: Ventilatory drive in normal man during semi-starvation, Chest 85:222-225, 1984.
18. Baker JP et al: Nutritional assessment: a comparison of clinical judgment and objective measurements, New Engl J Med 306:969-972, 1982.
19. Baker SS and Cohen HJ: Altered oxidative metabolism in selenium deficient rat granulocytes, J Immunol 130:2856-2860, 1983.
20. Baron DN: Serum transaminases and isocitrate dehydrogenase in kwashiorkor, J Clin Pathol 13:252-255, 1960.
21. Barrett PVD: Hyperbilirubinemia of fasting, JAMA 217:1349-1353, 1971.
22. Basu TK: Effects of protein malnutrition and ascorbic acid levels on drug metabolism, Can J Physiol Pharmacol 61:295-301, 1983.
23. Basu TK, Dickerson JWT, and Parke DV: Effects of protein/energy nutrition on rat plasma corticosteroids and liver microsomal hydroxylase activity, Nutr Metab 18:49-54, 1975.
24. Batuman V et al: Renal and electrolyte effects of total parenteral nutrition, JPEN 8:546-551, 1984.
25. Bender PR and Martin BJ: Ventilatory and treadmill endurance during acute starvation, J Appl Physiol 60:1823-1827, 1986.
26. Birkhahn RL et al: Effects of major skeletal trauma on whole body protein turnover in man measured by L-[1,14C]-leucine, Surgery 88:294-300, 1980.
27. Bistrian BR: Anthropometric norms used in the assessment of hospitalized patients, Am J Clin Nutr (letter)33:2211-2214, 1980.
28. Bistrian BR: Interaction of nutrition and infection in the hospital setting, Am J Clin Nutr 30:1228-1232, 1977.
29. Bistrian BR, Blackburn GL, and Hallowell E: Protein status of general surgical patients, JAMA 230:858-860, 1974.
30. Bistrian BR et al: Cellular immunity in adult marasmus, Arch Int Med 137:1408-1411, 1977.
31. Bistrian BR et al: Prevalence of malnutrition in general medical patients, JAMA 235:1567-1570, 1976.
32. Blackburn GL et al: Nutritional and metabolic assessment of the hospitalized patient, JPEN 1:11-22, 1977.
33. Blackburn WR and Rinijchiakul K: The pancreas in kwashiorkor: an electron microscopic study, Lab Invest 20:305-309, 1969.
34. Blair DGR, Yakimets W, and Tuba J: Rat intestinal sucrase ii. The effects of rat age and sex and of diet on sucrase activity, Can J Biochem Physiol 41:917-929, 1963.
35. Bloom WL: Fasting as an introduction to the treatment of obesity, Metabolism 8:214-237, 1959.
36. Bloom WL, Azar G, and Smith EG: Changes in heart size and plasma volume during fasting, Metabolism 15:409-413, 1966.
37. Bloom WL and Mitchell W, Jr: Salt excretion in fasting patients, Arch Int Med 106:321-326, 1960.
38. Boag F et al: Diminished creatinine clearance in

anorexia nervosa: reversal with weight gain, J Clin Pathol 38:60-63, 1985.

39. Bollet AJ and Owen SO: Evaluation of nutritional status of selected hospital patients, Am J Clin Nutr 26:931-938, 1973.

40. Boulter PR, Hoffman RS, and Arky RA: Pattern of sodium excretion accompanying starvation, Metabolism 22:675-683, 1973.

41. Bozzetti F, Inglese MG, and Terno G: Hypocurpremia in patients receiving total parenteral nutrition, JPEN 7:563-566, 1983.

42. Brass EP and Hoppel CL: Carnitine metabolism in the fasting rat, J Biol Chem 253:2688-2693, 1978.

43. Broom J, Fraser MH, and McKenzie K: The protein metabolic response to short-term starvation in men, Clin Nutr 5:63, 1986.

44. Brown HO, Levine ML, and Lipkin M: Inhibition of intestinal ephithelial renewal and migration induced by starvation, Am J Physiol 205:868-872, 1963.

45. Brown LAS, Bliss AS, and Longmore WJ: Effect of nutritional status on the lung surfactant system: food and caloric restriction, Exp Lung Res 6:133-147, 1984.

46. Buetler B and Cerami A: Cachectin (tumor necrosis factor): a macrophage hormone governing cellular metabolism and inflammatory response, Endocr Rev 9:57-66, 1988.

47. Burgert SL and Anderson CF: An evaluation of upper arm measurements used in nutritional assessment, Am J Clin Nutr 31:2136-2142, 1979.

48. Buzby GP et al: Prognostic nutritional index in gastrointestinal surgery, Am J Surg 139:160-167, 1980.

49. Buzby GP et al: Study protocol: a randomized clinical trial of total parenteral nutrition in malnourished surgical patients, Am J Clin Nutr 47(suppl):366-381, 1988.

50. Cerra FB: Hypermetabolism, organ failure and metabolic support, Surgery 101:1-14, 1987.

51. Cerra FB (editor): Pocket manual of surgical nutrition, St Louis, 1984, CV Mosby Co.

52. Chauhan S, Nayak NC, and Ramalingaswami V: The heart and skeletal muscle in experimental protein malnutrition in rhesus monkeys, J Path Bact 90:301-309, 1965.

53. Chinn RH et al: The natriuresis of fasting: relationship to changes in plasma renin and plasma aldosterone concentrations, Clin Sci 39:437-455, 1970.

54. Chopra JS et al: Effect of protein calorie malnutrition on peripheral nerves, Brain 109:307-323, 1986.

55. Christou NV, McLean APH, and Meakins JL: Host defense in blunt trauma: interrelationships of kinetics of anergy and depressed neutrophil function, nutritional status and sepsis, J Trauma 20:833-841, 1980.

56. Christou NV and Meakins JL: Neutrophil function in surgical patients: two inhibitors of granulocyte chemotaxis associated with sepsis, J Surg Res 26:355-364, 1979.

57. Christou NV, Meakins JL, and MacLean LD: The predictive role of delayed hypersensitivity in preoperative patients, Surg Gynecol Obstet 152:297-301, 1981.

58. Cizek LJ, Simchon S, and Nocenti MR: Effects of fasting on plasma volume and sodium exchange in male rabbits, Proc Soc Exp Biol Med 154:299-303, 1977.

59. Clarke RM: The effects of growth and of fasting on the number of villi and crypts in the small intestine of the albino rat, J Anat 112:27-33, 1972.

60. Cleri DJ, Corrado ML, and Seligman SJ: Quantitative culture of intravenous catheters and other intravenous inserts, J Infect Dis 141:781-786, 1980.

61. Clowes GHA, Jr et al: Effects of parenteral alimentation on amino acid metabolism in septic patients, Surgery 88:531-543, 1980.

62. Collins JP, McCarthy ID, and Hill G: Assessment of protein nutrition in surgical patients-the value of anthropometrics, Am J Clin Nutr 32:1527-1530, 1979.

63. Consolazio CF et al: Metabolic aspects of acute starvation in normal humans, Am J Clin Nutr 20:672-683, 1967.

64. Cox KL et al: Biochemical and ultrasonic abnormalities of the pancreas in anorexia nervosa, Dig Dis Sci 28:225-229, 1983.

65. Cruse PJE and Foord R: A five-year prospective study of 23649 surgical wounds, Arch Surg 107:206-210, 1973.

66. Cuthbertson D and Tilstone W: Metabolism during the post-injury period, Adv Clin Chem 12:1-55, 1977.

67. Dale G et al: The effects of surgical operation on venous plasma free amino acids, Surgery 81:295-301, 1977.

68. Daly JM, Dudrick SJ, and Copeland EM: Effects of protein depletion and repletion on cell-mediated immunity in experimental animals, Ann Surg 188:791-796, 1978.

69. D'Amours R, Clerch L, and Massaro D: Food deprivation and surfactant in adult rats, J Appl Physiol 55:1413-1417, 1983.

70. Datlof S et al: Ventricular dilation on CAT scans of patients with anorexia nervosa, Am J Psychiatry 143:96-98, 1986.

71. Desai ID: Regulation of lysomal enzymes. II. Reversible adaptation of intestinal acid hydrolases during starvation and refeeding, Can J Biochem 49:170-176, 1971.

72. Detsky AS et al: Evaluating the accuracy of nutritional assessment techniques applied to hospitalized patients: methodology and comparisons, JPEN 8:153-159, 1984.

73. Deutschman CS et al: Transient elevation of hepatic enzymes following resumption of gut feedings in ICU patients, Nutr Int 3:42-46, 1987.

74. Dionigi R et al: The effects of total parenteral nutrition on immunodepression due to malnutrition, Ann Surg 1985:467-474, 1977.

75. Diogeni R et al: Nutrition and infection, JPEN 3:62-68, 1979.

76. Dixit PK and Kuang HLC: Rat pancreatic B cells in protein deficiency: a study involving morphometric analysis and aloxan effect, J Nutr 115:375-381, 1985.

77. Doekel RC et al: Clinical semi-starvation; depression of hypoxic ventilatory response, N Engl J Med 295:358-361, 1976.

78. Duke JH, Jr et al: Contribution of protein to caloric expenditure following injury, Surgery 68:178-174, 1970.

79. Ecknauer R and Raffler H: Effect of starvation on small intestinal enzyme activity in germ-free rats, Digestion 18:45-55, 1978.

80. Edgren B and Wester PO: Impairment of glomerular filtration in fasting for obesity, Acta Med Scand 190:389-393, 1971.

81. Elia M et al: Effects of total starvation and very low calorie diets on intestinal permeability in man, Clin Sci 73:205-210, 1987.

82. Elia M et al: Energy metabolism during exercise in normal subjects undergoing total starvation, Hum Nutr Clin Nutr 38C:355-362, 1984.

83. Elwyn DH et al: Influence of increasing carbohydrate intake on glucose kinetics in injured patients, Ann Surg 190:117-127, 1979.

84. Faridy EE: Effect of food and water deprivation in the surface activity of lungs of rats, J Appl Physiol 29:493-498, 1970.

85. Fath JJ, Meguid MM, and Cerra FB: Hormonal and metabolic responses to surgery and stress. In Goldsmith HM (editor): Practice of surgery, New York, 1985, Harper & Row Publishers, Inc.

86. Feldman EJ et al: Effects of oral vs intravenous nutrition on intestinal adaptation after small bowel resection in the dog, Gastroenterology 70:712-719, 1976.

87. Fischer JE and Freund HR: Central alimentation. In Fischer JE (editor): Surgical nutrition, Boston, 1983, Little Brown & Co, Inc.

88. Fischer JW et al: Diminished bacterial defenses with intralipid, Lancet 2:819-820, 1980.

89. Fleck A: The acute phase response: implications for nutrition & recovery, Nutrition 4:109-117, 1988.

90. Fohlin L: Body composition, cardiovascular and renal function in adolescent patients with anorexia nervosa, Acta Paediatr Scand 268(suppl):6-63, 1977.

91. Forse RA and Shizgal HM: The assessment of malnutrition, Surgery 88:17-23, 1980.

92. Forse RA et al: Efficacy of total parenteral nutrition, Surg Forum 30:87-89, 1979.

93. Freeman JB and Fairfull-Smith RJ: Physiologic approach to peripheral parenteral nutrition. In Fischer JF: Surgical nutrition, Boston, 1983, Little Brown & Co, Inc.

94. Freund HR and Holroyde J: Cardiac function during protein malnutrition and refeeding in the isolated rat heart, JPEN 10:470-473, 1986.

95. Gail DB, Massaro GD, and Massaro D: Influence of fasting on the lung, J Appl Physiol 42:88-92, 1977.

96. Garbagni R et al: Effects of lipide loading and fasting on pulmonary surfactant, Respiration 25:458-564, 1968.

97. Garber AJ et al: Hepatic ketogenesis and gluconeogenesis in humans, J Clin Invest 54:981-989, 1974.

98. Garnett ES et al: Gross fragmentation of cardiac myofibrils after therapeutic starvation of obesity, Lancet 1:914-916, 1969.

99. Garnett ES et al: The roles of carbohydrate, renin and aldosterone in sodium retention during and after total starvation, Metabolism 22:867-874, 1973.

100. Gelman A et al: Starvation and renal function, Am J Med Sci 263:465-471, 1972.

101. Gjedde A and Crone C: Induction processes in blood-brain transfer of ketone bodies during starvation, Am J Physiol 229:1165-1169, 1975.

102. Golden MHN: Transport proteins as indices of nutritional status, Am J Clin Nutr 35:1159-1165, 1982.

103. Goodman MN et al: Sites of protein conservation and loss during starvation; influence of adiposity, Am J Physiol 246:E383-E390, 1984.

104. Gottdiener JS et al: Effects of self-induced starvation on cardiac size and function in anorexia nervosa, Circulation 58:425-433, 1978.

105. Grant JP, Curtas MS, and Kelvin KM: Fluoroscopic placement of nasojejunal feeding tubes with immediate feeding using a non-elemental formula, JPEN 7:299-303, 1983.

106. Grant JP, Custer PB, and Thurlow J: Current techniques of nutritional assessment, Surg Clin North Am 61:437-463, 1981.

107. Grant JP et al: Serum hepatic enzyme and bilirubin elevations during parenteral nutrition, Surg Gynecol Obstet 145:573-580, 1977.

108. Gray GE and Gray LK: Validity of anthropometric norms used in the assessment of hospitalized patients, JPEN 3:366, 1979.

109. Green GM and Kass EK: Factors influencing the clearance of bacteria by the lung, J Clin Invest 43:769-776, 1964.

110. Grimes CJC, Younathan MT, and Lee WC: The effects of preoperative total parenteral nutrition on surgery outcomes, J Am Diet Assoc 87:1202-1206, 1987.

111. Gross RL and Newberne PM: Role of nutrition in immunologic function, Physiol Rev 60:188-302, 1980.

112. Hageman JR and Hunt CE: Fat emulsions and lung function, Clin Chest Med 7:69-77, 1986.

113. Hamaway KJ, Moldawer LL, and Georggieff M: The effects of lipid emulsions on reticuloendothelial system function in the injured animal, JPEN 9:559-565, 1985.

114. Harkema JR et al: A comparison of starvation and elastase models of emphysema in the rat, Am Rev Respir Dis 129:584-591, 1984.

115. Harris JA and Cobb CG: Persistant gram-negative bacteremia: observations in twenty patients, Am J Surg 125:705-717, 1983.

116. Harvey KB et al: Biological measures of the formulation of a hospital prognostic index, Am J Clin Nutr 34:2013-2022, 1981.

117. Harvey KB et al: Hospital morbidity-mortality risk factors using nutritional assessment, J Clin Nutr 26:581A, 1978.

118. Heatley RV, Williams RHP, and Lewis MH: Preoperative intravenous feeding-a controlled trial, Postgrad Med J 55:541-545, 1979.

119. Hexhe JJ: Experimental undernutrition. 1. Its effect on cardiac output, Metabolism 12:1086-1091, 1967.

120. Heymsfield SB et al: Cardiac abnormalities in cachetic patients before and during nutritional repletion, Am Heart J 95:584-594, 1978.

121. Hiebert JM et al: The influence of catabolism on immunocompetence in burned patients, Surgery 86:242-247, 1979.

122. Hill GL: Editorial, Nutr Int 4:287-288, 1988.

123. Hill GL et al: Malnutrition in surgical patients: an unrecognized problem, Lancet 2:689-692, 1977.

124. Hindmarsh JT et al: Further studies on intestinal active transport during semistarvation, J Physiol 188:207-218, 1967.

125. Hirschfield JS and Kern F, Jr: Protein starvation and the small intestine. III. Incorporation of orally and intraperitoneally administered l-leucine 4,5-3H into mucosal protein of protein-deprived rats, J Clin Invest 48:1224-1229, 1969.

126. Hopper AF, Wannemacher RW, Jr, and McGovern PA: Cell population changes in the intestinal epithelium of the rat following starvation and protein-depletion, Proc Soc Exp Biol Med 128:695-698, 1968.

127. Imamura M et al: Liver metabolism and gluconeogenesis in trauma and sepsis, Surgery 868-880, 1975.

128. Ing AFM et al: Determinants of susceptability to sepsis and mortality: malnutrition vs anergy, J Surg Res 32:249-255, 1982.

129. Irvin TT and Goligher JC: Aetiology of disruption of intestinal anastamoses Brit J Surg 461-464, 1973.

130. Irvin TT and Hunt TK: Effect of malnutrition on colonic healing, Ann Surg 180:765-772, 1974.

131. Iseri LT, Freed J, and Bures AR: Magnesium deficiency and cardiac disorders, Am J Med 58:837-845, 1975.

132. Isner JM et al: Sudden unexpected death in avid dieters using liquid-protein-modified-fast diet, Circulation 60:1401-1412, 1979.

133. Jeejeebhoy KN and Marliss EB: Energy supply in total parenteral nutrition. In Fischer JE (editor) Surgical nutrition, Boston, 1983, Little Brown & Co, Inc.

134. Jeejeebhoy KN and Meguid MM: Assessment of nutritional status in the oncologic patient, Surg Clin North Am 66:1077-1090, 1986.

135. Jeejeebhoy KN et al: Chromium deficiency, glucose intolerance and neuropathy reversed by chromium supplementation in a patient receiving long-term total parenteral nutrition, Am J Clin Nutr 30:531-538, 1977.

136. Jeejeebhoy KN et al: Critical evaluation of the role of clinical assessment and body composition studies in patients with malnutrition and after total parenteral nutrition, Am J Clin Nutr 35:1117-1127, 1982.

137. Johnson WC et al: Role of delayed hypersensitivity in predicting postoperative morbidity and mortality, Am J Surg 137:536-542, 1979.

138. Jones WPT and Hay AM: Albumin metabolism: effect of nutritional state and dietary protein intake, J Clin Invest 47:1958-1972, 1968.

139. Ju JS and Nasset ES: Changes in total nitrogen content of some abdominal viscera in fasting and realimentation, J Nutr 68:633-645, 1959.

140. Kaminski MV et al: Correlation of mortality with serum transferrin and anergy, JPEN 1:27A, 1977.

141. Kelly SM et al: Inspiratory muscle strength and body composition in patients receiving total parenteral nutrition therapy, Am Rev Respir Dis 130:33-37, 1984.

142. Kelsen SG, Ference M, and Kapoor S: Effects of prolonged undernutrition on structure and function of the diaphragm, J Appl Physiol 58:1354-1359, 1985.

143. Kerr JS et al: Nutritional emphysema in the rat; influence of protein depletion and impaired lung growth, Am Rev Respir Dis 131:644-650, 1985.

144. Keys A, Henschel A, and Taylor HL: The size and function of the human heart at rest in semi-starvation and subsequent rehabilitation, Am J Physiol 50:153-169, 1947.

145. Keys A et al: The biology of human starvation, Minneapolis, 1950, University of Minnesota Press.

146. Kim YS et al: Alterations in the levels of peptide hydrolases and other enzymes in brush-border and soluble fractions of rat small intestine mucosa during starvation and refeeding, Biochem Biophys Acta 321:262-273, 1973.

147. King WWK et al: Nutritional efficacy and hepatic changes during intragastric, intravenous and prehapatic feeding in rats, JPEN 7:443-445, 1983.

148. Kinney JM: Indirect calorimetry in malnutrition: nutritional assessment or therapeutic reference? JPEN11:905-945, 1987.

149. Kinney JM and Weissman C: Forms of malnutrition in stressed and unstressed patients, Clin Chest Med 7:19-28, 1986.

150. Kirsch RE and Saunders SJ: Nutrition and the liver, S Afr Med J 46:2072-2978, 1972.

151. Klahr S and Alleyne GAO: Effects of chronic protein calorie malnutrition on the kidney, Kidney Int 3:129-141, 1973.

152. Klahr S and Tripathy K: Evaluation of renal function in malnutrition, Arch Int Med 118:322-325, 1966.

153. Klahr S, Tripathy K, and Lotero H: Renal regulation of acid-base balance in malnourished man, Am J Med 325-331, 1970.

154. Klahr S et al: On the nature of the renal concentrating defect in malnutrition, Am J Med 43:84-96, 1967.

155. Knochel JP: The pathophysiology and clinical characteristics of severe hypophosphatemia, Ann Intern Med 137:203-220, 1977.

156. Knudsen KB et al: Effect of fasting and refeeding on the histology and disaccharidase activity of the human intestine, Gastroenterology 55:46-51, 1968.

157. Kolanowski J, Desmecht P, and Crabbe J: Sodium balance and renal tubular sensitivity to aldosterone during total fast and carbohydrate refeeding in the obese, Eur J Clin Invest 6:75-83, 1976.

158. Kumar V, Deo MG, and Ramalingaswami V: Mechanisms of fatty liver in protein deficiency; an experimental study in rhesus monkeys, Gastroenterology 62:445-451, 1972.

159. Law DK, Dudrick SJ, and Abdou NI: The effects of dietary protein depletion on immunocompetence. The importance of nutritional repletion prior to immunologic induction, Ann Surg 179:168-173, 1974.

160. Law DK, Dudrick SJ, and Abdou NI: Immunocompetence of patients with protein-calorie malnutrition. The effects of nutritional repletion, Ann Int Med 79:545-550, 1973.

161. Lee PA et al: Endocrine and metabolic alterations with food and water deprivation, Am J Clin Nutr 30:1953-1962, 1977.

162. Lee PC, Brooks S, and Lebenthal E: Effect of fasting and refeeding on pancreatic enzymes and segretogogue responsiveness in rats, Am J Physiol 242:G215-221, 1982.

163. Letsou AP, Connaughton MC, and O'Donnell TF: Nutritional survey of a university hospital population, JPEN 1:40A, 1977.

164. Levenson SM and Seifter E: Starvation; metabolic and physiologic responses. In Fischer, JE (editor): Surgical nutrition, Boston, 1983, Little Brown & Co, Inc.

165. Levine GM, Deren JJ, and Steiger E: Role of oral intake in the maintenance of gut mass disaccharide activity, Gastroenterology 67:975-982, 1974.

166. Lewis M et al: The effects of malnutrition on diaphragmatic contractility and muscle fiber mophometry, Am Rev Respir Dis 131:A326, 1985.

167. Lichtenberger L, Welsh JD, and Johnson LR: Relationship between the changes in gastrin levels and intestinal properties in the starved rat, Dig Dis 21:33-38, 1976.

168. Long CL, Kinney JM, and Gieger JW: Nonsuppressability of gluconeogenesis by glucose in septic patients, Metabolism 25:193-201, 1976.

169. Lundvick J: Evaluation of a nutritional screen when used on oncology patients, JPEN 3:521A, 1979.

170. MacBurney M and Wilmore DW: Decision-making in nutritional care, Surg Clin North Am 61:571-582, 1981.

171. MacLean LD et al: Host resistance in sepsis and trauma, Ann Surg 182:207-217, 1975.

172. Marshall J and McLean AEM: The effects of oral phenobarbitone on hepatic microsomal cytochrome P-450 and demthylation in rats fed normal and low protein, Biochem Pharmacol 18:153-157, 1969.

173. Materese LE: Enteral nutrition. In Fischer JE: Surgical nutrition, Boston, 1983, Little Brown & Co, Inc.

174. McDonald ATJ, Phillips MJ, and Jeejeebhoy KN: Reversal of fatty liver by intralipid in patients on total parenteral alimentation, Gastroenterology 64:885-891, 1973.

175. McGarry JD and Foster DW: Regulation of ketogenesis and clinical aspects of the ketotic state, Metabolism 21:471-489, 1972.

176. McLaren DS: A fresh look at protein-energy malnutrition in the hospitalized patient, Nutrition 4:1-6, 1988.

177. McLaren DS, Bitar JG, and Nassar VH: Protein-calorie malnutrition and the liver, Prog Liver Dis 4:527-536, 1972.

178. McLaren DS and Meguid MM: Nutritional assessment at the crossroads, JPEN 7:575-581, 1983.

179. McLean AEM and McLean EK: The effect of diet and 1,1,1-trichloro-2,2-bis-(pchlorophenyl) ethane (DDT) on microsomal hydroxylating enzymes and on sensitivity of rats to carbon tetrachloride poisoning, Biochem J 100:564-571, 1966.

180. McLean AEM and Verschuuren HG: Effects of diet and microsomal enzyme induction on the toxicity of dimethylnitrosamine, Br J Exp Pathol 50:22-25, 1969.

181. McManus JPA and Isselbacher KJ: Effect of fasting versus feeding on the rat small intestine. Morphological, biochemical and functional differences, Gastroenterology 59:214-221, 1970.

182. Meakins JL et al: Delayed hypersensitivity; indicator of acquired failure of host devfenses in sepsis and trauma, Ann Surg 186:241-250, 1977.

183. Meguid MM et al: Reduced metabolic complications in total parenteral nutrition: pilot study using fat to replace one third of glucose calories, JPEN 6:304-307, 1984.

184. Messing B et al: Does total parenteral nutrition induce gall bladder sludge formation and lithiasis, Gastroenterology 84:1012-1019, 1983.

185. Miller CL: Immuniological assays as measurements of nutritional status: a review, JPEN 2:554-566, 1978.

186. Molloy DW et al: Hypomagnesemia and respiratory muscle power, Am Rev Respir Dis 129:497-498, 1984.

187. Moore FD et al: The body cell mass and it's supporting environment, Philadelphia, 1978, WB Saunders Co.

188. Moriguchu S, Sone S, and Kishino Y: Changes in alveolar macrophages in protein-deficient rats, J Nutr 113:40-46, 1983.

189. Mullen JL et al: Implications of malnutrition in the surgical patients, Arch Surg 114:121-125, 1979.

190. Mullen JL et al: Nutritional and immunological status of surgical patients, JPEN 1:39A, 1977.

191. Mullen JL et al: Prediction of operative morbidity and mortality by preoperative nutritional assessment, Surg Forum 30:80-82, 1979.

192. Mullen JL et al: Reduction of operative morbidity and mortality by combined preoperative and postoperative nutritional support, Ann Surg 192:604-613, 1980.

193. Muller JM et al: Preoperative parenteral feeding in patients with gastrointestinal carcinoma, Lancet I:68-71, 1982.

194. Myer BA et al: Protein deficiency: effects on lung mechanics and the accumulation of collagen and elastin in rat lung, J Nutr 113:2308-2315, 1983.

195. Nelson LM and Russell RI: Influence of the intake and composition of elemental diets on bile acid metabolism and hepatic lipids in the rat, JPEN 10:399-404, 1986.

196. Newey H, Sanford PA, and Smyth DH: Effects of fasting on intestinal transfer of sugars and amino acids in vitro, J Physiol 208:705-724, 1970.

197. Nohr CW et al: Malnutrition and humoral immunity: long-term protein deprivation, J Surg Res 40:432-437, 1986.

198. Nohr CW et al: Malnutrition and humoral immunity: short-term acute nutritional deprivation, Surgery 98:769-776, 1985.

199. Nordgren L and Von Scheele C: Hepatic and pancreatic dysfunction in anorexia nervosa: a report of two cases, Biol Psychiatry 12:681-686, 1977.

200. Nugent KE: Intralipid effects on reticuloendothelial function, J Leukocyte Biol 36:123-132, 1984.

201. Nutter DO et al: The effects of chronic protein-calorie undernutrition in the rat on myocardial function and cardiac function, Circ Res 45:144-152, 1979.

202. Obeyesekere I: Malnutrition among ceylonese adults, Am J Clin Nutr 18:38-45, 1977.

203. Ottow RT, Bruining HA, and Jeekel J: Clinical judgement versus delayed hypersensitivity skin testing for the prediction of postoperative sepsis and mortality, Surg Gynecol Obstet 159:475-477, 1984.

204. Owen OE et al: Energy expenditure in feasting and fasting, Adv Exp Med Biol 111:169, 1979.

205. Owen OE et al: Liver and kidney metabolism during prolonged starvation, J Clin Invest 48:574-483, 1969.

206. Pissaia O, Rossi MA, and Oliveira JSM: The heart in protein-calorie malnutrition in rats: morphological, electrophysiological and biochemical changes, J Nutr 110:2035-2044, 1980.

207. Pitchumoni CS: Pancreas in primary malnutrition disorders, Am J Clin Nutr 26:374-379, 1973.

208. Popp MB and Brennan MF: Metabolic response to trauma and infection. In Fischer JE: Surgical nutrition, Boston, 1983, Little Brown & Co, Inc.

209. Powell GK and McElveen MA: Effect of prolonged fasting on fatty acid reesterification in rat intestinal mucosa, Biochim Biophys Acta 369:8-15, 1974.

210. Prasad AS: Clinical, endocrinological and biochemical effects of zinc deficiency, Clin Endocrinol Metab 14:567-589, 1985.

211. Prevost EA and Butterworth CE: Nutritional care of hospitalized patients, Clin Res 22:579, 1974.

212. Pullman TN et al: The influence of protein intake on specific renal functions in normal man, J Lab Clin Med 44:320-332, 1954.

213. Rapaport A, From GLA, and Husdan H: Metabolic studies in prolonged fasting. I. Inorganic metabolism and kidney function, Metabolism 14:31-46, 1965.

214. Reinhardt GF et al: Incidence and mortality of hypoalbuminemic patients in hospitalized veterans, JPEN 4:357-359, 1980.

215. Ressel DM and Jeejeebhoy KN: Radionuclide assessment of nutritional depletion. In Wright RA, Heymsfield SB (editors): Nutritional assessment, London, 1984, Blackwell Scientific Publications Ltd.

216. Rhoades RA: Influence of starvation on the lung; effect on glucose and palmitate utilization, J Appl Physiol 38:513-516, 1975.

217. Rhoads JE and Alexander CE: Nutritional problems of surgical patients, Ann NY Acad Sci 63:268-275, 1955.

218. Rich AJ: The assessment of body composition in clinical conditions, Proc Nutr Soc 41:389-403, 1982.

219. Rochester DF: Malnutrition and the respiratory muscles, Clin Chest Med 7:91-99, 1986.

220. Rombeau JL et al: Preoperative total parenteral nutrition and surgical outcome in patients with inflammatory bowel disease, Am J Surg 143:139-143, 1982.

221. Rosenbaum SH et al: Respiratory patterns in profound nutritional depletion, Anesthesiology 51:S366, 1979.

222. Roy S et al: Ulstrstructure of skeletal muscle and peripheral nerve in experimental protein deficiency and its correlation with nerve condition studies, J Neurol Sci 17:399-409, 1972.

223. Royle GT and Kettlewell MGW: Liver function tests in surgical infection and malnutrition, Ann Surg 192:192-194, 1980.

224. Royle GT et al: Galactose and hepatice metabolism in malnutrition and septic man, Clin Sci Molec Med 55:199-204, 1978.

225. Roza AM, Tuitt D, and Shizgal HM: Transferrin-a poor measure of nutritional status, JPEN 8:523-528, 1984.

226. Rubin JW et al: Impaired pulmonary surfactant synthesis in starvation and severe non-thoracic sepsis, Am J Surg 123:461-467, 1972.

227. Russell GFM and Bruce JT: Impaired water diuresis in patients with anorexia nervosa, Am J Med 40:38-48, 1966.

228. Sahebjami H: Nutrition and the pulmonary parenchyma, Clin Chest Med 7:111-126, 1986.

229. Sahebjami H and MacGee J: Changes in connective tissue composition of the lung in starvation and refeeding, Am Rev Respir Dis 128:644-647, 1983.

230. Sahebjami H and MacGee J: Effects of starvation and refeeding on lung biochemistry in rats, Am Rev Respir Dis 126:483-487, 1982.

231. Sahebjami H and Vassallo CL: Effects of starvation and refeeding on lung mechanics and morphometry, Am Rev Respir Dis 119:443-451, 1979.

232. Sahebjami H and Vassallo CL: Influence of starvation on enzyme induced emphysema, J Appl Physiol 48:284-288, 1981.

233. Sahebjami H, Vassallo CL, and Wirman JA: Lung mechanics and ultrastructure in prolonged starvation, Am Rev Respir Dis 117:77-83, 1978.

234. Sahebjami H and Wirman JA: Emphysema like changes in the lungs of starved rats, Am Rev Respir Dis 124:619-624, 1981.

235. Sargent F and Johnson RE: The effects of diet on renal function in healthy men, Am J Clin Nutr 4:466-481, 1956.

236. Schlichtig R and Ayres SM: Nutritional support of the critically ill, Chicago, 1988, Year Book Medical Publishers.

237. Schloeder FX and Stinebaugh BJ: Renal tubular sites

238. Seltzer MH et al: Instant nutritional assessment, JPEN 3:157-159, 1979.

239. Sheldon GF, Petersen SR, and Saunders R: Hepatic dysfunction during hyperalimentation, Arch Surg 113:504-508, 1978.

240. Shennib H et al: Depression and delayed recovery of alveolar macrophage function during starvation and refeeding, Surg Gynecol Obstet 158:535-540, 1984.

241. Sherlock S and Walshe V: Effects of undernutrition in man on hepatic structure and function, Nature 161:604-629, 1948.

242. Shike M: Copper in parenteral nutrition, Bull NY Acad Med 60:132-143, 1984.

243. Shils ME, Jacobs DH, and Cunningham-Rundles S: Selenium deficiency and immune function in home TPN patients, Am J Clin Nutr 37:716-723, 1983.

244. Shizgal HM, Spanier AH, and Kurtz RS: Effects of parenteral nutrition on body composition in critically ill patients, Am J Surg 131:156-162, 1976.

245. Silvas SE and Paragas PD: Paresthesias, weakness, seizures and hypophosphatemia in patients receiving hyperalimentation, Gastroenterology 62:513-520, 1972.

246. Sima A: Studies on fibre size in developing sciatic nerve and spinal roots in normal, undernourished and rehabilitated rats, Acta Physiol Scand Suppl 406:3-55, 1974.

247. Simonson E, Henschel A, and Keys A: The electrocardiogram of man in semi-starvation and subsequent rehabilitation, Am Heart J 35:584-602, 1948.

248. Smale BF et al: The efficacy of nutritional assessment and support in cancer surgery, Cancer 47:2375-2381, 1981.

249. Smith R and Drenick EJ: Changes in body water and sodium during prolonged fasting for extreme obesity, Clin Sci 31:437-447, 1966.

250. Sobrado J et al: Lipid emulsions and reticuloendothelia system function in healthy and burned guinea pigs, Am J Clin Nutr 42:855-863, 1985.

251. Souba WW, Smith RJ, and Wilmore DW: Glutamine metabolism by the intestinal tract, JPEN 9:608-617, 1985.

252. Starker PM et al: Serum albumin levels as an index of nutritional support, Surgery 91:194-199, 1982.

253. Starker PM et al: The influence of preoperative total parenteral nutrition upon operative morbidity and mortality, Surg Gynecol Obstet 162:569-574, 1986.

254. Stein HD and Keiser HR: Collagen metabolism in granulating wounds, J Surg Res 11:277-283, 1971.

255. Steiner M et al: Effect of starvation on the tissue composition of the small intestine in the rat, Am J Physiol 215:75-77, 1968.

of natriuresis of fasting and glucose induced sodium conservation, Metabolism 19:1119-1128, 1970.

256. Studley HO: Percentage of weight loss: a basic indicator of surgical risk in patients with chronic peptic ulcer, JAMA 106:458-460, 1936.

257. Svoboda D, Grady H, and Higginson J: The effects of chronic protein deficiency in rats, Lab Invest 15:731-749, 1966.

258. Symreng T et al: Nutritional assessment and clinical course in 112 elective surgical patients, Acta Chir Scand 149:657-662, 1983.

259. Syndman DR et al: Total parenteral nutrition related infections: prospective epidemiological study using semiquantitative methods, Am J Med 73:695-699, 1984.

260. Temple WJ et al: Effect of nutrition, diet and suture material on long term wound healing, Ann Surg 182:93-97, 1975.

261. Thet LA and Alvarez H: Effect of hyperventilation and starvation on rat lung mechanics and surfactant, Am Rev Respir Dis 126:286-290, 1982.

262. Thompson BR, Julian TP, and Stremple JF: Perioperative total parenteral nutrition in patients with gastrointestinal cancer, J Surg Res 30:497-500, 1981.

263. Thompson CS et al: Effect of starvation on biochemical indices of renal function in the rat, Br J Exp Pathol 68:767-775, 1987.

264. Thompson JS et al: The effect of nutrient delivery on gut structure and diamine oxidase levels, JPEN 11:28-32, 1987.

265. Thurston J and Marks P: Electrocardiographic abnormalities in patients with anorexia nervosa, Br Heart J 36:719-723, 1974.

266. Train VM and Sath BT: Effect of starvation on renal function, Lancet II:620-622, 1973.

267. Twomey P, Ziegler D, and Rombeau J: Utility of skin testing in nutritional assessment: a critical review, JPEN 6:50-58, 1982.

268. Van den Berg G and Stam H: Metabolic respiratory effects of enteral nutrition in patients during mechanical ventilation, Inten Care Med 14:206-211, 1988.

269. Van Liew JB et al: Renal sodium conservation during starvation in the rat, J Lab Clin Med 91:560-659, 1978.

270. Vrbaski SR: The effects of long-term low protein intake on lipids of rat brain during adulthood, J Nutr 113:899-904, 1983.

271. Weisnier RL et al: Hospital malnutrition: a prospective evaluation of general medical patients during the course of hospitalization, Am J Clin Nutr 32:418-426, 1979.

272. Weiss HS and Jurrus E: Starvation on compliance and surfactant of the rat lung, Respir Physiol 12:123-129, 1971.

273. Widdowson EM, Dickerson JWT, and McCance RA: Severe undernutrition in growing and adult animals. 4. The impact of severe undernutrition on the chemical composition of the soft tissues in the pig, JPEN 1:25A, 1977.

274. Willicuts HD: Nutritional assessment of 1000 surgical patients in an affluent suburban community hospital, JPEN 1:25A, 1977.

275. Wilmore DW et al: Catecholamines: mediators of the hypermetabolic response to thermal injury, Ann Surg 180:653-699, 1974.

276. Wilmore DW et al: The gut: a central organ after surgical stress, Surgery 104:917-923, 1988.

277. Wood RJ, Bengoa JM, and Sitirin MD: Reduction of total parenteral nutrition induced urinary calcium loss by increasing the phosphorus in the total parenteral nutrition prescription, JPEN 10:188-190, 1986.

278. Yates B, Lopez A, and Jackson SS: Nutritional status of hospitalized patients, Clin Res 25:20, 1977.

279. Young GA, Chem C, and Hill GL: Assessment of protein calorie malnutrition in surgical patients from plasma proteins and anthropometric measurements, Am J Clin Nutr 31:429-435, 1978.

280. Zarchy TM, Lipman TO, and Finkelstein JD: Elevated transaminases associated with an elemental diet, Ann Intern Med 89:221-222, 1978.

Index

Page numbers in *italics* indicate boxed material or illustrations.
Page numbers followed by *t* indicate tables.